Laboratory Tests in Nursing Practice

Laboratory Tests in Nursing Practice

Jane Vincent Corbett, R.N., M.S.
Associate Professor
School of Nursing
University of San Francisco
San Francisco, California

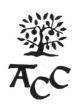

APPLETON-CENTURY-CROFTS/Norwalk, Connecticut

NOTICE. Our knowledge in the clinical sciences is constantly changing. As new information becomes available,
changes in treatment and in the use of drugs become
necessary. The author and the publisher of this volume
have, as far as it is possible to do so, taken care to make
certain that the doses of drugs and schedules of treatment
are correct and compatible with the standards generally
accepted at the time of publication. The reader is advised
to consult carefully the instruction and information material included in the package insert of each drug or therapeutic agent before administration in order to make certain
that the recommended dosage is correct and that there
have been no changes in the recommended dose of the
drug or in the indications or contraindications in its utilization. This advice is especially important when using new or
infrequently used drugs.

Prentice-Hall International, Inc., *London*
Prentice-Hall of Australia, Pty Ltd., *Sydney*
Prentice-Hall of Canada, Inc., *Toronto*
Prentice-Hall of India Private Limited, *New Delhi*
Prentice-Hall of Japan, Inc., *Tokyo*
Prentice-Hall of Southeast Asia (Pte.) Ltd., *Singapore*
Whitehall Books Ltd., *Wellington, New Zealand*

Library of Congress Cataloging in Publication Data

Corbett, Jane Vincent.
   Laboratory tests in nursing practice.

   Includes bibliographies and index.
   1. Nursing. 2. Diagnosis, Laboratory.   I. Title.
[DNLM: 1. Diagnosis, Laboratory—Nursing texts.
2. Diagnostic tests, Routine—Nursing texts.   QY 4
C789n]
RT48.C67   610.73   82-4080
ISBN 0-8385-5585-3   AACR2

Design: Jean M. Sabato

To Rod and Rhonda Jane,
who gave me the space and time
to make this book a reality and
whose contributions were invaluable

Contents

Preface

Written by a nurse, this book is intended to give other nurses and nursing students a better understanding of how to use the information about laboratory tests to improve patient care. Although written primarily for the nurse who is a generalist, the information in this book can also prove useful to clinical specialists and nurse-practitioners. Learning objectives at the beginning of each chapter outline the major points. The chapters present the following information for each test: clinical significance, procedures used, and patient preparation. The book emphasizes how laboratory data can be used above and beyond the specific care of the patient before and after tests. Throughout the text, the nurse's independent role is evident.

The pathophysiology that causes altered laboratory values is explained in an easy-to-understand format. Medical diagnoses and medical interventions are discussed when that information is pertinent to the nurse who may be assisting with treatment. A discussion of usual medical interventions for a particular set of circumstances is included to show how nursing use is related to and yet different from medical use of laboratory data.

Related tests are grouped so that general nursing implications for similar tests can be discussed and compared. Examples are used from various practice settings and for all age groups. Test questions at the end of each chapter feature patient-care examples. The nursing implications in this book are not listed in cookbook form. The nurse can read about the test and *possible* nursing implications, but then must apply the information to a specific clinical situation. The whole purpose of this book is to make nurses think more, not less.

It is intellectually challenging to broaden one's knowledge in a field, and in nursing we often have the added benefit of seeing that our increased knowledge is of direct benefit to the patient. My enthusiasm and sense of purpose in writing this book stem from my belief that students and practicing nurses will be able to use the practical information in the book to improve the care of many patients. I hope the reader finds the book informative, interesting, and useful in the practice of nursing.

Acknowledgments

The preliminary data collection for this book was done while I was on sabbatical from the University of San Francisco. A special thanks to the then-Dean of the USF School of Nursing, Sister Mary Geraldine, who gave me the encouragement and support to complete this book. To my colleagues, Mae Paulfrey, RN MS, and Terry Corwin, RN MS, who read and critiqued parts of this manuscript, thanks for the expert help.

I am also very grateful to the many nurses, physicians, and laboratory personnel at Kaiser Hospital, San Francisco, who willingly answered my many questions. Particularly helpful in obtaining information for me were: Carol Bailey, RN MS, Kaiser Home Care; Bruce Ettinger, M.D., Kaiser Permanente Medical Group.

A book of this sort must, of course, depend heavily on the previous writings of many. I am therefore indebted to many professionals whom I have met only through the printed page. References for each chapter give credit to the many resources that helped me obtain indepth knowledge about the subjects in this book.

I also acknowledge the help I have received from all the nursing students who have asked me over the years the questions that I am now answering in this book. I particularly acknowledge those students who asked the questions for which I had no answer! Various portions of this book have been used as independent study units at the University of San Francisco for the past three years; special thanks go to all the students who critiqued the drafts of the book used as study units in our curriculum.

To my typist, Debbie Fox, an official recognition for all the hard work—working with you was a pleasure. To Leslie Boyer and Jane Licht, my editors at Appleton-Century-Crofts, who were always there when I needed them —your encouragement and teamwork were of great benefit to me.

Laboratory Tests
in Nursing Practice

Introduction:
How to Use This Book

The first chapter of this book gives basic information about laboratory tests, but reading it is not an essential preliminary for the other chapters. All the chapters are individual units that can be read in any order. Objectives at the beginning of each chapter outline the chapter's most significant points while questions at the end are designed to test each of these important points. Thus the reader can quickly glance at the objectives and questions for each chapter to determine the content covered.

This book is designed to be used in three different ways:

1. It can be a textbook for students who are initially learning about laboratory tests. Students can study the objectives, read the chapter, and then be tested on the material. The information, which is basic, can be incorporated into two-year, three-year, or four-year nursing programs. Teachers in some types of educational programs may wish to expand on the material, but the information is relevant for all nursing programs. The student does need to have had supporting classes in science, as well as some fundamental knowledge of nursing techniques.

The book can probably best be used to supplement information about nursing care being presented in theory classes. The book's material lends itself well to inclusion in a nursing theory class in an integrated curriculum because it offers practical applications in a variety of settings.

Students can also use this book in the preparation of nursing care plans for all clinical areas. From the student's point of view, this may be the most prized quality of the book.

2. This book can also be used by practicing nurses who feel a need to gain more information about laboratory tests and the nurse's role. Nurses, or advanced students, can first test their knowledge by answering the questions at the chapter ends and then reviewing the material related to the questions that they miss. The text clearly spells out the answer to each question. Continuing education instructors may also give the test questions to students as a pre-test. The in-service class can then focus on what was confusing to the nurses.

3. This book is also designed to be used as a quick reference for nurses or nursing students in the clinical area. By consulting the index, the reader has access to any of the tests in the book. So to find out why an AFB has been ordered and whether there is any special technique in collecting the specimen, a nurse can quickly read about AFB. In fact, a universal recommendation of the nurses interviewed for this book is to have a simple, accurate book on laboratory tests available on all clinical units. By the same token, nurses who function in settings other than hospitals also expressed a desire for a book that would put useful nursing information at their fingertips when an unfamiliar laboratory test is ordered.

This book can also help direct nurses to other resources for self-learning. For example, they may look up information on why a patient with obstructive jaundice is having a PT (prothrombin time) done. When they look up the information on PT, they also find brief information about intolerance to fats and a lack of vitamin K. This synthesis of information can then motivate further study.

PURPOSE OF INTRODUCTION TO EACH CHAPTER

The introduction for each chapter provides an overview of the tests to be covered and why these specific tests have been grouped together. When necessary, some concepts from physiology or other basic information is briefly summarized at the beginning of the chapter so the reader can better understand the information about the specific tests. For example, Chapter 11 contains a summary of the pathway of bilirubin excretion.

After reading the summary, the reader can determine whether it is necessary to go to standard references on physiology, chemistry or pathophysiology to gain more background material. Specific references for background review are not included, since nurses or nursing students can use the books that are standard for their own schools. The overviews in the introduction are based on the assumption that none of the concepts is new since the reader has had basic science courses. Readers may skip the introduction if they are interested only in reading about one test in the chapter.

FORMAT OF TEST PRESENTATION

Definition and Purpose
After the introduction, the chapter is devoted to discussions of individual tests. The test's definition is geared to be meaningful to *nurses*. A brief description of the test outlines its outstanding points, such as why it is done only for a certain condition.

Preparation of Patient
and Collection of Sample
The general preparation of the patient for all the tests in a chapter is discussed at the beginning of the chapter. More specific patient preparation is included in the section on each test and it includes such items as whether medication, food and/or water should be withheld. Since the exact preparation of the patient, however, may vary from one laboratory to another, the reader may need to verify specific points. Appendix A also contains information on the collection of samples (the type of collection tube and so on).

Reference Values

Laboratory values in the literature are referred to as *normal reference values* or *reference values* and not as *normal values,* because each laboratory must determine what is "normal" for a test done in a specific laboratory. *The use of any of the reference values in this book may be hazardous to the well-being of patients unless values are verified by the local laboratory. No book can be the authority on what is normal for a specific laboratory.*

For the most part, the reference values used throughout this book are those periodically published in the *New England Journal of Medicine.* (See Appendix A for the address to write to obtain reprints of all the printed values.) These values, based on the ones used at Massachusetts General Hospital, have been periodically published since 1946. The reprint is of particular interest because it documents the source in the literature for each method of testing used. Reference values for some tests were gained from other literature and from Kaiser Hospital and Children's Hospital in San Francisco, California. Other sources for reference values are listed in each chapter and with the tables in the appendices.

Values vary not only due to the method of testing done, but also due to the population being tested. Chapter 1 discusses in detail the many factors that affect the "normal range" of laboratory values. It would be very tedious, and not of much benefit to nurses, to list all the variables that could affect each test. However, a few major variables need to be mentioned each time a reference value is listed, of which the most significant are sex (gender), age, and pregnancy. Thus each laboratory reference value in this book is reported with the significant variations for these factors. If only one value is given for a test, the reader may assume that there are not significant variations among different populations. For example, the level of serum sodium is essentially the same for all age groups, in both sexes and during pregnancy. (This is not to say that there is no variation, but it is not enough to make a difference in the clinical interpretation of reference values.) Appendices A, B, and C summarize some of the major changes in reference values due to gender and age. The normal changes in pregnancy are listed in Appendix D. If there are other significant variables besides the three major ones, these different values are also noted. For example, the RBC (red blood count) is different in Denver from San Francisco, because (besides gender, age, and pregnancy) altitude is an important variable for RBC.

Increased and Decreased Levels

Clinical Significance. The clinical significance of increases in values are covered separately from the clinical significances of decreases, to help the reader make clear distinctions between the two. This division also makes it easier to use the book as a quick reference when one is interested only in an increased value. It seemed necessary also to note when decreases are *not* significant, since beginning students sometimes waste time trying to figure out the pathological significance of a value that is below the normal reference values. For example, a low serum bilirubin is never of pathological significance, a fact that the novice may need to verify.

As much as possible, the clinical significance of changes are geared more toward the general pathophysiology exhibited rather than toward the names of specific medical diseases. This author's experience has been that information on laboratory test values becomes relevant to the student only if a reason is given for a change. For example, a simple listing of ten diseases where the Hct may be low is not very useful information for the nurse.

Possible Nursing Implications. The focus of the nursing implications section is on specific do's and don't's, as well as on more general information that may help the nurse plan overall nursing care. Some of the nursing implications on the care of the patient before or after a test are fairly specific. The nurse may need to observe for signs and symptoms that indicate a complication or a worsening of the condition. Yet it is a mistake to try to make a list of exactly what nursing actions "go with" each change in a laboratory test. There are commonalities when a laboratory test is altered, but the underlying pathophysiological condition causing the alteration may influence what should or should not be done. The section on nursing implications therefore contains helpful guidelines for nurses, so they can fashion care using the data. The suggestions are not to be taken as absolute directives. Clearly, the nursing care must be based on the total picture of the patient, not on *one* laboratory test seen in isolation.

When possible, nursing implications are grouped under headings such as "Assessments," "Interventions," or "Health Teaching" to help the reader fit the content into an overall nursing care plan. The use of laboratory data in the overall nursing process is further explored in Chapter 1.

CHAPTER ONE

Using Laboratory Data

Objectives

1. Describe how laboratory data can be used in the framework of the nursing process and how nursing use differs from the medical use of data.
2. Describe the traditional functions of nurses in relation to laboratory tests, including peripheral testing.
3. Identify the two nondisease factors that cause the greatest variations in normal reference values for laboratory tests.
4. Compare the meanings of the terms *specificity* and *sensitivity* in relation to diagnostic tests.
5. Explain in general terms how the normal curve and percentiles are used to establish normal reference ranges for laboratory tests.
6. Explain the meaning of the measurement symbols in the conventional laboratory system and in the SI system.
7. Describe the purpose of each of the four basic diagnostic screening tests recommended for asymptomatic adult populations.
8. Define how nurses can foster smooth working relationships with personnel in the laboratory department.

In discussing several issues that are pertinent to the nurse's utilization of laboratory data, this chapter touches briefly on the nursing process, on the differences between nursing care and medical care, and on the traditional roles of the nurse in relation to diagnostic tests. Emphasis is given to the many factors that influence test results, such as physiology, drug interference, and the statistical methods used to determine "normal" ranges. A comparison of conventional measurements and SI is included, and the purpose of screening tests is explored. The last section in the chapter discusses ways that the nurse can effectively work with personnel in other departments.

LABORATORY REPORTS AND
THE NURSING PROCESS

Up to the early seventies, problem-solving was emphasized as a way of thinking about the needs of patients. About that time, most nursing educators started turning to the nursing process, which is an elaboration of the problem-solving technique used by all disciplines. In essence, the *nursing process* is a way of systematically identifying the needs of patients and then logically planning the appropriate nursing actions to meet those needs. (The term "client" may be used for "patient," if one wishes.) Many practicing nurses use the nursing process even though they may be unsure about how to describe it step-by-step in writing. Yet, whether written out or not, the nursing process, as a way of thinking, helps the nurse to provide nursing care that is based on more than guesswork or generalizations about patients. This process is a deliberate way of using data to make the assessments and to identify the problems that are under the jurisdiction of the nurse. The evaluation and the modification of care are also essential components of the nursing process. The format for a written nursing care plan is shown in Table 1-1. Most hospitals have similar formats for use on the Kardex, but the collection of data is not written out.

Collection of Data

Nurses use a variety of ways to collect data, including physical assessment skills and interviewing techniques; laboratory data constitutes only one small part of the entire clinical picture. Consequently one can never use the laboratory data apart from other clinical data. For example, although an increased specific gravity is one objective sign of dehydration or a fluid volume deficit, the nurse must collect other data that may be relevant to this patient's situation. If the patient has just had diagnostic tests with radiopaque dye (Chapter 3), the specific gravity is not a meaningful contribution to data collection.

Nursing Diagnosis

Taking all the collected data, nurses must then formulate a *nursing diagnosis,* which is a problem within the scope of nursing practice. In a national conference, held in 1972, nurses identified a list of nursing diagnoses that were generally agreed to be under the control of the nurse (Gordon 1979). While many nurses use this official and quite specific list of nursing diagnoses others may prefer to use their own words to describe patient problems. The important point is that nurses must make sure the diagnosis or problem is truly within the scope of nursing.

    A nursing diagnosis is not the same as a medical diagnosis. While medicine is focused on the diagnosis and treatment of disease, nursing has to do primarily with the care, comfort, and support of people whose patterns of daily life are in some way threatened (Luckmann 1980). Nursing focuses on restorative support, nurturance, comfort measures, and health teaching (Schorr 1975:1979).

    Many patient problems can be identified by using the nursing process. For example, through assessment, the nurse may discover that Mr. Smith's urine has become concentrated because he cannot feed himself and no one has been offering him any fluids between meals. Thus the nursing diagnosis would be a fluid volume deficit due to an inability to obtain fluids. On the other hand, dehydration, or a fluid volume deficit may be due to a

TABLE 1-1. USE OF LABORATORY DATA IN NURSING PROCESS

Collection of Data	Nursing Diagnosis or Statement of Problem	Patient/Nurse Goals	Interventions (Nurse-to-Nurse Orders)	Evaluation and Modification Needed
Cannot use left arm to hold glass; mouth is dry; skin turgor poor; I&O for last 24 hours. I = 700 O = 600 s.g. 1.030	Fluid volume deficit due to inability to feed self.	Patient will remain hydrated with a s.g. no higher than 1.020. *Short-term:* Patient will drink at least 1,000 cc on the day shift and 600 cc on the evening shift.	Give mouth care at least once a shift. Ask patient what type of fluids are wanted— does not like *water.* Assist patient to drink out of glass—likes straw. In addition to meals, offer 250 ml fluids at: 10 AM 2 PM 4 PM 8 PM	Intake for 2-10: 7-3 PM 1,000 cc 3-11 PM 650 cc Patient's s.g. now 1.015 on 2-11. 2-11: Continue with plan.

serious medical problem such as ketoacidosis. The second case warrants medical interventions such as insulin administration and intravenous fluids. (See Chapter 8 on medical interventions for ketoacidosis.) As other examples:

1. An elevated direct bilirubin often causes itching in patients. What *comfort* measures by the nurse may be effective?
2. A patient has a low serum potassium level. What *health teaching* does the patient need about foods rich in potassium?
3. A woman is to have hormone tests as part of an infertility work-up. The nurse observes that the patient is very anxious. What can the nurse do to prepare the woman and to give her *nurturance?*
4. A young child has a low hemoglobin reading. What can the nurse teach the parents that would be *restorative support?*

The nursing process, however, is effective only if one knows the answers to go with the questions raised by the process. Hence the subsequent chapters provide the information necessary for planning individualized patient care.

Writing Goals or Patient Outcomes

With the nursing diagnosis, the nurse can write patient/nurse goals in behavioral terms. The goal should be acceptable to the patient and compatible with medical goals. For example, in Mr. Smith's case, an immediate short-term goal is to have him drink so many milliliters of fluid during each shift. The long-term goal is that he will not show any signs of dehydration, that is, his specific gravity will remain in a normal range.

Nursing Interventions

The nurse then plans what nursing actions or interventions are needed to reach the goals. She or he may consult with the patient about how to best achieve a mutually acceptable goal. Maybe Mr. Smith needs to be fed completely. Maybe he could feed himself and drink fluids if he were properly positioned. Maybe the patient would drink juice better than water. Collaboration with the physician and with other health team members (such as the dietician) is also necessary if medical interventions are needed too.

Nurses write goals and interventions in various ways. These interventions, called "nurse-to-nurse" orders, need to be written on the Kardex. The important point is to distinguish between actions that depend on physicians' orders and those that are independent nursing actions. Too often nurses do their own orders only by word of mouth from shift to shift. While nursing as a profession becomes more assured of its uniqueness, as something separate from medical care one hopes that nurse-to-nurse orders will become more common a practice.

Evaluation of Goals

Evaluation is necessary to see if the goals were met. If goals are not achieved, what needs to be modified? For example, a specific gravity measurement can be considered evidence that the patient has regained a normal fluid balance. "Responsibility" and "accountability" in nursing mean that nurses do take responsibility for the quality of patient care and that they are accountable if the care does not meet certain standards. Hence evaluation is an integral part of accountability.

NURSING FUNCTIONS IN LABORATORY TESTING

Gathering Information from Charts

In collecting data from a chart, nurses should always look at the latest laboratory data first to see the current status of the patient and to note trends in the data. One of the hardest things for novices to figure out is the meaning of the abbreviations used for many of the laboratory tests and diagnostic procedures. "ANA" on a chart, for example, has nothing to do with the American Nurses Association! It stands for antinuclear antibody test, which is a test done for systemic lupus erythematous (SLE). The standard abbreviations used to denote laboratory tests are listed in Appendix E. Learning them makes reading charts and collecting data much easier.

Transcribing Orders and Ordering Laboratory Tests

Generally, since the procedures for transcribing orders and making out laboratory requisitions vary from institution to institution, this skill is best learned by in-service or on-the-job training. In this book, the essential points to include on the laboratory requisitions are discussed in relation to each specific test. Ordering laboratory tests is a skill usually reserved for experienced nurse clinicians in special situations. In some clinical settings, however, nurses may order certain laboratory tests in accordance with the hospital's standardized orders.

Peripheral Testing by Nurses

Peripheral testing refers to testing that is done by nonlaboratory personnel, and it is often done by nurses whenever there is a need for quick results. Several simple tests require only a drop or two of blood or urine and no special equipment. Some of these tests include the dipsticks for urine chemistry, slide tests for occult blood, and simple procedures such as specific gravity reading by refractometers. (See Table 1–2.) In special care units, such as intensive care units or emergency rooms, nurses may also operate automated equipment that measures blood gases or hematocrits.

Nurses must be aware of the potential problems with administering such tests. For instance, the diagnostic test kits are reliable only if the nurses follow the instructions. It has been estimated that as many as 10% of all the readings of tests done with diagnostic kits are incorrect due to human error (Blatt 1975:30). Another problem is that test materials may not be properly cared for. Bottles are left open, materials get wet or hot, and the issue date of the test is unknown. Aides, inexperienced nurses, or interns may not do the test accurately, or the people doing the test may be color blind. (All laboratory people are tested for color blindness as a requirement for their jobs.) Too often the results of the test are recorded haphazardly on the chart.

Another interesting objection to peripheral testing is the cost to the hospital. Muschenheim (1979) makes the point that, right or wrong, many hospitals depend on the laboratory as one of the key services to generate income. So if laboratory tests are done outside the laboratory, the patient is not properly billed.

Quality control is another point of concern. The inspection standards of both the Joint Commission for Accreditation of Hospitals (JCAH) and the College of American Pathologists (CAP) state that the laboratory and the pathologist are charged with the responsibility for all clinical testing, inside and outside of the laboratory. Usually, with

TABLE 1-2. EXAMPLES OF COMMON TYPES OF PERIPHERAL TESTING

Specimen	Test For	Product Example	Discussed in
Urine	Glucose	Tes-Tape (3)*	Chaps. 2, 9
Serum	Glucose	Dextrostix (1)	Chap. 9
Urine	Glucose and other sugars	Clinitest (1)	Chaps. 2, 9
Serum and urine	Ketone bodies	Ketostix (1) Acetone tablets (1)	Chaps. 2, 9
Body secretions	pH of urine, vaginal secretions, naso-gastric contents	Nitrazine (1)	Chap. 2
Urine	Protein	Dipsticks Refractometer	Chap. 3
Urine	Specific gravity	Refractometer Urinometer	Chap. 3
Stool or other secretions	Occult blood	Guaiac tests Hematest (1) Hemoccult (6)	Chap. 13
Capillary blood	Hypothyroidism, galactesemia, and PKU in newborn	Heel stick on filter papers, various brands	Chap. 18
Urine	Phenylketonuria	Phenestix (1)	Chap. 18
Urine	Bilirubin	Icotest (1)	Chap. 11
Urine	Pregnancy	Various home kits	Chap. 18
Urine	Infection	Microstix (1) Unibac (2) Uricult (4) Clinicult (6) Bacturcult (7)	Chap. 16
Serum	Sickle cell screening	Sickledex (5)	Chap. 18

* Manufacturers:
 (1) Ames Laboratory, Elkhart, Indiana 46514
 (2) Bio-Dynamics, Irvine, California 92705
 (3) Eli Lilly Co., Indianapolis, Indiana 46206
 (4) Medical Technology, Hackensack, New Jersey 07606
 (5) Ortho Diagnostics, Raritan, New Jersey 08869
 (6) Smith Kline Diagnostics, Philadelphia, Pennsylvania 19101

Source: Blatt (1975) and product information from the seven companies listed above. Note that these companies have printed information to send to professionals.

peripheral tests, control by the laboratory is not very evident, but this circumstance may change in the future. Spark and Kundert (1979) have set up a comprehensive program to implement quality control of peripheral testing since the state of Arizona is requiring more stringent control. One of the key requirements of the program in Arizona is that all nurses take a "wet lab" session so that they can do the tests correctly.

The reader may be interested in finding out how a local hospital or clinic handles peripheral testing. Most institutions do not have formal training programs for peripheral testing. If nurses are not comfortable with the procedures used for peripheral testing, they should request in-service. Many of the manufacturers of diagnostic kits give free in-service to nurses and other health care workers. Also, many teaching aides about products may be obtained by writing directly to the manufacturer or by talking to the local sales representatives. Table (1–2) includes the addresses of some of the major manufacturers of products for peripheral testing.

Preparation of the Patient for the Laboratory Test

The nurse's role includes preparing the patient physically and psychologically. As a patient advocate, the nurse can make sure that the patient has adequate knowledge of what is to be done. As information giver or health teacher, the nurse can also seek additional input from other members of the health team so that the patient gives an informed consent. "The responsibilities of nurses in effecting the implementation of a doctrine of informed consent are related to her/his role within the health team, the facility wherein health care is given and the current law [CNA 1978:6]." In the past few years, there has been more emphasis on patients' rights as states have enacted laws to enforce the doctrine of informed consent.

Collection and Transportation of Specimens

Venous Samples. Experienced nurses often draw venous blood for blood work. When they do, they must avoid the following possible causes of hemolysis, which particularly invalidates tests such as potassium or LDH (Strand 1980:7):

1. skin too wet with antiseptic;
2. moisture in the syringe or collection tube;
3. prolonged use of a tourniquet;
4. use of a small gauge needle to withdraw a large volume of blood;
5. use of suction on the syringe;
6. vigorous shaking of the blood specimen;
7. not removing the needle from the syringe before expelling the blood into the collection tube; or
8. vigorous expulsion of blood from the syringe into the collection tube.

Other tips include not drawing blood on the arm where there is an intravenous because the values will be changed by the solution being infused. Appendix A includes notes for specific tests in relation to collection methods. The meanings of the various colors for tubes are also explained in a table in Appendix A. For example, a red top tube means "no additives." (Many venous blood samples for chemistry are collected without additives; see Chapter 13 for techniques for *arterial* blood samples.)

Finger and Heel Sticks. For some tests, such as hematocrits and blood sugars, finger sticks may be used rather than a venipuncture. The usual procedure is to cleanse with 70% alcohol, dry with a gauze sponge, and puncture with a sterile blade deep enough to get a free flow of blood. The first drop of blood is discarded, and enough blood is collected to fill a capillary tube supplied by the laboratory. Or a drop of blood may be put onto special filter paper. It is important not to squeeze to get capillary blood because the squeezing causes tissue fluids to dilute the sample. (If patients need to do finger sticks at home, they can buy from most surgical supply houses a small apparatus that automatically punctures the finger to the right depth.) In the infant, heel sticks are used for capillary blood. The foot is warmed for five minutes to dilate the capillaries and arterioles. The lateral aspects of the heel are used to avoid the plantar artery. A small adhesive band-aid is placed over the puncture site.

Urine and Other Specimens. The procedure for urine collection, including 24-hour testing, is detailed in Chapter 3. Chapter 16 gives explicit details on all the types of specimens collected for cultures.

After a specimen is collected, the way it is stored and transported to the laboratory can affect the test values. Some specimens, such as the serum for cold agglutinins must be carried to the laboratory in a 37°C bath. Other specimens, such as blood gases or anaerobic cultures, must not be exposed to the air. The nurse must check with the laboratory to determine if there are any special requirements about the transportation of specimens.

Seeing That Stat Tests Are Stat

The word "stat" means "at once." Because a stat request interrupts the normal laboratory routine, a test should be marked "stat" only when the results really do need to be known as soon as possible. In most stat situations, someone should hand-carry the specimen to the laboratory. The nurse should be familiar with the preparation needed and with the ex-

TABLE 1-3. TESTS MOST COMMONLY DONE AS STAT PROCEDURES*

Name of Test	Discussed in
Complete blood count (CBC)	Chap. 2
Urinalysis (UA)	Chap. 3
Blood urea nitrogen (BUN)	Chap. 4
Electrolytes (Na, K, Cl, Bicarb)	Chap. 5
Blood gases	Chap. 6
Calcium	Chap. 7
Glucose	Chap. 8
Acetone (serum)	Chap. 8
Bilirubin	Chap. 11
Amylase	Chap. 12
Prothrombin time (PT)	Chap. 13
Partial thromboplastin time (PTT)	Chap. 13
Platelet Count	Chap. 13
Fibrinogen	Chap. 13
Type and cross match	Chap. 14
Direct Coombs	Chap. 14
Transfusion reaction investigation	Chap. 14
Innoculate media for cultures	Chap. 16
Gram stains	Chap. 16
Alcohol	Chap. 17
Salicylates	Chap. 17
Cerebrospinal fluid (CSF)	Chap. 16

* Based on studies reported in Barnett (1978).

pected results of stat tests because these tests are done in emergency situations when there is little time to do reviews. Barnett (1978) did a study to find out which laboratory tests are most commonly done as stats in different hospitals. Table 1–3 lists 22 tests done as stats by at least 90% of the hospitals in that survey.

Action in the Event of Abnormal Test Results

Often the nurse is the first one to see the results of a laboratory report. In one study of 60 laboratories, 17 called the doctor to give the results of stats, 32 called the floor, and 11 carried the results to the floor (Barnett 1978). So nurses need to determine if a physician should be notified immediately or if the report is not urgent. The nurse may also need to alert other people to watch for symptoms or to take certain precautions. Although it is usually an abnormal report that requires immediate attention, a normal report may also have great diagnostic importance. For example, the clinician uses normal results to rule out the probability of certain disease entities (Gorry 1978). The significance of abnormal and normal results is discussed in detail with each specific test.

"NORMAL" REFERENCE VALUES AND THE VARIABILITY OF TEST RESULTS

Variable Techniques and Methods

The point already made in the introduction bears repeating: *No values in a book such as this can be used in the real clinical situation.* Each laboratory determines its own values. While some tests that are done by automation (such as the CBC by a Coulter counter) produce similar values in any laboratory, other tests (notably enzyme assays) have wide variations in normal ranges depending on the method used. Since one does need real numbers to discuss laboratory results, this book has used the reference values printed in the *New England Journal of Medicine* (Scully 1980).

Variables That Affect Test Results

Besides the obvious differences of technique and method, many other variables can influence laboratory reference values: Age and sex (gender) are the chief physiological factors that change the "norms." Pregnancy alters the normal reference values. Hytten (1975) is excellent for values in pregnancy. (See the tables in Appendices A, B, C, and D, for examples of changes in values in different populations.) Reference values for adults are better documented than those for children. Cherjan (1978) contains the expected variations for children. Other references are cited in the text and in the tables in the Appendices.

Other physiologic factors such as diet, the time of day, activity level, and stress may also alter what is "normal" for a test. For example, hormones (Chapter 15) have a diurnal variation; so the time of day must be noted when the specimen is drawn. Geographical location—including the altitude, temperature, and humidity—may also affect the results. Racial or ethnic variations can also cause different reference values for different groups (Galen 1979:465). Usually, however, ethnic or racial differences are not of much importance since a mixture of people is used to obtain values.

Drug Interferences

Drugs can change laboratory tests in two ways (Galen 1978):

1. They can change the patient's physiology. For example, birth control pills (Appendix D) cause changes in many of the laboratory tests by altering the woman's hormonal balance.
2. Drugs may have a direct interference with the method of chemical analysis. For example, the urine test for phenylketonuria (PKU) is not reliable if the infant has had salicylates or phenothiazines, either of which cause a reaction to the dipstick too (Chapter 18).

Often the reports in the literature on drug effects are in conflict. How significantly a drug alters a laboratory value may depend on the dosage, timing, physiology of the patient, and other variables such as the mixture of drugs. So the reader must consult pharmacology references or other more specialized texts than this for details on drug interactions, both from the physiological effects and the chemical effects on laboratory results. Galen (1979) has compiled a large list of drugs that can affect laboratory tests. Only the more common drug interferences are included in this text.

FALSE POSITIVE TESTS AND FALSE NEGATIVE TESTS

Specificity

If a test is 100% *specific,* it reacts positively only when the patient actually has the condition being tested. No laboratory test is 100% specific because there is always some factor, such as drugs, that can effect a false positive. For example, the radioimmunoassay (RIA) test for pregnancy is a very specific test because almost all women who have a positive result for the test are indeed pregnant. Still, other factors, such as the elevation of other hormones, can make the test a false positive. On the other hand, the VDRL, a test for syphilis, is not a highly specific test; that is, a significant number of people can have a positive VDRL even though they do not have syphilis. The danger of false positives is that the patient may receive additional tests and treatments that are unnecessary.

Sensitivity

The *sensitivity* of a test is the degree to which a test detects disease without yielding false negatives. No test is 100% sensitive, because there is always some possibility that the test will not reveal the abnormality even though it is present. For example, the direct agglutination technique of detecting pregnancy is not as sensitive as indirect agglutination methods, and neither is it as sensitive as the radioimmunoassay method (Chapter 18). So with the direct agglutination method, there are more false negatives than with the radioimmunoassay (RIA) method. That is, the patient *is* pregnant, but the direct method does not reveal it.

In disease states, false negative tests mean that patients are misclassified as not needing treatment or care when actually they *do* need treatment. For example, the electrocardiogram is not a sensitive test for coronary disease prior to a myocardial infarction.

In other words, coronary disease is not detected by this particular test. Thus a person may have a "normal" electrocardiogram (EKG) one day and a myocardial infarction the next.

New Tests

Specificity and sensitivity are important criteria when a new test is introduced into practice. Balint (1978:291) has suggested five questions to decide whether a new test or diagnostic procedure is worthwhile:

1. Does the new procedure provide a greater specificity and sensitivity than current methods?
2. Is the new information valuable in patient management?
3. Is the new approach as effective in routine clinical practice as it is in selected populations of a university center?
4. Would it provide answers not provided by clinical findings and established diagnostic procedures?
5. In light of the other four factors, is it cost effective?

ESTABLISHING THE "NORMAL" VALUE

It should be increasingly apparent that "blind faith" in the validity of laboratory tests is simply not realistic. In addition to the problems already discussed, even the so-called "normal" value can be misleading. The normal ranges are determined by testing a large sample of healthy individuals and then analyzing the results by statistical methods.

The Normal Curve

One such method is the so-called *normal curve* or *Gaussian distribution*. In this method a cutoff point, which usually consists of two standard deviations from the mean or average, is determined for each side of the curve. In other words, the lowest 2.5% and the highest 2.5% are outside the "normal" range (Dinham 1976:43). Even without a statistical background, the reader should be able to appreciate that any system with cutoff points automatically mean that some *healthy* people in the sample do not fall within the "normal" range. Also, if the distribution is not normal, the curve will be skewed. (Most students who have been exposed to grading by the bell curve know the situation where students who do exceptionally well are called "curve wreckers" by those on the other end of the curve.) Most physiological parameters do not fall in normal distributions, and so it is usually incorrect to speak of averages and normal curves in relationship to laboratory data (Elrebach 1970).

The Percentile Ranking System

The percentile ranking system is usually a better method since data that does not have a normal distribution can still be ranked. *All* the values are ranked, and a percentage is given for each value in relation to the other values. The value in the middle (the median) is at the 50th percentile. This means 50% of the scores are higher and 50% are lower (Dinham 1976:28). In way of analogy, note that National League for Nursing (NLN) test scores are ranked as percentiles. For example, a student who is at the 95th percentile has a score higher than 95% of the people who took the test. When laboratory data is ranked by percentiles, a cutoff point must be established to indicate an abnormality. Harwood (1978) explains in more detail the use of percentile rankings as criteria for normal and abnormal values. For example, values above the 95th percentile are usually considered beyond the ''normal'' reference values. Thus 5% of *healthy* people are *unhealthy* according to this statistical determination of ''normalcy.''

Nurses' Responsibility

Obviously nurses do not have to determine normal ranges or even understand the underlying statistics. They do, however, need to realize that a significant margin of error arises from the arbitrary setting of limits. In effect, with each laboratory test, the results *may* be outside the normal range due entirely to mathematical probability. If a laboratory test is considered normal up to the 95 percentile, then five times out of 100 a test will show an abnormality *even though the patient is not ill.* If the person has two tests done, the probability that both will be within the normal range is 0.95×0.95 or 90.25%. With three tests, the probability is $0.95 \times 0.95 \times 0.95$ or 85.7375%. The point is that, if a patient has a battery of tests, such as the SMA discussed at the end of this chapter, the possibility is great that some of the tests will be abnormal due purely to chance (Casscells 1978).

MEASUREMENTS IN LABORATORY REPORTS

Conventional Measurements

Probably most of the measurements used in laboratory reports, such as ''ml'' (milliliter) or ''mg'' (milligram), are already very familiar. A list of the common abbreviations used for metric measurements is included in Table 1–4, and a more complete list is included as Appendix F. Note that ''mg/dl'' means so many ''milligrams in a deciliter,'' which is 1/10 of a liter, or 100 milliliters. In other words, a blood sugar report of 90 mg/dl is the same as 90 mg per 100 ml.

The term *picogram* (pg) and *nanogram* (ng) are also becoming commonly used, now that radioimmunoassay (RIA) has made it possible to detect trace amounts of substances such as hormones or drugs in the serum (Chapter 15).

The measurement used for electrolytes is *milliequivalent* (mEq). This term's exact meaning, as well as how mg can be converted to mEq, is explained in Chapter 5. *Milliosmoles* (mOsm) are used to express the concentration of body fluids. (See Chapter 3 for a definition of milliosmoles in relation to urinary osmolality.) Note that m*Os*m is different from m*mo*l discussed next.

SI: A New Measurement System

SI units are based on a comprehensive modern form of the metric system called *Le Systeme Internationale* (hence ''SI''). The rationale for the adoption of this international system is to provide a common language for all the various disciplines all over the world (Young 1974). Used not just for the biological sciences but for all sciences, SI utilizes *moles* as the basic unit for the amount of a substance and *kilograms* for its mass. Length is still by *meter*.

TABLE 1–4. METRIC MEASUREMENTS USED IN LABORATORY REPORTS*

Length	Nonmetric Equivalent
Meter (m) ⟶	39.37 in
Centimeter (cm) 1/100 m ⟶	2.5 cm = 1 in
Millimeter (mm) 1/1000 m	
Weight	
Kilogram (kg) ⟶	2.2 lbs
Gram (g) ⟶	453 g = 1 lb
Milligram (mg) 1/1000 of a kg	
Microgram (mcg or μg) 1/1000 of a mg	
Nanogram (ng) 1/1000 of mcg	
Picogram (pg) 1/1000 of a ng	
Femtogram (fg) 1/1000 of a pg	
Volume	
Liter (1) = 1000 ml (or 1000 cc** or 1.05 qt)	
Deciliter (dl) = 100 ml or 1/10 of a liter	
Milliliter (ml) = 1 ml or 1/1000 of a liter	

* See Appendix F for an expanded list of measurement terms used in laboratory reports.
** Note that "ml" and "cc" are interchangeable, but "ml" is preferred since it is in the metric system.

The most profound change in laboratory reports effected by SI is that concentration is expressed as an amount per volume (moles or millimoles per liter) rather than as a mass per volume (grams or milligrams per 100 ml or dl). For some laboratory tests, the numbers stay the same even though the unit is new. For example, the normal range for potassium (K) in the conventional system is 3.5 to 5.0 *mEq/l* and 3.5 to 5.0 *mmol/l* in the new SI. Some of the other tests involve a radical change in numbers, so health workers must totally relearn the reference values. For example, the conventional reference value for glucose of *70 to 110 mg/dl* becomes *3.9 to 5.6 mmol/l* in the new SI.

Due to the drastic change in many of the laboratory reports, the conversion is taking place slowly in our country. At present, many laboratories report results in both conventional and SI units. Appendix A gives the reference values in both conventional and SI units.

SCREENING TESTS FOR ASYMPTOMATIC ADULT POPULATIONS

Biochemical profiles (BCPs) consist of a battery of tests, usually six or twelve, in which the patient's individual results are compared against the normals. BCP tests are provided by automatic analyzers from a number of manufacturers. The battery of tests is often called "SMA" because this was the first brand name commonly used: SMAC, for sequential multiple analysis computer by Technicon Corporation. More correctly, the test should be called a *biochemical profile* (BCP). The usual tests done by an automatic analyzer are listed in Table 1–5.

TABLE 1-5.   USUAL TESTS DONE BY AN AUTOMATIC ANALYZER

Name of Test	Described in
Total protein (TP)	Chap. 10
Albumin (Alb)	Chap. 10
Calcium (Ca)	Chap. 7
Phosphate (P)	Chap. 7
Glucose (RBS)	Chap. 8
Blood Urea Nitrogen (BUN) (creatinine can be substituted)	Chap. 4
Uric acid (optional)	Chap. 4
Total bilirubin	Chap. 11
Alkaline phosphatase	Chap. 12
LDH (optional)	Chap. 12
SGOT or AST	Chap. 12
Cholesterol (optional)	Chap. 9
Sodium (Na$^+$)	Chap. 5
Potassium (K$^+$)	Chap. 5
Chloride (Cl$^-$)	Chap. 5
Bicarbonate (HCO$_3^-$) or CO$_2$ content	Chap. 6

* *Automated measurement of 6 or 12 tests at once using a single sample of a few ml of serum. Check the brand of automatic analyzer for the exact amount needed. Hospitals may vary in the 6 or 12 tests chosen. Ahlvin (1970), Beeler (1977), Reece (1972), and Schaefer (1978) give examples of the use of automated screening in various settings.*

Reece and Hobbie (1972) developed a computer program that compared the patient's biochemical pattern of low and high test values with known patterns for at least seventy different pathological conditions. The computer was programmed to account for age and sex (gender) variations. The information that has been gained from studies with computer analysis have helped the physician focus on the most likely diagnoses of the patient. Available charts (Reece 1978) show the diagnostic possibilities when over fifty different serum tests are either high or low. Decision trees are also available to help with differential diagnosis (Beeler 1977).

Because such tests as the biochemical profile have become very easy to do in mass volume, screening tests have been used widely for many populations. The use of multi-screening tests for apparently healthy people was undertaken with the belief that many diseases could be detected early. However, the wide use of nondiscriminatory laboratory testing has not proven as valuable as once thought. In one typical study, 1,889 patients were tested by SMA 12 to determine the most common abnormalities in a nonsick population. The findings included 44 patients with increased blood sugar, 5 with increased calcium (Ca), 5 with increased SGOT, 3 with decreased sodium (Na), 2 with decreased potassium (K), and one with an increased bilirubin (Ahlvin 1970). The majority of such studies have concluded that it is seldom justified to do mass screening on asymptomatic populations (Schafer 1978). Kaiser Foundation had a multiphasic screening program for two decades (Kaiser Foundation Health Plan 1981). Over the years, all the screening tests were evaluated to see if each specific test was valuable in detecting a disease before the patient has symptoms. The study's conclusion at Kaiser and at other facilities is that only a few tests should be routinely done for all adults.

Blue Cross and Blue Shield have therefore recommended the phasing out of *routine* admission test panels. Biochemical profiles are done only on the order of the physician. Other tests that are not to be reimbursed, unless specifically justified, are Hgb (hemoglobin), UA (urinalysis), chest X-ray, and EKGs (Blue Cross/Blue Shield 1979). The point of these recommendations is that laboratory tests and other diagnostic procedures should be determined by the nature of the patient's problem, which must be discovered by careful history taking and physical examination.

The cost of testing compared to its usefulness is an issue that perplexes health care today. Skendzel (1978) explored how physicians use laboratory data differently in day-to-day practice. Laboratory tests seem to be sometimes overused or misused. Daniels (1977) found no relationship between laboratory use and the outcome of care. In summary, the use of a test does not always mean better patient care, but it does mean an increased cost. Health care workers must determine the cost, risk, and usefulness of any diagnostic procedure. The reader is encouraged to consult recent literature on the usefulness of diagnostic screening tests and on the cost to the individual.

Some health care workers may dispute the medical control of most diagnostic testing. Patients can go directly to private laboratories, where they can get multiphasic screening exams done and sent to the physician or to themselves. Self-help organizations may also encourage the use of some screening tests for preventive medicine.

Publications for lay people have stressed that the four critical screening tests and procedures for adults are:

1. blood pressure checks to detect hypertension,
2. tonometry to detect glaucoma,
3. stool for occult blood to detect cancer of the bowel, and
4. pap smears for women to detect cancer (Oppenheim 1980).

These four tests are routinely used at Kaiser Hospital—a large health maintenance organization (HMO).

(See Chapter 13 for guaiac tests for cancer of the bowel in people over 50.)

LABORATORY PERSONNEL

Who Works in a Clinical Laboratory?

The Pathologist. The laboratory is directed by a physician with a specialty in pathology, which focuses on the use and interpretation of laboratory tests in the diagnosis and treatment of disease. Many of the books listed as general references for this book were written by pathologists. Because they often interpret the results of laboratory tests to the attending physician, pathologists are often called the "doctor's doctors" (College of American Pathologists 1979).

Medical Technologist. The actual management of the laboratory is done by a medical technologist who has had additional training in management and administration. Usually the director of the laboratory sets up the policies and procedures that affect nursing. In most states, medical technologists have a bachelor's degree in a biological science, which includes a year or more study in a school of medical technology. States have their own medical technology examination, but a national examination is also available for certification. Licensing is not mandatory in all states.

Medical technologists typically become specialists in different areas, such as serology or hematology or bacteriology. Nurses should understand how the laboratory is organized well enough that they do not call the chemistry section, for example, for the results of a culture and sensitivity test.

Laboratory Technicians. The meaning of the commonly used term ''lab technician'', is not precise. Medical technologists want to be known as medical technologists since any lab assistant may be called a lab technician. Laboratory assistants have a high school diploma, along with some on-the-job experience or training in certain laboratory techniques. Laboratory assistants draw blood, process specimens, and assist in performing some of the more routine tests in the laboratory.

Cooperating with Laboratory Personnel
Too often nursing and laboratory personnel conflict with each other rather than cooperate for the good of the patient. Laboratory personnel complain that specimens are not marked correctly—that they are lost or otherwise ineptly handled by the nursing staff. Patients are not always correctly prepared for examinations, or the laboratory personnel are not informed of changes in orders. On the other hand, nurses complain that the laboratory is insensitive to the individual needs of the patient, late with stat requests, curt and demanding with nurses, and so forth. Unfortunately, both departments often have legitimate reasons for gripes, but poor communication between the departments often allows small problems to become major frustrations.

For their own part in this ongoing feud, nurses need to perform their own functions as accurately as possible. The information in the rest of this book should enable nurses to function better in preparing the patient for laboratory testing, as well as make them sensitive to what the laboratory personnel needs to know about any special problems with patients. For example, if the nurse knows a patient is disoriented and potentially combative, the laboratory personnel should be warned about this attitude before they go in to draw blood or to do other procedures. Nurses forget that they are often the only health professional that see the patient for more than 15 minutes at a time.

Nurses in hospitals also have to face a fact of hospital life: Although they often complain that they must always plan their care around the visits from physicians, laboratory personnel, X-ray personnel—who drop in for brief contacts with the patient—these people must have access to the patient. Whereas the emphasis in nursing is on caring and nurturing to meet not only the physical needs but also the psychosocial needs of the patient, such is not always the emphasis of other health workers who are trained to do more technical jobs. Hence nurses can foster smoother relationships with other health care workers by making the patient available whenever possible. At the same time, since they spend more time with the patient than the others, they can often be advocates for the sick patient who must deal with a host of other people in a fragmented way.

In general, nurses need to work in a spirit of cooperation with other health care personnel so that each can function well. If they have specific problems with the laboratory—stats not being done, lost reports, or whatever—nurses should collect written data about the problem and present this to the nursing supervisor so that some changes can be made. A lot of complaining to other nurses during a coffee break accomplishes little, if it goes no further than a gripe session.

Questions

1-1. Mrs. Rhoades has a specific gravity of 1.030 and other clinical signs of dehydration. In using the nursing process, the nurse should use this information about specific gravity not only to make an assessment of the problem but also to:

    a. diagnose the pathophysiology or underlying disease.

    b. initiate treatment for the disease.

    c. evaluate the effectiveness of nursing interventions.

    d. all of the above are parts of the nursing process.

1-2. The traditional functions of the nurse in relation to laboratory tests include all the following except:

    a. transcribing physician's orders and making out requisitions for the laboratory.

    b. collecting and transporting specimens to the laboratory.

    c. conducting peripheral testing on the unit.

    d. scheduling the times when tests are done by laboratory personnel on the unit.

1-3. Which of these two factors are generally the most common reasons for variations in normal reference values for laboratory tests?

    a. genetic factors and drugs.

    b. sex (gender) and age.

    c. activity levels and stress.

    d. geographic location and diet.

1-4. If a test yields too many false positives, the test is described as:

    a. "not very sensitive."

    b. "too sensitive."

    c. "not specific."

    d. "highly specific."

1-5. If the normal curve is used to establish normal references for laboratory values, the results of a large sample of healthy individuals are compiled and the normal range is designated as:

    a. 37.5% above and 37.5% below the average (75% of all scores)

    b. the lower half of the sample (50% of all scores).

    c. any value within the range (100% of all scores).

    d. two standard deviations above and below the average (95% of all scores).

1-6. In conventional laboratory reports, the smallest amount of a substance would be measured by weight as a:

    a. ng.

    b. pg.

    c. dl.

    d. mg.

1-7. Laboratory results measured in SI units are reported as amount per volume as expressed by:

    a. milliequivalents (mEq).

    b. milliosmoles (mOsm).

    c. millimoles (mmol).

    d. milligrams (mg).

1-8. Which of the following is of questionable value as a *basic* screening test for *asymptomatic* adult populations?

    a. biochemical profile (BCP) or SMA-12.

    b. checking stools for occult blood (guaiac tests).

    c. checking for increased intraocular pressure (Tonometry).

    d. blood pressure checks.

1-9. Nurses can foster smooth working relationships with personnel in laboratory departments by all the following measures *except:*

    a. calling the laboratory to seek information about patient preparation for an unfamiliar test.

    b. seeing that stat specimens are hand delivered to the laboratory and that only real emergencies are marked stat.

    c. making sure that special needs of the patient are conveyed to personnel from other departments who must interact with the patient.

    d. complaining only to other nurses about the mistakes made by the laboratory personnel.

REFERENCES

Ahlvin, Robert. "Biochemical Screening—A Critique." *New England Journal of Medicine* (November 12, 1970): 1084–1086.

Balint, John. "When is a New Test a Valid Test?" *American Journal of Digestive Diseases* 23 (April 1978): 291–292.

Barnett, Roy *et al.* "Medical Usefulness of STAT Tests." *American Journal of Clinical Pathology* 69 (May 1978): 520–523.

Beeler, Myrton. "Interpretation of the Diagnostic Biochemical Profile." *Southern Medical Journal* 70 (December 1977): 1425–1427.

Blatt, George *et al.* "Diagnostic Kits: Product Survey." *Nursing 75* 5 (April 1975): 28–33.

Blue Cross of Northern California. "Medical Necessity Project." *Update—A Report to Administrators of Health Care Facilities* No. 30 (March 1978).

"Blue Cross/Blue Shield Limits Admission Test Payments," *American Journal of Nursing* 79 (April 1979): 572.

California Nurses Association (CNA), *Position Paper on Informed Consent.* San Francisco, Cal.: California Nurses Association, 1978.

Casscells, Ward *et al.* "Interpretation by Physicians of Clinical Laboratory Results." *New England Journal of Medicine* 229 (November 2, 1978): 999–1000.

Cherjan, George and Hill, Gilbert. "Percentile Estimates of Reference Values for 14 Chemical Constituents in Sera of Child and Adolescents." *American Journal of Clinical Pathology* 69 (January 1978): 24–31.

College of American Pathologists (CAP), *Why Do You Need a Laboratory Test?* (Patient Information Booklet) Skokie, Ill.: College of American Pathologists, 1979.

Daniels, Marcia and Schroder, Steve. "Variations Among Physicians in Use of Laboratory Tests, Relation to Clinical Productivity and Outcomes of Care," *Medical Care* 15 (June 1977): 482–487.

Dinham, Sarah. *Exploring Statistics.* Monterey, Cal.: Brooks/Cole Publishing Co., 1976.

Elrebach, L. R. *et al.* "Health, Normality and the Ghost of Gauss," *JAMA* 211 (1970): 69–75.

Galen, Robert. "True or False? Drugs Significantly Affect Clinical Laboratory Tests." *Diagnostic Medicine* 1 (November 1978): 99–100.

Galen, Robert. "Predictive Value of Laboratory Testing." *Orthopedic Clinics of North America* 10 (April 1979): 465–494.

Gordon, Marjory. "The Concept of Nursing Diagnosis," *Nursing Clinics of North America* 14 (September 1979): 487–495.

Gorry, Anthony. "The Diagnostic Importance of the Normal Finding." *New England Journal of Medicine* 298 (March 2, 1978): 486–489.

Harwood, Steven J. "Reference Values Based on Hospital Admission Laboratory Data," *JAMA* 240 (July 21, 1978): 270–274.

Hytten, Frank and Lind, Tom *Diagnostic Indices in Pregnancy.* Summit, N.J.: Ciba-Geigy Corp., 1975.

Kaiser Foundation Health Plan, "Adult Health Screening," *Planning for Health* 23 (January 1981): 1.

Luckmann, Joan and Sorenson, Karen. *Medical-Surgical Nursing: A Pathophysiological Approach.* 2nd ed. Philadelphia: W. B. Saunders Co., 1980.

Muschenheim, Frederick and Przada, Sandra. "We Banned Peripheral Testing in Our Hospital," *Medical Laboratory Observer 11* (May 1979): 143–145.

Oppenheim, Mike. "Medical Tests—How Useful Are They?" *Woman's Day* 43 (February 12, 1980): 58.

Reece, Richard and Hobbie, Russell. "Computer Evaluation of Chemistry Values." *American Journal of Clinical Pathology* 57 (May 1972): 664–675.

Reece, Richard and Hobbie, Russell. "Diagnostic Clues in Abnormal Test Patterns." *Patient Care* 12 (January 30, 1978): 74–77.

Schaefer, Steven and Dickman, Jones. "Automated Laboratory Screening: An Analysis of Value in a Nursing Home Population." *Wisconsin Medical Journal* 77 (August 1978): 81–82.

Schorr, Thelma. Editorial, *American Journal of Nursing* 75 (November 1975): 1979.

Scully, R. E., ed., Case Records of Massachusetts General Hospital. "Normal Reference Laboratory Values." *New England Journal of Medicine* 302 (January 3, 1980): 37–48.

Skendzel, Laurence. "How Physicians Use Laboratory Tests." *JAMA* 239 (March 13, 1978): 1077–1980.

Spark, Ronald and Kundert, Linda. "Control of Peripheral Testing by the Laboratory." *Medical Laboratory Observer* 11 (April 1979): 112–129.

Strand, Marcella and Strand, Lucille. *Clinical Laboratory Tests: A Manual for Nurses,* 2nd ed. St. Louis, Mo.: C. V. Mosby Co., 1980.

Young, D. S. "Standardized Reporting of Laboratory Data: The Desirability of Using SI Units," *New England Journal of Medicine* 290 (February 14, 1974): 368–373.

CHAPTER TWO

Hematology Tests

Objectives

1. Describe the purpose for each of the seven different tests done by the Coulter counter.
2. Plan appropriate patient care goals for patients with increased and decreased hemoglobin and RBC levels.
3. Anticipate how a change in the hydration status of a patient affects hematocrit (Hct) results.
4. Describe how acute and chronic blood loss, iron deficiency anemia, and pernicious anemia change the erythrocyte indices (MCV, MCH, and MCHC).
5. Prepare teaching plans, which include specific information on drugs and diet, for patients with abnormal serum folic acid, B_{12}, iron or G-6-PD levels.
6. Give examples of patient care situations in which an elevated reticulocyte count is an expected physiological response.
7. Plan appropriate nursing interventions for a patient with rheumatoid arthritis who has an increasing erythrocyte sedimentation rate (sed rate or ESR).
8. Compare and contrast reference values for the WBC differential count in children, in adults, and in pregnancy.
9. Define the meaning of the phrase "shift to the left" with regard to the WBC differential count.
10. Plan appropriate nursing interventions for patients with increased and decreased levels of the different types of leukocytes.

The five components of the complete blood count (CBC) are:

1. the red blood cell count (RBC),
2. the hematocrit (Hct or Crit),
3. the hemoglobin (Hb or Hgb),
4. the white blood count (WBC), and
5. the differential white count (Diff).

TABLE 2-1.   SEVEN TESTS DONE AUTOMATICALLY BY COULTER COUNTER*

Hct	Hematocrit
Hb	Hemoglobin
WBC	Leukocyte or white blood cells (differential requires separate test)
RBC	Erythrocyte or red blood cells
MCV	Mean corpuscular volume
MCH	Mean corpuscular hemoglobin
MCHC	Mean corpuscular hemoglobin concentration

*Can do all tests on 1 ml of blood. Blood is collected in a vacutainer with EDTA as anticoagulant (lavender top). See Appendix A.

Sometimes only one component of the CBC is needed. For example, if the primary concern is assessing blood loss, a Hct done a few hours after the bleeding gives an index of the severity of the blood loss. With an undiagnosed anemia, it would be important to have RBC, Hb, and Hct readings. These three different measurements of the erythrocytes (red blood cells) are the figures used to compute the erythrocyte indices: (1) mean corpuscular volume (MCV), (2) mean corpuscular hemoglobin (MCH), and (3) mean corpuscular hemoglobin concentration (MCHC).

Routine hematology tests can be done by automatic counters so the results are more reliable than the older method of counting under a microscope. See Table 2–1 for the seven tests routinely done by a Coulter counter, a standard instrument in almost all laboratories. If the WBC is abnormal, it is necessary to know which of the five types of white blood cells are increased or decreased. The test of the five WBC types is called a *differential*. In some laboratories, differentials are still done by hand, but certain machines can also stain and count the various types of normal white blood cells. Abnormal cells must be examined by microscope.

A reticulocyte count gives an indication of the rate of production of red blood cells. One test that involves erythrocytes and that is discussed in this chapter is the sed rate, or ESR (erythrocyte sedimentation rate), but it really has nothing to do with erythrocyte production or function. The sed rate or ESR is a test for inflammatory reactions. A peripheral smear of blood is done to look for abnormal blood cells. This chapter mentions some of the common terms used on laboratory reports of peripheral smears. Related hematology tests (such as serum iron levels, folic acid, B_{12} levels and G-6-PD) are also mentioned because they may be needed to assess a persistent and unexplained anemic state. Although platelets are formed by the bone marrow, these fragments of tissue are not really blood cells in the true sense of the word. Platelets are covered with tests of clotting factors in Chapter 13.

RED BLOOD CELL COUNT (RBC)

The RBC is a count of the number of red blood cells per cubic millimeter (mm^3) of blood. In addition to other less understood mechanisms, a hormone named erythropoietin is secreted by the kidney and stimulates the production of red blood cells by the red bone marrow. Tissue hypoia causes an increased secretion of erythropoietin.

Preparation of Patient
And Collection of Sample

There is no special preparation of the patient for this test, which requires 1 ml of venous blood. EDTA is used as the anticoagulant (Lavender top vacutainer.)

Reference Values

Male adult	4.6-6.2 million (or 10^6)/mm^3
Female adult	4.2-5.4 million/mm^3
Pregnancy	Slightly lower
Newborns	5.5-6, gradually decreases
Children	4.6-4.8, varies with age

Note also that values increase at high altitudes.

Increased RBC (Polycythemia)

Clinical Significance. Physiological increases of RBC's occur with a move to high altitude or after increased physical training. In both instances, the underlying reason is a response to an increased need for oxygen. At high altitude there is less oxygen in the atmosphere, so the bone marrow increases the production of red blood cells. In the event of prolonged physical training, the increased muscle mass requires more oxygen.

The RBC may be elevated also for many pathological reasons. One is a disease of unknown origin called polycythemia vera, whose name implies that it is a true (''vera'') increase in RBC. The increase in this case is not due to an oxygen need, as it is in all other cases of polycythemia, which are termed *secondary*. Two very common clinical examples of secondary polycythemia are patients with chronic lung diseases and children with congenital heart defects that display cyanosis. Secondary polycythemia is an attempt to compensate for the chronic hypoxia brought on by the disease state.

Possible Nursing Implications.

Differentiating between Primary and Secondary Polycythemia. In caring for a patient with an elevated RBC, the nurse must differentiate primary from secondary polycythemia. In the event of primary polycythemia, medical treatment is geared to slowing the overactive bone marrow. More commonly, the polycythemia is secondary to a state of chronic hypoxia, and so therapeutic measures are geared toward correcting the cause of the hypoxia. For example, when will the child with a congenital heart defect have surgery? In the meantime, how much activity is optimal? What can the nurse do to help improve the lung functioning of a patient with chronic lung disease?

Maintaining Adequate Hydration. One of the basic problems that occurs with polycythemia, regardless of the cause, is that the blood becomes more viscous, and this increased viscosity makes the patient more susceptible for the formation of venous thrombi. A key nursing implication for the patient with polycythemia is therefore to maintain adequate hydration of the patient. In some cases, it may be desirable to increase fluids to a set level, such as a minimum of 2,000 ml a day for an adult. Before assuming that fluids need to be increased, assess the overall status of the patient, particularly the cardiovascular status. Both children with congenital heart defects and adults with chronic lung disease may often be on the verge of congestive heart failure. Confer with the physician to determine the optimal hydration state for individual patients. It is important that any patient with polycythemia not become dehydrated. For example, it may be harmful for the patient to be kept NPO for an extended time for tests.

Encouraging Activity. The patient with polycythemia needs as much activity as possible so that venous stasis does not contribute to the potential problem of venous thrombosis.

Assisting with Medical Interventions. Sometimes a phlebotomy (the opening of a vein) is done for the patient with too many red blood cells. Usually about a pint of blood is removed at one time for an adult and less for a child. The procedure is very similar to taking a pint of blood from a donor, except that the collection bottle does not have anticoagulant chemicals because the removed blood is never used for transfusions. In time, however, the red bone marrow replaces the red blood cells, so a phlebotomy is a temporary alleviation. Myelosuppressive agents, such as radioactive phosphorus (P^{32}) or nitrogen mustard compounds, may be administered for polycythemia vera. Luckman (1980: 1055) discusses the various treatments for polycythemia.

Decreased RBC

Clinical Significance. A low red blood cell count can result from:

1. an abnormal loss of erythrocytes,
2. abnormal destruction of erythrocytes,
3. a lack of needed elements or hormones for erythrocyte production, or
4. bone marrow suppression.

The term "anemia" is a nonspecific term that can mean a decrease either in the total number of red blood cells, in the hemoglobin level of red blood cells, or in both the number and the hemoglobin content of red blood cells. Thus if the RBC count is low, looking at hemoglobin levels is also important in order to classify the type of anemia. The classification of different types of anemia is covered under the section on erythrocyte indices.

Possible Nursing Implications. It is not necessary for an RBC count to be used routinely to check for bleeding because the hematocrit (Hct) can be done more quickly. Refer to the section on hematocrit to see the nursing implications when the low RBC is due to blood loss.

If the low RBC is caused by some condition other than blood loss, then hemoglobin levels and a peripheral smear that identifies the shape and size of erythrocytes may be necessary to identify the type of anemia. Refer to the sections on hemoglobin and on erythrocyte indices for related nursing implications in different types of anemias.

HEMATOCRIT (Hct, PCV, or Crit)

The hematocrit is a fast way to determine the percentage of red blood cells in the plasma. When the serum is centrifuged, the white blood cells and platelets rise to the top in what is called the Buffy coat. Since the heavier red blood cells are packed in the bottom, the hematocrit is sometimes also called the PCV or packed cell volume. The hematocrit is reported as a percentage because it is the proportion of red blood cells to the plasma. Note that the results are based on the assumptions that the plasma volume is normal. A hematocrit is useful as a measurement of the red blood cell count *only if the hydration of the patient is normal*. The newer technique of microhematocrits, which takes only a few milliliters of blood, is generally as accurate as the older macrohematocrit or Wintrobe technique of centrifuging a larger amount of blood. (Ravel 1978:2).

Preparation of Patient
And Collection of Sample

There is no special preparation of the patient. Since the Hct can be done on capillary blood, a patient may have a finger stick (or heel stick for infants) rather than a venipuncture. (See Chapter I for the procedure for heel and finger sticks.) The first drop of blood is discarded, enough blood is collected to fill a capillary tube supplied by the laboratory, and a small band-aid can be placed over the site. The stick method should be noted on the laboratory requisition because capillary values may be 5 to 10% higher than values by venipuncture. Do *not* squeeze the tissue to get capillary blood because doing so adds tissue fluids, which dilute the sample.

Reference Values

Adult:	Male	45–52%
	Female	37–48%
Pregnancy		Decreases, particularly in last trimester as serum volume increases (Hytten 1975)
Newborn		Up to 60%
Children		Varies with age

Note that capillary blood may be 5–10% higher. Values are increased in high altitudes.

Relation to Hemoglobin Levels

If the RBC and Hb are both normal, the Hct is about three times the Hb. So a patient whose Hct is 45% would be expected to have a Hb of about 15 g.

Increased Hematocrit

Clinical Significance. Since the hematocrit is a proportion (or percentage) of red blood cells to volume, any decrease in the volume of plasma causes an increase in the hematocrit, even though the red blood cells have not increased. Any kind of severe dehydration makes the Hct abnormally high. For example, in the patient with a burn, plasma can be lost in large amounts through damaged capillaries in the burned area. The loss of fluid from the vascular space makes the blood very concentrated, and hence the Hct may be as high as 60 or 65%.

If the patient's hydration status is normal, an elevated hematocrit signifies a true increase of red blood cells. Reasons for an increased red blood cell count (polycythemia) were discussed under the section on RBC.

Possible Nursing Implications. When caring for a patient with an increased hematocrit, it is essential to find out if this is a reflection of (1) decreased plasma volume or (2) a true increase in red blood cells. If all clinical assessments point to lack of volume, measures to increase the plasma volume are needed. Medical orders may include a plan to give fluids intravenously. For example, parenteral fluid replacement is an essential part of the treatment for a patient with severe burns. In other, less severe situations, it may be sufficient to increase fluids orally to overcome dehydration.

If the elevated hematocrit reflects an increased number of red blood cells, some additional fluids may be appropriate to decrease the blood viscosity. The precautions for overhydrating the patient with polycythemia were mentioned in the previous section on increased RBC counts.

Decreased Hematocrit

Clinical Significance. A decreased hematocrit can be due to either (1) an overhydration of the patient, which increases the plasma volume, or (2) a true decrease in the number of red blood cells. The second reason for the low hematocrit is much more common. See the previous discussion on RBC for the causes of decreased RBC's.

Possible Nursing Implications. In the rare situation where the low hematocrit reflects an increased plasma volume, the patient may show some other signs and symptoms of excess fluid. Therapeutic measures may include a decrease in fluid intake. However, the hematocrit test is not a key assessment tool for volume expansion. (See the discussion on low serum sodium levels, Chapter 5, as a test for overhydration.)

One of the major uses for the hematocrit is assessing the magnitude of blood loss. It is important for nurses to realize that a hematocrit drawn immediately after a massive blood loss will probably be normal because both plasma and red cells have been lost in equal proportions. Within a few hours after a bleeding episode, assuming the patient has adequate fluid balance, the plasma volume returns to normal by a shift of some interstitial fluid into the plasma. The red blood cells, however, cannot be replaced so quickly. The bone marrow takes about seven days to make new cells, and those cells need another four days to mature. So a few hours after the bleeding episode, the plasma volume is back to normal and the hematocrit becomes low because the red blood cells that were lost in the hemorrhage are still missing. *A hematocrit reading must always be interpreted in relationship to the time drawn and to the probable hydration status of the patient at the time.*

Assessing for Associated Symptoms. Paleness of the skin, particularly of the conjunctiva, is a clue that there has been a significant blood loss. Checking for pallor of the conjunctiva is particularly helpful for assessing black patients. Since the plasma volume is usually replaced within a few hours after a bleeding episode, patients with low hematocrits have normal blood pressures. If there is not enough fluid to shift in the vascular space to make up the loss, the blood pressure falls and the patient shows signs of shock. However, if the blood loss is not severe enough to create shock, the pulse may still give a clue to the magnitude of blood loss: The pulse increases when the patient sits up—the "tilt" test. The pulse may become even more elevated if much exercise is attempted because the oxygen-carrying capacity of the blood is diminished. When the hematocrit is as low as 28%, the cardiac rate may be increased even at rest. Monitoring the pulse before and after activity helps to assess the effect of the low hematocrit on the individual patient.

Preventing Fatigue. Weakness and fatigue on exertion should be taken into account when planning activities. It may be better not to do the patient's bathing, bed-changing,and mobilization all at once. If a low Hct continues to drop, then a key nursing implication is to assess for signs of continued bleeding. A detailed description of nursing assessments for occult (hidden) bleeding is covered in Chapter 13 on clotting factors.

Differences Between Acute and Chronically Low Hematocrits. The effect of the low hematocrit on the patient not only depends on how low the hematocrit is, but also on whether the loss is acute or chronic. If the hematocrit is low due to a sudden blood loss, the patient may quickly develop signs of shock. A patient with a chronically low hemato-crit may have only a few symptoms because the body has had time to adjust to the low number of red blood cells. For example, patients on renal dialysis often tolerate a hematocrit as low as 18%. (The low hematocrit in renal failure is partially due to a lack of the hormone erythropoietin that is normally produced by the kidney.) A patient with sickle cell anemia is another example of a patient who may have few symptoms related to a hematocrit as low as 18 to 20%. (In sickle cell anemia the red blood cells have an abnormal type of hemoglobin, which decreases the life of the red blood cells.) The essential point to remember about interpreting low hematocrits is to understand not just the reason for the low hematocrit, but also whether the drop is acute or chronic.

Patient Teaching on Iron and Protein Intake. The patient with a low hematocrit needs adequate iron and protein in the diet so that the bone marrow can manufacture additional red blood cells. If oral intake is possible, the nurse may help the patient choose foods that are high in protein and iron. Iron derived from animal products, called *heme iron,* is readily available for absorption. Iron from all other sources, called *nonheme iron,* is often not absorbed well due to dietary inhibitors. Recent studies have shown that ascorbic acid is one of the most powerful promoters of nonheme iron absorption (Lynch 1980). The person who also has a lack of protein may produce less protein hormones such as erythropoietin (Price 1976:170). A dietician can be useful to help plan optimal meals for the severely malnourished.

Once a patient is deficient in iron, as happens with a chronic blood loss, it may be difficult to increase iron intake by diet alone. Sometimes the patient is put on iron supplements. Patients need to be aware that iron supplements cause the feces to be a dark greenish-black in color and that iron can be constipating. Iron is better absorbed in a acidic stomach but some iron combinations are better tolerated with food. The patient should not take antacids and iron together since the iron is much less soluble in an alkaline medium. Other drugs, such as tetracycline and cholesterol-lowering drugs, also significantly reduce iron absorption (Rodman 1981: 65). The usual therapeutic plan is to continue iron supple-ments for about three months after the hematocrit is back to normal because the body takes this long to build up a reserve of iron (Wood 1977). Patients are usually quite interested in knowing the change in hematocrit reading, and their inquiry can be a good occasion to explain why iron is needed. Serial hematocrits are used to assess whether the amount of red blood cells have returned to normal.

Assisting with Blood Transfusions. If the hematocrit is below 25 to 30%, a physician may order blood, usually in the form of packed cells, to replace the erythrocytes. Packed cells are used when the patient needs the red blood cells but not additional plasma. No set figure means the patient needs blood. As discussed earlier, some patients have chronically low hematocrits with few symptoms. Depending on the symptoms of the patient and on the individual circumstances, blood may be given before patients have hematocrits as low as 25 or 30%. For example, if a patient is going to surgery, it is important that the hematocrit not be too low—"too low" usually meaning under 30%. Because blood transfusions can create additional problems, such as allergic reactions or hepatitis, the physician may choose to let the body replenish erythrocytes normally whenever this is feasible. (See Chapter 14 for a discussion on transfusion reactions.) As a rough guideline, a unit of whole blood or packed cells raises the hematocrit about 3% in an adult (Ravel 1978:100).

HEMOGLOBIN (Hb or Hgb)

Hemoglobin is composed of a pigment (*heme*), which contains iron and a protein part (*globin*). If each erythrocyte has the normal amount of hemoglobin, the hematocrit is roughly three times the hemoglobin level. A hematocrit of 45% would indicate around 15 g of hemoglobin. It is not necessary to do both tests to assess for bleeding. As already discussed, the hematocrit is a simpler test to monitor blood loss. If red blood cells are abnormal in size or shape, or if hemoglobin is not being produced normally, the hemoglobin level cannot be estimated from the hematocrit reading. Hemoglobin levels are necessary as part of the assessment for various types of anemia. See the erythrocyte indices for an explanation of how the hemoglobin level is used with hematocrit and RBC tests to get a clearer picture of erythrocyte abnormalities.

Preparation of Patient
And Collection of Sample
There is no special preparation of patient. Venous blood is used for the test. EDTA (lavender top Vacutainer) is used as the anticoagulant in the collection tube.

Reference Values

Adult:	Male	13.0–18.0 g/100 ml
	Female	12–16 g/100 ml
Pregnancy		11–12 g/100 ml
Newborn		17–19 g/100 ml
		(80% fetal hemoglobin) (Jensen 1981)
Children		14–17, depending on age

Values increase in high altitudes.

Increased Hemoglobin

Clinical Significance. Since a normal red blood cell already contains the optimum amount of hemoglobin, any increase in hemoglobin levels must be looked at in relation to the number and size of the erythrocytes. See the discussion on erythrocyte indices for an explanation of how the hemoglobin level is used with the hematocrit and RBC to determine if the erythrocyte is hypochromic (less color), normochromic, or (very rarely) hyperchromic.

Related Nursing Implications. See section on increased RBC.

Decreased Hemoglobin

Clinical Significance. Since hemoglobin is a component of the red blood cell, all the conditions that cause a low RBC naturally result in a low hemoglobin level too. Some of the common conditions for a low RBC would be blood loss, hemolytic anemias, and any type of bone marrow suppression.

Hemoglobin levels are low in persons who have abnormal types of hemoglobin or hemoglobinopathies. Red blood cells with abnormal types of hemoglobin tend to be fragile and easily destroyed in the vascular system. The normal hemoglobin in adults is almost all adult hemoglobin (HbA) with only a very small amount (0–2%) of fetal hemoglobin (HbF). A process called *hemoglobin electrophoresis* can identify the specific type of abnormal hemoglobin that is present. Over 200 hemoglobins can be identified, but only a few cause symptoms (McFarlane 1977).

In thalassemia major, the person has an unusual amount of fetal hemoglobin and abnormalities in the synthesis of hemoglobin. The abnormal red blood cells can be identified by a peripheral blood smear. In sickle cell anemia, the person has an abnormal hemoglobin called *sickle hemoglobin* (HbS). (See Chapter 18 for screening tests for sickle cell anemia and for thalassemia, which are both genetically determined.)

It is possible to have a normal RBC count with a low hemoglobin level. For example, with an iron deficiency anemia, the count may be near normal but each cell has less hemoglobin than normal. This is called a *hypochromic* (less than normal color) anemia. The cells also tend to be *microcytic* (smaller than normal). Women in general need more iron than men due to the loss of iron in the menstrual flow, and women who have heavy menses may be prone to low hemoglobin levels. The demand for iron is increased in pregnancy. If a woman begins pregnancy with low iron reserves, she may become severely anemic as the pregnancy progresses. It is recommended that a pregnant woman be tested for hemoglobin levels at the beginning of pregnancy, about mid-pregnancy, and during the month prior to delivery (Connell 1979). Since there is a normal drop in hemoglobin levels in the last trimester, due to the expanded plasma volume, some lowering in hemoglobin levels is "normal." This lowering is sometimes called the *physiological anemia of pregnancy.*

Possible Nursing Implications. Most of the nursing implications for the patient with a low hemoglobin level have already been covered in the section on low Hct. Additional insights about the significance of low hemoglobin levels are covered in the section on erythrocyte indices. See the section on MCH (mean corpuscular hemoglobin) and MCHC (mean corpuscular hemoglobin concentration) for nursing implications for hypochromic and normochromic anemias.

ERYTHROCYTE INDICES

To make the nonspecific term "anemia" more meaningful, it is necessary to see whether the individual red cells are their normal size and whether they have the normal amount of hemoglobin concentration. The determinations can be made by comparing the results of the Hb, Hct, and RBC. In laboratories that use automated counters—and almost all of them do now—the indices are automatically figured as part of the CBC. Nurses never need to figure out the indices, but the formula for each is given, because they make it easy to explain the meaning of the results. In the examples used, the patient has a Hct of 40%. a Hb of 13.5 g, and a RBC of 4.5 million/mm^3. Note that with these figures all the indices would, of course, be normal.

Preparation of Patient
And Collection of Sample
There is no need to draw additional blood since the indices are derived from the Hct, Hb, and RBC.

MEAN CORPUSCULAR VOLUME (MCV)

The mean corpuscular volume (MCV) describes the mean or average size of the individual red blood cell in cubic microns. The hematocrit is divided by the RBC to obtain the MCV.

Reference Value and Example

Reference Value	80–94 cubic microns
Formula	$MCV = \dfrac{Hct \% \times 10}{RBC \ (millions/mm^3)}$
Patient Example	$\dfrac{Hct \ 40\% \times 10}{RBC \ 4.5} = 89$ microns

Change in the MCV

Clinical Significance. The MCV is an indicator of the size of the red blood cells. If the MCV is lower than 80 cubic microns, the erythrocytes are *microcytic,* or smaller than normal. Red blood cells are microcytic in certain types of anemia such as iron deficiency anemia. Thalassemia minor and thalassemia major (Cooley's anemia), which are genetic diseases, also cause microcytosis. (See Chapter 18 on screening tests for the thalassemias.) If the MCV is higher than 94 cubic microns, the erythrocytes are *macrocytic,* or larger than normal. Macrocytic red blood cells are characteristic of pernicious anemia and folic acid deficiencies. If the MCV is within normal reference range, the erythrocytes are *normocytic,* or of normal size. Anemia from an acute blood loss would result in a normocytic anemia. Also, sickle cell anemia may have normal size cells.

Obviously the size of the red blood cells is not enough to diagnose the reason for the anemia, but, with other indices (MCH and MCHC), the anemia can be classified by size and color. Other tests, such as the peripheral blood smear, can identify the characteristic cell shapes of various pathologies.

MCH(Mean Corpuscular Hemoglobin)

These two parts of the erythrocyte indices are discussed together because both are ways to determine whether the erythrocytes are *normochromic* (normal color), *hypochromic* (less than normal color), or *hyperchromic* (more than normal color). The MCH is the amount of hemoglobin present in a single cell. The result is reported by weight in picograms. The weight of hemoglobin in the average cell is obtained by dividing the hemoglobin by the RBC.

Reference Value and Example

Reference Value	MCH 27–32 pg (picogram)
Formula	$MCH = \dfrac{Hb\ (g/100\ ml) \times 10}{RBC\ (in\ millions/ml^3)}$
Patient Example	$\dfrac{13.5\ g \times 10}{4.5} = 30\ pg$

MCHC (Mean Corpuscular Concentration)

The mean corpuscular hemoglobin concentration (MCHC) is the proportion of each cell occupied by hemoglobin. Since this is a proportion, the results are reported in percentages. To get the percentage, the hemoglobin is divided by the Hct and multiplied by 100.

Reference Value and Example

Reference Value	32 to 36%
Formula	$MCHC = \dfrac{Hb\ (g/100\ ml)}{Hct} \times 100$
Patient Example	$\dfrac{13.5\ g \times 100}{40\%} = 33.8\%$

Changes in MCH and MCHC

Clinical Significance. The MCHC is more useful than just the MCH in determining the actual hemoglobin concentration in the cells. A decreased MCHC below 32% (or a MCH below 17 pg) indicates that the erythrocytes have a decrease in hemoglobin concentration (hypochromic). Iron deficiency anemia is the most common type of hypochromic anemia. Chronic conditions that cause anemia may show some hypochromia, but they are usually not as marked as when there is a true deficiency of iron. Certain genetically caused anemias such as thalassemia (Cooley's anemia) cause hypochromia too. With many types of anemia, the remaining cells have the normal amount of hemoglobin and hence are called normochromic. Hyperchromia (an abnormally high MCHC) is not seen except for a rare genetic condition called *hereditary spherocytosis*. As a general rule, normal red blood cells can hold only so much hemoglobin so the cells cannot be hyperchromic.

Possible Nursing Implications. It is important for the nurse to understand that abnormal erythrocyte indices are useful in classifying types of anemia, but they are not enough to establish a definite medical diagnosis. The history of the patient, physical assessment findings, and other tests are needed to determine the cause for the anemia. The specific nursing interventions depend on the reason for the anemia. Some general nursing implications for patients with anemia were discussed under the sections on RBC, Hb, and Hct. Other general nursing implications can be classified under the three categories of anemia. (See Table 2–2 for a list of the three categories and common pathology that could cause each type.)

Microcytic, Hypochromic Anemias. Most likely this type of anemia is due to an iron deficiency, if other causes are ruled out (Crosby 1979). The serum iron level can be measured, as well as the iron binding capacity. (These two tests are discussed next.) As discussed earlier in the section on Hb, it is hard to correct an iron deficiency with diet alone. (See the section on hemoglobin for what to teach a patient about iron therapy.)

Normocytic, Normochromic Anemias. As discussed, the cause could range from acute blood loss to a chronic genetic problem such as sickle cell disease. With a normocytic anemia, iron supplements may not be needed, but the nurse should make sure that the patient has adequate protein and iron in the diet since there is a continuing need for an increased production of red blood cells. If the anemia is of genetic origin, the nurse's role centers on helping the patient and family adjust to a chronic disease (see Chapter 18 on genetic screening). Anemia is but one sign of a larger pathological problem.

Macrocytic Anemias. This type of anemia may be hypochromic, normochromic, or very rarely hyperchromic. The two most common reasons for macrocytic anemias are vitamin B_{12} deficiency and folic acid deficiency. These two anemias are also called *megaloblastic anemias.* "Megaloblastic" refers to the appearance of a certain type of red blood cell precursor in the bone marrow and often in the bloodstream. It is very important

TABLE 2–2. CLASSIFICATION OF ANEMIAS BY ERYTHROCYTE INDICES*

Laboratory Results	Classification	Example of Common Pathology
MCV, MCH, and MCHC all normal	Normocytic, normochromic anemias	Acute blood loss
Decreased MCV, decreased MCH, and decreased MCHC	Microcytic, hypochromic anemias	Iron deficiency
Increased MCV, variable MCH and MCHC	Macrocytic anemia	B_{12} deficiency Folate deficiency

See text for explanation and Crosby (1979) for more details.

that the exact cause of the macrocytic anemia be identified since folic acid replacements can reverse the anemia, but folic acid cannot prevent the degeneration in the spinal cord from a persisting vitamin B_{12} deficiency due to pernicious anemia (Wood 1977).

Patient Teaching about Pernicious Anemia. Pernicious anemia (a type of macrocytic anemia) refers to a pathological inability of the body to absorb vitamin B_{12} due to the lack of the intrinsic factor in the stomach. (The Schilling test is a test for B_{12} absorption.) Nurses can help patients understand that not all types of "tired blood" can be treated with over-the-counter vitamin and iron mixtures. Patients often do not understand that anemia is only a symptom. The underlying pathological reason for the anemia must be determined to ensure its successful treatment. For example, if the macrocytic anemia turns out to be due to pernicious anemia, the patient needs vitamin B_{12} shots for the rest of his or her life. So the nurse will probably be involved in helping the patient and a member of the family learn to give injections.

Preventing Folic Acid Deficiencies. Since vitamin B_{12} is present in all animal protein, rarely do people in this country develop a true deficiency. However, unless vegetables are fresh, folic acid deficiency can develop since most of the folic acid is destroyed by heat.

Pregnancy and the use of oral contraceptives are situations where a macrocytic anemia may occur due to an increased need for folic acid in the diet (Aftergood 1980). Oral contraceptives may also cause a decrease in vitamin B_{12} (see Appendix D). Folic acid antagonists, such as methotrexate used for cancer treatment, may also deplete the patient of folic acid. It may be necessary for some patients to have oral supplemental vitamin preparations that are high in folic acid. Orange juice is a good natural source of folate. Folic acid can also be given subcutaneously if malabsorption is a problem (Loebel 1977:655).

Alcohol abuse may contribute to the development of a macrocytic anemia due not only to folate and/or B_{12} deficiency, but also to other unknown factors (Crosby 1979). In such cases, diet teaching is of little avail until other problems are addressed. It is important for the nurse to see abnormal indices in relation to the patient's total picture.

SERUM FOLIC ACID AND VITAMIN B_{12}

Both B_{12} and folate can be measured in the serum when the initial laboratory results show macrocytosis (elevated MCV), a low reticulocyte count (discussed later), and hypersegmented neutrophils. These tests are used to help in diagnosing a macrocytic anemia that may be due to dietary deficiency or malabsorption.

Reference Values

Folic acid	Greater than 1.9 ng/ml (Borderline 1.0-1.9 ng/ml)
Vitamin B_{12}	90-280 pg/ml (Borderline 70-90)

Preparation of Patient
And Collection of Sample

Check with the laboratory about food or drug interference. No special preparation of patient is necessary. The test for folic acid requires 1 ml of serum. The test for vitamin B_{12} requires 12 ml of serum.

Deficiencies

Clinical Significance. See the previous discussion on macrocytic anemias. Note that the Schilling test is a specific test for a lack of vitamin B_{12} absorption.

SERUM IRON (Fe) LEVELS,
TOTAL IRON BINDING CAPACITY (TIBC),
AND SERUM FERRITIN LEVELS

The measurement of serum iron is used to assess the adequacy of iron in the body. A small amount of ferritin, the major iron-storage protein, is normally present in the serum. In healthy adults, serum ferritin concentrations are directly related to iron stores (Jacobs 1975). Transferin is the iron-transporting plasma protein; normally about one-third of this plasma protein transports iron. The total iron-binding capacity (TIBC) is a measurement of the transferin available to bind more iron.

These three tests are not *routine* for all patients who are put on iron supplements. Rather, they are reserved for further evaluation of patients with microcytic hypochromic anemia who do not respond to iron therapy. These tests may also be used to help diagnose iron depletion in renal failure or in iron storage problems of the liver.

Preparation of Patient
And Collection of Sample

The patient should be fasting but can have water. The tests of iron and TIBC require 5 ml of serum. Special iron-free tubes and needles are required. (Vacutainers with brown tops have minimal lead content.) Check with the laboratory for specific methods for ferritin levels.

Reference Values

Serum iron	50–150μg/dl (higher in males)
Serum ferritin	20–400 ng/l
	Values vary depending on techniques. Mean for men is around 120, and 55 for women.
Total iron-binding capacity (TIBC)	250–410 μg/dl

Changes in Iron Levels

Clinical Significance. A low serum iron and a high TIBC suggest the need for continued iron replacement. A high or normal serum iron and a normal TIBC are evidence that the hematological problem is not due to iron deficiency. Pathological conditions such as liver necrosis, leukemia, and Hodgkin's disease all falsely elevate iron levels. Diseases such as hemochromatosis can cause elevated iron stores. The measurement of ferritin gives additional information about the adequacy of iron storage. Less than 20 ng of ferritin indicates iron deficiency and above 400 ng is a sign of iron excess.

GLUCOSE-6-PHOSPHATE-DEHYDROGENASE (G-6-PD)

Glucose-6-phosphate-dehydrogenase (G-6-PD) is one of many enzymes normally present in the erythrocytes. Some people have a lack of this enzyme due to a genetic defect. Such persons may develop hemolytic anemia if exposed to certain drugs, infections, or an acidotic state. Drugs that cause hemolysis of erythrocytes in susceptible people are the sulfas, nitrofurantoin (Furadantin), aspirin, and phenacetin (Ravel 1978:32). Several laboratory tests detect a deficiency of this enzyme. Since there are two common types of G-6-PD deficiencies known as African and Mediterranean variance, some drugs may cause hemolysis only in one or the other (Prchal 1980:41).

Preparation of Patient
And Collection of Sample

There is no special preparation of the patient. The test requires 9 ml of venous blood collected in a tube with a special anticoagulant (ACD). Note that various laboratories may do other types of testing that require only a few milliliters of blood with other anticoagulants.

Reference Values

All groups 5-15 U/g Hb

G-6-PD Deficiencies

Clinical Significance. The G-6-PD test may be used to determine if a hemolytic anemia is due to a lack of this specific enzyme. Other enzymes, such as pyruvate kinase, may also be deficient in the erythrocytes and cause anemia, but a lack of G 6 PD is more common. The lack of the enzyme is a sex-linked recessive trait carried on the X chromosomes. The effect is more pronounced in males. (See Chapter 18 for a discussion on genetic diseases.) Unless the person either is exposed to drugs that cause the hemolysis or has a severe infection or an acidiotic state, he or she is typically unaware of the defect.

Possible Nursing Implications. The person who has a lack of G-6-PD must not be given any of the drugs that can cause hemolysis. Patients need health teaching about exactly which drugs are to be avoided. Certain foods, such as fava beans, are not tolerated if the defect is the Mediterranean variant (Prchal 1980).

RETICULOCYTE COUNT (Retic Count)

Reticulocytes are the less mature type of red blood cells in the bloodstream. They are called reticulocytes because they show a fine network (reticulum) when stained. After about four days in the bloodstream, the cell loses this reticulum and becomes a mature red blood cell. The reticulocyte count is valuable because it is a measure of bone marrow function.

Preparation of Patient
And Collection of Sample

There is no special preparation of the patient. Laboratory needs less than a ml of blood.

Reference Values

Adults	0.5-1.5% of the total RBC
Pregnancy	Slight increase
Newborns	Increased first week 3-5%

Increased Reticulocyte Count

Clinical Significance. An increase in the percentage of reticulocytes indicates that the release of red blood cells into the bloodstream is occurring more rapidly than usual. Since this is a physiological response to the need for more red blood cells, the retic count may be as high as 10% after an acute blood loss. Such an increase is also expected when the appropriate treatment is begun for a specific type of anemia. For example, when the patient with iron deficiency anemia is given iron supplements, the retic count may go as high as 32%.

Possible Nursing Implications. An increase in the retic count after therapy for anemia has begun is an encouraging sign that the bone marrow is responding to the treatment. The nurse can use this test as one part of an assessment of an improving clinical situation.

Decreased Reticulocyte Count

Clinical Significance. In certain macrocytic anemias (see the discussion under erythrocyte indices), cell development is arrested before the reticulocyte stage. For example, in pernicious anemia, the ineffective production of red blood cells leads to a low reticulocyte count.

Possible Nursing Implications. A decrease in reticulocytes, particularly after a bleeding episode, indicates an abnormal response of the bone marrow. The patient needs further medical evaluation to determine the reason for this lack of erythrocyte production. In certain macrocytic anemias, such as pernicious anemia, red blood cell development is arrested before the reticulocyte stage. However, once effective treatment is begun, the reticulocyte count should increase. If the count does not rise after treatment, the patient needs further medical evaluation as to the cause of the anemia.

PERIPHERAL BLOOD SMEAR

The peripheral blood smear is useful for the identification of abnormalities in erythrocytes, leukocytes, and platelets. If necessary, a bone marrow may be done as a follow-up for abnormal results. A review of hematology studies by Byrne (1976) includes technical details about red cell morphology.

Only the more common terms that may appear on laboratory reports are included here:

Descriptive Terms for RBC

1. *Anisocytosis* means that the cells vary in size.
2. *Poikilocytosis* means that the cells are irregular in shape.
3. *Rouleaux formation* is a laboratory phenomenon in which red blood cells stick to one another. (Note that this is the basis for the sedimentation rate.)
4. *Basophilic stipplings*—certain abnormalities of hemoglobin synthesis give a characteristic pattern of dark spots. This phenomenon is seen in lead poisoning and severe anemias.

Descriptive Terms for WBC

1. *Atypical lymphocytes* (Downey cells) are characteristic of infectious mononucleosis, hepatitis, and certain other viral and allergic reactions. Also present with certain malignancies of the bone marrow.
2. *Myelocytes* and *Metamyelocytes* are two stages of immature leukocytes that are normally in the bone marrow, not in the bloodstream. Pathological conditions in bone marrow production may cause the release of various immature forms into the bloodstream.
3. *Blasts* are very primitive cells. Found in certain malignancies involving the bone marrow.

Descriptive Terms for Platelets

1. *Thrombocytopathy* means abnormal-looking platelets. (See Chapter 13 for a discussion on platelet counts.)

ERYTHROCYTE SEDIMENTATION RATE
(ESR or Sed Rate)

The sed rate measures the speed with which red blood cells settle in a tube of anticoagulated blood. The results are expressed as millimeters in an hour (mm/hr). An increase in plasma globulins or fibrinogen causes the cells to stick together (Rouleaux formation) and thus to fall faster than normally. If the cells are smaller than normal (microcytic), they also fall faster than normally. And if they are larger than normal (macrocytic), they fall more slowly than normally. The laboratory takes into account any change in the size of the erythrocyte and corrects for this.

Because so many different conditions can cause an increase in globulins, fibrinogen, or other substances that can cause erythrocytes to clump together, the sed rate is a very nonspecific test. (See the discussion on c-reactive protein, Chapter 14, for another test of inflammation.) Both the sed rate and the c-reactive protein indicate a pathological condition, but they do not identify the source. Sometimes the sed rate is explained as "showing how hot the fire (inflammation) is, but not where it is."

Preparation of Patient And Collection of Sample

There is no special preparation of the patient. The test requires a minimum of 5 cc of anticoagulated blood. EDTA is used as the anticoagulant (the lavender top vacutainer).

Reference Values

Adult:	Male	1–13 mm/hr
	Female	1–20 mm/hr
Pregnancy		44–114 mm/hr
Aged:		
	Males over 50	1–20 mm/hr
	Females over 50	1–30 mm/hr

Z-Sed Rate

The Zeta Sed rate, a mechanical technique, uses a centrifuge to cause red cells to clump quickly. The results are obtained in 5 minutes instead of an hour. Check with the laboratory for reference values since some laboratories may do both Z-sed rates and the conventional sed rates as comparisons.

Increased Sed Rate

Clinical Significance. A marked increase in the sedimentation rate during pregnancy is a normal occurrence because there is an increase in globulins and in the fibrinogen level in pregnancy. A pathological reason for an increased sedimentation rate is usually an inflammation or tissue injury. For sed rates above 100 mm (in the nonpregnant patient, of course), the most likely causes are infections, malignancies, or collagen vascular diseases (Wyler 1977). The sedimentation rate is often used to monitor the course of rheumatoid arthritis.

Possible Nursing Implications. If the sed rate is used as a screening device, the results may not be very useful in planning nursing care since an abnormal sed rate requires more testing to determine the underlying pathophysiology. If the disease process is known, then the results of the sed rate are helpful in assessing the acuteness of the inflammatory process. For example, a patient with rheumatoid arthritis may exhibit an increasing sed rate, which is one clue that the patient may need therapeutic interventions to control the inflammation, as well as bed rest to permit inflamed joints to rest.

A decreasing sed rate is indicative of a lessening of the inflammatory response. The change in the sed rate should alert the nurse to confer with the physician about reevaluating limitations placed on the patient.

Approximately 85% of patients with rheumatoid arthritis can manage their disease if they readjust their life style, learn to rest, do their exercises and take their aspirin or other prescribed medication. These patients can be managed well under the watchful eye of a knowledgeable nurse [Brown-Skeers 1979: 31].

Decreased Sed Rate

Clinical Significance. Since the range of values begins with zero, a low rate is not clinically significant. Cells with greater surface area settle more slowly, but the rate may still be within the reference values.

TOTAL WHITE BLOOD CELL COUNT (WBC) AND DIFFERENTIAL (Diff)

Two measurements of the white blood cells are commonly done. One is the count of the total number of white blood cells in a cubic millimeter of blood (WBC). The other is the determination of the proportion of each of the five types of white blood cells in a sample of 100 white blood cells (differential). The first measurement, the WBC, is an absolute number of so many thousand WBC per cubic millimeter (/mm^3). The second measurement, the differential count (diff) is in percentages because it is a report of the proportion of each type cell in a sample of 100.

It is important to understand that the diff is reported in percentages because an increase in the percentage of one type of cell always means a decrease in the percentage of another type *even though* the absolute number for the second type of cell does not decrease. For example, a man has a normal WBC of 10,000/mm^3, with a neutrophil count of 60% and a lymphocyte count of 30%. Although the laboratory report does not report the actual number of lymphocytes, one can figure out that the man has 3,000 lymphocytes per cubic millimeter (10,000 total × 30%). If this man gets a severe bacterial infection, his total WBC may rise to 20,000/mm^3. In a severe bacterial infection, almost all of the increase in WBC will be due to an increase in neutrophils. The differential count now shows 75% neutrophils and only 15% lymphocytes, but this does not mean the man has fewer lymphocytes. He has 15% of 20,000 or 3,000 lymphocytes per cubic millimeter, just as before. Only the proportions have changed. Absolute numbers may change, and the proportions of each type of WBC may change, but the percentages must always add up to 100%. Neutrophils, lymphocytes, and the three types of WBC that make up the other 10% of the WBC will be discussed in a separate section.

Adult Male and Female Total WBC	4,500–11,500/mm³
Bands or stabs (young neutrophils)	3–5%
Polymorphonuclears or Granulocytes	
Neutrophils or segs	51–67%
Eosinophils	1–4%
Basophils	0–1%
Mononuclear or non-granular leukocytes	
Lymphocytes	25–33%
Monocytes	2–6%
Differential adds up to 100%.*	
Pregnancy	The leukocytosis of pregnancy (up to 16,000/mm³ is due mostly to an increase in the neutrophils with only a slight increase in lymphocytes.
Newborns	Day of birth 18,000–40,000/mm³. Drops to adult levels within two weeks. Reference values for differential have wide ranges depending on time after birth. Neutrophils predominate for first few days, but eventually lymphocyte predominance is seen (Crist 1980: 33).
Children	Until about age 5–8, lymphocytes are more prominant than neutrophils. WBC up to 14,500/mm³ may be in normal range depending on age. Consult specific laboratory for relative values for the differential at different ages.
Aged	Some sources suggest total WBC may decrease slightly with age, but this has not been well documented.

Note if the laboratory uses certain automated instruments to count the WBC, some large cells may not take the stain properly. These large unstained cells (LUC) may make up to 3% of the normal specimen. If there are more than 3% unstained cells, the laboratory will perform a microscopic examination (peripheral smear) to identify the abnormal cells.

Increase in Neutrophils and Bands (Neutrophilia)

Clinical Significance. Neutrophils, classified as polymorphonuclear leukocytes (PMN's), seem to be the body's first defense against bacterial infection and severe stress. Normally most of the circulating neutrophils are in the mature form, which the laboratory can identify by the way the nucleus of the cell is segmented. Hence some laboratories call mature neutrophils *segs* or segmented neutrophils. In contrast, the nucleus of the less mature neutrophil is not in segments, but still in a band, so the lab calls these immature neutrophils *bands*. Another name for bands are *stabs*, a name that comes from the German for rod.

Notice that there are at least four names for mature neutrophils (segs, segmented neutrophils, polymorphonuclear leukocytes, or PMNs) and two names for immature neu-

TABLE 2-3. COMPARISON OF NORMAL DIFFERENTIAL TO A "SHIFT TO THE LEFT" IN AN ADULT WITH AN ACUTE BACTERIAL INFECTION

	Stabs or Bands	Neutrophils or Segs	Eosino-phils	Baso-phils	Lympho-cytes	Mono-cytes
Normal differential— total WBC 9,400	3%	61%	4%	1%	26%	5%
"Shift to the left"— total WBC 14,300	10% ↑	70% ↑	3%	1%	12% ↓	4%

trophils (bands or stabs). An increased need for neutrophils will cause an increase in both the segs (mature neutrophils) and the bands (immature or young neutrophils). The greater the demand for neutrophils, the higher the number of immature neutrophils in the bloodstream.

When a patient may possibly have appendicitis, one of the questions is, "Does the patient have a shift to the left?" When laboratory reports were written out by hand, the bands or stabs were written first on the left-hand side of the page. Hence, a "shift to the left" means that the bands or stabs have increased. Table 2-3 demonstrates what a shift to the left would look like in comparison to a normal differential in *an adult*.

Although with a shift to the left, the lymphocytes appear to have decreased, as explained earlier, the diff count is only a percentage. The total number of lymphocytes has not changed, but the neutrophils have increased. In bacterial infections the total WBC does increase, and an examination of the differential enables one to determine that the increase is due to an increase in both immature and mature forms of neutrophils.

The slang "shift to the right" is rarely if ever used to describe the alteration toward the other side of the neutrophil differential. A shift to the right is used to imply that there are abnormal hypersegmented neutrophils, seen in certain anemias and in liver disease.

Besides bacterial infections, an increase in neutrophils can be due to various inflammatory processes, physical stress, or tissue necrosis such as that in myocardial infarction or in severe burns. Childbirth, as well as many drugs and toxins, increase the neutrophil count. Neutrophils are increased in granulocytic leukemia and in many other malignancies. Emotional stress can also increase the neutrophil count, but usually not as dramatically as a physical stress.

Possible Nursing Implications.

Assessing for Infection. When a patient has an elevated neutrophil count, one of the first things to determine is whether the patient has an infection. If so, should he or she be isolated to protect others? Although infection is not the only reason for an increased neutrophil count with a "shift to the left," it should always be considered along with other factors (see Chapter 16 for culture collections). For example, a beginning nursing student once explained that her patient had a high neutrophil count probably because of emotional stress. The emotional stress (as perceived by the student) was that the man had been given a bed bath by a female. Whether or not the bath had been distressing, the student overlooked the fact that the man had a very severe infection developing in his foot. In the absence of any signs of infection, the nurse can assess whether there has been some other assault to the body that has caused the bone marrow to increase the number of neutrophils.

Measures to Promote Recovery. The increase in neutrophils is actually a healthy response—a defense mechanism against an insult to body integrity. The nurse can help patients maximize their defense against assaults by promoting rest, adequate nutrition, and plenty of fluids. As the body successfully overcomes the assault, bacterial or otherwise, the neutrophil count will fall back to normal. This falling neutrophil count is an objective assessment that therapeutic measures have been successful.

Decreased Neutrophil Count (Neutropenia)

Clinical Significance. Although most bacterial infections cause an increase in the neutrophil count, some bacterial infections (such as typhoid, tularemia, or brucelosis) cause a decreased neutrophil count (neutropenia). (See Chapter 14 on the febrile agglutinization tests for these diseases.) Many of the viral diseases such as hepatitis, influenza, measles, mumps, and rubella also cause a decreased neutrophil count. (Most of these viruses cause a lymphocytosis.) An overwhelming infection of any type may completely exhaust the bone marrow and cause a neutropenia. Certain drugs, particularly those used to treat cancer, can cause severe bone marrow depression. Radiation therapy also carries the risk of neutropenia. Antibiotics such as nafcillin, penicillins, and cephalasporins can also induce neutropenia, as can psychotropic drugs such as lithium and the phenothiazines.

The diagnosis of neutropenia in the pediatric population is fairly common. Most neutropenia observed in children is mild and occurs during viral infections. More severe forms of neutropenia may be hereditary or due to serious pathology such as collagen vascular disease (Crist 1980).

Possible Nursing Implications.

Protecting from Infection. There are two major concerns for the patient with a low neutrophil count. First, the patient must be protected from sources of infection, and, if the etiology is known, the agent that caused the neutropenia must be avoided. Protective measures may need to be as strict as reverse isolation, depending on the circumstances. The problem is that, since the patient is often infected by organisms that are normally present in the body, preventing infection may be very hard. Most authorities do not stress isolation as much as meticulous hand washing.

Mackey (1980) discusses how to use drugs to keep infections down when a patient's neutrophil count is very low (1,000/mm³). Besides the usual hygiene measures to protect the patient from infection, nonabsorbable antibiotics are given as a prophylaxis. The rationale is that this reduces the number of organisms in the patient's gastrointestinal tract that are often the source of the infection in the severely neutropenic patient. It is very important to recognize the beginning of the drop in neutrophils before the situation becomes critical. An infection needs to be treated immediately with antibiotics. Fever is usually the most reliable sign of an infection. (See Chapter 16 on tips for collecting cultures.)

Preventing Neutropenia from Developing. The nurse must always check the last WBC before giving drugs that may cause neutropenia. For patients on chemotherapy for cancer, the WBC and diff may be ordered daily. Some nurses become "chemotherapy specialists" and, under the supervision of a physician, take over the functions of cancer drug preparation and administration, patient education, and monitoring of side effects including the effects on the hematologic system. These nurses usually specialize in the care of oncology patients (Zehlevitt 1980).

For patients on long-term drugs known to induce neutropenia, a WBC and diff may be ordered periodically. The nurse must confer with the physician so that the drug may be withheld if the neutrophil count drops below a certain number. Since in the adult the majority of white blood cells are neutrophils, the change in neutrophils most affects the total count. But neutropenia may be present even with a normal number of other types of WBC.

Increased Eosinophil Count (Eosinophilia)

Clinical Significance. The actual function of the eosinophils is not clearly understood, but they are associated with antigen–antibody reactions. The most common reasons for an increase in eosinophils (eosinophilia) are allergic reactions such as asthma, hay fever, or hypersensitivity to a drug. Parasitic infestations, such as round worms, are another reason for an eosinophil increase. Other conditions where eosinophils increase are certain skin diseases and neoplasms.

Possible Nursing Implications. If an increased eosinophil count has been attributed to a specific allergen, the nurse may be involved in helping the patient learn to avoid the allergen. Otherwise the eosinophil count may just be useful as an indication that the patient is likely to give a history of allergies; this fact should then be taken into account in planning diets and so on. If the elevated eosinophil count is due to a possible parasitic infection, the nurse should question whether stool precautions are necessary. (See Chapter 16 for the collection of stool specimens for parasites.)

Decreased Eosinophil Count

Clinical Significance. Increased levels of adrenal steroids decrease the number of circulating eosinophils. Before the refinement of tests to measure corticosteroid levels directly, a drop in the eosinophil count after an injection of ACTH (Thorn test) was an indirect measure of functioning adrenal glands. (See Chapter 15 for cortisol measurements.)

Possible Nursing Implications. A decrease in eosinophils is not clinically useful, but it is interesting to note the drop in eosinophil count for an allergic patient who is begun on corticosteroid therapy.

Changes in the Basophil Count

Clinical Significance of Increase of Basophils. The purpose of basophils in the bloodstream is not known. Very few conditions seem to increase this relatively rare type of white blood cell. Leukemias and other pathological alterations in bone marrow production may give rise to an increase in basophils. If a basophil count is elevated, several repeats may be done to determine whether it is a true increase.

Clinical Significance of Decrease in Basophils. Since the normal basophil count is considered to be 0–2%, a decline is not likely to be detected unless absolute counts are done. Corticosteroids, allergic reactions, and acute infections may all lower the basophil rate, but this information is not usually clinically useful.

Possible Nursing Implications. Since the basophil count is usually not of clinical significance, nurses do not need to be concerned with any special implications for this part of the WBC.

Increased Lymphocyte Count (Lymphocytosis)

Clinical Significance. Lymphocytes are the principal components of the body's immune system, but only a small proportion of them circulate in the bloodstream. (See Chapter 10 for a discussion on the T and B lymphocytes.) In the differential count (diff), T and B lymphocytes are grouped together. In adults, lymphocytes are the second most common type of white blood cell, after neutrophils. In children up to at least the age of 5 to 8, the lymphocytes are more numerous than the neutrophils. Even in older children, the percentage of lymphocytes nearly equals or even surpasses the percentage of neutrophils (Byrne 1976).

Lymphocytes increase in many viral infections, such as mumps or infectious hepatitis; they also increase with pertussis, with infectious mononucleosis, and often with tuberculosis. (See Chapter 14 for serological tests for infectious mononucleosis.) *Chronic* bacterial infections cause an increase in lymphocytes. A common reason for a very marked lymphocytosis (80–90%) is lymphocytic leukemia. Ninety percent of all leukemias, both acute and chronic, are lymphocytic. Acute lymphocytic leukemia is much more common in children, while chronic lymphocytic leukemia is most common in older adults. Children also have a rather benign disease called infectious lymphocytosis where the lymph count is quite high.

Possible Nursing Implications.

Lymphocytes Are Increased Due to Leukemia. If the lymphocyte count is extremely high, the physician orders other tests to establish the possible existence of leukemia. The nurse needs to be aware of the specific type of leukemia diagnosed, since treatment measures and prognosis differ for different subcategories of the disease. The peripheral blood smear, maybe along with a bone marrow biopsy, is needed to clearly differentiate the type of abnormal white cells. Three potentially lethal complications in the leukemic patient are (1) infection due to the lack of normal white blood cells, (2) hemorrhage due to the lack of platelets, and (3) hyperuricemia due to the increase of uric acid from cell destruction (Pochedly 1978:1714). (See Chapter 4 for a discussion about high serum uric acid levels in certain malignancies such as leukemia. See Chapter 13 for a discussion on low platelet counts, or thrombocytopenia.)

Promoting Recovery. If the lymphocyte count is not due to a malignancy, the important question is whether the patient has an infection that may be transmitted to others. Other measures, discussed under increased neutrophil counts, also apply since the nurse needs to help the person resist some type of assault that has triggered an immunoresponse. The increased lymphocyte count is needed for a defense against certain viral or chronic bacterial infections.

Decreased Lymphocyte Count (Lymphopenia)

Clinical Significance. Very few conditions cause the actual number of lymphocytes to decrease. Adrenal corticosteroids and other immunosuppressive drugs do cause some decrease. Severe malnutrition will decrease the absolute number too. There will be a percentage of decrease in lymphocytes any time the percentage of neutrophils increase. Since increases in neutrophils occur for many reasons, decreased lymphocyte counts may often be explained by changes in the neutrophils. Review the discussion in the beginning of this chapter if it is not clear why a marked increase in the percentage of neutrophils always causes a decrease in the percentage of lymphocytes, even though the absolute number of lymphocytes has not decreased.

Possible Nursing Implications. First of all, the nurse must determine whether the patient has an absolute or relative decrease in the lymphocyte count. If the decrease is relative, then the nursing implications are those discussed under increased neutrophil counts.

On the other hand, a patient with a true (or absolute or actual) decrease in the number of lymphocytes is immunodeficient. This patient may need very extensive protection from sources of infection. Also, if an immunodeficient patient does get an infection, there may be few signs or symptoms that this assault is occurring. So the nurse needs to use very careful assessment techniques to detect early infections in the absence of the classical signs, such as fever and the like. For example, patients on chronic steroid therapy may have lower-than-normal levels of lymphocytes, and so it should not be surprising that these patients sometimes develop tuberculosis.

Nurses can often help patients with chronic lowered resistance to find ways to enhance their health by diet, rest, and all the measures too often overlooked as "simple" health habits. Sometimes the objective sign of a laboratory test can prompt the nurse to evaluate the total health of the patient. Smith (1981:6) recommends a complete metabolic evaluation for patients who have a total lymphocyte count less than $1,800/mm^3$.

Increased Monocyte Count

Clinical Significance. Like the basophils and eosinophils, the monocytes are but a small percentage of the total WBC. It is thought that monocytes act as phagocytes in certain chronic inflammatory diseases. A significant increase of monocytes, for example, accompanies tuberculosis. Some protozoan infections such as malaria, as well as some rickettsial infections such as Rocky Mountain spotted fever, cause increases in the monocyte count. (See Chapter 14 on tests for rickettsial infections.) Monocytic leukemia, acute or chronic, also causes an increased count, but monocytic leukemia is far less common than the lymphocytic type. Chronic ulcerative colitis and regional enteritis both cause an increased monocyte count, as do some collagen diseases.

Possible Nursing Implications. As a general rule, the condition that causes increased monocytes is more likely to be a chronic condition, but further investigation for a specific pathology is necessary to make the monocytic count useful clinically.

**Clinical Significance of a
Decrease in the Monocyte Count**
A decreased monocyte is not clinically significant.

Questions

2-1. A complete blood count (CBC) would include tests for:

  a. Hb, Hct, RBC, and WBC with differential.

  b. RBC, WBC, platelets.

  c. RBC, Hb, Hct, and erythrocyte indices.

  d. Hematology and electrolyte panel.

2-2. Mrs. Landy lost a large amount of blood during surgery for a mastectomy. A hematocrit (Hct) drawn in the recovery room was 43%. It is now twelve hours after surgery, and the Hct just done is 37%. Which action by the nurse is appropriate?

  a. Take her blood pressure and call the physician immediately since Mrs. Landy is most likely bleeding again.

  b. Slow down the intravenous rate until the physician can be notified because Mrs. Landy is probably overhydrated.

  c. Consult the physician for further fluid orders because Mrs. Landy is probably slightly dehydrated.

  d. Notify the physician of the lab report when rounds are made in a couple of hours because this drop in Hct is expected due to a fluid shift from the interstitial space.

2-3. The test that is most frequently done to assess for loss of blood is the:

  a. RBC   **b.** Hb   **c.** Hct   **d.** CBC

2-4. The practice of being NPO for routine tests is likely to be detrimental for an adult female patient who has a:

  a. hemoglobin (Hb) of 10 g/100 ml.

  b. red blood cell count (RBC) of 6 million/mm^3.

  c. hematocrit (Hct) of 30%.

  d. all of the above.

2-5. A low RBC would be expected for a patient who is known to have:

  a. low levels of erythropoietin.   **c.** hemolysis.

  b. bone marrow depression.   **d.** all of the above.

2–6. As a rough guide, each unit of packed cells given to an adult raises the hematocrit about:

    a. 3%.   **b.** 6%.   **c.** 9%.   **d.** 12%.

2–7. Assuming that the erythrocyte indices are normal, the estimated hemoglobin level (Hb) for a patient whose Hct is 30% would be around:

    a. 6 g.   **b.** 8 g.   **c.** 10 g.   **d.** 12 g.

2–8. Mrs. London has a Hb of 11 g due to a continuing blood loss from a heavy menstrual flow. Which of the following nursing actions is the most appropriate?

    a. Encourage additional fluids to prevent thrombus formation.

    b. Explain that increased physical activity stimulates increased production of red blood cells.

    c. Assess her dietary intake of protein and iron.

    d. Prepare the patient for the eventual need for blood transfusions to correct the anemia.

2–9. Anemia due to a recent blood loss would most likely be:

    a. microcytic ($\downarrow$MCV), hypochromic ($\downarrow$MCHC).

    b. macrocytic ($\uparrow$MCV), normochromic (normal MCHC).

    c. normocytic (normal MCV), hypochromic ($\downarrow$MCHC).

    d. normocytic (normal MCV), normochromic (normal MCHC).

2–10. An increased MCV (mean cell volume) would be part of the clinical picture of the patient with:

    a. pernicious anemia.   **c.** both of the above.

    b. folic acid deficiency.   **d.** neither of the above.

2–11. A decreased mean corpuscular hemoglobin concentration (MCHC) is characteristic of:

    a. chronic blood loss.   **c.** both of the above.

    b. iron deficiency anemia.   **d.** neither of the above.

2–12. A reticulocyte count above 2% would be expected for all the following patients *except:*

    a. Mr. Joseph, who has an untreated macrocytic anemia due to B_{12} deficiency.

    b. Mrs. Lars, who has been receiving iron supplements for iron deficiency anemia.

    c. Timmy Logon, who recently moved to a high altitude.

    d. Ms. Garfield, who had an acute blood loss last week after a miscarriage.

2-13. Mrs. Toby has rheumatoid arthritis that flares up occasionally. Her sedimentation rate (sed rate) is higher than it has been. The visiting nurse is planning a home visit to evaluate the need for a change in care. In regard to this lab test, the nurse should consult with the physician about teaching Mrs. Toby to:

a. take additional fluids to prevent dehydration.

b. decrease fluid intake to prevent circulatory overload.

c. increase her activity to promote the full range of motion of all joints.

d. decrease her activity to promote the rest of joints, which are actively inflammed at the present.

2-14. In an acute bacterial infection, which type of immature WBC is elevated when the patient has a "shift to the left"?

a. lymphocytes. **c.** basophils.

b. neutrophils. **d.** eosinophils.

2-15. If the *absolute* number of lymphocytes is increased, what is the effect on the lymphocyte and neutrophil counts in the *differential?*

a. Lymphocytes and neutrophils remain the same in percentages.

b. Neutrophils show a percentage decrease, and lymphocytes show a percentage increase.

c. Lymphocytes show a percentage increase, and neutrophil percentage stays the same.

d. Any of the above can be produced depending on how much the lymphocytes increase.

2-16. Mr. Jelco is receiving chemotherapy for treatment of cancer of the bowel. His last white blood count (WBC) was 3,000/mm³. Based on this laboratory report, a nursing care plan must include nursing interventions to:

a. protect from infection. **c.** prevent stasis of circulation.

b. protect from stressful situations. **d.** prevent dehydration.

2-17. Mrs. Jaboni is receiving an antibiotic that can cause neutropenia. Which of these laboratory reports would be an indication to withhold the antibiotic until the physician can be consulted?

a. WBC of 15,000/mm³ with a normal diff.

b. WBC of 15,000/mm³ with a marked shift to the left.

c. WBC of 5,000/mm³ with a normal diff.

d. WBC of 5,000/mm³ with a marked increase in lymphocytes on the diff.

2-18. Eosinophil counts are usually elevated when the patient:

a. has had an allergic reaction. **c.** has a viral infection.

b. is on corticosteroid therapy. **d.** experiences any of the above.

2-19. Which of the following tests is used to check for a lack of an enzyme in the RBC?

    a. TIBC (total iron binding capacity).   **c.** G-6-PD.

    b. Serum ferritin level.   **d.** Serum B_{12} or folic acid levels.

2-20. Which of the following laboratory reports gives the strongest indication that the patient is likely to be immunodeficient?

    a. Increased neutrophils.   **c.** Decreased neutrophils.

    b. Increased lymphocytes.   **d.** Decreased lymphocytes.

2-21. An increased lymphocyte count is expected when the patient has:

    a. viral infections such as mumps or hepatitis.

    b. chronic bacterial infections such as tuberculosis.

    c. chronic lymphocytic leukemia.

    d. all of the above.

2-22. In adults, the most common type of WBC in the differential is the neutrophil. In children of age 3 or 4, the most common type of WBC is the:

    a. neutrophil.   **c.** immature neutrophil.

    b. lymphocyte.   **d.** monocyte.

2-23. The vast majority of leukemias, whether acute or chronic, show a marked increase in:

    a. neutrophils.   **c.** eosinophils.

    b. lymphocytes.   **d.** monocytes.

2-24. The presence of abnormal white blood cells is confirmed by the:

    a. reticulocyte count.   **c.** G-6-PD.

    b. WBC diff.   **d.** peripheral blood smear.

REFERENCES

Aftergood, Lilla and Alfin-Slater, Roslyn. "Women and Nutrition." *Contemporary Nutrition* 5:3 (March 1980).

Brown-Skeers, Vicki. "How the Nurse Practitioner Manages the Rheumatoid Arthritis Patient," *Nursing 79* 9 (June 1979): 26–35.

Byrne, Judith. "Hematology Studies, Part II: The Differential White Cell Count," *Nursing 76* 6 (November 1976): 15–17.

Byrne, Judith. "Hematology Studies, Part III: Stained Red Cell Examination," *Nursing 76* 6 (December 1976): 15.

Connell, Elizabeth. *Anemia During Pregnancy* (Patient Information Booklet). Chicago: American College of Obstetricians and Gynecologists, 1979.

Crist, William and Dearth, James. "Neutropenia in Childhood," *Continuing Education for the Family Physician* 13 (July 1980): 33–36.

Crosby, William. "Red Cell Indices," *Archives of Internal Medicine* 139 (January 1979): 23–24.

Hytten, Frank and Lind, Tom. *Diagnostic Indices in Pregnancy.* Summit, N.J.: Ciba-Geigy Corporation, 1975.

Jacobs, A. and Worwood, M. "Ferritin in Serum." *New England Journal of Medicine* 292 (May 1, 1975): 951–956.

Jensen, Margaret *et al. Maternity Care: The Nurse and the Family,* 2nd ed. St. Louis: The C.V. Mosby Co., 1981.

Loebel, Suzanne *et al. The Nurses' Drug Handbook.* New York: John Wiley & Sons, Inc., 1977.

Luckmann, Joan and Sorensen, Karen. *Medical–Surgical Nursing: A Psychophysiologic Approach,* 2nd ed. Philadelphia: W. B. Saunders Company, 1980.

Lynch, Sean. "Ascorbic Acid and Iron Nutrition," *Contemporary Nutrition* 5:9 (September 1980).

McFarlane, Judith. "Sickle Cell Disorders," *American Journal of Nursing* 77 (December 1977): 1948–1954.

Mackey, Christine and Hopefl, Alan. "Keeping Infections Down When Risks Go Up," *Nursing 80* 10 (June 1980): 69–73.

Pochedly, Carl. "Acute Lymphoid Leukemia in Children," *American Journal of Nursing* 78 (October 1978): 1714–1716.

Prchal, James. "Red Cell Enzymes: An Overview." *Continuing Education for the Family Physician* 13 (July 1980): 41–50.

Price, Sylvia and Wilson, Lorraine. *Pathophysiology: Clinical Concepts of Disease Processes.* New York: McGraw-Hill Book Company, 1978.

Ravel, Richard. *Clinical Laboratory Medicine,* 3rd ed. Chicago: Year Book Medical Publishers, Inc., 1978.

Rodman, Morton. "The Drug Interactions We All Overlook," *RN* 44 (April 1981): 61–65.

Smith, Lynn. "Implications of Malnutrition in the Surgical Patient," *Point of View* 18 (July 1981): 6–7.

Wood, Camilla. "Macrocytic Megalobastic Anemias," *Nurse Practitioner* 2:6 (July –August 1977): 33–35.

Wood, Camilla. "Iron Deficiency Anemia," *Nurse Practitioner* 2:5 (May-June 1977): 24–29.

Wyler, David. "Diagnostic Implications of Markedly Elevated Erythrocyte Sedimentation Rate: A Re-Evaluation," *Southern Medical Journal* 70:12 (December 1977): 1428–1430.

Zehlevitt, Doreen. "Cancer Chemotherapy," *RN* 43 (June 1980): 53–56.

CHAPTER THREE

Routine Urinalysis And Other Urine Tests

Objectives

1. State three important nursing considerations in obtaining urine for routine urinalysis and for random testing.
2. Recognize findings on a routine urinalysis report that may have pathological significance.
3. Summarize important points about the various types of dipsticks and other reagents used by the nurse for urine testing.
4. Explain when periodic tests of urine pH, specific gravity, protein, sugar, and ketones may be useful in planning and modifying nursing goals.
5. Describe what should be taught to a patient about any 24-hour urine collection.
6. Give examples of common tests and the types of preservatives used for 24-hour urine specimens.

A routine urinalysis includes tests for:

1. pH,
2. specific gravity,
3. glucose,
4. ketones,
5. and protein.

It also involves a microscopic examination for:

1. red blood cells (RBC),
2. white blood cells (WBC),
3. casts,

4. crystals, and

5. bacteria and certain fungi, which may also be seen in the microscopic examination.

Color and odor are usually not noted on a laboratory report unless abnormal. Yet, since the nurse usually collects the specimen, some common reasons for color and odor changes are included in this chapter.

Because a routine urinalysis is indeed routine for almost every patient, the nurse needs to fully understand the meaning of each component of the urinalysis. All these tests are screening tests that may indicate the need for a more thorough assessment.

Since several of the components of the urinalysis are sometimes done by nurses in the clinical unit, the discussion on specific gravity includes directions on the two methods for obtaining a specific gravity on the clinical unit. Several of the other tests can be done quickly with the use of chemically impregnated paper strips that can be dipped into a urine specimen. In some situations, the nurse may do this "dipstick" method as one part of the assessment of the patient. It is important to make sure that the materials for testing are fresh (note the date on the container) and that the directions are followed exactly. Some strips must be read within a certain time limit, and specific directions should always be included with the testing equipment. Since color changes are the basis for the results of the dipstick test, a good light is needed and personnel need to be checked for color blindness. Some laboratories have set up special training sessions for nurses so that they can do the tests accurately. (See Chapter 1 on peripheral testing.)

Specific techniques to do each component of the dipstick (glucose, protein, pH, hemoglobin, and ketone) will be covered with each component of the test. (See Table 3–1 for a summary about reagent strips for urinalysis.) Specific tips on the two methods of testing for glucose in the urine will also be covered in regard to the special points to note when nurses are actually doing the tests.

The second part of the chapter includes information on urine tests for nitrites, porphyrins, occult blood, bilirubin, ascorbic acid, delta-aminolevulinic acid, and 5-HIAA. Information on reagent strips for some of these tests is included. This last part of the chapter also presents the correct procedure for collecting 24-hour urine specimens. The final table (Table 3–7) lists the usual substances tested by 24-hour specimens, whether any preservatives are needed, and where the test is covered in detail in later chapters.

COLLECTION OF URINE SPECIMENS

For a routine urinalysis, the laboratory needs about 30 ml of urine. The perineal area in the woman or the end of the penis in the male should be cleaned before the urine is collected. For a female patient, collecting midstream urine lessens the contamination of the urine from vaginal secretions or menstrual flow; use of a vaginal tampon also helps in this respect. Most laboratories have disposable cups with covers for collecting routine urine specimens.

If a *culture and sensitivity* are to be done in addition to the routine urinalysis, the urine has to be in a sterile container. In that case, collecting a clean catch urine sample will

TABLE 3-1.   N-MULTISTIX C—REAGENT STRIPS FOR URINALYSIS*

Substance Tested and Tips on Interpreting	Further Discussion in Addition to Chapter 3
pH—Colors range from orange through yellow and green to blue to cover entire range of urinary pH. Make sure not to let urine remain on test strip, or the acid reagent from neighboring protein may run over and make pH acid or more acid.	Chap. 7 on respiratory and metabolic alkalosis and acidosis
Protein—Detects as little as 5 to 20 mg albumin/dl. May get false positive with alkaline urine. Does not test for Bence-Jones protein.	Chap. 10 on protein electrophoresis
Glucose—Enzyme method specific for glucose only. So need reduction method (Clinitest) for any other types of sugar. May be affected by ascorbic acid. Large quantities of ketone may depress color.	Chap. 8 on tests for galactosemia
Ketone—Provides results as small, moderate, and large. Reacts with acetoacetic acid and acetone but not beta-hydroxybutyric. PKU, BSP, or L-dopa can cause false positive.	Chap. 8 for serum ketone tests
Bilirubin—Sensitive to 0.2–0.4 mg bilirubin/dl. Icotest tablets are more sensitive. May be affected by chlorpromazine (Thorazine), phenazopyridine (Pyridium), ethoxazene (Serenium), or ascorbic acid.	Chap. 11 for tests of bilirubin
Occult blood—More sensitive to hemoglobin and myoglobin than intact erythrocytes. Complements the microscopic exam. Affected by ascorbic acid and some infections that produce peroxidase.	Chap. 13 for detecting occult bleeding
Nitrates—Any pink color suggests urinary infection, but a negative result does not provide sufficient proof of no bacteria since some bacteria do not produce nitrates. Affected by ascorbic acid. High specific gravity may inhibit.	Chap. 16 on urine cultures
Urobilinogen—False positive with porphobilinogen, P-aminosalicylic acid or azo dyes, such as phenazopyridine found in Azo Gantrisin or Pyridium.	Chap. 11 for more on urobilinogen
Ascorbic Acid—If ascorbic acid is as high as 25 mg/dl, the strip turns purple. Alerts that glucose, nitrite, occult blood, and bilirubin may not be accurate due to interference from ascorbic acid.	

* *Information compiled from Product Profile, Ames Division, Elkhart, Indiana (1980). Complete information on all testing products is available by contacting Ames. These tests are also available in separate dipsticks or in other combinations such as Keto-Diastixs for glucose and ketone or Uristix for nitrite, glucose, and protein. See Chapter 1 for the addresses of the major companies that make diagnostic kits.*

necessitate the use of an antiseptic solution as well as cleansing of the area. Urine for culture and sensitivity is discussed in Chapter 16.

If the patient is instructed to bring in a urine specimen from home, any small clean jar with a tight-fitting nonrusty lid may be used. The first voided specimen in the morning is the ideal for a routine urinalysis because the urine is concentrated and any abnormalities will be more pronounced in the screening tests.

Urine specimens need to be examined within two hours. Urine that is left standing too long becomes alkaline because bacteria begin to split urea into ammonia. Visualization of microscopic casts and the test for protein are inaccurate if the urine has undergone a conversion to a high pH (that is, if it has become alkaline). Urine should be refrigerated if the specimen cannot be sent to the laboratory within two hours.

Reference Values

pH	4.3 to 8 with an average of around 6 (depends on diet)
Specific gravity (s.g.):	
Adult	Range of 1.001–1.040. Random sample usually around 1.015–1.025.
Infant to 2 years	Range of 1.001–1.018.
Aged	May have a lowered range due to decreasing concentrating ability.
Protein	Usually negative, a few healthy people may have orthostatic proteinuria.
Sugar	Usually negative, may be trace in normal pregnancy. Lactosuria common in last trimester.
Ketone	Should be negative.
Microscopic sediment:	
Crystals	Usually have little significance, see discussion.
Casts	Most are pathological, a few hyaline casts are considered normal.
WBC	Should be only a few white blood cells in the urine (less than 4–5 per high power-field).
RBC	Only an occasional red blood cell is expected (less than 2–3 per high power-field).

COLOR OF URINE

Normally the color of the urine, from light yellow to dark amber, depends on its concentration. *Urechrome* is the name of the pigment that gives urine the characteristic yellow color. Any time urine has an unusual color, it is a good idea to save a specimen of it for the physician to see, as well as sending the urine to the laboratory. When the reason for a color abnormality is not known, the laboratory must do a chemical analysis to discover the cause. Usually the nurse or the patient first notes that something is wrong with the urine color. Such changes should always be called to the attention of the physician and recorded in the nurses' notes.

A number of things can cause a change in the color of urine. If the patient is known to be on a medication that causes color changes in the urine, this information should be written on the laboratory slip. It is also important that patients be told about expected color changes in the urine so they do not become unnecessarily concerned. For example, phenazopyridine (Pyridium) a drug used as a urinary tract analgesic, causes the urine to turn orange. (See Table 3–2 for 26 other drugs that can color urine.) Certain foods, such as beets or rhubarb, may cause color changes in the urine, as do certain dyes used in food. Purulent matter in the urine gives urine a cloudy appearance. Blood makes the urine dark and ''smokey'' looking. Pseudomonas infections of the bladder may give the urine a greenish color. Bilirubin turns the urine a dark orange that foams on shaking. (The other reason that urine may foam is the presence of large amounts of protein.)

TABLE 3–2.   DRUGS THAT CAN COLOR URINE*

Generic Name and Brand Name of Drug	Color Produced in Urine
Amitriptyline (multisource)	Blue-green (rare)
Anisindione (Miradon)	Orange in alkaline urine
Cascara (multisource)	Red in alkaline urine, red-brown in acid
Chloroquine (Aralen)	Rusty yellow
Chlorzoxazone (Paraflex)	Orange or purple-red (rare)
Danthron (multisource)	Pink in alkaline urine
Deferoxamine (Desferal)	Red
Ethoxazene (Serenium)	Orange-red
Furazolidone (Furoxone)	Brown
Iron preparations (multisource)	Dark brown or black on standing
Levodopa (multisource)	Dark brown on standing, red or brown in hypochlorite toilet bleach
Methocarbamol (multisource)	Brown, black, or green on standing
Metronidazole (Flagyl)	Dark brown on standing (rare)
Nitrofurantoin (multisource)	Brown
Phenazopyridine (Pyridium also in Azo-Gantrisin)	Orange-red
Phenindione (multisource)	Orange-red in alkaline urine
Phenolphthalein (multisource)	Pink-red in alkaline urine
Phenothiazine (multisource)	Pink, red, red-brown
Phensuximide (Milontin)	Pink, red, red-brown
Phenytoin (Dilantin)	Pink, red, red-brown
Primaquine	Rusty yellow (red or dark brown a sign of inherited hemolytic anemia reaction)
Quinacrine (Atabrine)	Intense yellow, especially in acid urine
Riboflavin	Intense yellow
Rifampin (multisource)	Red-orange
Sulfasalazine (multisource)	Orange-yellow in alkaline urine
Triamterene (Dyrenium)	Pale blue fluorescence

* Compiled from Slawson (1980: 40), Ravel (1978: 107), and Shapter (1976).

ODOR OF URINE

Old urine has the very characteristic smell of ammonia because bacteria split the urea molecules into ammonia. If a freshly voided urine specimen has a foul odor, there may be a urinary tract infection; that is, bacteria are converting urea to ammonia in the bladder.

A foul odor in freshly voided urine, however, may also be due to drugs or food. Asparagus gives a distinct smell to the urine. The unusual odor should be charted and called to the laboratory's attention for any needed further investigations. Note that certain metabolic abnormalities due to genetic defects can cause a peculiar odor in the urine of newborns. (See Chapter 18 on tests for genetic defects.)

pH OF THE URINE

A "higher pH" means "toward the alkaline side," and "lower pH" means "toward the acid side." Normally the pH of urine tends to be "lower" or acidic, largely due to diet. Meat and eggs contribute much of the acid metabolic wastes, while most fruits and vegetables, including citrus fruits, contribute to an alkaline urine. Thus a meatless diet would be one reason why the pH of the urine may be higher than usual.

Most of the bacteria that cause urinary tract infections, with the exception of *Escherichia coli* (*E. coli*), create alkaline urine because the bacteria split urea into ammonia and other products. The urea-splitting properties of many bacteria also explains why urine left standing at room temperature for a couple of hours usually turns alkaline from bacterial contamination.

The urine pH varies in different types of acidosis and alkalosis. Generally all forms of acidosis cause a strongly acid urine because the body is trying to compensate for the acidotic state by excreting hydrogen ions. If the acidotic problem is renal in origin, however, the kidneys may not be able to secrete those large amounts of hydrogen ions; so the urine will not be strongly acid. One might expect that in alkalosis the urine would become alkaline because the body would tend to retain hydrogen ions to compensate for the alkalotic state. Yet the pH of the urine often remains acid even with severe types of alkalosis because the kidneys are obligated to excrete hydrogen ions if potassium ions are not available. The relationship of potassium levels, acid–base balance, and urine and blood pH levels are discussed in detail in Chapter 7 on blood gases.

Possible Nursing Implications.
Usually changes in the pH of the urine are not very important since the pH fluctuates with food and with the metabolic state of the person. Sometimes, however, it may be necessary to see that the urine remains alkaline or acid. For example, if the patient has a tendency to form uric acid stones, it may be desirable to keep the urine alkaline or at least as high as 6.5. Sometimes medications are given to achieve an alkaline urine. The nurse may need to teach the patient to monitor the pH of the urine to see that it remains alkaline. This teaching is made easy by means of the dipstick method. (See Table 3–1 for one example of a dipstick (for pH.)

In other situations it may be desirable that the urine pH remain strongly acid. The two common clinical justifications for not letting the urine ever be alkaline are:

1. alkaline urine promotes the growth of certain organisms in the urine, and
2. alkaline urine promotes the formation of calcium renal stones in susceptible patients.

For example, quadriplegic patients are very prone for the formation of renal stones due to the higher calcium content in the urine that results from their lack of mobility. Such patients are also very prone to urinary tract infections because of urinary stasis due to loss of bladder control. Increasing the acidity of the urine may help prevent both infections and calcium stones. Often such patients are given cranberry juice several times a day to increase the acidity of their urine. Milk products may be limited, as well as citrus fruits which leave an alkaline ash. Of course, the volume of urine is an important consideration, and worrying about the pH is secondary to the concern for making sure that the person receives enough fluid to keep the urine dilute.

Testing the pH of Vaginal Secretions
Note that dipsticks may also be used on vaginal secretions. The vaginal secretions are usually acidic, but the presence of amniotic fluid makes an alkaline reaction. The pH is a test to assess if the amniotic "bag of waters" has broken.

Dipsticks for the pH of Gastric Contents
The pH of the gastric contents is strongly acid, while the contents below the pylorus are alkaline. A dipstick test of secretions from a long gastrointestinal tube, such as a Cantor, helps assess if the tube has progressed through the pylorus.

SPECIFIC GRAVITY OF URINE

The specific gravity is a measure of the density of urine compared with the density of water, which is 1.000: the higher the number, the more concentrated the urine unless there are certain abnormal constituents in the urine. The adult has a very wide range from very dilute to very concentrated. In infants, the upper limits for specific gravity are much lower than the adult limits because the young kidneys are not able to concentrate urine as effectively as mature kidneys. Often nurses may do the specific gravity as part of an assessment of fluid balance, using both the urinometer and the refractometer.

Two Methods for Testing Specific Gravity

Urinometer. An older method to test specific gravity uses a float called a urinometer or hydrometer. The float has been calibrated to the 1.000 mark when floating in distilled water at 20° C (68° F).

Each degree above 20° C will cause an increase of 0.001 of the specific gravity. Thus urine tested should be at 20° C (68° F), which is usually about room temperature. Refrigerated urine will have a pseudo low specific gravity when tested by the urinometer. A test tube is filled with 20 ml of urine, and the float is placed into the liquid. The higher the density of the urine, the more the float rises in the urine. The calibrated mark on the float that the urine covers is the specific gravity reading. Reading the marks exactly is sometimes difficult since the numbers are very small and close together. However, a reading of 1.011 or 1.012 would be acceptable since only wide variations are significant.

Refractometer. A newer technique, the refractometer looks like a small telescope. Only a drop of urine is needed. This drop is placed on a slide at the end of the scope, and the refractor is held up to a light. The instrument must be kept level. The density of the particles in the urine determine the direction of the beam of light through the eye of the scope. The refractor is calibrated to translate the refractive index into the standard way of reporting the specific gravity. For example, if the light beam is at the 1.026 mark, this figure is then recorded as the specific gravity of the urine.

The refractor has an added advantage of measuring the protein content in the same drop of urine. The protein measurements are on the right side of the scale. Knowledge about the presence of protein in the urine is important when doing a specific gravity because protein in the urine is one of the things that makes the specific gravity falsely high. The temperature of the urine does not change the results of the refractometer as it does the test for specific gravity with the urinometer.

Reference Values

Adults	Range of 1.001–1.040 with random samples around 1.015–1.025.
Infants to 2 years old	1.001–1.018
Aged	May have a decrease in concentrating power so that upper limits are lowered.

Increase in Specific Gravity

Clinical Significance. The specific gravity is falsely high if glucose, protein, or a dye used for diagnostic purposes is in the urine. Urine above 20° C (68° F) will have a falsely elevated specific gravity. All these abnormal constituents increase the density of the urine. If they are not present, the high specific gravity means the kidneys are putting out very concentrated urine, for which there are two reasons: (1) Either the patient is lacking in fluids, or (2) there is an increased secretion of antidiuretic hormone (ADH), which causes a decrease in urine volume. Trauma and stress reactions cause an increased ADH secretion (Condon 1975:192).

Possible Nursing Implications. Assuming the urine does not contain protein, glucose, or dyes, a high urine specific gravity most often indicates that the patient needs additional fluids. It is much rarer that a high specific gravity would be due to an increased secretion of ADH (antidiuretic hormone).

Nurses should understand, however, the nature of a phenomenon called *surgical diuresis*. In a patient who has been under a lot of stress, such as a major surgical procedure, the urine specific gravity is higher than normal because additional fluid is being held in reserve in the vascular system due to the presence of extra ADH and other hormones. As the stress lessens, the ADH and other hormones such as the glucocorticosteroids return to normal levels, and the fluid that was held in reserve is then excreted. This excretion of extra urine a few days after surgery is sometimes referred to as "surgical diuresis." It is important for nurses to understand the nature of this kind of fluid retention so that they do not overload patients with fluids because the specific gravity is a little higher than normal.

Frequent monitoring of the volume of urine output and of the specific gravity of each voiding help assess a patient's fluid needs. A specific gravity that continues to increase or that remains high when stress is not an overriding factor is a very clear indication that the patient is not receiving adequate fluid intake. In acutely ill patients, this condition necessitates medical orders for increased intravenous fluids. In the nursing home setting or for patients with chronic problems, it may be up to the nurse to devise ways to get adequate oral fluids into the patient. A specific gravity that drops back to normal is an objective evaluation that the patient is no longer dehydrated. Specific gravity readings are more objective than just charting "concentrated" urine.

The nurse also needs to be aware of patients who could be dehydrated due to a shift of fluid into a "third space." The normal two spaces are intracellular fluid and extracellular fluid compartments. A third space is any fluid collection that is physiologically useless, such as edema or ascites. Twombly (1978) discusses in detail the concept of third spacing and the potential for hypovolemia and decreased renal output.

Decreased Specific Gravity

Clinical Significance. Refrigerated urine will have a lower than normal specific gravity. Otherwise a low specific gravity is indicative of dilute urine. Dilute urine (a low specific gravity) is normal if the patient has had a lot of fluids. Diuretics cause a large urine output with a low specific gravity too. Chapter 4 contains a discussion of tests for serum and urine osmolality. These tests are much more accurate in determining the actual dilution or concentration of the urine as compared to the dilution or concentration of the plasma. Specific gravity readings are only crude indicators of fluid imbalances in serious conditions.

Sometimes a patient has a *fixed specific gravity* around 1.010. (This reading is usually pronounced as "ten-ten" since "one-point-zero-one-zero" is much harder to say.) A fixed specific gravity does not change even when the patient becomes dehydrated. This continually low specific gravity indicates that the kidneys have lost the ability to concentrate urine. The fixed specific gravity is always around 1.010 because 1.010 is the density of the plasma (Widmann 1979:563).

Another rarer reason for a continually low specific gravity is a deficiency of ADH (antidiuretic hormone). If not enough ADH is being secreted by the posterior pituitary gland, the kidneys excrete too much water. This condition is called *diabetes insipidus.*

Possible Nursing Implications. Often a careful assessment of the patient's total fluid intake uncovers the explanation for a low specific gravity. If the intake is larger than normal, it may be necessary to evaluate the possibility that the patient is in danger of a fluid overload. For example, patients may be on intravenous fluids in addition to oral intake. Also note whether the patient is on diuretics since this could explain the persistently low specific gravity. Intake and output records should be automatically maintained for any patient when there is any possibility of overload or dehydration. A persistently low specific gravity when the fluid intake is not high is a potentially serious sign that needs medical evaluation. A low specific gravity on a routine early morning specimen indicates the need for a thorough assessment of the renal system and an evaluation of ADH (antidiuretic hormone) secretion, if the physician deems it necessary. Persons with fixed low specific gravities (1.010) may have difficulty getting medical insurance because they are considered high risk patients for future renal problems.

A patient who is known to have a fixed specific gravity of 1.010 needs to be kept well hydrated so that the kidneys can effectively remove the waste products. Keeping this patient NPO for tests and the like may cause an increase in the blood urea nitrogen (BUN). A patient with a fixed low specific gravity needs to be taught always to maintain an adequate intake. As kidney disease progresses, fluid restrictions and other interventions are needed. The two common tests for renal function, BUN and creatinine, and the nursing implications of each are covered in Chapter 4.

PROTEIN IN THE URINE (PROTEINURIA)

Qualitative Method

Most often protein in the urine is checked by the dipstick method. This method, which uses bromnophenol paper, does not detect the presence of abnormal proteins such as the globulins and the Bence-Jones protein of myelomas. For most screening purposes, however, the dipstick method is adequate. (See Table 3-1 for one type of dipstick.) Nurses often use it for testing for albumin in the urine of prenatal patients. If there is a need to check the urine for protein other than albumin, the laboratory uses other agents such as sulfosalicyclic acid. Since the dipsticks are designed to be used with acid urine, there may be a false positive for protein if the urine is highly alkaline. Time is not critical in reading the results. The deepening shades of green (Multistix) indicate increasing amounts of protein. Note the exact color chart for each particular brand.

Reference Values (Qualitative Method)

Trace	As little as 5–30 mg/dl
1+	30 mg/dl protein
2+	100 mg/dl protein
3+	300 mg/dl protein
4+	over 1,000 mg/dl protein

Quantitative Method

The finding on one random sample should be negative. For persons who may have orthostatic or postural proteinuria, a second urine sample should be collected before arising from bed. If random samples are persistently positive for protein, a quantitative

(24-hour) sample may be done. A 24-hour specimen should show less than 150 mg of protein. See Table 3–7 for the details about collection.

Clinical Significance. Severe stress can cause proteinuria, but this is usually a temporary occurrence. Persistent protein in the urine is a common characteristic of renal dysfunction. Almost all types of kidney disease cause mild to moderate protein leakage into the urine. Moderate proteinuria is 500 to 4000 mg a day. Some people have proteinuria that is called orthostatic or postural because it occurs only when the person is in the upright position. Usually no renal abnormalities are associated with this apparently benign condition. Preeclampsia and the toxemia of pregnancy cause massive loss of protein in the urine. In what is called the nephrotic syndrome, which may be the end result of many diseases that cause kidney dysfunction, the protein loss is as much as 4000 mg a day. Albumin is the primary protein lost in all these conditions. Myelomas and certain other malignancies cause large protein losses, too, but since these proteins are abnormal it is necessary for the laboratory to use special quantitative methods to determine the presences of these proteins (Shapter 1976).

Possible Nursing Implications. Persistent protein in the urine is an indication for further assessment of the renal system. The nurse may be the one to explain to the patient how to get another specimen that is collected before the patient gets out of bed. If the proteinuria is due to renal dysfunction, other laboratory tests should be looked at to assess the degree of impairment. See the section on renal function tests in Chapter 4.

For the pregnant patient, a check for protein in the urine is a routine part of each prenatal visit. Nurses usually perform this test. Ideally the protein should be negative in pregnancy too. In the event that the pregnant patient begins to show protein in the urine, it is important to assess carefully for hypertension and edema. Proteinuria, hypertension, and edema are the classical triad for preeclampsia (Hytten 1975). The appearance of this triad is an indication for immediate medical assessment and medical interventions.

SUGAR IN THE URINE (GLYCOSURIA)

There are two different methods of screening for glucose in the urine.

1. Dipsticks (TesTapes, Clinistix, and the like) change color in the presence of glucose due to the reaction of an enzyme, glucose oxidase.
2. Tablets (Clinitest) use the reducing properties of cupric oxide to cause a color change in the presence of glucose *and* of other sugars.

Since nurses frequently test the urine for sugar it is necessary to understand how the two methods differ.

Dipstick (Enzymatic) Method
The dipstick or enzymatic method is very easy: A tape is just dipped into the urine and read for color changes after one minute. With TesTape (Lilly), a yellow color means the urine is glucose-free. If there is a color change on the darkest area, one should wait an

TABLE 3-3.   DRUGS THAT CAN AFFECT GLUCOSE TESTING*

Reduction Method	

Clinitest (Ames product)
    False positive
	Ascorbic Acid
	Cephalosporing (Keflin, Ancef, etc.)
	Chloramphenicol (Chloromycetin)
	Levo-dopa
	Methyl-dopa (Aldomet)
	Nalidixic acid (Neg Gram)
	Probenecid (Benemid)
	Penicillin
	Salicylates (high dosages)
	Sulfonomides
	Tetracylines
	Sugars other than glucose, i.e., lactose, frustose,
	    galactose, and pentoses

Enzyme Methods	
TesTape (Lilly product) Clinistix (Ames product) False positive or negative	Phenazopyridine (Pyridium, Azo-Gantrisin)
False negative	Ascorbic acid Levo-dopa (only Clinistix) Methyldopa Salicylates (high dosages) (only Clinistix) Cancer metabolites

Information compiled from Lundin (1978), Ames Products (1980), and Ravel (1978: 111). See Chapter 1 for the addresses of Ames and Lilly.

additional minute to make the final comparison with the color chart. Patients often use this at home. The enzyme method is also used for multistix testing (Table 3–1).

The tapes should not be used if they are outdated. The activity of the tape or tablet can be checked by doing a mock test of a cola drink, since commercial beverages (except for diet ones!) all contain more than 2% glucose. The tapes should not be stored in a hot or humid room (such as the bathroom).

Since the enzyme method is specific for glucose *only*, this method should be used if the patient is on any of the drugs that may make a false positive with the reducing method (Clinitest tablets). Such drugs are salicylates, penicillin, cephalosporins, ascorbic acid, and probenecid. (See Table 3–3 for a summary of drug effects on both methods.)

Tablets (Reducing) Method

Sometimes it is necessary to check for the presence of sugars other than glucose. The reducing method detects the presence of fructose, galactose, lactose, or the pentoses. For example, in screening the urine of an infant for potential abnormal sugars in the urine it would be essential to use Clinitest tablets (Ames) and not TesTapes or other enzyme tests. (See Chapter 8 on galactosemia and lactose intolerances.)

In what is called the *five-drop method,* five drops of urine and ten drops of water are added to a test tube. When the Clinitest tablet is added, a boiling action occurs. This chemical reaction makes the bottom of the test tube hot. After the boiling stops, wait fifteen seconds and then gently shake the tube. Then compare the sample with a chart. Urine that is free of sugar remains blue. There may be a whitish sediment in the urine, but this is not significant. Increasing amounts of glucose turn the urine from green to brown to orange.

As the boiling reaction is taking place, it is important to watch because the color may go very quickly to a dark brown color, which signifies more than 2% sugar. If so, this change is called a *pass-through reaction,* and it should be recorded as over 2%. Otherwise the dark color that occurs *after* the initial reading at fifteen seconds should be ignored. Only the color change at fifteen seconds is compared to the chart.

The *two-drop method* uses the same tablet and amount of water but only two drops of urine. The two drop method, by making the urine more dilute, avoids the "pass through" effect. Use the specific color chart for each method (Ames Products).

Reporting Test Results

Unfortunately, the same readings on two different scales do not necessarily mean the same thing. For instance, a "1 + " by one method does not mean the same as a "1 + " by another method. Even enzyme methods from two different companies may use different scales (Lundin 1978). So it is much better to report the amount of sugar as a percentage. To illustrate the differences in the scales, three methods are compared in Table 3–4. This table shows that a urine sugar of 2 + could mean ¼%, ½%, or ¾% sugar depending on which commercial preparation is used. Obviously reporting the results in a percentage decreases the confusion when more than one method is used in a given situation. Note that for 2% sugar in the urine all methods report this as "4 + ." The American Diabetic Association has recommended that all manufacturers change the color charts to percentage readings so patients (and health care workers!) are not confused by the various meanings of sugar reported in so many pluses.

TABLE 3–4.   THE MEANING OF THE PLUSES FOR URINE GLUCOSE TESTING

	No Sugar	1/10%	1/4%	1/2%	3/4%	1%	2%
TesTape (enzyme method)	neg	+	+ +	+ + +			+ + + +
Lab Stick (enzyme method)	neg	trace	+	+ +		+ + +	+ + + +
Clinitest (reducing method)	neg	neg	trace	+	+ +	+ + +	+ + + +

Example of Sliding Scale Coverage for Positive Sugar and Acetone

Sample Orders:	(Use Clinitest tablets)
for 1+:	No insulin
for 2+:	5 units regular insulin
for 3+:	10 units regular insulin
for 4+:	15 units regular insulin

Call House Officer if acetone present

Increased Glucose in the Urine (Glycosuria)

Clinical Significance. Glucose in the urine signifies either (1) hyperglycemia (see Chapter 8 for a detailed discussion of the causes of hyperglycemia) or (2) a decreased renal threshold for glucose.

The *renal threshold* for glucose is usually around 160 to 190 mg/100 ml of blood; in other words, no sugar is spilled into the urine until the blood sugar rises above this level. Various situations, including diabetes, may cause a blood glucose level higher than 160 mg, as well as alter the renal threshold for glucose. For example, in pregnancy the renal threshold for glucose may be lowered so that small amounts of glycosuria may be present and are usually not considered abnormal. Lactosuria is common in the third trimester. Patients on hyperalimentation have glycosuria if the intravenous solution (which has very concentrated sugar) is going faster than the pancreas can produce insulin. Hereditary defects, such as galactose intolerance, cause a positive Clinitest, since a positive result with the reducing method is capable of also indicating the presence of sugars other than glucose. But such defects do not effect a positive result with TesTape or other enzyme dipsticks.

Possible Nursing Implications. Sugar in the urine on a random specimen of urine is an indication that the patient needs to be observed for continued spilling of sugar into the urine. It is important to not jump immediately to the conclusion that such patients are diabetic since many factors may cause transient glycosuria. (See Chapter 8 for the nursing implications for patients who have elevated blood sugar levels.) These patients may be checked routinely for sugar and acetone in the urine while other assessments are being done.

Because nurses are responsible for doing routine checking for sugar and acetone in the urine, it is important that they understand the method used. (Refer to the beginning of this section for the specific steps for each method.) Besides testing for sugar, diabetic patients are taught to check also for acetone. The significance of a positive acetone is discussed in the next section. The nurse should allow patients to do the testing several times in the hospital so that they completely understand the technique. It is also a good idea to allow diabetic patients to continue testing their urine when they are admitted to the hospital if conditions permit. This is not only an opportunity to assess the level of the patient's understanding, but also a way to promote a level of independence. Nurses in clinics or those who make home visits should also watch patients perform the urine testing. Guthrie (1980) has excellent tips on how to help the diabetic do urine testing and to manage self-care.

A double-voided specimen for periodically testing for sugar in urine is desirable. The patient empties the bladder and then voids again as soon as possible. From a practical point of view, getting two specimens from a patient may not be possible; so it is always wise to test the first voiding too. With this procedure one is sure that the urine reflects the current status, which is a particularly important condition if insulin is ordered—as is sometimes done—to cover any glycosuria. The insulin order is on a "sliding-scale" basis with a typical pattern as shown in Table 3-4. See Chapter 8 for other tests such as Dextrostix (Ames) which patients may use at home for blood glucose levels.

If the glycosuria is due to too fast a rate of hyperalimentation fluids, this condition must be remedied immediately. Continual glycosuria wastes the needed sugar in the intravenous solution and causes extra water to be lost in the urine. A high concentration of sugar in the blood acts as an osmotic diuretic; so water is excreted as the sugar spills into the urine. The presence of glycosuria, from any cause, alerts the nurse to the fact that the patient needs additional fluid intake and could undergo severe dehydration if the glycosuria is allowed to continue. (See Chapter 8 for a discussion on hyperglycemic hyperosmolar nonketotic coma [HHNK].) If the glycosuria is due to hyperalimentation therapy, the physician may eliminate the spilling of glucose in two different ways: (1) Either slow down the rate of the concentrated sugar solution, or (2) order insulin to help the body utilize the large load of glucose.

In the diabetic patient a continued spilling of sugar leads not only to severe dehydration, but also to ketonuria and eventually to ketoacidosis as the ketone bodies build up in the serum. The nurse needs to be aware that the presence of a positive acetone with a positive sugar indicates a need for immediate medical intervention.

KETONES IN THE URINE

Ketones are metabolic end-products of fat and protein metabolism. When the body does not have sufficient glucose to use for energy, the excretion of ketones increases. The three ketone bodies in the urine are acetone, acetoacetic acid, and betahydroxybutyric acid. Test strips and tablets check only for acetone and acetoacetic acid, but this is sufficient since a change in the small amount of acetone signifies the same degree of change in the other ketones. Acetoacetate and acetone can also be measured in the serum (see Chapter 8).

The usual procedure is to test for both sugar and acetone in the urine when there is any question about glucose metabolism. As in the tests for sugar, acetone can be tested either by a dipstick or by a tablet. (Refer to the section on glycosuria, on obtaining a double-voided urine specimen.) Both methods show a deepening purple color when acetone is present. The scale indicates small, moderate, or large amounts of acetone. Symptomatic ketosis occurs at levels of about 50 mg/dl or when the patient has moderate acetone in urine testing. Urine containing bromsulfalein (BSP dye, Chapter 11), phenyl-ketones (PKU, Chapter 18), or L-dopa metabolites may give false positive results.

Reference Values

Normally urine should not contain enough ketones to give a positive reading.

Small	20 mg/dl of ketones
Moderate	30–40 mg/dl of ketones
Large	80 mg or above

Clinical Significance. The presence of ketones in the urine signifies that the body is using fat as the major source of energy. Fats are used when glucose is unavailable to the cells. The unavailability of glucose may be because glucose is not being transported to the cells, as in diabetes, or because glucose is lacking in the body due to starvation, fasting, or an all-protein diet.

Possible Nursing Implications. The presence of ketones in the urine alerts the nurse to the fact that the metabolic state of the patient is precarious. If the ketone bodies continue to build up in the bloodstream, the patient will develop a type of metabolic acidosis called *ketoacidosis.* Ketones are acidic and use up the buffers in the bloodstream. The presence of acetone signifies the move toward ketoacidosis.

If the patient is a known diabetic, ketonuria (a positive acetone by testing) indicates that the insulin and glucose balance is not satisfactory. There is an abundance of glucose in the bloodstream, as evidenced by the 2% sugar in the urine, but it is unavailable to the cells. The diabetic patient with a positive acetone has switched to using fats as the primary source of energy because the lack of insulin prohibits the transport of glucose to the cells. This patient usually has regular insulin ordered in the form of a sliding scale that varies depending on the amount of glucose spillage and the appearance of acetone. The patient needs this insulin so that glucose can reach the cells and be used as the primary source of energy. (See Chapter 8 for more information about ketoacidosis.)

If the acetone is positive due to a starvation state, the positive ketone is associated with a *negative* glucose in the urine. If the patient is not diabetic, a search must be made for other reasons why the cells do not have glucose. Questions to be asked would be:

1. Has the patient had a reduced amount of food?
2. Has there been a lot of vomiting?
3. Is the patient trying to lose weight by being on an all-protein diet?

Depending on the circumstances, the patient needs glucose in some form so that fats and/or proteins do not continue to be the primary source of energy. The person also needs extra fluids so that the ketones can be excreted by the kidneys. Patients on tube feedings that are very high in protein may show ketones in the urine unless they also receive adequate glucose in the feeding, along with plenty of water to rid the bloodstream of the ketones.

A patient who goes on an all-protein diet in an attempt to lose weight should be under careful supervision. The patient should check the urine for the amount of ketones that build up. Sufficient fluids must be taken to prevent ketone toxicity. All-protein diets are controversial due to the possible danger to the physiological balance of the body.

EXAMINATION OF URINE SEDIMENT

As the last part of a routine analysis, the urine sediment is centrifuged and examined microscopically for crystals, casts, RBC (red blood cells), WBC (white blood cells), and bacteria or yeast. Table 3–5 contains a brief summary of the meaning of each of these findings.

TABLE 3-5.   A SUMMARY OF URINE SEDIMENT FINDINGS

WBC	Normally there should not be more than a few white blood cells in the urine (4-5 per high power field). Infections or inflammations anywhere along the urinary tract cause an increase of white blood cells in the urine. Urinary tract infections occur in 1 to 2% of all pregnancies (Connell 1979).
RBC	Normally there should be only an occasional red blood cell in the urine (2-3 per high power field). An increased number of red blood cells in the urine indicate bleeding somewhere in the urinary system, which may be due to renal disease, trauma, or a bleeding disorder. In females it is important to make sure that the urine was not contaminated by the menstrual flow. Insertion of a tampon and a collection of midstream urine are ways to prevent this contamination.
Crystals	Most crystals have little clinical significance. If the patient is on drugs that may cause crystallization in the urine, such as some of the sulfa drugs, this finding may be clinically important.
Casts	A few hyaline casts are considered normal, but all other casts need to be evaluated by the physician. Unlike crystals, casts are suggestive of actual kidney disease. Casts are a compacted collection of protein, cells, and debris that are formed in the tubules of the kidneys. Those that form in the distal tubule have a narrow caliber. Those that form in the collecting tubules tend to be very broad. Broad granular casts are sometimes called *renal failure casts* because they indicate major renal destruction. The width and composition of the cast has great significance in the diagnosis and prognosis of renal diseases (Schuman 1978).
Bacteria or Yeast	Often the presence of a few bacteria or yeast is indicative only of contamination from the perineal area, but a culture and sensitivity may need to be done if a large amount of bacteria is noted on routine screening. Chapter 16 discusses the nursing implications for obtaining a urine specimen for a culture and sensitivity or for a smear. See the test for nitrates discussed in this chapter.

INDIVIDUAL URINE TESTS

Random urine specimens may be needed for various other tests besides a routine urinalysis; Table 3-6 shows some tests that are done on a single specimen. A multitude of tests can be done on one dipstick. Table 3-1 gives some tips about factors that can affect the N-Multistix C (Ames), which tests nine substances. Note that these dipsticks are also available in different combinations for specific testing of one or more urine constituents. Information about nitrates, porphyrins, delta-aminolevulinic acid, and 5-HIAA is included next since these tests are not covered in other chapters.

NITRITES

Most species of bacteria, if present in the urine, cause the conversion of nitrates, which are derived from dietary metabolites, to nitrites. Thus a dipstick test for nitrites is a check for urinary infections.

TABLE 3-6. EXAMPLES OF TESTS ON URINE (other than routine urinalysis or **24**-hour urine specimens)

Test	Reference Value	Specimen	Information About Test
Bence-Jones protein	Negative	First morning specimen	Chap. 10
Human chorionic gonadotropin (HCG)	Negative (unless pregnant)	First morning specimen	Chap. 18
Tests for occult blood Hematest—Ames Hemastix—Ames Hemoccult—Smith, Kline, French	Negative	Random	Chap. 11 on tests to detect bleeding. Note microscopic exam is more sensitive test.
Porphobilinogens	Negative	Freshly voided specimen	This chapter.
Bilirubin	Negative	Random	Chap. 11
Urobilinogen	0.3–1.0 Ehrlich units/2 hr	2-hr specimen 1–3 P.M.	Chap. 11
Nitrites	No pink color	Clean catch or midstream specimen	This chapter and Chap. 16.

Preparation of Patient
And Collection of Sample

Optimal results are obtained by using a first morning urine sample that has been "incubating" in the bladder for four or more hours. The urine should be done by a clean catch midstream technique (see Chapter 16 on clean catch urine specimens), and it should be tested within an hour of voiding. As an alternative to the clean catch method, the patient may wet the strip by holding it in the urinary stream.

A specialized dipstick for nitrites, Microstix-3 (Ames Products) can also be used for a culture. Immediately after the strip is read, it is put into a transparent bag. The dipstick has two miniaturized culture areas that support both gram-positive and gram-negative bacteria. If the dipstick is to be cultured, it must not be touched. The dipstick in the bag is put into an incubator for a minimum of 18 hours. Results are ready within 18 to 24 hours. Various other companies make diagnostic culture kits (see Chapter 16).

Reference Values

Nitrate reagent	Turns pink if bacteria are present. The pink color is *not* quantitative in relation to the number of bacteria present. Ascorbic acid or a high specific gravity may invalidate the results. Blood, or other pigments in the urine, can interfere with the color changes.
Cultures	Usually growth of 100,000 per ml is considered evidence of a bacterial infection (see Chapter 16 on culture reports).

Note: A negative nitrite test or negative culture does not provide proof that the urine is free of all bacteria, particularly if there are clinical symptoms to the contrary. Some bacteria, such as streptococci and gonococci, do not produce nitrites.

URINARY PORPHYRINS

Porphobilinogen, coproporphyrins and uroporphyrins are intermediaries in the synthesis, of heme, which is part of hemoglobin and of several enzymes. Delta-aminolevulinic acid (Δ-ALA) is an important enzyme for the formation of porphobilinogen. Abnormalities of porphyrin metabolism may be either genetic or due to drug intoxication, usually lead (Free 1979:71). Several tests can be done to demonstrate an abnormality in the metabolism of heme. Since the porphyrins are precursors of the pigment (heme), the urine may be burgundy color or pink when exposed to black light.

Special Preparation of Patient
And Collection of Sample

Coproporphyria and uroporphyrin require a 24-hour urine specimen. As the preservative, use 5 g of sodium carbonate. Porphobilinogen is done on a random urine specimen, consisting of 10 ml of freshly voided urine. (See instructions at the end of this chapter on collecting 24-hour specimens.)

Reference Values

Coproporphyrin	50–250 ug/d
Uroporphyrin	0
Porphobilinogen	0

Abnormal Porphyrins

Clinical Significance. Elevations of these tests are indications of one of the porphyrias, which are several different diseases that may be acute or chronic. Acute intermittent porphyria, the most common, can be precipitated by barbituates. Coproporphyrins may document toxicity to lead (see Chapter 17).

Possible Nursing Implications. O'Conner (1981) describes in detail the many nursing needs of a patient with acute intermittent porphyria. The disease may be very hard to diagnose because it mimics so many other conditions. At the present time treatment is symptomatic.

DELTA-AMINOLEVULINIC ACID (ΔALA)

Delta-aminolevulic acid (ΔALA) is an enzyme that is needed for the proper conversion to porphobilinogen in the metabolic formation of heme. ΔALA is not present in the urine of healthy subjects, but it is present in lead intoxication. ΔALA may also be elevated in certain kinds of genetic deficiencies of porphyrin metabolism (the porphyrias).

Preparation of Patient
And Collection of Sample
Collect a 24-hour urine sample. See instructions at the end of this chapter.

Reference Value

1–7 mg/d

Clinical Significance. See Chapter 17 for the use of this test in relation to lead poisoning. O'Conner (1981) discusses the nursing needs for patients with acute intermittent porphyria.

URINARY 5-HIAA
(5-HYDROXYINDOLEACETIC ACID)

Glands in the gastrointestinal tract secrete the hormone serotonin. Carried in the platelets, serotonin is a vasoconstrictor that is especially important to small arterioles after tissue injury. It is also a regulator of smooth muscle contraction, such as in peristalsis. The chief metabolite of serotonin, excreted in the urine, is 5-hydroxyindoleacetic acid (5-HIAA). Certain tumors, called carcinoid tumors, of the argentaffin cells in the gastrointestinal tract may begin to secrete abnormal amounts of serotonin. Hence a measurement of the amount of 5-HIAA in the urine is a help in diagnosing carcinoid tumors (Ravel 1978:396).

Preparation of Patient and Collection of Sample

The patient must not eat foods such as bananas, tomatoes, plums, avocados, eggplants, or pineapples because all these foods contain a significant amount of serotonin (Ravel 1978: 471). Since many drugs may also affect the test results, the patient should not take any medication during the test. The nurse must check with the laboratory about specific drug interactions. Except for the foods mentioned, a normal diet can be taken during the test. The urine is collected in a special container with 10 ml of HCl. Follow the procedure for a collection of 24-hour specimen (discussed at the end of this chapter).

Reference Values

24-hour screening test	Negative
Quantitative test	2-9 mg/d— women lower than men

Clinical Significance. An elevated level of 5-HIAA in the urine is evidence of increased serotonin, which may be due to carcinoid tumors. These tumors may be either benign or malignant. Note that tumors in other organs may sometimes produce serotonin. (See Chapter 15 on ectopic hormone production by tumors.)

Possible Nursing Implications. The symptoms of serotonin excess may include cyanotic episodes, flushing of the skin, diarrhea, abdominal cramps, and bronchial constriction. The nurse should note and record any type of symptoms that occur during the time the patient is being worked up for a possible carcinoid tumor. The major clinical manifestations of the syndrome are due to biologically active agents released by the tumor. In addition to the release of serotonin, bradykinin, histamine, and ACTH, other substances are also released (Taub 1980:53). Treatment involves the surgical removal of the tumor.

COLLECTION OF 24-HOUR URINE SPECIMEN

These collections are useful only if *all* the urine is collected for 24 hours. Even if "just one specimen" is discarded, the test is not valid. The nurse must make sure that the patient fully understands the importance of saving all the urine. On account of the problem with incomplete urine collections, laboratories sometimes check the creatinine present in the urine to validate that the urine is representative of a full 24 hours. Assuming the patient does not have renal problems, a creatinine value below the normal range of 25 mg/kg of body weight suggests an incomplete collection (Ravel 1978:499).

To begin the 24-hour urine collection, the patient voids and *discards* the urine so that the urine from the previous night is not included. Then all the urine for the next 24

TABLE 3-7. 24-HOUR URINE SPECIMENS*

Substance Tested	Reference Values d = 24-Hour Day	Preservative Needed	Information about Test
Aldosterone	2-23 μg/d	Refrigerate	Chap. 15
Amylase	24-76 U/ml	None	Chap. 12—may do for only two hours
Calcium	150 mg/d or less	Need 10 ml of HCl	See Sulkowitch test (Chap. 7) for random tests of urine calcium
Catecholamines Epinephrine Norepinephrine	Under 20 μg/d Under 100 μg/d	Need 12 ml of HCl (pH kept 2-3)	Chap. 15
Coproporphyrin	50-250 μg/d Children under 80 lb: 0-75 μg/d	5 g of Na carbonate	See this chapter.
Creatinine	15-25 mg/kg of body weight	None	Chap. 4
Creatinine clearance	Male 95-135 ml/min Female 85-125 ml/min	None	Need serum creatinine too (Chap. 4).
Delta-aminolevulinic acid	1-7 mg/d	None	See this chapter and Chap. 17.
FSH	Varies with sex and age	None	Chap. 15
5-HIAA	2-9 mg/d women lower than men	10 ml of HCl	See this chapter.

	Reference value	Preservative	Notes
Lead	120 μg or less/d	None	Make sure lead-free container Chap. 17.
Pregnanetriol	Male 1–2 mg/d Female 0.5–2 mg/d Children less than 0.5 mg/dl	Refrigerate	Chap. 15
Phosphorus	1 g/d—varies with intake	10 ml of HCl	Chap. 7
Potassium	40–80 mEq	None	Chap. 5
Pregnanediol	Male less than 1 mg/d Female 1–8 mg/d	Refrigerate	Chap. 15
Protein	Less than 150 mg/d	None	See quantitative and qualitative tests in this chapter.
Sodium	40–220 mEq/d	None	Chap. 5
17-Ketosteroids	Varies with age and sex	None	Chap. 15
17-Hydroxysteroids	Varies with age and sex	None	Chap. 15
Urea Nitrogen	6–17 g/d	None	Chap. 4
Uroporphyrin	Negative	5 g of Na carbonate	See this chapter.
VMA (vanilylmandelic acid)	Up to 9 mg/d	12 ml of HCl	Chap. 15

* Reference values: Sculley (1980) and Modern Chemistry (1978: 78). Note that most laboratories prefer all 24-hour urine specimens iced. Check with the laboratory for the specific technique used. Also see Appendix A, Table 2 for urine values in SI units.

hours is saved and put into a large collection bottle. If a patient voids and discards the urine at, say, 8:20 A.M., the test ends at 8:20 A.M. the next day. The patient should do a final voiding as close to 8:20 A.M. as possible so that the last urine in the bladder can be included. The urine specimen should be sent to the laboratory as soon as possible. Some laboratories may want only 25 ml of the total, but this quantity must be verified with the laboratory. The times for beginning and ending the urine collection should be noted on the requisition.

The laboratory will supply the collection bottle, along with any preservative needed (Table 3–7 for common 24-hour urine specimens and the preparations needed). The laboratory should also notify the nurse or the patient if certain drugs or foods invalidate the test. (See the discussions in the various chapters of specific points for each test.) If a preservative is not used, a few specimens, such as those for hormones, must be refrigerated. Usually refrigeration is preferred for most urine tests but the nurse should validate this requirement with the laboratory. The rationale for refrigeration is to inhibit bacterial growth, which may interfere with some tests.

For toddlers, when a diaper is used at night, a 12-hour specimen may have to suffice. For infants, urine may be collected in disposable paste on collection bags. Rarely, it may be necessary to insert a Foley catheter to get a 24-hour urine collection from a child. The danger of a urinary tract infection is a drawback.

Questions

3-1. A specimen of urine for a routine urinalysis should be:

    a. at least 120 ml.

    b. put into a sterile container.

    c. an early morning specimen, if possible.

    d. sent to the laboratory as a stat procedure.

3-2. Which of the following foods tend to make the urine pH higher?

    a. Meat.   **c.** Cranberry juice.

    b. Eggs   **d.** Citrus juices.

3-3. Mrs. Leggins may have a pseudomonas infection of the bladder. Which of the following urinalysis findings is/are suggestive of this type of urinary tract infection?

    a. More than 5 WBC in the microscopic exam of urinary sediment.

    b. Urine pH of 6.

    c. Presence of casts.

    d. All of the above.

3-4. In interpreting the meaning of specific gravity of a urinalysis for a child under two, it is important for the nurse to realize that in a child this young, the maximum specific gravity is:

    a. much lower than for an adult.

    b. higher than for an adult.

    c. essentially the same as the adult range.

    d. fixed at 1.010.

3-5. Which of the following patients demonstrates the concept of a ''fixed'' specific gravity (s.g.)?

    a. Mrs. Jung, who has a s.g. around 1.025 on three early morning urine specimens.

    b. Mr. Louis, who has a s.g. of 1.010 on a random urine specimen.

    c. Mr. Tagelino, whose s.g. remains around 1.008 while he is on diuretics.

    d. Mrs. Foley whose s.g. was 1.010 during a prolonged period of fluid restriction.

3-6. A patient is asked to obtain a urine specimen before arising to rule out orthostatic or postural:

    a. glycosuria.   **c.** proteinuria.

    b. ketonuria.   **d.** all of the above.

3-7. Which of the following conditions is considered a nonpathological reason for proteinuria?

    a. Diet high in protein.   **c.** Pregnancy.

    b. Orthostatic or postural proteinuria.   **d.** Any of the above.

3-8. The nurse in a prenatal clinic has just tested Mrs. Ames' urine and found it to be ½% for glucose and 3+ for protein by the dipstick method. There will be a 30- to 40-minute delay before the patient sees the doctor. She says she is ''feeling okay'' so she wishes to have her appointment rescheduled. Which action by the nurse would be the most appropriate?

    a. Reschedule her appointment for another day since glucose and protein in the urine are not uncommon in the third trimester of pregnancy.

    b. Say nothing about the urine test but insist that she wait to see the physician because the clinic schedule is always full.

    c. Do a nursing history on the patient and tell her the glucose in her urine needs investigation by the physician since she may be diabetic.

    d. Take her blood pressure, check her ankles, and explain why it is necessary to make these assessments to help the physician evaluate the seriousness of the proteinuria. Insist that she wait to see the physician.

3-9. For a newborn, when the purpose of testing the urine for sugar is to detect the spilling of sugars other than glucose, the test that detects this is:

  a. TesTape

  b. Clinistix.

  c. Clinitest.

  d. All of the above.

3-10 The enzyme method (TesTape) for testing for sugar in the urine is different from the reducing method (Clinitest) in that the enzyme method:

  a. detects smaller amounts of glucose.

  b. is specific for glucose only.

  c. is not affected by drugs such as the cephalosporins.

  d. all of the above are true.

3-11. Marilyn is a 19-year-old college freshman who is quite obese. She has come to the campus health clinic because she feels very tired. A routine CBC and urinalysis were normal except for a trace of acetone. (Urine sugar was negative.) Based on these laboratory findings, which question by the nurse will most likely help to discover the reason for the abnormal ketones?

  a. Have you been eating a lot of fats lately?

  b. Have you been under a lot of stress?

  c. Is there a history of diabetes in your family?

  d. Have you been on a strict reducing diet lately?

3-12. Renal tubular damage is most clearly documented by the presence of which element in the microscopic exam of urine sediment?

  a. Casts.   **b.** Crystals.   **c.** RBC's.   **d.** WBC's.

3-13. Mrs. Zorba is in the last trimester of her pregnancy. A dipstick test for nitrites in the urine was positive (pink color). Her specific gravity was normal. A positive reaction is evidence of:

  a. preeclampsia.

  b. normal dietary metabolites of protein.

  c. possible urinary tract infection.

  d. possible lack of ascorbic acid in her diet.

3-14. Mr. Bowdin is to collect a 24-hour specimen for urine coproporphyrins for possible lead toxicity. He has been given a container with the necessary preservative. Which of the following instructions by the nurse is correct?

  a. Begin the test exactly at 8 A.M. and collect all urine until 8 A.M. the next day.

b. Discard the first urine specimen tomorrow morning and then collect all the urine for the next 24 hours.

c. Discarding only one specimen will not create a problem if he can estimate the amount lost.

d. If urine cannot be added to the bottle immediately after voiding, keep it on ice.

REFERENCES

Condon, Robert and Nyhus, Lloyd. *Manual of Surgical Therapeutics*. Boston: Little, Brown & Co., 1975.

Connell, Elizabeth. *Changes in the Urinary Tract During Pregnancy* (Patient Information Booklet). Chicago: American College of Obstetricians and Gynecologists, 1979.

Free, Alfred and Free, Helen. *Urodynamics: Concepts Relating to Routine Urine Chemistry*. Elkhart, Indiana: Ames Division, Miles Laboratories, 1979.

Guthrie, Diana. "Helping the Diabetic Manage His Self-Care," *Nursing 80* 10 (February 1980): 57–65.

Hytten, Frank and Lind, Tom. *Diagnostic Indices in Pregnancy*. Summit: N.J.: Ciba-Geigy Corporation, 1975.

Lundin, Dorothy. "Reporting Urine Test Results: Switch from + to %," *American Journal of Nursing* 78 (May 1978): 876–879.

Modern Urine Chemistry: A Guide to the Diagnosis of Urinary Tract Disorders and Metabolic Disorders. Elkhart, Indiana: Ames Division, Miles Laboratories, 1978.

O'Connor, Louise. "Acute Intermittent Porphyria," *American Journal of Nursing* 81 (June 1981): 1184–1186.

Product Profiles on N-Multistix (Reagent Strips for Urinalysis). Elkhart, Indiana: Ames Division, Miles Laboratories, 1980.

Ravel, Richard. *Clinical Laboratory Medicine*, 3rd ed. Chicago: Yearbook Medical Publishers, Inc., 1978.

Schumann, Berry *et al.* "An Improved Technique for Examining Urinary Casts and a Review of Their Significance," *American Journal of Clinical Pathology* 69:1 (January 1978): 18–23.

Shapter, Robert. *The Art of Urinalysis*. Summit, N.J.: Ciba-Geigy Corporation, 1976.

Slawson, Michele. "Thirty-Three Drugs that Discolor Urine and/or Stools," *RN* 43 (January 1980): 40–41.

Taub, Sheldon. "Identifying Malignant Carcinoid Syndrome," *Hospital Medicine* 16 (July 1980): 53–54.

Twombly, Marilyn. "The Shift into Third Space," *Nursing 78* 8 (June 1978): 38–41.

Widmann, Frances. *Clinical Interpretation of Laboratory Tests*, 8th ed. Philadelphia: F. A. Davis Co., 1979.

CHAPTER FOUR

Renal Function Tests

Objectives

1. Compare and contrast the factors that affect the BUN and serum creatinine levels.
2. Explain the rationale for checking BUN and/or serum creatinine levels before administration of certain antibiotics.
3. Describe the nursing assessments and interventions that are appropriate when a patient has markedly elevated BUN and serum creatinine levels.
4. Compare the usefulness of urine osmolality to the measurement of urine specific gravity.
5. Given various changes in serum and urine osmolality, plan appropriate nursing interventions.
6. Prepare a teaching plan that helps a patient with high serum uric acid levels to decrease the possibility of renal stones.
7. Describe the role of the nurse in preparing patients for creatinine clearance and PSP tests.

This chapter focuses on the common laboratory tests related to renal function or dysfunction:

1. blood urea nitrogen (BUN),
2. serum and urine creatinine levels,
3. serum creatine levels,
4. serum and urine osmolality,
5. uric acid levels, and
6. phenosulfonphtalein (PSP) excretion test.

Some of these tests are used only for renal assessment, while others have several purposes. For example, serum creatinine levels, urine creatinine levels, and the creatinine clearance tests are all used only to evaluate renal function, and only renal dysfunction changes the result. (A brief discussion of *creatine* is covered so that this test is not confused with the *creatinine* tests.) On the other hand, the blood urea nitrogen (BUN), also used primarily to assess renal function, can be affected by many factors. Tests for serum and urine osmolality are newer tests that are useful not only in assessing renal function, but also for assessing fluid requirements and fluid imbalances. The discussions on urine osmolality should be read after one has read about specific gravity measurements in the previous chapter. One test covered in this chapter, uric acid, is not really a test for renal dysfunction at all, but uric acid is likely to be elevated in severe renal dysfunction. Therefore the discussion on uric acid fits into a general discussion about renal dysfunction, even though it is not used as an assessment tool for the severity of the dysfunction. An older test of renal function, the PSP excretion test, is discussed at the end of the chapter.

BLOOD UREA NITROGEN (BUN)

The blood urea nitrogen test measures the amount of urea nitrogen in the blood. Urea, a waste product of protein metabolism, is formed by the liver and carried via the blood to the kidneys for excretion. Because urea is cleared from the bloodstream by the kidneys, the BUN can be used as a test of renal function. However, protein breakdown, dehydration, overhydration, and liver failure all invalidate the BUN as a test for renal dysfunction.

Preparation of Patient And Collection of Sample
There is no special preparation of the patient. The laboratory needs 1 ml of blood or serum for the test. Certain drugs, such as streptomycin, chloramphenicol, or mercurial diuretics, may interfere with test results.

Reference Values

Adults	8-25 mg/100 ml. Males may be slightly higher than females.
Pregnancy	Values may decrease about 25%.
Newborns	Values tend to be slightly lower than adult ranges.
Aged	Values may be slightly increased due to lack of renal concentration.

Increased BUN

Clinical Significance. Any situation that causes impaired renal function results in a rise in the BUN. Diseased or damaged kidneys cause an elevated BUN because the kidneys are no longer able to rid the blood of the waste product, urea. Even if the kidneys are not diseased or damaged, conditions where renal perfusion is decreased result in an increase of urea in the blood. Thus either a patient in shock or one in congestive heart failure may have higher-than-normal BUN levels due to poor circulation to the kidneys. A patient who is severely dehydrated may also have an elevated BUN due to the lack of volume for normal urine output. Because urea is an end-product of protein metabolism, a diet that is very high in protein may cause some increase in the BUN level. Bleeding into the gastrointestinal tract and tube feedings of concentrated protein are two ways that the urea level may be increased in the bloodstream. Increased protein metabolism, coupled with dehydration, would make the rise in BUN even more likely. When blood is broken down in the gastrointestinal tract, this becomes a source of protein. For example, loss of 1,000 ml of blood into the gastrointestinal tract may elevate the BUN to 40 mg/dl.

Since creatinine is changed only by renal dysfunction, a comparison of the BUN with the serum creatinine is useful. Normally, the ratio of BUN to creatinine is about 15:1 (Ravel 1978). A patient with a BUN of 15 mg would be expected to have a serum creatinine level around 1.0 mg. If the patient becomes dehydrated or breaks down more protein (such as with gastrointestinal bleeding), the BUN increases while the creatinine does not; so the ratio of 15:1 is increased in dehydration or protein breakdown. On the other hand, a ratio of BUN to creatinine would be less than 15:1 in low-protein intake, overhydration, or severe liver failure, which reduce the BUN but not the creatinine.

Possible Nursing Implications.

Assessing for a Need for More Fluids. Because an increased BUN may be due to anything that causes poor renal perfusion or renal dysfunction, it is important to look at the BUN in relation to the pathophysical process for the individual patient. If the BUN is due to poor renal perfusion, the focus is on increasing renal flow. For example, if the patient has a dehydration problem, this must be corrected. However, if the elevated BUN reflects actual renal damage, then fluids may have to be restricted. The nurse must discover the necessary fluid requirements or other restrictions in light of an increasing BUN that is due to actual renal damage. See Table 4–1 for a comparison of BUN and creatinine in various stages of renal disease.

TABLE 4–1.   POSSIBLE CONTINUUM OF CHRONIC RENAL DISEASE*

Reduced or diminished renal reserve	BUN may be slightly high or high-normal, but no problems unless stress (infections, surgery, emotional crisis, etc.) challenges limited reserve. Creatinine levels within normal range.
Renal insufficiency	BUN mildly elevated. May not tolerate high-protein intake. Impaired urine concentration (see serum osmolality). Mild anemia. Stress easily impairs renal function. Creatinine level beginning to rise (see Table 4–2).
Renal failure	Both creatinine and BUN are elevated. Levels vary with severity *and* other factors. Other abnormal tests may be hypernatremia, hyperkalemia (Chapter 5), anemia (Chapter 2), hypocalcemia, hyperphosphatemia (Chapter 7).
End-stage renal disease	Serum creatinine above 10 mg/d. BUN rise somewhat proportionately. Other tests mentioned are increasingly abnormal.

* See text, Stark (1980), and Oestreich (1979) for more details.

If the elevated BUN can be traced to a great increase in protein in the diet, a reduction of protein and/or an increase of fluid intake will help the kidneys get rid of the excess urea. For example, increased fluids will be needed with high protein supplements.

Balancing the Problem Nutrients of Potassium, Sodium, and Protein. Since urea is not the only substance that is increasing in the bloodstream as renal dysfunction persists, the nurse must be alert to which medications and food may be contraindicated. Sodium and potassium are excreted by the kidneys. Sodium may need to be restricted, and supplemental potassium is contraindicated in the patient who has progressive renal dysfunction. See Chapter 5 on hyperkalemia and hypernatremia. Usually protein in the diet is not restricted for mild renal insufficiency, but one would question a high-protein diet, which would tend to increase the BUN even more. The protein level may need to be adjusted to maintain lean body mass and still not cause a high BUN (Luke 1979). See Chapter 7 for the discussion on supplemental calcium and the restriction of phosphorus in renal disease.

The child and adolescent in renal failure present additional nutritional problems due to the needs of their growing bodies. Few infants are placed on fluid restrictions. Yet as with adults, sodium, potassium, and protein are the problem nutrients (Hetrick 1979: 2152). Infants may be undergoing a life-threatening hyperkalemia (high potassium level), even though the BUN is not over 35 (Jones 1979).

Preparing the Patient for Possible Dialysis or Other Interventions. Azotemia means an increase of nitrogenous waste products in the serum. *Uremia* is the broader name given to the toxic condition in which the kidneys are not able to excrete urea and other substances, such as potassium, creatinine, and organic acids. In the days before the advent of peritoneal and renal dialysis, patients with high levels of BUN would develop a condition called *uremic frost,* which consisted of urea crystals that were being excreted through the sweat glands. Fortunately urea levels can be lowered now with dialysis before patients develop toxic uremia. Once the patient is on dialysis, severe dietary and fluid restrictions may not be as necessary since the dialysis substitutes for renal function (Luke 1979). BUN and creatinine levels are done frequently for all patients on dialysis to monitor the effectiveness of the treatment program.

Not all patients with increasing BUN levels have dialysis. Sometimes the BUN remains elevated only for a brief time until the underlying pathophysiology is corrected.

Assessing for Symptoms of Azotemia. Patients with a mild gradual increase in the BUN level may not have many symptoms. The level of BUN that causes symptoms in patients varies tremendously (Oestreich 1979). As BUN levels continue to rise, the patient is likely to experience fatigue, muscle weakness, and some nausea and vomiting. There may be a decline in mental awareness, drowsiness or confusion. Nurses need to assess the mental and physical capabilities of any patients with increased BUNs to ensure their safe care. Patients who may be slightly confused or unsteady on their feet need careful watching.

Using BUN Levels to Monitor Aminoglycoside Therapy. BUN and creatinine levels are also used to monitor patients who are receiving drugs known to be potentially nephrotoxic, such as the antibiotics classified as aminoglycosides. Some of the aminoglycosides are gentamicin (Garamycin), kanamycin (Kantrex), tobramycin (Tobricin), and an older antibiotic, streptomycin. Before administering a drug that is known to be potentially nephrotoxic, nurses should look at the patient's BUN and/or creatinine levels. If either level is higher than the reference range, they should withhold the drug until consulting the physician. Since aminoglycosides tend also to be toxic to the eighth cranial nerve, assessments of auditory and vestibular functions are ways to monitor for neurotoxicity. The impaired hearing or dizziness that may occur is more likely if the drug is continued when there is renal dysfunction (Goodman 1975:1175). More and more hospitals now do measurements of the levels of drugs in the serum so that a therapeutic level can be maintained. (See Chapter 17 for a discussion about the measurement of serum levels of aminoglycosides, such as gentamicin.) It is important to keep the patient well hydrated when aminoglycosides are used because they are excreted almost unchanged in the urine (Langslet 1981).

Decreased BUN

Clinical Significance. Just as dehydration may cause an elevated BUN, overhydration causes a decreased BUN. Thus plasma volume increases, such as in pregnancy, reduce the BUN level. A marked decrease in protein breakdown also tends to lower the BUN. Usually a BUN that is slightly lower than the reference values has little clinical significance (Burke 1978). Because urea is synthesized by the liver, severe liver failure causes a reduction of urea in the serum. Yet the inability of the liver to form urea results in an increase of other nitrogen products, such as ammonia, so that tests for ammonia levels are much more clinically significant in liver dysfunction than are lowered BUN levels. (See Chapter 10 on ammonia levels.)

Possible Nursing Implications. Since a decreased BUN raises the possibility of expanded plasma fluid volume, some attention should be paid to the overall hydration status of the patient. Yet the test by itself is not that helpful in identifying plasma dilution. (See Chapter 5 on the serum sodium as a test for plasma dilution.)

CREATINE AND CREATININE LEVELS IN SERUM

Creatinine is the waste product of creatine phosphate, a high-energy compound found in skeletal muscle tissue. The measurement of serum *creatinine* is useful in evaluating any type of renal dysfunction where a large number of nephrons have been destroyed. On the other hand, the measurement of serum *creatine* is useful in evaluating certain degenerative diseases of muscles such as muscular dystrophy; serum creatine levels in muscular disorders rise above the reference range for creatine of 0.5 to 0.9 mg/dl. It is important for the nurses to realize that there are laboratory tests for both crea*tine* and crea*tinine*. This discussion focuses on creatinine because this is the much more common laboratory test of the two.

Preparation of Patient And Collection of Sample
The laboratory needs 1 ml of venous blood. High doses of ascorbic acid, PSP dye, or barbituates may distort the results. Ketone bodies and cephalosporin antibiotics may elevate the results (Ravel 1978:133).

Reference Values

Adults:	Males 0.6–1.5 mg/100 ml. Females 0.6–1.1 mg/100ml Values tend to be slightly higher for males because of their larger muscle mass.
Pregnancy	Values are reduced in pregnancy, presumably because creatinine clearance is markedly increased.
Newborns	Lower than children.
Children	Slight increases with age because values are proportional to body mass. After puberty, males slightly higher.

Increased Creatinine Level

Clinical Significance. The only pathological condition that causes a significant increase in the serum creatinine level is damage to a large number of nephrons (Table 4–2). Unlike the BUN, the serum creatinine level is not affected by protein metabolism, and little if at all, by the hydration state of the patient. Certain muscular diseases may cause a slight increase in the creatinine, but if muscular disease is suspected, then the creatine, rather than the creatinine, test is used for assessment.

Possible Nursing Implications.

Nursing Care for Renal Insufficiency. Most of the nursing implications discussed for patients with an elevated BUN also apply to those with an elevated creatinine because, if both tests are elevated, they have some renal insufficiency (Table 4–1). As discussed in the section on BUN, a change in the BUN/creatinine ratio may be useful in pinpointing the primary factor that needs correction. Since the creatinine is not increased until at least half of the nephrons are nonfunctioning, it is not elevated in reduced or diminished renal reserve as is the BUN. Thus patients with an increased creatinine are most likely to have potentially severe renal impairment. Nursing care is geared toward the myriad manifestations of renal insufficiency or failure.

Using Creatinine Levels to Monitor Drug Therapy, Dialysis, and Renal Transplants. Like the BUN, serum creatinine is used to detect potential renal damage when nephrotoxic

TABLE 4–2. RELATIONSHIP OF CREATININE LEVELS TO ESTIMATED AMOUNT OF NEPHRON LOSS*

Creatinine Level	Estimated Loss of Nephron Function
Normal creatinine (0.6–1.5 mg/dl)	Up to 50% loss
Creatinine level above 1.5 mg/dl	Over 50% nephron function loss
Creatinine level of 4.8 mg/dl	As much as 75% nephron function loss
Creatinine level about 10 mg/dl	90% loss of nephron function—end-stage kidney disease

* *Modified from Stark (1980: 36).*

drugs, such as the aminoglyoside antibiotics, are used. Serum creatinine levels are also routinely done for all dialysis patients and for patients who have had renal transplants. Nurses must recognize any elevations of creatinine so that the development of uremia can be halted. Since creatinine levels rise and fall more slowly than BUN levels, creatinine levels are often preferred for long-term assessment of renal function.

Decreased Creatinine Level

Clinical Significance. A decreased serum creatinine level may indicate atrophy of muscle tissue. However, if skeletal muscle problems are suspected, the serum creatine is used. Note also that the creatine phosphokinase (CPK) is an important enzyme test for muscular disease. (See Chapter 12 on CPK.)

CREATININE CLEARANCE TEST

The creatinine clearance test is used as an indication of the glomerular filtration rate (GFR). The test compares the serum creatinine level with the amount of creatinine excreted in a volume of urine for a specified time period. The time period may be for 2, 12, or 24 hours. A 24-hour collection is most common. At the beginning of the test, the patient empties his or her bladder, and this urine is discarded. Thereafter, all the urine voided during the specified time period is collected. (See Chapter 3 on 24-hour urine collections. No preservative is needed.)

Sometime during the test period, usually about in the middle, a blood sample is drawn to determine the serum creatinine. The rate of creatinine clearance is thus determined by the following formula:

$$\frac{\text{Urine creatinine} \times \text{Urine Volume}}{\text{Creatinine in serum}} = \text{Creatinine clearance rate}$$

—expressed as so many milliliters per minute per 1.72 m² of body surface—

Although nurses are never responsible for calculating the creatinine clearance rate, they should have more insight into the laboratory's report if they have a basic understanding of how the reference values are obtained.

Reference Values

Adult males	95–135 ml/minute. Varies with the amount of lean body mass; so muscular males are usually in the upper limits of the range.
Females	85–125 ml/minute.
Pregnancy	May be as high as 150 to 200 ml/minute.
Aged	Values diminish slightly with age even if no renal disease exists. May be as low as 50 ml/min in the elderly (Ravel 1978:131).

Decreased Creatinine Clearance

Clinical Significance. A decreased creatinine clearance rate is an indication of decreased glomerular function. In preeclampsia, the creatinine clearance drops (Hytten 1975). The creatinine clearance detects renal dysfunction in the early stage. The creatinine clearance rate is a more sensitive indication of renal dysfunction than the serum creatinine alone because the serum creatinine may remain normal until the creatinine clearance is less than half than normal. Creatinine clearance is also used to evaluate the progression of renal disease. A minimum creatinine clearance of around 10 ml/minute is necessary to maintain life without the use of renal or peritoneal dialysis (Condon 1975:149).

Nursing Implications. The results of the creatinine clearance test, together with other assessments of renal dysfunction, help to determine the severity of renal disease. Nursing implications depend on the severity of the renal disease and on the long-term plans for the patient. These patients may have repeated creatinine clearance tests since the changes in the results may be more significant when compared over a period of time. Nurses usually have the responsibility for instructing patients on their role in the tests. When they are well informed, patients are less likely to inadvertently discard urine specimens.

SERUM AND URINE OSMOLALITY

The osmolality of serum, urine, or any other fluid depends on the number of active ions or molecules in a solution. The osmolality of a solution reflects the total *number* of osmotically active particles in the solution, without regard to the size or weight of the particles. In laboratory reports osmolality is expressed as so many milliosmols per kilogram of water (mOsm/kg water).

Although nurses do not need to know how to calculate milliosmols, they may find it helpful to conceptually understand the meaning of a milliosmole (mOsm). A milliosmole is 1/1000 of an osmole. *Osmols* are a standard of measurement based on the freezing point of a solution: As the number of osmotically active particles in a solution increases, the freezing point decreases. For example, a lower temperature is needed to freeze a salt solution than to freeze plain water. As a standard of measurement, one osmole is the amount of a particular solute that lowers the freezing point of one kilogram of water by 1.86° Centigrade. With a standard measurement of osmols, and of milliosmols for clinical studies, the precise concentration of active solutes in the serum and urine can be calculated. While sodium is the major constituent of serum osmolality, urea nitrogen is one of the major factors in urine osmolality (Ravel 1978:292).

Urine osmolality, like specific gravity, is a measurement of the concentration of the urine. (See Chapter 3 on the specific gravity of urine.) Urine osmolality reflects the total number of osmotically active particles in the urine, without regard to the *size* or *weight* of the particles. As a result, high sugar concentrations, proteins, or dyes do not raise the urine osmolality as they do the specific gravity of the urine (Smithline 1976). The urine osmolality test has at least three other advantages over the specific gravity:

1. The temperature variable is controlled with the osmolality determination, so that the results are more accurate.
2. Also, since the osmolality test is a more sensitive measurement, a small change in the amount of solutes is evident with the osmolality test, but not with the specific gravity.
3. The urine osmolality can be compared to the serum osmolality to get a more definitive picture of the fluid balance or imbalance.

The urine osmolality may eventually replace specific gravity as part of a routine urinalysis.

The disadvantage of the osmolality test is that it cannot be done immediately by the nurse as can the specific gravity.

Preparation of Patient
And Collection of Sample
There is no special preparation of the patient for the test. Depending on the type of machine used, the laboratory can perform an osmolality on as little as 2–5 ml of serum or urine.

Reference Values

Serum osmolality	Range 282–295 mOsm/kg water. Usually around 285 (290 mOsm = 1.010 specific gravity).
Urine osmolality	Extreme range of 50–1400 mOsm/kg water but average is around 500–800 mOsm. (800 mOsm = 1.022 specific gravity). After an overnight fast (12 hours), the urine osmolality should be at least three times the serum osmolality or more than 800 mOsm/kg water.

Increased or High Urine Osmolality

Clinical Significance. A high urine osmolality, when the serum osmolality is normal or increased, indicates that the kidneys are conserving water. As the serum osmolality rises, due to the presence of abnormal solutes or to hemoconcentration, the urine osmolality should also rise: the higher the number of milliosmoles in the urine, the more concentrated the urine. This is the expected physiological response to a lack of fluids for metabolic needs.

A less-than-normal serum osmolality and a high urine osmolality do not constitute a normal physiological response. For some reason the plasma is remaining dilute. An increased level of the antidiuretic hormone (ADH) causes a dilution of the plasma and a more concentrated urine. Certain drugs, trauma, or stress reactions may cause an increased production of ADH, but this reaction is usually transitory.

Possible Nursing Implications. A very high urine osmolality means that the patient is dehydrated. A moderately high urine osmolality is probably also due to a lack of fluids, as long as it is not due to some fluid retention resulting from an increased antidiuretic hormone (ADH). The urine osmolality should be used as only one part of the data base about the fluid balance of the patient. Other factors, such as clinical signs of dehydration, total intake and output, weight gain or loss, and the pathological state of the patient, must all be taken into account. The serum osmolality, if available, helps to determine the amount of dehydration present. The type and method of fluid replacement depends on the cause and severity of fluid loss.

If the patient's retention of fluids is possibly due to an increased level of antidiuretic hormone (ADH), then extra fluids may not be warranted even though the urine osmolality is a little high. For example, in the postoperative patient, concentrated urine may be normal for two or three days after surgery, since ADH is holding some extra fluid in the plasma (Luckmann 1980:413). As the stress level decreases, hormone levels return to normal, and the extra fluid is released. This is sometimes called *surgical diuresis*. A similar diuresis occurs after other kinds of stress, such as a major burn (Condon 1975:206).

A comparison of serum and urine osmolality may be very helpful in distinguishing a slightly increased urine osmolality that is due to fluid retention from one that continues to increase due to a basic lack of fluids. It is important neither to overload patients with fluids nor to let them become dehydrated. Nurses can use the serum osmolality as one objective measurement to add to their data collection tools.

Low Urine Osmolality

Clinical Significance. Urine osmolality should always be higher than serum osmolality unless there is a known reason for the excretion of dilute urine, such as increased fluid intake or the use of diuretics. In the case of either, the serum osmolality is expected to be within normal range as the excess fluid is excreted. What is not expected is a continuing low urine osmolality when the serum osmolality begins to increase. With the patient in a dehydrated state, the urine osmolality should be quite high. If the serum osmolality is normal and the urine osmolality remains around 280 mOsm/kg water, this set of conditions indicates an inability to concentrate urine, which may be an early sign of renal damage. Or it may be due to a lack of secretion of the antidiuretic hormone (ADH), which causes the patient to have very dilute urine all the time. This pathological lack of ADH is called *diabetes insipidus*.

Possible Nursing Implications. Since dilute urine is expected in patients on diuretic therapy, the major nursing concern is to monitor their fluid balance so that not too much fluid is lost. A low urine osmolality is also expected if the goal is to force fluids to make the urine dilute. Urine osmolality can be an objective evaluation that an increased fluid intake is having the desired results. (Recall that a patient who is not getting enough fluids has a consistently high urine osmolality.)

The main concern about a low urine osmolality is when it persists even when the patient is not well hydrated. For example, an early morning urine specimen should have an osmolality of around 800 or 900 mOsm/kg water. So should the urine specimen of a patient who has been NPO for tests. If urine osmolality remains low under fluid restrictions, the kidney may be losing the ability to concentrate urine. Further medical assessments are needed to rule out the possibility of renal dysfunction.

Eventually with renal dysfunction, the urine osmolality may remain the same as the plasma level, which is around 290 mOsm/kg water. Chapter 3 explained why a "fixed" urine specific gravity is always around 1.010 because this is the specific gravity of the plasma. The comparison of urine and plasma osmolalities is a more sensitive measurement of this same concept. Nursing implications for patients with an inability to concentrate urine include a careful assessment of the amount of fluids they need to excrete waste products. Dehydration must be avoided.

Much more rarely, a decreased urine osmolality may be related to a lack of antidiuretic hormone, in which case nurses would observe that the patient is excreting huge amounts of urine. Antidiuretic hormone levels (ADH) can be measured by immunoassay. Medical treatment includes the prescribing of ADH replacement, either by the intramuscular route or by nasal spray. Nurses may be responsible for teaching the patient how to take the drug and how to observe any side effects or complications (Luckmann 1980:1620).

URIC ACID

Uric acid is the end-product of purine metabolism. Purines, which are in the nucleoproteins of all cells, are obtained from both dietary sources and from the breakdown of body proteins. The kidneys excrete uric acid as a waste product.

The exact level of uric acid that is considered pathological is controversial. In recent years it has been generally recognized that the so-called "normal" ranges of uric acid are quite wide. In light of this ambiguity, and since uric acid levels show day-to-day and seasonal variations in the same individual, clinicians usually order several uric acid levels over a period of time.

Special Preparation of Patient And Collection of Sample
There is no special preparation of the patient. To do the test, the laboratory needs 1 ml of serum which has to be sent immediately to the laboratory. It may be useful to ask about a dietary history of intake of purine-rich foods. Levo-dopa and diuretics lead to distortion in results.

References Values

Adults	
Male	2–7.5 mg/dl
Female	2–6.5 mg/dl
Pregnancy	In early pregnancy, the levels fall by about one-third, but may rise to nonpregnant levels by term.
Children (ages 10–18)	
Males	3.6–5.5 mg/dl

(*continued*)

Reference Values (*continued*)

Females	3.6–4 mg/dl
	Striking rise in males 12–14 coincides with puberty. Rise in females may be before age 12 (Harlan 1979).
Aged	
Male over 40	2–8.5 mg/dl
Female over 40	2–8.0 mg/dl
	Rise in women is related to menopause.

Note uric acid levels tend to vary from day to day.

Increased Uric Acid Level (Hyperuricemia)

Clinical Significance. Although gout is the specific disease associated with consistently high serum uric acid levels, several other conditions commonly cause uricemia.

1. The most common is renal impairment since the kidneys normally excrete uric acid. However, since the level of the uric acid increase does not correlate with the severity of the renal disease, serum uric acid is not used as a test of renal function. (The BUN and creatinine tests are the two basic blood tests for renal function.)
2. A variety of drugs, such as the thiazides and some other diuretics, can cause an abnormal elevation of serum uric acid by impairing uric acid clearance by the kidneys.
3. In preeclampsia and particularly in eclampsia, serum uric acid levels are quite high, partially due to the reduced glomerular filtration rate (Hytten 1975).
4. Another common reason is abnormal cell destruction, such as that associated with neoplasms. In neoplastic disease, the utilization of chemotherapy or radiation therapy may further elevate serum uric acid levels due to the accelerated destruction of cells.
5. With prolonged fasting or chronic malnutrition, uric acid levels are higher than normal, due to the breakdown of cells.

Possible Nursing Implications.

Assessing for Joint Pain. Since many patients with hyperuricemia are asymptomatic, the basic nursing assessments are not always a clue that they have a problem with uric acid. The symptoms characteristic of gout are due to deposit of urate crystals in the joint. For gout patients, the warning symptom may be minor discomfort from the bedspread resting on a toe or some swelling and pain in one joint.

Ensuring Adequate Hydration. Whatever the reason for the high uric acid level, the danger is that uric acid, in the form of urates, will crystallize in an acid urine and form renal stones. In the absence of some contraindication, patients with high serum uric acid levels need a liberal intake of fluids to prevent renal stones. A ''liberal intake of fluids'' or ''force fluids'' should be put into specific terms, such as enough fluid to maintain a urine output of 2,000 ml per day. The specific gravity test (Chapter 3) or the urine osmolality covered in this chapter are ways to measure whether the urine is dilute enough.

TABLE 4-3.   EXAMPLES OF FOODS HIGH IN PURINES

Liver	Lentils
Sardines	Mushrooms
Anchovies	Spinach
Kidneys	Asparagus
Sweetbreads	

Dietary Restrictions. Dietary restrictions are usually not emphasized because drugs are used to reduce persistently high serum uric acid levels. However, foods that are high in purines (such as sardines, anchovies, and organ meats) should probably be completely eliminated from the diet (Table 4-3); the nurse can also find out whether other meats, poultry, or fish should be restricted in their total amounts. It is important that patients with high serum uric acid levels have adequate nutrition, since fasting or starvation diets cause more of an increase in the serum acid levels. Any needed weight reduction must be done gradually. Maintaining adequate nutrition for a patient on chemotherapy may be very difficult; failure to do so may compound the serum uric acid problem.

Assisting with Medications. Depending on the level of the serum uric acid level and the underlying pathophysiological condition, the physician may order:

1. drugs that interfere with the production of uric acid levels, such as allopurinal (Zyloprim);
2. uricosuric agents, which promote the elimination of urate salts by the kidneys such as probenecid (Benamid); or
3. for acute attacks of gout, colchicine, which does not seem to affect uric acid metabolism but which does decrease urate crystal deposition (Goodman 1975).

Refer to a pharmacology book for detailed nursing implications for each type of drug.

Promoting Alkaline Urine. In addition to hydration and medications, a third factor may be helpful in decreasing the possibility of renal stones from hyperuricemia: an alkaline urine (Rastegar 1972). Normal urine has an acid pH because cheese, eggs, bread, meat, fish, poultry, and a few fruits and vegetables contribute to acid waste products. An acidic urine may contribute to urate crystallization. On the other hand, foods that leave an alkaline ash include milk, most fruits (except cranberries, plums, and prunes), and almost all vegetables (except corn and lentils). Hence an alkaline urine is sometimes achieved as a result of a strict vegetarian diet.

Since one cannot routinely achieve alkalinization of the urine without severe dietary restrictions, medication such as sodium bicarbonate or potassium citrate—may be used to make the urine pH higher or closer to the alkaline side (Spataro 1978).

The effectiveness of either dietary modifications and/or drug treatments should be periodically evaluated by testing the pH of the urine. This is easily done by using the dipstick method described in Chapter 3. Nurses can quickly teach patients to test their own urine.

Special Needs for Renal Dysfunction. If the increased serum uric level is due to renal dysfunction, nursing implications would include those discussed earlier in this chapter for the patient with elevated creatinine and BUN levels.

Decreased Serum Uric Acid Level

Clinical Significance. A decreased serum uric acid level is not clinically significant. Decreased levels usually reflect some increase in plasma volume.

PHENOSULFONPHTHALEIN (PSP) EXCRETION TEST

The PSP test is a test of renal function. One ml (6 mg) of a dye, phenosulfonphthalein (PSP) is given intravenously. Then urine is collected at certain time intervals to determine whether glomerular and tubular functions are normal. Patients must have normal cardiovascular function—that is, they may not be in congestive heart failure—for the test to be valid. In general, since the results give about the same clinical information as the creatinine clearance (discussed earlier in this chapter), creatinine clearance is replacing the PSP, which is the older test (Ravel 1978:133).

Preparation of Patient
And Collection of Sample
The nurse should inquire about drugs that should not be given for at least 24 hours before the test. Drugs that may interfere with PSP excretion include salicylates, penicillins, some diuretics, radiographic contrast media, and other dyes. The patient should be aware that PSP may color the urine pinkish (in alkaline urine). Before any dye is given intravenously, it is important to ask the patient about any known allergies. An emergency tray, complete with adrenalin, must be available for the possibility of anaphylactic reactions to the phenol red dye.

The patient should be well hydrated *before* the dye is injected intravenously. If the patient has the urge to void *before* the dye is given, it will be possible to get the 15-minute specimen. The exact time of administration of the dye is noted, and urine specimens are collected after 15 minutes, 30 minutes, and 2 hours. Patients can have water during the test, but they must not drink so much liquid that they cannot hold the urine for the 2-hour specimen. An exact amount of urine is not needed—only that the bladder is emptied each time so all the dye excreted can be measured. The exact time of each specimen must be noted. All specimens are sent to the laboratory in separate containers, even though the voidings may have been a little earlier or later than the specified times. The urine does not need refrigeration or any preservative.

Reference Values

Percentage of Dye Excreted in Urine	
15 minutes	25%
30 minutes	40%
2 hours	60–80%

Clinical Significance. Only the amount of the dye excreted for the 15-minute specimen may be abnormally low in early renal disease. When kidney function is moderately to considerably decreased, the amounts at the 30-minute and 2-hour intervals are also diminished.

Nursing Implications. See the discussion under elevated creatinine levels for the nursing implications when a patient has renal insufficiency or renal failure.

Note that the IVP (intravenous pyelogram) is a diagnostic test that uses radiopaque dye to assess the structure of the urinary tract. The IVP may be done in conjunction with tests for renal function, but the use of dyes must be done with caution if renal excretion is not optimal.

Questions

4-1. An increase of *both* the BUN and serum creatinine is characteristic of which of the following?

    a. Dehydration.   **c.** Chronic renal failure.

    b. High-protein diets.   **d.** All of the above.

4-2. Mrs. Balboa is a patient with congestive heart failure who has a slightly elevated BUN. What is the most likely explanation for the abnormal BUN?

    a. Plasma dilution due to aldosterone increase.

    b. Increased protein breakdown due to stress.

    c. Poor renal perfusion.

    d. Impaired liver function.

4-3. Because certain antibiotics may be nephrotoxic, BUN and creatinine levels should be checked before the administration of antibiotics, which are classified as which of the following?

    a. Aminoglycosides, such as gentimicin.

    b. Cephalosporins, such a cephadyl.

    c. Penicillins, such as penicillin G.

    d. Tetracyclines, such as terramycin.

4-4. Mr. Tod's latest lab reports show a BUN of 75 mg and a creatinine level of 6.0 mg. (Reference values for the hospital are BUN 8–25 mg/dl and creatinine 0.6–1.5 mg/dl.) Which nursing action would be appropriate based on the lab information?

    a. Put the patient on 2-hour vital signs.

    b. Question whether potassium should be continued in the IV solution.

    c. Encourage the intake of protein foods in the diet.

    d. Encourage more active ambulation.

4–5. Serum creatine (not serum creatinine) is clinically useful as an assessment of which of the following?

    a. Renal dysfunction.   **c.** Liver dysfunction.

    b. Fluid imbalances.   **d.** Skeletal muscle disorders.

4–6. Mr. Bobbins is to have a 24-hour creatinine clearance test begun this morning. He has just emptied his bladder. For this test, what should he be instructed to do?

    a. Save a urine sample each time he urinates so this can be compared to serum creatinine levels drawn every four hours.

    b. Save all the urine voided in the next 24 hours after he is given a dose of creatinine intravenously.

    c. Not eat any food or drink any fluids while the urine is being collected as a 24-hour specimen.

    d. Save all urine for 24 hours and expect to have blood drawn during the middle of the test for a serum creatinine level.

4–7. For testing for renal function and fluid balance, urine osmolality is a superior test to urine specific gravity because urine osmolality:

    a. Can be done faster on the clinical unit.

    b. Detects the presence of specific electrolytes.

    c. Is not changed much by sugar, protein, or X-ray dyes.

    d. All of the above.

4–8. When there is an increased level of ADH (antidiuretic hormone) in response to severe stress, which of the following are the lab reports for serum and urine osmolality most likely to reflect?

    a. A slight increase in serum and urine osmolality.

    b. A slight decrease in serum osmolality and an increase in urine osmolality.

    c. A slight decrease serum and urine osmolality.

    d. A slight increase serum osmolality and decrease in urine osmolality.

4–9. Mrs. Regola has a serum osmolality of 290 mOsm/kg and a urine osmolality of 1,400 mOsm/kg. Based on this information, the nurse should assess this patient for effects of which of the following?

    a. Fluid overload.   **c.** Lack of antidiuretic hormone.

    b. Dehydration.   **d.** Renal dysfunction.

4–10. A urine osmolality of 300 mOsm/kg or a specific gravity of 1.010 on a first voided morning urine specimen is an indication that the patient needs to be further assessed for which of the following?

    a. Dehydration.   **c.** Renal dysfunction.

    b. Circulatory overload.   **d.** Nothing (this is a normal finding).

4-11. Higher-than-normal serum uric acid levels are likely for all these patients *except* which of the following?

    a. Jackie, age 8, who is undergoing chemotherapy for leukemia.

    b. Mrs. Dillon, age 63, who has rheumatoid arthritis.

    c. Jennifer, age 21, who is on a starvation diet to lose weight.

    d. Mrs. Benidito, age 34, who is showing signs of preeclampsia.

4-12. Which of the following foods are highest in purine content?

    a. Dairy products.   **c.** Grains.

    b. Organ meats.   **d.** Citrus fruits.

4-13. What are the two measures, other than drug therapy, that help reduce the possibility of the formation of uric acid renal stones?

    a. Forcing fluids and keeping urine alkaline.

    b. Exercise and forcing fluids.

    c. Exercise and keeping urine acid.

    d. Forcing fluids and keeping urine acid.

4-14. Uric acid levels are not used as a test of renal function because uric acid levels:

    a. are not affected by renal impairment.

    b. vary considerably due to the dietary intake.

    c. are often elevated without any symptoms.

    d. do not correlate with the severity of the renal disease.

4-15. Mr. Jellystone is to have a PSP done this AM. The nurse should prepare the patient for the test by teaching him all of the following *except:*

    a. The PSP dye will be given intravenously.

    b. He needs to drink several glasses of water before the test begins.

    c. The dye may turn the urine pink or reddish.

    d. All urine must be saved for 24 hours.

REFERENCES

Burke, Desmond *et al.* "Laboratory Studies: When to Act on Unexpected Test Results," *Patient Care* 12 (January 30, 1978): 14–87.

Condon, Robert and Nyhus, Lloyd. *Manual of Surgical Therapeutics.* Boston: Little, Brown & Company, 1975.

Goodman, Louis and Gilman, Alfred. *The Pharmacological Basis of Therapeutics.* New York: Macmillan, Inc., 1975.

Harlan, William *et al.* "Physiologic Determinants of Serum Urate Levels in Adolescence," *Pediatrics* 63 (April 1979): 564–577.

Hetrick, Anne. ''Nutrition in Renal Disease: When the Patient is a Child,'' *American Journal of Nursing* 79 (December 1979): 2152–2154.

Hytten, Frank and Lind, Tom. *Diagnostic Indices in Pregnancy*. Summit, N.J.: Ciba-Geigy Corporation, 1975.

Jones, Alan *et al*. ''Renal Failure in the Newborn,'' *Clinical Pediatrics* 18 (May 1979): 286–291.

Langslet, Julie and Habel, Maureen. ''The Aminoglycoside Antibiotics.'' *American Journal of Nursing* 81 (June 1981): 1144–1146.

Luckmann, Joan and Sorenson, Karen. *Medical–Surgical Nursing: A Psychophysiologic Approach,* 2nd ed. Philadelphia: W. B. Saunders Company, 1980.

Luke, Barbara. ''Nutrition in Renal Disease: The Adult on Dialysis,'' *American Journal of Nursing* 79 (December 1979): 2155–2157.

Oestreich, Sandy. ''Rational Nursing Care in Chronic Renal Disease,'' *American Journal of Nursing* 79 (June 1979): 1096–1099.

Ravel, Richard. *Clinical Laboratory Medicine,* 3rd ed. Chicago: Yearbook Publishers, Inc., 1978.

Rastegar, Asynan and Thier Samuel. ''The Physiologic Approach to Hyperuricemia,'' *New England Journal of Medicine* 286: 9 (March 2, 1972): 470–476.

Spataro, Robert *et al*. ''The Use of Percutaneous Nephrostomy and Urinary Alkalinization in the Dissolution of Obstructing Uric Acid Stones,'' *Radiology* 129 (December 1978): 629–632.

Stark, June. ''BUN/Creatinine: Your Keys to Kidney Function,'' *Nursing 80* 10 (May 1980): 33–38.

Smithline, Neil and Gardner, Kenneth. ''Gaps—Anionic and Osmolal,'' *JAMA* 236 (October 4, 1976): 1594–1597.

CHAPTER FIVE

Four Commonly Measured Electrolytes

Objectives

1. State which of the four commonly measured electrolytes show significant variation in different age groups and in pregnancy.
2. Differentiate between milligrams (mg) and milliequivalents (mEq) in relation to measurements of electrolytes in the serum and in replacement therapy.
3. Give examples of how the serum cations and anions are kept in electrical neutrality by the kidney and by shifts into and out of cells.
4. Explain the effect of water deficit and water overload on serum sodium levels.
5. Describe nursing assessments that might detect patients with increased and decreased serum sodium levels.
6. Describe the nurse's role in the treatment of hypernatremia and hyponatremia.
7. Explain why serum potassium levels may not accurately reflect the total body potassium levels.
8. Describe the nursing assessments that might detect patients with increased or decreased serum potassium levels.
9. Describe the nurse's role in assisting with the various treatments for hyperkalemia and hypokalemia.
10. Explain the clinical significance of the relationship of serum chloride to serum bicarbonate.
11. Describe how chlorides are usually replaced in therapy.

Although many electrolytes are in the blood, when electrolytes (or "lytes") are ordered as a laboratory test, the test is only for:

1. sodium (Na+),
2. potassium (K+),

3. chloride (Cl−), and

4. bicarbonate (HCO_3−) ions.

Laboratory evaluations of these four basic electrolytes are critical in the assessment of fluid and electrolyte balance as well as acid-base balance.

This chapter focuses primarily on the serum levels of the first three, as well as on the urine levels of sodium and potassium. Since the reference values for these three electrolytes are essentially the same for all populations after the newborn period, it is expedient for nurses to memorize them. Only bicarbonate is significantly changed according to age and pregnancy.

Bicarbonates will be discussed in the next chapter, in relation to acid–base balance and arterial blood gases. The discussion will explain why some laboratories may report serum bicarbonate levels with a test called the ''CO_2 content.''

The three less commonly measured electrolytes—calcium (Ca++), magnesium (Mg++), and phosphate (PO_4)—are covered in Chapter 7.

INTERPRETING SERUM ELECTROLYTE REPORTS

When interpreting the reports of serum electrolytes, one must always keep in mind that the laboratory report reflects only *serum* levels. It may not be an accurate reflection of the body's total electrolyte level. Generally, the level of electrolytes in the serum is very close to the electrolyte levels in the interstitial fluid with one major exception. Interstitial fluid does not have the plasma proteins found in serum. Since the electrolytes can shift readily from plasma to interstitial fluid, or vice versa, the extracellular fluid remains similar in substances other than the plasma proteins.

But the electrolytic compositions of extracellular (serum and interstitial) fluid and intracellular (cell) fluid are strikingly different. Sodium (Na+) and chloride (Cl−) are the two major electrolytes in the extracellular fluid, while potassium (K+), magnesium (Mg+), and phosphate (PO_4−) are major intracellular ions (see Table 5-1). Shifts of

TABLE 5-1. COMPOSITION OF ELECTROLYTES IN SERUM, INTERSTITIAL FLUIDS, AND CELLS

Fluid	Major Electrolytes	
Extracellular:		
Serum	Na+	Sodium
	Cl−	Chloride
	HCO_3 −	Bicarbonate
Interstitial	Almost the same as plasma (note no plasma proteins).	
Intracellular:		
Cellular	K+	Potassium
	MG++	Magnesium
	PO_4^-	Phosphate

See Metheny (1979).

electrolytes do occur between the cells and the extracellular fluid, but not in major amounts. So the measurement only of serum levels cannot always accurately reflect the status of the electrolytes in the individual cells. For example, during a pathological state such as acidosis, more potassium may shift out of the cells because more hydrogen (H+) ions are moving into the cell. Thus the serum level may seem normal or even high, yet the cells are becoming deficient in their main electrolyte, potassium.

Serum sodium and chloride levels rarely reflect the total sodium or chloride content in the body because a change in these levels causes a corresponding change in the volume of the plasma (Widmann 1979:374). Sodium and chloride are responsible for most of the osmotic pressure in extracellular fluids. So if the sodium and chloride ions increase in the plasma, they retain more water in the plasma. Hence the concentration of sodium is still reported as 135 to 145 mEq and the chloride as 100 to 106 mEq, both *per liter of fluid*. More sodium and chloride (that is, more salt) in the plasma holds more water in the vascular system and eventually in the interstitial spaces (edema).

MEASUREMENT BY MILLIEQUIVALENTS (mEq)

Eletrolytes are reported in measurements of milliequivalents (mEq) rather than in milligrams (mg). The reason is that milligrams measure only the weight of the chemical element, and equal weights do not mean equal chemical activity. For example, it takes 39 mg of potassium (K+) to equal 23 mg of sodium (Na+) in a measurement of chemical activity based on a common standard (Table 5-2). The standard of equivalents is based on how many grams of an element or compound liberate or combine with one gram of hydrogen (Holum 1979:179). Since it takes 23 g of sodium to liberate 1 g of hydrogen, the equivalent weight of sodium is 23 g. *A milliequivalent*, the term used in lab reports, is one one-thousandth (1/1,000) of an equivalent. If it takes 23 *g* to make 1 equivalent, 23 *mg* equals 1 mEq.

The important point to remember about the standard of equivalents and milliequivalents is that 1 mEq of one element always has the same chemical activity as 1 mEq of another element. If milligrams or grams are used to measure the amount of electrolytes in diets or medications, a conversion to the amount of electrolyte milliequivalents must be done to discuss the physiological effect of the drugs or diet. For example, a diet of 1,000 mg of sodium (not sodium chloride) would provide about 43 mEq of sodium. This figure is derived from the fact that it takes 23 mg of sodium to make 1 mEq: 1,000 mg divided by 23 mg equals 43 mEq. A more detailed discussion about sodium and salt is covered under the section on sodium. Usually sodium is measured in milligrams.

Potassium is the other electrolyte that may sometimes be measured in milligrams in medication or diet prescriptions. A diet that contains 1,560 mg of potassium supplies 40 mEq of potassium (since it takes 39 mg of potassium to equal one mEq: 1,560 mg divided by 39 equals 40 mEq). Medications such as potassium chloride may be marked in both milligrams and milliequivalents. It is much easier to understand the physiological effect of electrolytes when the dosage is noted in milliequivalents as well as in milligrams or volume. Although medications list the electrolyte composition clearly, doctors sometimes order—and nurses sometimes record—only that the patient took a teaspoon of a potassium supplement and not how many mEq are contained in the teaspoon.

TABLE 5-2. CONVERSION OF MILLIGRAMS (mg) TO MILLIEQUIVALENTS (mEq)

Measurement of Weight	Measurement of Chemical Activity*
23 mg of sodium (Na+)	1 mEq
39 mg of potassium (K+)	1 mEq
35.5 mg of chloride (Cl−)	1 mEq
30 mg of bicarbonate (HCO_3 −)	1 mEq

Problem #1
    1,000 mg of sodium = _____ mEq
    Solution: 1,000 ÷ 23 = 43.4 mEq

Problem #2
    40 mEq of potassium = _____ mg
    Solution: 40 × 39 = 1,560 mg

*See text and Holum (1979: 178).

CHEMICAL ELECTRICAL NEUTRALITY

All electrolytes in the serum carry either negative charges (*anions*) or positive charges (*cations*). These negative and positive charges must always be in perfect balance so that the serum remains neutral. The cations must always balance the anions. The electrical neutrality of the serum is essential in understanding why certain electrolytes may be lost or retained in the serum, even though this upsets acid–base balance.

One way for the body to always maintain an equal number of positive and negative ions in the serum is shifting of electrolytes from the cells or vice versa. For example, when bicarbonate (HCO_3 −) levels are reduced in the serum, other negative ions must replace the missing negative bicarbonate ions. To keep the electrical balance in the serum neutral, chloride can shift out of the erythrocytes (Chan 1978: 507); this *chloride shift* is discussed in detail later. Another example involves the relationship of the positive ions potassium (K+) and hydrogen (H+). When the level of serum potassium (K+) falls, there is an increased shift of potassium out of the cells to keep the serum potassium (K+) normal (Stroot 1977). As potassium comes out of the cell, hydrogen (H+) diffuses into the cell to replace the loss of positive ions intracellularly. This shifting of electrolytes from plasma to cells and vice versa is actually a more complex situation, because the kidneys are also working to remove any excess ions from the bloodstream.

Since sodium (Na+), hydrogen (H+), and potassium (K+) are all positive ions, a change in one means some change in the others. In the distal tubules of the kidney, sodium (Na+) is usually reabsorbed in exchange for either potassium (K+) or hydrogen (H+) ions. If there is an abundance of hydrogen (H+) ions to excrete, the kidney does not excrete many potassium ions. On the other hand, if the potassium level in the serum is low, the kidneys have to continue to excrete hydrogen (H+) ions even when the hydrogen (H) is needed to maintain the acid–base balance of the serum. The relationship of increased potassium levels to acidosis, as well as that of decreased potassium levels to alkalosis, is discussed in the section on potassium.

When the sodium (Na+) ion is reabsorbed by the kidney, a negative ion of either chloride (Cl−) or bicarbonate (HCO_3−) must be reabsorbed also. If one of these two negative ions is low in the serum, more of the other must be absorbed to maintain the proper amount of anions (negative ions). This inverse relationship of chloride (Cl−) and bicarbonate (HCO_3 −) is an important consideration in many types of metabolic acid–base imbalances (Kaplan 1979).

THE ANION GAP

Table 5–3 shows the amount of the positive ions (Na+ and K+) compared to the amount of negative ions (Cl− and HCO_3 −). For the two cations (positive ions) and two anions (negative ions) that are measured in the serum, there seems to be more positive ions than negative ions, because some of the anions are not measured. This difference between the number of cations and the number of measured anions is called the *anion gap* (Smithline 1976). Actually, this gap (of 14 mEq in Table 5–3) is made up of unmeasured anions such as sulfates, phosphates, and organic acids. Usually these unmeasured anions are around 10 to 14 mEq, depending on the particular references used by a laboratory (Widmann 1979:334).

The importance of the anion gap is that it is increased in the types of metabolic acidosis where organic or inorganic acids are increased in the bloodstream. This increase in the anion gap is helpful in identifying the type of acidosis present. If there is no change in the unmeasured anions in metabolic acidosis, the decreased bicarbonate level (a negative ion) is replaced by an increased serum chloride (Cl−) level (another negative ion). Other much rarer situations may cause some changes in the anion gap, but for general purposes, nurses use only the concept of the anion gap in caring for patients with metabolic acidosis. Narins (1977) gives examples of how the anion gap is useful in complicated acid–base imbalances.

By this point, the reader may be a little bewildered by so many references to acid–base balance when this chapter is supposed to be on electrolytes. Obviously, electrolyte disturbances and acid–base imbalances are so intimately connected that it is hard to learn about one and not the other. Following the summary of acid–base balances in the next chapter, a chart gives general guidelines of how each electrolyte is changed in the four different types of acid–base imbalance. The concept of the anion gap is also explored further in Chapter 6, in the discussion on the three types of metabolic acidosis.

TABLE 5-3. CATIONS AND ANIONS IN SERUM

Positive Ions (Cations)		Negative Ions (Anions)		Unmeasured Anions
Sodium	140 mEq	Chloride	103 mEq	Phosphates
Potassium	4 mEq	Bicarbonate	27 mEq	Sulfates
				Organic Acids
Total	144 mEq	Total	130 mEq	(Gap of 14 mEq)
		144 − 130 = Gap of 14 mEq*		

*See text for explanation of this anion gap and Smithline (1976).

Preparation of Patient
And Collection of Sample

Most laboratories require about 8 cc of blood to do all four electrolytes. If electrolytes are done as part of a total chemical profile, the laboratory may need a larger sample. If the electrolytes are done by an automatic analyzer, only 2.5 ml may be needed (see SMA in Chapter 1). Usually all four are done routinely, but sometimes only one is ordered, particularly just the potassium. Just one test requires only about 2 ml of serum. It is particularly important that the blood sample not be traumatized because hemolysis of cells makes the potassium report inaccurate. (Recall that potassium is an intracellular ion.) The serum is obtained by venipuncture. The patient does not need to be fasting.

Reference Values

Sodium (Na+)	135-145 mEq/l
Potassium (K+)	3.5-5.0 mEq/l (slightly more in newborns)
Chloride (Cl-)	100-106 mEq/l
Bicarbonate (HCO_3 -) (measured as CO_2 content)	
Adults	24-30 mEq/l
Pregnancy	19-20 mEq/l (see pCO_2 levels in Chapter 6 for explanation of reason for lower bicarbonate levels in pregnancy).
Infants	20-26 mEq/l
Children	Slightly lower than references for adults.

Note that all four electrolytes may be reported in moles per liter (mmol/l) rather than mEq if the Systeme International (SI) is adopted by a particular laboratory. Since there is no change in basic numbers for these four electrolytes, 24 mEq of HCO_3 - is 24 mmol/l (see Chapter 1 on SI).

SERUM SODIUM (Na+)

Sodium has the highest concentration of all the electrolytes measured in the serum, and yet changes in its level are not commonly seen, because its concentration is always correlated with fluid balance. Since sodium is the primary factor in maintaining osmotic pressure in the extracellular fluid, changes in sodium are hidden because "water goes where salt is." So one must always interpret a change in serum sodium levels in relationship to possible fluid overload or dehydration. A rough estimate of the plasma osmolality (discussed in Chapter 4) can be calculated from the sodium level by multiplying the sodium by 2. A normal serum sodium of 140 mEq/l times 2 would equal a normal plasma osmolality of around 280 mOsm/kg water.

The serum level of sodium is not totally dependent on diet because the kidneys can conserve sodium when necessary. The hormone aldosterone causes a conservation of sodium and chloride and a release of more potassium. The daily requirement of sodium for an adult is about 100 mEq or 2.3 g. In children, the usual requirement is around 3 mEq/kg

TABLE 5–4.   RELATIVE SODIUM CONTENT OF FOODS

A. *Foods with about 500 mg sodium (21 mEq)* ¼ scant tsp salt (40% of salt is sodium) ¾ tsp monosodium glutamate ½ boullion cube 1 cup tomato juice average serving of cooked cereal 1 hotdog 1½ oz ham	B. *Foods with about 250 mg sodium (about 11 mEq)* 1 oz canned tuna ⅔ cup buttermilk 5 salted crackers C. *Foods with about 200 mg sodium (about 9 mEq)* 1 slice bread 2 slices bacon 3 oz shrimp ½ oz cheese 1 tbsp catsup

Source: Sodium Restricted Diets, *AHA 1977. Note that processed food, such as a Big Mac from McDonald's Restaurant, has 1,510 mg of sodium and a Heinz pickle, 1,137 mg of sodium (Hill 1979).*

daily (Chan 1978). Many American diets contain much more than these daily minimums. Some authorities estimate that the average diet may contain as much as 6 to 10 g (or 260 to 435 mEq) of sodium. (As explained in the introduction, it takes 23 mg of sodium to equal 1 mEq.)

It is necessary to measure sodium, not just sodium chloride, in the diet because sodium is present in forms other than salt. For example, monosodium glutamate is added to many foods in the American diet. Most American diets can be substantially reduced in sodium by avoiding very salty foods and not adding extra salt to foods at the table. One gram of NaCl is about 0.6 g chloride and about 0.4 g, or 17 mEq, of sodium (400 mg divided by 23 equals 17.39 mEq). See Table 5–4 for the amount of sodium in different proportions of salt and food substances.

Reference Values

Adult   135–145 mEq/l

The same reference values are used for all age groups. Pregnancy may cause a drop of 2–3 mEq, but the range is still within general values.

Increased Serum Sodium Level (Hypernatremia)

Clinical Significance. An increase in the serum sodium level becomes apparent only when there is not sufficient water in the body to balance the increasing sodium level. Because sodium has an osmotic action, an increase in serum sodium pulls water into the vascular system from the interstitial spaces and the cells. When the laboratory test for *serum* sodium level is elevated, the patient is depleted in water, not only in the extracellular compartment, but also in the cells. Thus many cases of an increase in *total body* sodium do not cause an increased *serum* sodium level. For example, patients with congestive heart failure have sodium retention due to the action of the hormone aldosterone. However, the retention of sodium means an equal retention of water, so the serum sodium level remains around 140 mEq per *liter* of fluid.

For the serum sodium level to be increased on a laboratory report, it is necessary that either (1) there is a large increase in sodium *without* a proportional increase in water, or (2) there has been a loss of a large amount of water *without* a proportional loss of salt. Under most circumstances, increasing sodium intake without increasing water intake is hard because an increased sodium intake makes a person very thirsty. If the person is receiving intravenous fluid, such as normal saline, that contains a relatively large amount of sodium, it may be possible to overload with sodium. Intravenous solutions of normal saline contain 0.9% NaCl, that is, 0.9 g of salt in a 100 cc or 90 g in 1,000 cc. This percentage is 154 mEq of sodium and 154 mEq of chloride per liter (Metheny 1979). Infants who receive exchange transfusions with stored bank blood may become hypernatremic because stored blood has high sodium levels. An intravenous of Dextrose 5% in water is given to prevent overload of sodium.

The much more common reason for an increased serum sodium level is a loss of a large amount of water without a proportional loss of sodium. For example, diarrhea or vomiting may cause a severe decrease in total body water, particularly in infants (Chan 1978:505). Not all dehydration results in an increased sodium level, however, because just as much sodium may be lost as water; this loss of equal amounts of sodium and water is called *isotonic dehydration*. In dehydration due to a loss of water or a lack of water intake, the sodium loss is not proportional and hence the dehydration is *hypertonic*. Even in the early stages of hypertonic dehydration, the serum sodium level is not elevated because water is pulled from the interstitial spaces to keep the sodium at a normal dilution in the serum.

When the serum sodium level begins to rise above normal, this is a sign of a very serious deficit of water that has extended to the cellular level. Another term for this type of dehydration is *hyperosmolar dehydration*. The serum is increased in osmolality, not because of a total sodium increase, but because of a total body water deficit. Luckman (1980:177) discusses in detail the differences between hyperosmolar, hyposmolar, and isotonic imbalances of sodium and water.

TABLE 5-5. CLINICAL SITUATIONS COMMONLY ASSOCIATED WITH SERUM SODIUM ABNORMALITIES*

Hypernatremia—serum Na increased (↑) 145 mEq/l
  1. Dehydration is the most frequent cause.
  2. Overuse of Intravenous saline solutions.
  3. Exchange transfusion with stored blood.
  4. Impaired renal function.
Hyponatremia—serum Na decreased (↓) 135 mEq/l
  1. Excessive water—"dilutional" hyponatremia.
  2. Loss of sodium by vomiting, diarrhea, GI suctioning, or sweating.
  3. Use of diuretics, diabetic acidosis, Addison's disease, or renal disease, which all cause increased loss of sodium via urine.

---

* See text for explanation of why fluid volume changes are usually the underlying cause for changes in serum sodium levels. Ravel (1978: 283), Stroot (1977), and Metheny (1979) give more details on uncommon reasons for serum sodium changes.

Possible Nursing Implications.

Assessing for Hypernatremia. The initial symptom of hypernatremia is likely to be thirst, which, if the person is unconscious, confused, or very young, is a subjective symptom that is not communicated to the nurse. Other clinical assessments that correlate with a high serum sodium level include elevated temperature, dry, sticky mucous membranes, and little or no urine output. The specific gravity of the urine is high if the kidneys are still able to concentrate urine. The hematocrit is increased when the water deficit is severe. In the infant, a high-pitched cry and depressed fontanels are other signs of severe water deficit. Hyperactive reflexes and irritability may lead to seizures in infants with high sodium levels.

For the adult, each 3 mEq of serum sodium above the usual reference range represents a deficit of about one liter of fluid. Thus a serum sodium (Na+) level of 157 mEq would be about 12 mEq above the reference of 135 to 145 mEq. This excess indicates a deficit of about 4 l of fluid. Since 1 l of water weighs 1 K (2.2 lbs), a loss of 4 l would mean a weight loss of nearly 9 lbs. Obviously this would be very severe dehydration. In a small child, the loss of even a liter of fluid would be severe dehydration because a loss of 2.2 lbs may be 10% of the total weight of the child. The most accurate measurement of the amount of water deficit is the patient's loss of weight. Daily weights should be part of the nursing assessment for any patients experiencing fluid losses.

Assisting with Treatments. For hypernatremia due to a water deficit, the therapeutic interventions focus on replacing the lost water. If oral intake is not possible, physicians order intravenous fluids to hydrate the patient—usually dextrose 5%, which is the best hydrating solution because it contains no sodium. The fluid deficit may need to be corrected very gradually, since changing the sodium level too quickly may be dangerous, particularly for infants. The deficit may need to be replaced over two to four days if the sodium concentration is above 160 mEq/l. This slow reduction of the sodium level is necessary to prevent cerebral hemorrhage, which may occur with the rapid correction of hypernatremia (Chan 1978:505). Fluid orders may need to be changed every few hours depending on the response of the patient. If the dehydration was due to gastrointestinal problems, food is gradually added back to the diet. The BRAT diet (*B*ananas, *R*ice cereal, *A*pplesauce, and *T*ea or *T*oast) is easy on the gastrointestinal tract.

Preventing Sodium Overload. Often the nurse may be able to prevent hypernatremia due to water deficit from developing by careful observation of patients at risk. For instance, patients who are not taking enough oral fluids may become water deficient. Those who are receiving normal saline solutions (0.9% NaCl) should be checked for any signs of hypernatremia. Intravenous solutions for maintenance are usually only one-half normal saline (0.45% NaCl) or even one-fourth normal saline (0.25% NaCl). Normal saline solutions (0.9% NaCl) are not used for maintenance solutions unless the patient has hyponatremia (Metheny 1979). Infants who receive blood exchange usually have a peripheral line for infusion of dextrose 5% in water, since the stored blood is high in sodium.

Assessing for Symptoms of Excess Sodium and Excess Water. When both sodium and water are retained in excessive amounts, the symptoms are very different from when sodium is in excess. The signs and symptoms of increased total body sodium levels are weight gain, elevated blood pressure, dyspnea and pitting edema (the common signs of fluid retention). In the adult, edema becomes apparent only after about 3 l of water are retained; this amount of water retention would mean 3 Kg or 6.6 lbs of weight gain before the edema shows. Thus weight gain is the most sensitive detector of early fluid retention (Pflaum 1979).

Teaching About Salt Restriction. The patient with both sodium and water retention is often on diuretics and/or a low-sodium diet. A "restricted sodium" diet would mean less than the 2.3 g or 100 mEq as a basic requirement. Thus the most mild restriction of sodium is a 2-g (87-mEq) sodium diet. A moderate restriction of sodium is 1,000 mg (43 mEq). A diet of 500 mg is very restrictive since this amount allows only 21 mEq of sodium a day (500 mg divided by 23 mg equals 21.1 mEq). A teaspoon of salt has 2,000 mg of sodium or 87 mEq.

The effectiveness of sodium restriction is determined by the absence of fluid retention, *not by the serum sodium level.* Nurses may need to go over this point several times with patients. It may be hard for patients to see a need to restrict sodium and salt intake when the laboratory report is "normal" for sodium. Hill (1979) gives some practical tips on how nurses can help patients control their sodium intake. The American Heart Association has excellent teaching material about low-sodium diets.

Decreased Serum Sodium Level (Hyponatremia)

Clinical Significance. Like serum sodium increases, serum sodium (Na+) decreases are not accurate reflections of total body sodium levels because sodium is usually lost with water. The most common reason for a low serum sodium (Na+) on a laboratory test is an excess of water in the body. The water excess can be caused by giving salt-free intravenous fluids. Also, in stress and severe illness, there may be an increased production of antidiuretic hormone (ADH), which causes an increase in total body water (Metheny 1978). Most cases of water excess are usually terminated by an increased urine output, which restores the sodium and water balance.

Although a real water excess is the more common reason for a low serum sodium level, actual sodium depletion can also be a cause of a low serum sodium level. Ordinarily, the hormone aldosterone conserves sodium, but a continual loss of sodium with only water replacement and no sodium replacement eventually leads to a true sodium depletion. For example, a patient who is on diuretics and a restricted sodium diet may experience massive sodium depletion from the body. Excessive sodium loss also occurs:

1. in some types of renal failure, in which there is "salt wasting";
2. in diabetic acidosis, in which case polyuria contributes to a great loss of sodium;
3. particularly in young children, in whom vomiting and diarrhea can lead to hyponatremia if gastrointestinal losses are replaced only with water; and
4. in exercise, in which perspiration can deplete sodium.

Patients with a lack of adrenal corticosteroids (Addison's disease) suffer from hyponatremia or low serum sodium levels. The severe hypotension of an Addisonian crisis occurs because the total body sodium is not enough to keep fluid in the vascular system (see Chapter 15 on cortisone tests). Any low serum sodium level due to a true loss of sodium means a lack of sodium not only in the extracellular fluid, but also in the intracellular compartment.

Possible Nursing Implications. Although this discussion distinguishes the symptoms of hyponatremia (low sodium level) due to fluid excess from those due to a true sodium deficit, the clinical picture is usually not so clear-cut. Since low serum sodium levels denote several imbalances in fluids, most likely other electrolyte imbalances and pathology make the clinical picture more complicated than just looking for a few key signs of each type of sodium decrease.

Assessing for Water Intoxication. When the low serum sodium level is due to just an excess of body water, there may be few clinical signs.

One sign is that the patient has a weight gain that is equal to the amount of excess liters retained. For example, a patient who is maintained on routine intravenous fluids should not be gaining weight because the caloric intake is minimal. (A bottle of 1,000 cc of dextrose 5% contains only 50 g of dextrose.) In fact, an adult patient who is being maintained on intravenous fluids of dextrose 5% usually loses about half a pound a day. So if the patient is gaining weight at all, this weight has to be water. A gain of a pound means the retention of over 500 ml of fluid. (Every nurse should memorize the fact that a liter of water weighs 1 Kg or 2.2 lbs. or a pound for every pint.)

The other symptom of water excess is an increased urine output. If the water excess continues, and if the kidneys cannot get rid of the excess water, the water diffuses into the interstitial spaces and eventually into the cells. The edema that develops is generalized; it is not contained in dependent areas such as the feet. So, for example, the face may look a little puffy. Edema of brain cells causes nausea and vomiting and eventually convulsions when the serum sodium (Na+) is as low as 120 mEq. This condition is a hyposmolar imbalance (Luckmann 1980).

Careful nursing assessment of the intake and output records, as well as of weight gains, for patients who are susceptible to fluid overload can do much to prevent severe water intoxication.

Assisting with Treatment. The treatment for water excess is just to restrict fluid intake for a while. To objectively evaluate that the fluid balance is returning to normal, one must keep accurate records of intake, output, and weight loss.

Preventing and Assessing for Sodium Depletion. Nurses need to be aware of patients who may be developing a true depletion of sodium, because this type of low serum sodium level can often be prevented if early symptoms of sodium depletion are noted. With mild to moderate depletions of sodium, the serum sodium (Na) level remains within the normal reference range. Yet this condition is still an isotonic imbalance, and the urine sodium becomes low. (See the next section on urine sodium levels.) As the total sodium becomes low, the patient has anorexia, apathy, and sometimes a sense of impending doom. Confusion may occur, particularly in elderly patients. Muscle cramps, weakness, and diarrhea reflect the lack of sodium for normal muscle contractions. Eventually the low serum sodium leads to hypotension and shock because there is a loss of osmotic pressure in the vascular system. Infants, although they may be lethargic, may also be asymptomatic until the sodium level is low enough to cause edema and seizures.

Assisting with Sodium Replacement. The therapeutic measures for a true sodium depletion are geared toward replacing both sodium and the lost fluid. Usually the intravenous solution used for replacement would be normal saline (0.9% NaCl), although in extreme cases, a hypertonic (3% NaCl) saline solution may be used. Nurses must carefully monitor patients who are receiving hypertonic intravenous fluids, since too rapid an infusion of a hypertonic solution is very dangerous. The hypertonic solution cannot only cause hemolysis of red blood cells, but it can also pull a large amount of fluid into the vascular space, leading to circulatory overload. No more than 200 or 300 ml of 3% NaCl should be given in four hours (White 1979:61). The hypertonic solutions of salt are rarely used now. Either normal saline (0.9% NaCl) or Ringer's Lactate (another isotonic solution) can supply enough sodium to make up the deficiency more safely.

Patient Teaching. Because the body can conserve sodium, it is not necessary to instruct patients to eat high-sodium content food over a long period. Yet patients who may become sodium-depleted due to vomiting, diarrhea, or vigorous exercise should drink some salty replacement fluids, such as broths instead of just water. For infants, special formulas of electrolytes are used to replace gastrointestinal losses. Athletes who do vigorous exercises know to replace lost fluids with special oral electrolyte preparations that are commmercially available. In the past, salt tablets were often used by people who engaged in intense physical activity; it is now generally recommended to replace salt more gradually by dietary increases or salty fluids (Darby 1980). Note that one cup of tomato juice has 486 mg of sodium (Table 5-7).

As mentioned, the American diet usually contains more than enough sodium. But sometimes patients may follow too restricted a sodium diet. For example, nurses may need to assess the dietary habits of elderly patients to make sure that their sodium restrictions are not too severe, particularly if they are started on diuretics. Also, patients who are on nasogastric suctioning can lose significant amounts of sodium and thus become hyponatremic if replacements of sodium are not begun. Irrigations of nasogastric tubes should always be with normal saline, not with water, which would increase sodium loss. Children with cystic fibrosis lose extra sodium in their sweat. (See Chapter 18 on the sweat test for CF.) Patients on lithium must also have plenty of sodium in the diet. (See Chapter 17 on lithium toxicity.)

URINE SODIUM LEVELS

Normally the amount of sodium excreted in the urine varies with the sodium intake. Increased amounts of aldosterone in the serum cause a decreased secretion of urine sodium. (See Chapter 15 on serum aldosterone levels.) Conversely, a decreased level of aldosterone activity causes an increased loss of sodium in the urine. Diabetic acidosis and diuretics also cause an increased loss of sodium. Various types of renal failure may cause either increased losses or retention of sodium.

Urinary excretion of sodium may be utilized for differential diagnosis of the different varieties of acute renal failure (Chan 1978). The values of the urine sodium must be interpreted in view of the total clinical picture.

Preparation of Patient
And Collection of Sample
See Chapter 3 on 24-hour urine collections. No special preservative is needed. The diet of the patient should be noted as to the amount of sodium intake.

Reference Values

40–220 mEq/24 hrs   or   30 mEq/l

SERUM POTASSIUM (K+) LEVELS

Potassium is primarily an intracellular ion, but the small amount that is in the serum is essential for normal neuromuscular and cardiac function. Small changes in the serum potassium (K+) level can have profound effects on the cardiac muscle. In a normal state of health, adequate potassium is easily obtained by eating a variety of foods. The intake of potassium, which is probably around 40 to 80 mEq a day for an adult, needs to be on a daily basis because potassium, unlike sodium, is not conserved well by the body. The kidneys continue to excrete 40 to 80 mEq a day even when there is no intake.

Although potassium can also be lost in gastrointestinal drainage, the kidneys excrete almost all of the potassium. The renal mechanism for potassium (K+) ion excretion is shared with another positive ion hydrogen (H+). Either a potassium (K+) or hydrogen (H+) ion is excreted when a sodium (Na+) ion is reabsorbed by the kidney. This relationship partially explains why potassium levels are increased in acidosis and decreased in alkalosis. The shifting of potassium (K+) and hydrogen (H+) ions into and out of the cells in acid–base imbalances also contributes to marked changes in potassium levels. (See Chapter 6 on acid–base balances.)

Reference Values

3.5–5.0 mEq/l

In pregnancy there may be a fall of about 0.2 to 0.3 mEq due to increased volume. Slightly higher in newborns due to hemolysis.

TABLE 5–6.   CLINICAL SITUATIONS COMMONLY ASSOCIATED WITH SERUM POTASSIUM ABNORMALITIES*

Hyperkalemia—serum K increased (↑) 5 mEq/l (or above 6.5 in newborns)
  1. Renal failure.
  2. Too rapid intravenous infusion of K+ replacement.
  3. Initial reaction to massive tissue damage.
  4. Associated with metabolic acidosis (see Chapter 6).
Hypokalemia—serum K decreased (↓) 3.5 mEq/l
  1. Diuretics, particularly thiazides.
  2. Inadequate intake when NPO, vomiting, or on K-free intravenous feedings.
  3. Large doses of corticosteroids.
  4. Aftermath of tissue destruction or high stress.
  5. Associated with metabolic alkalosis (see Chapter 6).

See text and references at end of chapter for further details –Stroot (1977), Metheny (1979), and Luckmann (1980). Newborn references from Children's Hospital San Francisco, California.

Increased Serum Potassium Level (Hyperkalemia)

Clinical Significance. The major reason for an increased serum potassium level (hyperkalemia) is inadequate renal output. Thus hyperkalemia is always a problem in the oliguric phase of renal failure unless potassium intake is limited. (See Chapter 4 for the distinction between renal insufficiency and renal failure.)

The intake of too much potassium in medications can also cause an increased serum potassium (K+) level. An overdose from oral supplements of potassium is unlikely, but the danger is very real with intravenous use of potassium in high concentrations. Other medications such as penicillin K, which contains potassium ions, can cause hyperkalemia if renal output is not adequate. (See Chapter 4 on BUN and creatinine levels as assessments of renal function.)

Since potassium is primarily an intracellular ion, anything that causes massive cell destruction increases the serum potassium level. Thus massive tissue injury or a burn causes the release of potassium from damaged cells. Although the serum potassium level may increase after cellular damage, the actual total body potassium is decreased. Thus the hyperkalemia that occurs with a burn or injury is followed by hypokalemia.

Because aldosterone and other steroids cause a retention of sodium and an increased secretion of potassium, conditions in which hormones are decreased may cause an increased serum potassium level. For example, in Addison's disease, a malfunctioning of the adrenal cortex reduces the corticosteroid level. The serum sodium (Na+) levels are decreased and the potassium (K+) serum levels may be increased. (See Chapter 15 on laboratory tests for cortisone.)

Although almost all diuretics cause an increased loss of potassium, there are two exceptions. Spironolactone (Aldactone) is an aldosterone antagonist and thus causes increased retention of potassium. Triamterene (Dyrenium) does not affect aldosterone, but it too is a diuretic that may cause hyperkalmia. Triomerene acts directly on the distal tubules to cause excretion of Na+ and retention of K+ (Govoni 1978:721).

Hyperkalemia is often associated with metabolic acidotic states. In acidosis, the kidney must excrete more hydrogen ions, which means less secretion of potassium ions by the renal selection mechanism. In addition, an abundance of hydrogen ions in the serum means that some of these ions go into the cells, which drives potassium out of the cells. Thus, in acidotic states, the total body potassium is not increased, but more potassium ions are in the serum. If the acidotic state is due to diabetic ketoacidosis, the lack of insulin compounds the problem of hyperkalemia because potassium needs insulin, as does glucose, to be transported into the cell (Reed 1974:24).

Possible Nursing Implications.
Assessment for Hyperkalemia. Probably the most important thing to remember about checking for symptoms of increasing serum potassium (K+) levels is that many of the symptoms are nonspecific. Potassium is important to nerve and muscle function but so are most of the other electrolytes. Early symptoms of hyperkalemia may be irritability, nausea, diarrhea, and abdominal cramping. Later symptoms may include skeletal muscle weakness. The muscle weakness can progress to a flaccid-type paralysis with difficulty in speaking and breathing.

Hyperkalemia is usually an emergency situation because, a high serum potassium level can cause cardiac arrhythmias that can lead to cardiac arrest: The heart stops in diastole. Since the clinical signs of hyperkalemia can be confused with other conditions (hypokalemia can cause paralysis too), the level of serum potassium must be assessed by the laboratory report, not just by physical symptoms. Remember that the serum laboratory test may not reflect the total body potassium. The electrocardiograph is a very sensitive indicator of intracellular potassium, even when the serum potassium still seems normal. High-peaked T waves, a prolonged QRS interval, a decreased amplitude of P and R waves, and depressed ST segments are typical electrocardiographic findings that suggest high potassium levels (Reed 1974:22).

Assisting with Medical Interventions. Although there is not a *specific* antidote for hyperkalemia, several different medications may be used to treat a high serum potassium level.

1. Sometimes calcium gluconate is given intravenously to lessen cardiac toxicity. Calcium may be particularly useful if the calcium levels were intially low or borderline. It is not used if the patient is on digitalis, because digitalis and calcium have a synergistic effect on the heart.
2. Sodium bicarbonate may be given intravenously if the pH of the blood is low. As the pH of the blood returns to normal, potassium shifts back into the cells. Also, when the pH is normal, the kidney can secrete more potassium ions because there is not a demand to excrete so many hydrogen ions.
3. Intravenous solutions with glucose and insulin help promote the reentry of potassium into the cells, even for patients who are not diabetic.

Because there is no specific antidote for a high serum potassium level, all of these drugs are indirect methods to reduce the serum potassium level. Since they may be ordered in an emergency or near-emergency state, nurses must carefully monitor the effects of the drug on the patient's total status. Govoni (1978) lists the separate nursing implications for each of the drugs discussed.

In more chronic states of hyperkalemia, certain other drugs may be used to increase potassium excretion via the bowel. Sodium polystyrene sulfonate (Kayexalate), given orally or by enemas, is a sodium–potassium exchange resin. The nurse responsible for giving the medication must follow specific directions on how to use the drug to gain maximal effectiveness. The drug may cause constipation.

For the patient with chronically high potassium levels, usually due to renal failure, the treatment may include peritoneal dialysis or hemodialysis.

Patient Teaching. The nurse needs to find out whether the hyperkalemia is likely to be a chronic or recurring situation. If so, the patient needs to be taught to read the labels on foods and medications, to determine whether they are high in potassium. For example, most salt substitutes are composed of large amounts of potassium. Instant coffee and other prepared foods may have potassium as one of the ingredients.

Dietary teaching about eliminating potassium may also need to be done. To reinforce patient behavior, a contract may be written between the nurse and patient to keep potassium levels low through diet adherence. Sheckel (1980:1596) has used graphs of potassium levels posted at the foot of the beds of dialysis patients as one way to reinforce diet selections. Thus potassium levels can be one evaluative tool of effective teaching. (See Table 5–7 for foods particularly high in potassium.)

Assessing for Hypokalemia. The last nursing implication for patients with hyperkalemia may sound a little paradoxical at first. Often they may need to be observed for hypokalemia or low serum potassium (K+) levels, which may follow hyperkalemia. If the high serum levels of potassium were due to metabolic shifts in acidosis, the potassium shifts back into the cells when the pH is returned to normal, and patients may have a serum deficit. Also, if the serum potassium level was increased due to cell damage, the potassium lost from injured cells results in a total body deficit. Always consider the possibility that the hyperkalemia of today could result in hypokalemia tomorrow. (See the discussion on nursing implications of hypokalemia.)

Decreased Serum Potassium Levels (Hypokalemia)

Clinical Significance. Because potassium is not conserved well in the body, an inadequate intake results in a low serum level. However, since the daily need of potassium for an adult is only about 80 mEq insufficient oral intake is usually not the cause for a low potassium unless the person is totally NPO. Even in fasting states, the serum potassium level may not drop immediately, because the breakdown of cells for energy causes the release of potassium.

More commonly, hypokalemia results from an excessive loss of potassium. Any loss of fluid from the gastrointestinal tract causes a loss of potassium. Almost all diuretics cause an increased excretion of potassium, except spironolactone (Aldactone) and triamterene (Dyrenium). Certain hormonal changes also contribute to an excessive excretion of potassium. Since the corticosteroids cause sodium retention and excretion is increased. Certain tumors may produce hormones that act much like the steroids and thus increase potassium excretion. (See Chapter 15 on ectopic hormone production.) Also, patients may be on high doses of corticosteroids for treatment of various disease states. All such patients are prone to the development of hypokalemia. (See Chapter 15 on cortisone measurements.)

An alkalotic serum pH (pH above 7.4) is another reason for a lowered serum potassium. In alkalosis, hydrogen ions (H+) shift out of the cell in an attempt to lower the pH of the serum to normal. When hydrogen (H+) shifts out of the cell, more potassium shifts into the cell to replace the missing positive ions. Conversely, a low serum potassium level also contributes directly to the development of an alkalotic state because, when serum potassium levels are low, the kidneys must excrete more hydrogen ions in exchange for the reabsorption of sodium by the distal tubule. So either alkalosis may be the cause of hypokalemia, or hypokalemia may contribute to the development of metabolic alkalosis (Stroot 1977). The role of hypokalemia in the development of metabolic alkalosis is covered in Chapter 6 under the section on bicarbonate changes in acid–base balance.

Possible Nursing Implications.

Assessing for Hypokalemia. Nurses need to be aware of patients who may be having extra losses of potassium so they can assess for potential hypokalemia. The only objective assessment for a low serum potassium level is the laboratory test, along with the electrocardiograph changes. Although certain clinical symptoms are caused by hypokalemia, these symptoms can also be caused by other clinical abnormalities. Patients with a low serum potassium level may have anorexia, muscle weakness, a decrease in bowel sounds, and abdominal distention due to decreased peristalsis (ileus). Ileus and lethargy are key symptoms of hypokalemia in the newborn too. Flaccid paralysis may develop with more severe hypokalemia, as well as with hyperkalemia, because both potassium imbalances alter the resting potential of muscle cells (Felver 1980:1591). Low serum potassium levels make respiratory effort difficult, and they can lead to paroxysmal tachycardia, premature contractions, and other arrhythmias. For patients on digitalis, hypokalemia is quite dangerous because the toxic effects of digitalis are more likely to occur when the serum potassium level drops quickly. The typical electrocardiograph in hypokalemia has prominent U waves, and the T waves are flat or even inverted. (In hyperkalemia, the T waves are just the reverse, very peaked.) Sometimes the replacement of severe potassium losses is monitored by electrographic readings because the EKG is a very sensitive indicator of not just serum potassium levels, but also of intracellular potassium levels.

Assisting with Potassium Replacement. Depending on the severity of the hypokalemia, potassium may be replaced in three ways: (1) intravenously, (2) by oral supplements, or (3) by diet.

1. *Intravenous potassium* is usually prepared and monitored by the nurse. Most preparations of potassium chloride (KCl) for intravenous use are marketed as 2 mEq per 1 ml. Thus, for a dose of 40 mEq, the nurse would add 20 ml to the intravenous fluid. Potassium must *always be diluted*. Potassium chloride is never given directly by intravenous push no matter how severe the deficiency. Usually no more than 40 mEq of potassium is added to a 1,000 ml of intravenous fluids although sometimes as much as 80 mEq are added to a liter. Patients should usually not be given more than 10–20 mEq in an hour, although some authorities say 30–40 mEq an hour is safe in severe deficiencies. For example, if the serum potassium is less than 2 mEq, with electrocardiographic changes and paralysis, up to 40 mEq may be given within an hour (Travenol Product Information, 1979). The determination of the dosage and the rate of the infusion are the physician's responsibilities, but the nurse must know the limits of safety. As mentioned, EKG monitoring is a useful assessment tool when high levels of potassium are given. Many patients complain of burning at the site of the infusion when more than 40 mEq are added to a liter of intravenous fluid. If the intravenous must be slowed down because of the burning sensation, the solution needs to be made more dilute or a larger vein used for infusion.

Any patient who is receiving potassium must have adequate urinary output. In the adult, "adequate" means at least 30 ml an hour. Newborns should produce 1 cc of urine per kilogram per hour. Thus a newborn who weighs 4 Kg (8.8 lbs) should produce about 4 ml/hr. In older children, 1–2 ml/k/hr is a minimum output. The urinary output should always be assessed before potassium is added to an intravenous. Once the intravenous is infusing, nurses must continue to make sure that urinary output remains adequate. Otherwise hyperkalemia can develop rapidly.

2. *Oral preparations* of potassium chloride may come marked in various strengths, such as 10 or 20% solutions, or as so many milligrams per teaspoon. On the bottle, however, the dosage in mEq is also given, and this is the dosage form that should be used. One teaspoon of potassium chloride elixir is not as precise as 20 mEq. Every patient should be told the dosage exactly in mEq, not just to take a certain amount by volume.

TABLE 5-7.   FOODS HIGH IN POTASSIUM AND CORRESPONDING Na CONTENT

Potassium at Least 10 mEq or More by Serving	Sodium (mg)
Avocado ½	5
Banana, 1 medium	1
Cantalope, 1 cup	19
Dates, 10	1
Figs, 5	10
Instant coffee, 3 g	
Molasses, 2 tbsp	3
Orange juice, 1 cup	2
Potato, baked	2
Prunes, 10 (high calories)	9
Salt substitutes (varies, but may be 30–40 mEq in tsp)	Varies. Check label.
Soybeans, ½ cup	2
Tomato juice, canned, 1 cup	486! (not good if on low-sodium diet)

Source: Facts About Potassium, *AHA 1977. Note that the American Heart Association has patient information cards as well as pamphlets about potassium content in foods.*

The oral preparations of potassium come in various forms of elixirs and tablets, some that fizz when mixed with juice. Since the major problem with oral supplements of potassium is the gastrointestinal upsets they can cause, nurses should teach patients not to take potassium supplements on an empty stomach. Solutions may be put in orange juice, a good vehicle, because it has a high potassium level. Overdoses of oral potassium supplements are not common, but it is important that the urinary output always be adequate.

Potassium replacement can also be done with a relatively inexpensive salt substitute that contains potassium chloride (Felver 1980). See Table 5-7 on the potassium in salt substitutes.

3. *The dietary intake of potassium* is usually around 40 to 80 mEq for adults. For patients who are on diuretics or who for other reasons need a higher intake of potassium, it may be wise to assess their dietary habits to see if they can gain extra potassium by dietary intake. Table 5-7 shows the amount of potassium in some common foods. By including some of the potassium-rich foods, patients may be able to reduce or eliminate the need to take potassium supplements. However, the serum potassium levels for patients on long-term diuretics should be checked periodically to make sure that dietary intake of potassium is adequate to balance an increased potassium loss.

URINE POTASSIUM LEVELS

The amount of potassium in the urine varies with the diet. It also varies with an increased amount of serum aldosterone or cortisol, which causes an increased excretion of potassium. Further, extra potassium is lost in diabetic acidosis and with thiazide diuretics, but a serum potassium is a better measurement of the need for replacement after diuresis. Renal failure causes a decreased excretion of potassium. Ravel (1978:461) states the primary use for a 24-hour urine potassium is to assess hormonal functioning. (See Chapter 15 on aldosterone and cortisol levels.) Urine potassium levels are also used sometimes in research studies as one indication of the stress level of the body.

Preparation of Patient
And Collection of Sample

See Chapter 3 for 24-hour urine collections. No preservative is needed.

Reference Values

40–80 mEq/24 hrs

SERUM CHLORIDE LEVELS (Cl−)

Chloride, the major negative ion in the extracellular fluid, is very important, in combination with sodium, for maintaining the osmotic pressure in the serum. A loss or a gain of chloride is often due to the factors that also cause a loss or gain of sodium. For example, in fluid imbalances, the chloride, like the sodium, is not changed in the serum until the total body water is decreased or increased. Except for acid–base imbalances, in which bicarbonate levels decrease or increase, chloride levels rise and fall in relationship to the rise and fall of sodium levels. In acid–base balances, the relationship is inverse between chloride (Cl−) and bicarbonate (HCO_3−), the other major negative ion in the plasma. An increase in bicarbonate (HCO_3−) causes a decrease in chloride Cl−) and vice versa. The role of the unmeasured negative ions in relation to chloride levels is covered in the section on bicarbonate. (See "chloride shift" in Chapter 6.)

Chloride is found in a variety of foods, usually in combination with sodium. A diet restricted in sodium causes a reduction of chloride intake, too, but not to an inadequate level. The kidneys selectively secrete chloride or bicarbonate ions depending on the acid–base balance. In certain types of renal failure, chloride excretion may be impaired.

Reference Values

All age groups 100–106 mEq.   Falls little if at all, in pregnancy

Increased Serum Chloride Level (Hyperchloremia)

Clinical Significance. "Hyperchloremia" is a term that is rarely used clinically. An increase in chlorides in the serum is not a primary focus since the increase must always be looked at in relationship to (1) an increase in sodium (Na+) levels, or (2) a decrease in the serum bicarbonate (HCO_3−) level.

Aldosterone, a mineral corticosteroid, causes retention of both sodium (Na+) and chloride (Cl−). In most cases, a proportional increase in water retention makes the electrolytes in the serum appear not to be increased. For the sodium and chloride levels to be elevated, there must be a deficit of water or a large intake of sodium chloride. Since in these situations, the chloride level parallels the rise or fall of the sodium level, the sodium level is used to monitor fluid deficits.

In a couple of clinical situations, the rise in chlorides may be even greater than the rise in sodium levels. In certain types of renal failure, the kidneys are unable to excrete chlorides properly; this inability leads to a type of acidosis called *renal hyperchloremic acidosis*. Chlorides may also be greatly increased in the bloodstream if large amounts of normal saline (0.9% NaCl) are infused over several days. "Normal saline" is not really normal in relation to the sodium and chloride content of the serum, even though it is classified as an isotonic solution. Normal saline contains 154 mEq of sodium (Na+) ions and 154 mEq of chloride (Cl−) ions per liter. This is a little higher than the serum level of 135 to 145 mEq for sodium (Na+) ions and a great deal higher than the 100–106 mEq for serum chloride (Cl−) (White 1979).

Chloride levels are increased in most types of acidosis because the chloride is needed to replace the loss of another negative ion, bicarbonate (HCO₃−), from the serum. If the metabolic acidosis is due to an increase of other negative ions, such as ketoacids, the chlorides are not increased—and may actually decrease—due to diuresis. The changes in the bicarbonate level, in the chloride level, and in the unmeasured negative ions (the anion gap) give useful information about what is causing the acidotic state. The most important thing to remember about the relationship of a high serum chloride level to acidosis is that, if the chlorides are higher than normal, this condition causes a drop in the serum bicarbonate level because there is room for only a set amount of negative ions. If the serum bicarbonate level drops first, then chlorides may be increased to keep the correct number of negative ions in the serum. Increased chloride levels can be either a cause or a result of metabolic acidosis (Widmann 1980).

Possible Nursing Implications. Since changes in chloride levels always take place in combination with changes in other electrolytes, assessments depend on nurses' understanding of the basic reason for the increased chloride level. For example, if the chloride level is related to an increased sodium level, then the nursing implications for sodium are to be followed. If the increased chloride level is causing, or was caused, by acidosis, then the symptoms exhibited are those of acidosis. (The care in metabolic acidosis is covered in the section of bicarbonate levels in Chapter 6.)

Chloride levels return to normal when fluid balance is accomplished if the problem is due to a sodium–chloride–water imbalance. If the chloride levels are high due to acidosis, the restoration of the serum bicarbonate level to normal automatically insures the return of chlorides to normal. (Key nursing implications when sodium bicarbonate is given intravenously are covered under the section on bicarbonate deficiencies in Chapter 6.)

Decrease in Serum Chloride Level (Hypochloremia)

Clinical Significance. Decreases in the serum chloride level are commonly due to loss from vomiting, gastric suction, diarrhea, and the use of diuretics (Metheny 1978).

Since sodium, hydrogen, and potassium ions are usually lost with the chlorides, a chloride drain is only part of a larger problem. For example, the loss of chlorides from the serum means that more bicarbonate must be retained to replace the lack of negative ions, thus contributing to the development of metabolic alkalosis. The loss of potassium or of hydrogen ions also contributes to the development of metabolic alkalosis. Conversely, alkalotic states can cause a low chloride level. In any alkalotic state, the bicarbonate level in the serum increases, so the other major negative ion, chloride, must decrease in the bloodstream. (By now the inverse relationship between the negative ions, bicarbonate, and chloride should be clearly apparent!)

As explained in Chapter 6, patients with chronic lung disease often have high serum bicarbonate levels to balance an increase pCO_2 level in the bloodstream. This chronically elevated serum bicarbonate level also causes a decreased serum chloride level. This condition would be considered a normal compensation in patients with chronic lung disease.

Possible Nursing Implications. If the chloride level is low due simply to water excess, the nursing implications would be those for low serum sodium levels. If the chloride level is low due to a continual loss of chlorides, then the nursing implications are those for metabolic alkalosis, which is an acid–base disorder covered in the next chapter.

Preventing Chloride Losses. Nurses need always to be aware of patients who may be losing abnormal amounts of chlorides, so that replacement therapy can begin before alkalotic states develop. For example, patients who are on gastrointestinal suctioning are losing not only chlorides, but also potassium and hydrogen ions. All three losses contribute to the development of metabolic alkalosis. Since potassium supplements contain chloride, the use of potassium chloride is one way that lost chlorides are replaced. If necessary, the physician may order some normal saline (0.9% NaCl) to be given intravenously to replace large chloride losses. The use of oral electrolyte solutions for infants or salty broths for adults to replace sodium losses was already mentioned. Nurses must always keep in mind that a loss of electrolytes usually involves several electrolytes and never just chlorides alone.

SERUM BICARBONATE LEVELS (HCO_3-)

Serum bicarbonate levels (HCO_3-) are routinely part of both "electrolytes" and arterial blood gases. Because changes in the serum bicarbonate level always signify some change in the acid–base balance, the relationship of bicarbonate to the measured carbon dioxide in the serum (pCO_2) is important to note. This bicarbonate-to-carbonic-acid (as measured by the pCO_2) ratio of 20 to 1 is the most important buffer in the serum. The 20:1 ratio is fundamental to understanding the clinical significance of changes in serum bicarbonate levels. The next chapter includes a summary of this ratio before discussing how serum bicarbonate levels decrease and increase in acid–base imbalances.

Questions

5-1. The only one of the four commonly measured electrolytes that shows significant variation in pregnancy and in different age groups is which of the following?

    a. Na+.   **c.** Cl−.

    b. K+.   **d.** HCO_3-.

5-2. Which one of the following electrolytes has a greater concentration in the plasma than in intracellular fluid?

a. Cl−.   c. PO−.

b. K+.   d. Mg++.

5-3. Serum electrolytes are measured in milliequivalents (mEq) rather than in milligrams (mg) because milliequivalents are:

a. more precise for small concentrations of electrolytes in the serum.

b. easier to compute in an automated laboratory.

c. not dependent on the metric system.

d. based on a measurement of chemical activity, not of weight.

5-4. Given the fact that 39 mg of K+ equals 1 mEq, compute how many mg of K+ are needed to give a dose of 40 mEq.

a. 1.56 g or 1,560 mg.   c. 3.9 g or 3,900 mg.

b. 0.56 g or 560 mg.   d. 1.4 g or 1,400 mg.

5-5. A loss of serum chloride (Cl−) causes an increase in serum bicarbonate (HCO_3−) due to which of the following reasons?

a. the fluid balance changes unless electrolytes are shifted into the cell.

b. bicarbonate is a negative ion needed to keep the electrical balance of the serum neutral.

c. bicarbonate helps stabilize the acid–base balance.

d. the kidneys usually secrete the two ions together.

5-6. Hydrogens ions (H+) shift into the cell when serum potassium (K+) levels drop because, as more K+ diffuses out of the cell:

a. the fluid balance changes unless electrolytes are shifted into the cell.

b. another positive ion must enter the cell to keep the electrical charges neutral.

c. the acid–base balance must be maintained by decreasing serum H+ ions.

d. there is a lack of positive ions to be excreted by the kidney.

5-7. When the total amount of serum Na+ and K+ ions (cations) are compared to the total amount of serum Cl− and HCO_3− ions (anions), there are fewer anions. This "anion gap" is due to which of the following facts?

a. There are always more cations (positive ions) then anions (negative ions) in the serum.

b. Some anions, such as organic acids, are not measured.

c. The electrical balance is not always neutral in acid–base imbalances.

d. The loss of electrolytes decreases the total number of anions in the serum.

5-8. When a patient has an abnormal serum sodium (Na+) report, the most useful nursing assessment to help explore the reason for the sodium imbalance would be which of the following?

    a. Dietary intake pattern of salt and sodium-containing foods.

    b. Intake and output records and daily weights.

    c. Vital signs over last 24 hours.

    d. Record of all medications given.

5-9. The laboratory measurement of serum sodium (Na+) levels does not accurately indicate increases of total body sodium due to which of the following reasons?

    a. Serum sodium is kept constant by the kidney.

    b. The laboratory procedure to determine serum sodium is not very accurate.

    c. Total body sodium is not necessarily influenced by serum sodium levels.

    d. An increased serum sodium causes an increased retention of water in the vascular system.

5-10. A laboratory report of an increased serum sodium level would most likely be part of the clinical findings for a patient:

    a. with severe congestive heart failure who has pitting edema of the ankles.

    b. on corticosteroid therapy for several months for rheumatoid arthritis.

    c. having diarrhea and unable to take fluids by mouth.

    d. maintained on intravenous fluids of dextrose 5% in 0.45% sodium chloride for several days after surgery.

5-11. A laboratory report of a slightly low serum sodium (Na+) could be due to all of the following conditions *except* which?

    a. Diet containing no more than 2.3 g (100 mEq) of sodium daily.

    b. Maintenance intravenous solutions of 5% dextrose in water (D_5W) for several days.

    c. Drinking large amounts of water after strenuous exercise.

    d. Use of a diuretic that is an aldosterone blocking agent.

5-12. Characteristic assessments expected for a patient with a high serum sodium (Na+) level due to a water deficit would include all but which of the following?

    a. Hypertension.   **c.** Weight loss.

    b. Thirst.   **d.** Elevated temperature.

5-13. Characteristic assessments for a patient with a low serum sodium (Na+) level due to total body sodium depletion would include all but which of the following?

    a. Confusion.   **c.** Weight gain.

    b. Hypotension.   **d.** Muscle cramps.

5-14. Characteristic assessments for a patient with a serum sodium level below 120 mEq due to excess water intake would include all but which of the following?

a. Weight loss.

b. Nausea and vomiting.

c. Convulsions.

d. Edema.

5-15. An increase in serum sodium (Na+) levels is usually an indication that the patient needs which of the following?

a. Less sodium in the diet.

b. Less fluid intake.

c. More fluid intake.

d. Both sodium and water restrictions.

5-16. In the patient whose low serum sodium (Na+) level is not due to a decrease in total body sodium, the usual treatment is to:

a. encourage additional fluids, that are salty in content, such as broth.

b. give extra water.

c. limit water intake.

d. give intravenous replacement of 0.9% Na chloride.

5-17. The primary reason why the total body potassium level cannot be accurately measured by the serum potassium concentration is because:

a. Methods differ from lab to lab, so "normals" cannot be compared.

b. Different age groups have different amounts of total body potassium (K+).

c. The extracellular potassium (K+) tends to be bound to other ions such as chloride (Cl−).

d. The bulk of the body's store of potassium (K+) is intracellular.

5-18. Which of the following patients is the *least* likely to have an elevated serum K level?

a. Mary Burden who is in renal failure.

b. Baby Lois who suffered extensive burns today.

c. Candy Phillips who is in metabolic alkalosis.

d. Jack Brown who has Addison's disease.

5-19. A low serum potassium (K+) may be a potential problem for all these patients *except* which?

a. Mr. Rhodes who is on long-term diuretic therapy with thiazides.

b. Mary Rogers who has severe morning sickness with vomiting.

c. Jackie, age 8, who is on corticosteroid therapy as part of the treatment for leukemia.

d. Mrs. Cabrillo who has a severe respiratory infection and who is not taking much fluid.

5-20. Serum potassium levels may be lowered by all but which of the following treatments?

    a. Glucose and insulin, intravenously.

    b. Sodium bicarbonate, intravenously.

    c. Sodium–potassium exchange resin, rectally.

    d. Sodium chloride, intravenously.

5-21. Which of the following signs or symptoms is the most suggestive of hyperkalemia?

    a. Paralytic ileus (lack of bowel sounds).

    b. Peaked T waves on the cardiac monitor.

    c. Skeletal muscle cramps.

    d. Depressed T waves on the cardiac monitor.

5-22. Mrs. Forrest, who is scheduled for a cholecystectomy tomorrow, has a serum K+ of 2.3 mEq. (She has been on thiazide diuretics.) The nurse is to monitor the potassium replacement, which Mrs. Forrest is to receive intravenously. Which of these guidelines about potassium is correct?

    a. Urine output should be at least 100 cc an hour.

    b. No more than 10 mEq of KCl should be given in an hour.

    c. No more than 80 mEq of KCl should be added to 1,000 cc bottle.

    d. KCl is given IV push only in extreme cases where the serum K+ is below 2.5 mEq.

5-23. Mrs. Forrest is going home on hydrochlorathiazide (Hydrodiuril) due to hypertension. The doctor has prescribed a potassium chloride (KCl) supplement to be taken in liquid form t.i.d. The nurse should instruct the patient to:

    a. dilute the KCl in water, but not in juice.

    b. never take the KCl at the same time as any other medicine.

    c. not take the KCl on an empty stomach.

    d. keep the KCl in the refrigerator.

5-24. Mrs. Forrest asks the nurse about foods that are high in potassium. What item does not contain at least 10 mEq of potassium?

    a. Orange juice, 1 cup.   **c.** Instant coffee, 3 g.

    b. Cranberry juice, 1 cup.   **d.** Potato, 1 baked.

5-25. All of the following patients are likely to have low serum chloride (Cl−) levels *except* which?

    a. Mr. Hagan who has an elevated serum bicarbonate (HCO_3−) level due to ingestion of baking soda.

b. Baby Raggio who has had severe vomiting.

c. Mrs. Rhodes who is on loop diuretics and a low-sodium diet.

d. Mrs. Nicholls who is in renal failure.

5-26. The usual methods of replacing serum chloride levels would include all *except* which of the following?

a. Potassium chloride (KCl) supplements.

b. Intravenous solutions of normal saline (NaCl 0.9%).

c. Ammonium chloride tablets (NH_4Cl).

d. Salty broths or electrolyte solutions containing chlorides.

5-27. The main function of the bicarbonate (HCO_3-) ion in the bloodstream is to maintain which of the following?

a. The buffer system with carbonic acid at a 20:1 ratio.

b. Neural and muscular function of the cellular membrane.

c. Fluid balance by replacing lost chlorides.

d. A neutral electrical charge by balancing sodium ions.

REFERENCES

American Heart Association. *Facts About Potassium, How to Meet Your Potassium Requirements.* American Heart Association, 1977.

American Heart Association. *Sodium Restricted Diets, 1000 Milligrams and 500 Milligrams.* American Heart Association, 1977.

Chan, James. "Clinical Disorders of Sodium, Potassium, Chloride and Sulfur Metabolism: Diagnostic Approach to Children," *Urology* 12 (November 1978): 504–508.

Darby, William. "Why Salt? How Much?" *Contemporary Nutrition* 5 (June 1980): 6.

Felver, Linda. "Understanding the Electrolyte Maze." *American Journal of Nursing.* 80 (September 1980): 1591–1595.

Govoni, Laure and Hayes, Janice. *Drugs and Nursing Implications,* 3rd ed. New York: Appleton-Century-Crofts, 1978.

Hill, Martha. "Helping the Hypertensive Patient Control Sodium Intake," *American Journal of Nursing* 79 (May 1979): 907–909.

Holum, John. *Elements of General and Biological Chemistry,* 5th ed. New York: John Wiley & Sons, Inc., 1979.

Kaplan, Alex and Szabo, LaVerne. *Clinical Chemistry: Interpretation and Techniques.* Philadelphia: Lea and Tebiger, 1979.

Luckmann, Joan and Sorensen, Karen. *Medical–Surgical Nursing: A Psychophysiological Approach,* 2nd ed. Philadelphia: W. B. Saunders Company, 1980.

Metheny, Norma and Snively, William. "Peri-Operative Fluids and Electrolytes," *American Journal of Nursing* 78 (May 1978): 840–845.

Metheny, Norma and Snively, William. *Nurses' Handbook of Fluid Balance,* 3rd ed. Philadelphia: J. B. Lippincott Company, 1979.

Narins, Robert *et al.* "The Anion Gap" (Letters to the Editor), *Lancet* 1304 (June 18, 1977).

Pflaum, Sandra. "Investigation of Intake–Output as a Means of Assessing Body Fluid Balance," *Heart–Lung* 8 (May–June 1979): 495–498.

Potassium Chloride Injection, Package Insert. Morton Grove, Ill.: Travenol Laboratories, Inc., 1979.

Ravel, Richard. *Clinical Laboratory Medicine,* 3rd ed. Chicago: Yearbook Publishers, Inc., 1978.

Reed, Gretchen. "Confused About Potassium? Here's a Clear, Concise Guide," *Nursing 74* 4 (March 1974): 20–27.

Reed, Gretchen and Sheppard, Vincent. *Regulation of Fluid and Electrolyte Balance: A Programmed Instruction in Clinical Physiology,* 2nd ed. Philadelphia: W. B. Saunders Company, 1977.

Sheckel, Susan. "Contracting with Patient-Selecting Reinforcers," *American Journal of Nursing* 80 (September 1980): 1596–1599.

Smithline, Neil and Gardner, Kenneth. "Gaps—Anionic and Osmolal," *JAMA* 236 (October 4, 1976): 1594–1597.

Stroot, Violet; Lee, Carla; and Schaper, Ann. *Fluid and Electrolytes: A Practical Approach,* 2nd ed. Philadelphia: F. A. Davis Co., 1977.

White, Sara, "IV Fluids and Electrolytes: How to Head Off the Risks," *RN* 42 (November 1979): 60–63.

Widmann, Frances. *Clinical Interpretation of Laboratory Tests,* 8th ed. Philadelphia: F. A. Davis Co., 1979.

CHAPTER SIX

Arterial Blood Gases (ABG)

Objectives

1. Demonstrate the four-step sequence in interpreting the meaning of arterial blood gas reports to determine the four primary acid–base imbalances.
2. Explain how the buffering system, the lungs, and the kidneys maintain the serum bicarbonate to carbonic acid ratio of 20:1.
3. Describe the nurse's role when arterial blood gases are drawn.
4. Explain why reference values for blood gases are altered in pregnancy and in the newborn period.
5. Explain the physiological basis for the symptoms of acidosis and alkalosis, both metabolic and respiratory in origin.
6. Describe the possible nursing implications for patients with increased and decreased pCO_2 levels (respiratory alkalosis and acidosis).
7. Describe the possible nursing implications for patients with increased or decreased serum bicarbonate levels (metabolic alkalosis and acidosis).
8. Explain how electrolytes alter and are altered by changes in the acid–base balance.
9. Explain the concept of the anion gap in relationship to the various kinds of metabolic acidosis.
10. Explain why high concentrations of oxygen may be dangerous for the patient with a low pO_2 and a high pCO_2.
11. Demonstrate how pO_2 and pCO_2 levels are utilized by the nurse to assist with treatment of respiratory problems.

This chapter begins with an introductory section about acid–base imbalances. Several charts help to show the fundamental differences in the four primary acid–base imbalances. After this general discussion, pH, pCO_2, and bicarbonate tests are presented first due to their major significance in acid–base imbalances. The last part of the chapter discusses pO_2 and O_2 saturation.

Each laboratory measurement is discussed as a separate test so that the reader can better understand the clinical significance of both increases and decreases in each value. As in other chapters, nursing implications for each change in laboratory test are discussed after the clinical significance.

PURPOSE OF BLOOD GASES

Only the pO_2 and the pCO_2 measurements actually measure blood gases. The "p" before the O_2 and CO_2 stands for the partial pressure of the gases. The respiratory gases include nitrogen, oxygen, carbon dioxide, and water vapor. Dalton's *law of partial pressure* states that the total pressure exerted by a mixture of gases is the sum of the individual partial pressure (Boyce 1976). Table 6-1 shows the percentage of gases in the blood and how this determines the partial pressure of each.

Blood gases are used to determine the respiratory status and/or the acid-base balance of the patient. If the primary focus is to evaluate the respiratory status of the patient, then the pO_2, pCO_2, and pH levels, as well as sometimes the oxygen saturation, are the most important to evaluate. If the primary focus is to evaluate a metabolic acid-base imbalance, then the pO_2 has little significance. By looking first at the pH, then the pCO_2, and then the HCO_3-, one can figure out whether the acidosis is primarily either respiratory or metabolic in origin (Worthington 1979). In some confusing clinical situations, patients may have a combination of acid-base disorders, but this chapter focuses on the four basic types. Table 6-2 summarizes the way to interpret blood gas results to determine the primary acid-base imbalance. The last part of the chapter discusses hypoxic states that are not directly related to acid-base imbalances.

SUMMARY OF ACID-BASE BALANCE

The normal pH of arterial blood is between 7.35 and 7.45, with 7.4 taken as the average. Varying a little from this narrow range can be disasterous. Many chemical reactions in the

TABLE 6-1.   FOUR GASES IN ARTERIAL BLOOD AT SEA LEVEL*

Gas	Percentage of Gas	Partial Pressure (mm Hg)
Nitrogen (not measured)	75.5%	574 mm Hg
Oxygen	13.0%	99 mm Hg—venous drops to 40 mm Hg
Carbon dioxide	5.3%	40 mm Hg—venous rises to 46 mm Hg
Water vapor (not measured)	6.2%	47 mm Hg
Totals	100.00%	760 mm Hg

Note that the total pressure exerted by a mixture of gases is the sum of the individual partial pressures. See Holum (1979: 84) and Miller (1977, 1978: Parts I, II, and III) for measurements of gases in atmosphere and in alveolar air.

TABLE 6-2.   FOUR STEPS TO DETERMINE THE FOUR PRIMARY ACID-BASE IMBALANCES*

Step 1: *Look at pH.*	Is the pH above 7.45? If so, the patient is alkalotic. Go to Step 2. Is the pH below 7.35? If so, the patient is acidotic. Go to Step 3.
Step 2: When the pH is elevated.	Is the pCO_2 below 40 mm Hg? If so, the alkalosis is respiratory in origin. Is the pCO_2 above 40 mm Hg or in the normal range? If so, the alkalosis is not respiratory in origin. Look for metabolic causes. Go to Step 4.
Step 3: When the pH is decreased.	Is the pCO_2 above 40 mm Hg? If so, the acidosis is respiratory. Is the pCO_2 below 40 mm Hg or normal? If so, the acidosis is metabolic in origin. Go to Step 4.
Step 4: Looking at the bicarbonate in relation to the pH.	Note that in metabolic acidosis, both the pH and the bicarbonate level are decreased. In metabolic alkalosis, both the pH and the bicarbonate are elevated. (See Table 6-4 for compensation.)

Worthington (1979) includes several case studies as practice for determining acid-base imbalances by looking at laboratory reports in a systematic manner.

body do not function normally if the pH of the blood is not in the normal range (Holum 1979). If the pH is below 7.35, this condition is called *acidosis*. If the pH is above 7.45, it is called *alkalosis*. As demonstrated in Table 6-2, if the increased or decreased pH is due to a marked change in the pCO_2, then the acid-base imbalance is respiratory in origin; all other acid-base imbalances are considered metabolic. The *American Journal of Nursing* (Miller 1977; 1978) has an excellent programmed instruction on the physiological principles underlying acid-base.

Understanding how pCO_2 and bicarbonate ($HCO_3 -$) function in the buffering system of the body is necessary if one is to be able to interpret the meaning of abnormal blood gas values. Buffer systems act as chemical sponges, which can give off or absorb hydrogen ions. There are minor buffers in the bloodstream, such as the phosphates and proteins, but these are not measured in evaluating the acid-base balance. The major buffer system is the carbonic acid-bicarbonate buffer system. The carbonic acid level is measured indirectly by the pCO_2 level and the bicarbonate level by the bicarbonate level or the total carbon dioxide content. (Table 6-3). This carbonic acid-bicarbonate buffer system is often referred to as the *20:1 ratio*, which means one part of carbonic acid for each twenty parts of bicarbonate.

Note that, although the carbonic acid level is not measured directly, it can be figured out because it is always 3% of the pCO_2. Hence a pCO_2 of 40 mm Hg indicates 1.2 mEq of carbonic acid in the serum, which must be balanced by 20 parts of bicarbonate or 24 mEq (Shrake 1979). As long as this ratio is maintained, whether it is 40 to 2 or 10 to 0.5, the pH of the blood stays in the normal range (Miller 1977). Thus if the carbonic acid level changes, the kidneys try to compensate by changing the bicarbonate level. For example, since a pCO_2 of 34 reflects a carbonic acid level of 1 mEq (34 times 3% equals 1.02), the bicarbonate level must drop to 20 mEq to keep a 20:1 ratio. If the bicarbonate level changes, the lungs change the carbonic acid level, but this type of compensation is more limited because the lungs must continue to function for oxygen exchange too.

TABLE 6-3. THREE LABORATORY TESTS THAT MEASURE THE BICARBONATE-CARBONIC ACID BUFFER SYSTEM*

$CO_2 + H_2O$	$\rightleftarrows$	H_2CO_3	$\rightleftarrows$	H	+	HCO_3^-
$\downarrow$		$\downarrow$		$\downarrow$		$\downarrow$

Carbon dioxide measured by pCO_2 (40 mm Hg) ★Test #2	Carbonic acid not measured directly but is always 3% of pCO_2 or 3% × 40mm = 1.2 mEq	Concentration of hydrogen ions measured by pH (7.35-7.45) ★Test #1	Bicarbonate level measured by serum bicar-bonate (24 mEq) ★Test #3
pCO_2 controlled by lungs		Hydrogen, bicarbonate, and other electrolytes controlled by kidneys	

★Test #1: pH
Test #2: pCO_2
Test #3: serum bicarbonate

* A bicarbonate level of 24 mEq and a pCO_2 of 40 mm Hg (carbonic acid of 1.2 mEq) is the desirable 20:1 ratio that maintains the pH of the serum between 7.35 and 7.45.
Modified from diagrams in Shrake (1979), Miller (1977), and Holum (1979).

TABLE 6-4. CHANGES IN pH, pCO_2, AND HCO_3^- AND THE COMPENSATORY MECHANISMS IN ACID-BASE IMBALANCES*

	pH	pCO_2	HCO_3^-	Compensation
Respiratory alkalosis	$\uparrow$	$\downarrow$	Normal until compensation.	Kidneys will eventually reduce HCO_3^- (takes few days to complete).
Metabolic alkalosis	$\uparrow$	Normal unless lungs compensate.	$\uparrow$	Lungs will try to increase pCO_2 slightly. Can do quickly.
Respiratory acidosis	$\downarrow$	$\uparrow$	Normal until kidneys compensate.	Kidneys will eventually retain more HCO_3^-. Takes a few days to complete.
Metabolic acidosis	$\downarrow$	Normal until lungs compensate.	$\downarrow$	Lungs will usually reduce pCO_2. Can do quickly.

* See text for full explanation. Note that:
  1. in respiratory alkalosis and respiratory acidosis, the pH and pCO_2 vary inversely;
  2. in metabolic alkalosis and metabolic acidosis, the pH and HCO_3^- rise or fall together;
  3. the kidneys try to compensate for respiratory imbalances, but the compensation takes several days; and
  4. the lungs try to compensate for metabolic imbalances, and their compensation is accomplished in a few minutes—but it is limited.

Only the lungs control the regulation of pCO_2. In the bloodstream, carbon dioxide combines with water to form carbonic acid. If more pCO_2 is retained, this condition results in more carbonic acid and hence the person tends toward acidosis. If more carbon dioxide is blown off (hyperventilation), there is less carbonic acid in the bloodstream and the person tends toward alkalosis. By this mechanism, the lungs can shift the pH of the blood in just a few minutes.

The kidneys are also instrumental in the regulation of the pH of the bloodstream. Not only do the kidneys constantly excrete hydrogen ions, but they also control the serum bicarbonate level, as well as retaining or excreting sodium, potassium, and chloride ions. For major corrective shifts, it may take the kidneys several days to restore the pH to normal (Kaplan 1979).

If all these regulatory mechanisms—buffer systems, lungs, and kidneys—are not successful in restoring the pH, patients go with varying speeds, either into acidosis, leading to coma and death, or into alkalosis with irritability, tetany, and sometimes death. As a general rule, acidotic states are usually more life threatening than alkalotic states (Engberg 1976).

By looking at three laboratory tests, one can usually determine whether the acid–base imbalance is respiratory or metabolic in origin. Table 6-4 shows the laboratory findings for each of the four basic types of acid–base imbalance *before* compensation occurs, and

TABLE 6–5.   COMMON REASONS FOR ACID-BASE IMBALANCES*

Primary Acid–Base Imbalance	Description of Imbalance	Common Reasons for Imbalance
Respiratory alkalosis	Decrease in pCO_2 due to hyperventilation.	Anxiety. Fever, pain, hypoxia. Improperly adjusted respirator.
Respiratory acidosis	Increase in pCO_2 due to hypoventilation.	Chronic lung disease which causes CO_2 retention. Respiratory depression from drugs or anesthesia.
Metabolic alkalosis	Increase in serum bicarbonate (HCO_3) due to increased intake of bicarbonate or increased loss of chlorides, hydrogen, or potassium ions.	Vomiting or gastric suctioning, which causes loss of hydrogen, chloride, and potassium ions. Ingestion or infusion of soda bicarbonate.
Metabolic acidosis	Decrease in serum bicarbonate due to excess acid production, loss of bicarbonate, or increase in serum chloride levels.	Excess acids such as ketone bodies in diabetic acidosis or lactic acid in cardiac arrest. Loss of bicarbonate via intestines. Increase in serum chloride level— renal failure.

* See text for explanations.

how compensation changes the laboratory tests. In the actual clinical situation, because the patient may have more than one imbalance, a chart does not always pinpoint the origin of the difficulty.

Table 6-4 makes the fundamental difference between respiratory and metabolic acid–base imbalances easy to see. If there is a marked increase or decrease in the pCO_2, the acid–base imbalance is respiratory in origin. Otherwise, the imbalance is metabolic, and the change in the bicarbonate level has shifted the pH. Table 6-5 summarizes the common reasons for each type of acid–base imbalance.

If the acidosis or alkalosis is metabolic in origin, or if the respiratory problem is chronic enough for the kidneys to be involved, it is also important to look at the laboratory tests for electrolytes. [Refer to Chapter 5 to review (1) the inverse relationship between chloride (Cl−) and the bicarbonate (HCO_3−) ions, (2) the concept about the anion gap, and (3) why hyperkalemia is associated with acidotic states and hypokalemia with alkalotic states. In Chapter 3 there is a discussion about the changes of the urine pH in the different types of acidosis and alkalosis.] Table 6-6 shows the usual electrolyte abnormalities for each of the four primary types of acid–base imbalances.

TABLE 6-6. POSSIBLE CHANGES IN ELECTROLYTES AND URINE pH FOR ACID–BASE IMBALANCES

	Sodium (Na+)	Potassium (K+)	Chloride (Cl−)	Urine pH
Respiratory alkalosis	Usually not changed.	May be low if alkalosis persists.	Will be increased when HCO_3^- decreases for compensation.	High if chronic problem.
Metabolic alkalosis	Usually not changed.	Low	Low	High or paradoxically pH may continue low.
Respiratory acidosis	Usually not changed.	May be a little increased.	In compensation, the increase in HCO_3^- causes decrease in Cl.	Low. Many H+ ions excreted.
Metabolic acidosis	Total Na+ is low if diuresis as in diabetic acidosis, serum levels may be normal in some states.	May be high although cellular deficit of K+.	May increase to replace lost HCO_3^-. If unmeasured anions are high, Cl− may decrease or be normal.	Very low pH as kidneys try to excrete H+ ions

See Chapter 5 for discussion on electrolytes and Chapter 3 for urine pH. Also see Chan (1978), Narins (1977), and Smithline (1976) for more details.

ARTERIAL BLOOD GASES IN GENERAL

Preparation of Patient And Collection of Sample

The physician or someone skilled in arterial puncture must collect the blood sample, which can be drawn from the radial, brachial, or femoral arteries. In most hospitals only physicians are allowed to do femoral punctures, while nurses with special training may do radial or brachial punctures.

Sumner (1980) gives tips for nurses on how to do arterial punctures. The site must be disinfected and allowed to dry. Patients need to be told that the stick will be momentarily painful. If they are very afraid of the procedure or if the attempt to obtain a specimen is prolonged, patients may hyperventilate due to anxiety, and they can thus alter test results. If arterial blood samples are needed frequently, patients usually have an arterial catheter in place. Nurses usually obtain specimens from an arterial line. In neonates, arterial sampling can be done via an umbilical catheter.

After being collected in an airtight, heparinized syringe, the blood must be packed in ice for transport to the laboratory. (Special care units may have facilities for testing the sample immediately in the unit.) The airtight container and the ice help to prevent the loss of gases from the sample.

The amount of blood needed for arterial blood gases depends on the technique used. Although some of the blood gas analyzers can test less than 0.5 ml of blood, accuracy is more assured with a minimum of 3 ml. Some laboratories may require 5 to 10 ml of blood. Check with the individual laboratory as to how much heparin should be in the syringe. Too much heparin with a small sample causes inaccurate results.

After the sample is drawn, continuous pressure should be applied to the puncture site for at least five minutes if the radial artery is used and ten minutes for the femoral. If the patient has any bleeding problems, the pressure dressing should be taped on and left for several hours.

It is important to note on the laboratory slip whether the patient was receiving oxygen at the time the sample was drawn, since there may be quite a difference in pO_2 if the patient is having oxygen therapy as opposed to breathing room air. The nurse should note how long the patient has been on a specific amount of oxygen, such as ''25 minutes on 2 liters by nasal cannula.'' If the patient is on assisted ventilation, the settings for the respirator should be noted in case changes need to be made later. The temperature of the patient should also be noted since a fever increases the metabolic rate.

If arterial blood cannot be obtained, capillary blood samples may be used. The area should be warmed for five minutes before the sample is taken. The warmed ear site is used in children and adults, while the warmed heel is used for infants. (See Chapter 1 for the heel stick technique.)

Continuously Monitoring Oxygen Levels With Electrodes

Recently a skin surface electrode has been developed that can continuously monitor the oxygen level in the blood. Dingle (1980) describes this monitoring method for the neonate. The monitor (a Hutch electrode) measures the amount of oxygen diffusing through the skin, since this skin measurement correlates closely with arterial blood samples. The monitor is more accurate for newborns because the infant's skin is thin and there is little subcutaneous fat as compared to an adult's.

The rest of this chapter is devoted to a discussion of the meaning of each component of the blood gases. Discussed first are pH, pCO_2, and serum bicarbonate due to their importance in the acid–base balance. Then pO_2 and O_2 saturations are discussed at the end of the chapter. The nursing implications for each alteration are also discussed.

pH OF THE BLOOD

The pH test measures the alkalinity or acidity of the blood. For chemical solutions, a pH of 7 is the neutral point; above 7 is alkaline and below 7 is acid (Holum 1978). For the blood pH, the neutral point is 7.4. It is critical that the blood pH remain within a narrow range because many enzymes and other physiological processes do not function normally when the pH is altered.

Reference Values

Adults	7.35–7.45
Newborns	7.3–7.4
	See Table 6-7 for pH in newborns.

Increased pH of Arterial Blood (Alkalosis)

Clinical Significance. An increased serum pH indicates that the patient is in a state of alkalosis. To determine whether the alkalosis is respiratory or metabolic in origin, it is necessary to look at the pCO_2 and the serum bicarbonate (HCO_3^-) level. If the alkalosis is respiratory in origin, the pCO_2 is markedly decreased. If the alkalosis is metabolic in origin, the serum bicarbonate (HCO_3^-) level is markedly elevated. The common clinical situations that would cause these changes and the reference value are discussed under the pCO_2 and the $HCO_3 -$ tests.

Possible Nursing Implications.
    Assessing. Nursing implications depend on whether the alkalosis is respiratory or metabolic in origin. Some general symptoms of both types of alkalosis include tingling in the extremities or nose, facial twitching, light-headedness, muscle tremors, and tetany. The neuromuscular irritability in alkalotic states occurs because calcium is less soluble in an alkaline medium. Many of the symptoms of alkalosis are those of hypocalcemia. (See Chapter 7 on hypocalcemia.)
    One other important point: In respiratory alkalosis the respiratory rate is high because hyperventilation is the cause of the alkalosis. Factors causing hyperventilation are discussed in the section on pCO_2 levels. In metabolic alkalosis the respiratory rate is normal to slightly depressed, with slow and shallow breaths. The depressed respirations in

metabolic alkalosis is an attempt by the lungs to retain more pCO_2 to balance the increased serum bicarbonate level.

Decreased pH of Arterial Blood (Acidosis)

Clinical Significance. A decreased serum pH indicates that the patient is in a state of acidosis. To determine whether the adicosis is respiratory or metabolic in origin, it is necessary to look at the pCO_2 and the serum bicarbonate (HCO_3-) level. In respiratory acidosis the pCO_2 is increased. In metabolic acidosis the serum bicarbonate level is lower than normal. Each type of acidosis is covered in the discussion about pCO_2 and serum bicarbonate levels. Note in Table 6-7 that newborns with low Apgar scores have a proportionately low pH.

TABLE 6-7.   RELATIONSHIP OF APGAR SCORES IN NEWBORN TO pH LEVEL

Sign	Score 0	Score 1	Score 2
Heart rate	Absent	Below 100	Over 100
Respiratory rate	Absent	Slow, irregular, hypoventilate	Good, crying lustily
Muscle tone	Flaccid	Some flexion of extremities	Active motion/well flexed
Reflexes	No response	Cry, some motion, grimace	Vigorous cry
Color	Blue, pale	Body pink/hands and feet blue	Completely pink

Apgar Score	Estimate of pH
9–10	7.3–7.4
7–8	7.2–7.29
5–6	7.10–7.19
3–4	7.0–7.09
0–2	Below 7

The Apgar score is a simple and practical method to assess the overall physical status of the infant immediately after delivery. It is done at 1 minute and 5 minutes after birth (Jensen 1981:466).

Possible Nursing Implications.

Assessing. The nursing implications depend on whether the acidosis is respiratory or metabolic in nature. General symptoms for both types of acidosis include headaches, weakness, lethargy, and confusion. The level of consciousness is depressed as the acidotic state worsens. Unless the acidotic state is corrected, drowsiness leads from a stuporous state, to coma, and eventually to death. As with alkalotic states, the respiratory patterns are exactly the opposite for the two types of acidosis. In respiratory acidosis, the respiratory rate is depressed because hypoventilation is the cause of respiratory acidosis. In metabolic acidosis, the respiratory rate is faster and deeper than normal (Kussmaul's respirations) because the lungs are trying to compensate for the decreased serum pH by blowing off more carbon dioxide.

pCO_2 (ARTERIAL)

The pCO_2 test measures the partial pressure of carbon dioxide in the arterial blood. When carbon dioxide is transported in serum, much of it is combined with water to form carbonic acid (H_2CO_3), which dissociates into bicarbonate (HCO_3^-) and hydrogen (H^+) ions. The actual carbonic acid level in the serum is not measured, but it can always be determined by multiplying the pCO_2 by 3%. A pCO_2 of 40 mm Hg is 1.2 mEq of carbonic acid ($40 \times 3\%$) (Shrake 1979). Because the end result is an increase in the amount of free hydrogen ions, an increase in the pCO_2 causes the blood pH to drop below 7.4. The special preparation for obtaining blood gases was covered earlier in this chapter.

Reference Values

All patients	35–45 mm Hg (millimeters of mercury)
Pregnancy	Values may be as low as 30 mm Hg by the end of the second trimester. 30–37 mm Hg is normal for pregnancy because of hyperventilation. The kidneys compensate by excreting more bicarbonate, so that the pH of around 7.4 is maintained. Research studies have suggested that progesterone may be the cause of the hyperventilation in pregnancy (Milne 1979: 319).
Altitude	At higher altitudes the atmospheric pressure is less, so the partial pressure of carbon dioxide is proportionally reduced. (See discussion for pO_2 values.)

Increased pCO_2 (Hypercarbia or Hypercapnia)

Clinical Significance. An increased pCO_2 level indicates that the normal amount of carbon dioxide is not being blown off. Any situation that causes hypoventilation, such as a drug overdose that results in respiratory depression, causes an elevated pCO_2. Higher-than-normal pCO_2 levels are also present in certain chronic lung conditions where the exchange of carbon dioxide and oxygen is impaired. Patients with chronic obstructive lung disease may have both hypoxia and hypercarbia (elevated pCO_2), although the latter is not always associated with hypoxia. Some acute lung dysfunctions, such as pneumonia, may cause hypoxia but not an elevated pCO_2. Hypoxia does not always lead to a retention of carbon dioxide for two basic reasons: First, carbon dioxide diffuses more readily across alveolar surfaces than does oxygen, so an impairment of respiratory function results in a fall of pO_2 before the pCO_2 changes. Second, hypoxia is a stimulus for breathing (Pavlin 1978). If the lungs can respond to the low oxygen level by increasing the respiratory rate, the carbon dioxide level may stay normal or drop to below normal due to the hyperventilation.

The type of hypoventilation that causes an increased pCO_2 can be very transitory and self-limiting, such as when the breath is held. The resultant high level of pCO_2 cannot be maintained because it becomes an overpowering stimulus for taking a breath—one cannot commit suicide by holding one's breath. Patients with chronic lung disease who have high carbon dioxide levels no longer use carbon dioxide as a stimulus for breathing. Instead, hypoxia becomes the primary stimulus for breathing, and the kidneys compensate for the gradual increase in pCO_2 level by increasing the serum bicarbonate level. The normal blood pH is maintained as long as the kidneys can keep the 20:1 ratio of bicarbonate to carbonic acid. It takes the kidneys several days to compensate for increasing pCO_2 levels, so a quick increase in pCO_2, or acute respiratory failure, leads to respiratory acidosis.

Just as the kidneys try to compensate for lung malfunction, the lungs try to compensate for metabolic acid–base imbalances. In metabolic alkalosis, the pCO_2 is usually more than 40 mm Hg because the lungs are attempting to reestablish the bicarbonate–carbonic acid ratio by increasing the carbonic acid to match the increased serum bicarbonate. This compensatory hypoventilation is not very effective because the respiratory rate cannot be depressed very much without creating hypoxia (Lee 1975). To summarize, elevated pCO_2 levels can be the cause of respiratory acidosis or a compensatory attempt for metabolic alkalosis, but the compensatory effect is very slight.

Possible Nursing Implications.

Assessing for CO_2 Narcosis. Nurses must always be aware of the early signs of increasing pCO_2 levels. The term CO_2 "narcosis," another name for respiratory acidosis, gives a clue that carbon dioxide can be a central nervous system depressant. Early signs of increased pCO_2 may be headache, dizziness, and confusion. The confusion may progress to decreasing levels of consciousness until the patient is comatose.

The seriousness of an elevated pCO_2 level can be evaluated only in relation to the amount of compensation that has occurred. For example, patients with chronic lung disease may have a higher-than-normal pCO_2 with a higher-than-normal bicarbonate level and a resulting normal pH. So they may not be in immediate danger. (In addition to looking at these three lab results, also look at the chloride level, which is lower than normal because the negative ion bicarbonate (HCO_3-) is increased in the serum. See Chapter 5.) A drug that depresses the respiratory center, a respiratory infection, or some treatment that causes a lot of exertion may throw such compensated patients into respiratory acidosis, or CO_2 narcosis.

Potential Danger of Oxygen and Sedatives. High doses of oxygen can be lethal for patients who have a chronically high pCO_2 because hypoxia has become the respiratory stimulus for the patient. The medullary center no longer responds to high levels of pCO_2, which is normally the primary stimulus for respiration, because the chronically elevated pCO_2 has made the center insensitive to carbon dioxide as a stimulus for breathing. The only stimulus for breathing is hypoxia. For patients with advanced emphysema, a pO_2 of 50 to 60 mm Hg is "normal." Their color may improve as the hypoxia is eliminated, but their respirations become slower and slower since they no longer have a stimulus to breathe. If these patients are not stimulated to breathe, the pCO_2 level rises even higher, and they may die in respiratory acidosis.

Note also that very small doses of drugs such as morphine or diazepam (Valium) can also depress respirations to a serious degree, because the response to hypoxia is depressed (Paulin 1978:3). (See the discussion under pO_2 on ways to assess and intervene for hypoxia in both the patient with acute and chronic respiratory problems.)

Assisting with Medical Interventions. The treatment for respiratory depression may include assisted ventilation until the underlying pathophysiology can be medically treated. Nursing interventions are geared toward improving the respiratory status. Frequent arterial blood gases help to monitor the improvement of the patient and ensure that increasing carbon dioxide levels are not occurring.

Decreased pCO_2

Clinical Significance. Just as hypoventilation leads to an increased pCO_2 level, hyperventilation leads to a decreased pCO_2 level. (The terms "hypocarbia" or "hypocapnia" are rarely used.) Often hyperventilation is due to severe anxiety. Hysterical or semihysterical people tend to breathe very fast and deeply, with a lot of sighing. Physical conditions such as fever, pain, or hypoxia can also cause hyperventilation. No matter what the stimulus, the end result is that, if enough carbon dioxide is blown off to lower the pCO_2, the person will be in respiratory alkalosis.

Some patients may have a slightly low pCO_2 most of the time, but usually this form of chronic hyperventilation is not noticed until the person has an acute anxiety attack (Waites 1978). It is unusual to see compensation for respiratory alkalosis because severe hyperventilation typically does not last long enough for the kidneys to begin to excrete extra bicarbonate. An exception, however, is the patient on a respirator: An improperly adjusted respirator can be responsible for hyperventilation that continues over a long period of time.

A lower-than-normal pCO_2 can also be a compensatory mechanism for metabolic acidosis. For example, patients in diabetic acidosis use up much of the bicarbonate buffer in their bloodstreams to buffer the ketone bodies. The lungs try to restore the 20:1 ratio by reducing the pCO_2 and hence the carbonic acid part of the ratio (Kussmaul's respirations), but this compensation cannot offset the severe metabolic acidosis. To summarize, decreased pCO_2 levels can be the cause of respiratory alkalosis or part of the compensation for metabolic acidosis.

Possible Nursing Implications. *Assessing for Decreased pCO_2 Levels.* A decreased pCO_2 is not nearly as serious as an increased pCO_2 because once the person stops hyperventilating, the pCO_2 quickly returns to normal. (A lowered pCO_2 in acidotic states is not considered in this discussion.)

Most of the symptoms that result from a lowered pCO_2, which can be alarming to the patient and to the nurse, can be explained on the basis of the effect of an alkaline pH on serum calcium levels. Since calcium is less soluble in an alkaline medium, less ionized calcium is available when the blood pH rises above normal. Hence the patient has symptoms of hypocalcemia. (See Chapter 7 for the symptoms of hypocalcemia.) There may be tingling of the fingers, twitching, muscle tremors, carpopedal spasms, and even tetany. The person may feel light-headed and dizzy. If the hyperventilation is less severe and more of a chronic problem, the person may have only such symptoms as chronic exhaustion or diffuse weakness.

Nurses in emergency rooms or outpatient clinics are the ones most likely to see people who are seeking treatment because of hyperventilating (Sandvik 1977). Recognizing that the patient is hyperventilating is easy, but assessing whether it is due to anxiety or to physical causes may not be so easy. Ruling out fever, pain, or hypoxia as reason for the hyperventilation is important. (If the hyperventilation is due to an underlying metabolic acidosis, there will be no symptoms of alkalosis because the pH remains acid from the metabolic problem.)

Interventions to Decrease Hyperventiliation. If the hyperventilation is due to functional anxiety, nursing interventions can be instrumental in stopping the hyperventilation. The person needs to be reassured that slower breathing will decrease the symptoms. Breathing into a paper bag helps to increase the pCO_2 level. The nurse needs to maintain a calm, soothing environment so the person can gain control and reduce the feeling of anxiety. Hyperventilating may be a recurring problem that warrants a referral for counseling to help the person learn ways to deal with anxiety. If the anxiety level is high, the physician may order drugs to reduce the anxiety. Sometimes the patient may need to be taught the proper way to do diaphragmatic breathing. The long-term goal is to help the person deal with the anxiety and to see how the anxiety has caused the breathing problem.

Preventing Hyperventilation. The nurse needs to be aware of other situations where hyperventilating may occur. For example, a patient in labor may not be doing the breathing exercises correctly and thus go into respiratory alkalosis. Also, patients on respirators need careful monitoring to make sure that the ventilation rate is not too fast. If hyperventilation is due to a stimulus such as fever, then therapeutic measures to reduce the fever will eliminate the hyperventilation.

SERUM BICARBONATE LEVELS (HCO_3-)

Bicarbonate functions as a very important buffer in the bloodstream. To keep the bloodstream's pH between 7.35 to 7.45, the bicarbonate in it is kept at a 20:1 ratio to carbonic acid. The section on pCO_2 explained how changes in the pCO_2 cause changes in the bicarbonate level. Since bicarbonate and chloride are both negative ions in the serum, an increased retention of serum chloride means less retention of bicarbonate (Miller 1978). Thus serum bicarbonate measurements are useful in both acid–base imbalances and electrolyte imbalances, and they are therefore a routine part of laboratory tests for either ''electrolytes'' or ''arterial blood gases.''

Bicarbonate is ingested in food and in medications. Large amounts of baking soda (soda bicarbonate) can actually increase the serum level of bicarbonate. All gastrointestinal secretions below the pylorus are rich in sodium bicarbonate. In contrast, above the pylorus, secretions of the stomach have a very acid content (Lee 1977). When sodium is reabsorbed into the distal tubule, either a chloride (Cl) or bicarbonate (HCO_3-) ion is retained. The kidney secretes or retains bicarbonate depending on the overall need for chloride or bicarbonate in the serum (Miller 1977).

Direct and Indirect Methods to Measure Bicarbonate
There are several different laboratory methods to measure the serum bicarbonate level. Some laboratories may do direct measurements of the bicarbonate and report it as such. One indirect method involves measuring the total carbon dioxide content of the serum and calculating the bicarbonate level from this figure. An older method involves measuring the CO_2 combining power of the serum.

Nurses do not need to understand the technicalities of how these various tests are done, but it is important to use the reference values that correspond to the exact method used by a specific laboratory. There is less standardization of bicarbonate measurement than with the other electrolytes. If a laboratory report does not have any item marked ''bicarbonate,'' look for something called ''carbon dioxide content'' or ''carbon dioxide capacity,'' which reflect the bicarbonate component of the blood.

Meaning of ''Base Excess'' or ''Base Deficit''
Some laboratories also measure the total buffer base of the body and report this as a ''base deficit'' or a ''base excess.'' The *buffer base* refers to all the buffer ions in the serum, including not only bicarbonate but also phosphates, hemoglobin, and plasma proteins. The total buffers are usually around 50 mEq/l, but the laboratory just reports so many

minus or plus milliequivalents. The normal would be a −2 mEq to a +2 mEq. More than a −2 mEq means a *base deficit,* which correlates to a decrease in bicarbonate levels. A result of over 2 mEq signifies a *base excess,* which correlates to an increased bicarbonate level.

Reference Values

Bicarbonate Levels measured by carbon dioxide content.

Adults	24–30 mEq/l
Pregnancy	Falls early in pregnancy by an amount consistent with the fall in the pCO_2. A pCO_2 of 34 mm Hg is balanced with a HCO_3 of around 20 mEq to keep the pH around 7.4.
Newborns	20–26 mEq/l (Prematures may have even lower reference values.)
Children	Slightly lower references than those for adults.
Base excess or base deficit	−2 to +2 mEq/l

Increased Serum Bicarbonate Level (Base Excess)

Clinical Significance. The loss of hydrogen, potassium, and chloride ions all contribute to the development of metabolic alkalosis. First of all, any loss of hydrogen ions causes a proportional increase in the bicarbonate side of the bicarbonate–carbonic acid buffering system. Second, as discussed in Chapter 5, when potassium is low in the serum, the kidneys are unable to excrete bicarbonate normally. Third, when chloride, a negative ion, is decreased in the bloodstream, another negative ion is needed to keep the positive and negative ions balanced in the serum (Chan 1978). Thus the kidneys cause a retention of bicarbonate to replace the missing chloride.

The most common reason for an increase in the bicarbonate level is a loss of gastric contents. Patients who vomit or who have nasogastric suctioning without proper potassium chloride replacement (KCl) are prone to have high bicarbonate levels. Patients on diuretics may also lose abnormal amounts of chloride and potassium.

An increase in the serum bicarbonate level can also occur with the ingestion of large amounts of sodium bicarbonate. As a home remedy, patients may take baking soda (soda bicarbonate), which is systemically absorbed. Commercial antacids, such as Maalox, are usually not systemically absorbed, so they do not cause alkalosis, but they may contribute to metabolic alkalosis if there is inadequate renal function. Alkalosis can also occur from overdosage with intravenous soda bicarbonate to treat acidosis. Usually this rebound effect is not a serious problem.

The third major reason for an increased serum bicarbonate level is an increase as a compensatory mechanism for the elevated pCO_2 of the patient with chronic lung disease. In this last situation, the serum chloride is decreased because the negative ion bicarbonate is increased. The increased bicarbonate level is necessary to keep the pH of the serum normal.

Possible Nursing Implications.

Assessing. Usually patients in metabolic alkalosis do not have many symptoms directly related to the acid–base imbalance. Their respirations may be a little slow because their lungs are trying to compensate by conserving some carbon dioxide. The change in their respiratory rate may be too slight to be clinically significant. Other symptoms would be related to the decreased solubility of calcium in an alkaline pH. As with respiratory alkalosis, patients may experience neuromuscular irritability, tingling in the fingers, twitching of the nose or lips, and even tetany or convulsions if the alkalosis is not corrected. Since the alkalotic patient is susceptible to atrial tachycardia, the pulse rate should be carefully monitored (Lee 1975).

Assisting with Medical Interventions. Corrective measures, as well as the appropriate nursing actions, depend on what has caused the elevated serum bicarbonate. If the patient has a history of either vomiting, nasogastric suctioning, or diuretic loss, he or she may need both potassium and chloride replacement. (Table 6–5). Nursing implications for potassium chloride administration were covered in the last chapter. The patient may also be given isotonic solutions to intravenously replenish the loss of chlorides. Fruit juices and broth may be given in less severe depletions of chloride and potassium.

If the patient has a history of increased intake of soda bicarbonate, then stopping the ingestion is usually enough. Patients need to be taught that baking soda is not a desirable antacid because it is absorbed into the bloodstream. If they have had a lot of sodium bicarbonate intravenously for the treatment of an acidotic state, the nurse must look for a rebound effect. Ammonium chloride, although a systemic acidifier, is rarely used to counteract alkalosis. Determining and correcting the reason for the increased bicarbonate is usually sufficient.

Recognizing Compensatory Mechanisms. If the elevated serum bicarbonate level is a compensatory mechanism for chronic lung disease, the elevated bicarbonate is needed to keep the blood pH within normal ranges. Specific nursing precautions for the patient with a chronically elevated pCO_2 were covered earlier in this chapter. The nursing implications are those for the patient with chronic lung disease.

Decreased Serum Bicarbonate Level (Base Deficit)

Clinical Significance. Unless the patient has a low pCO_2, and thus a low serum bicarbonate level as compensation, a decrease in the serum bicarbonate level is an indication that the patient has some type of metabolic acidosis. The severity of the acidotic state depends on how low the blood pH has dropped. The decrease in serum bicarbonate levels that occurs in metabolic acidotic states can be due to:

1. utilization of the bicarbonate to buffer acids such as excessive lactate, ketone bodies, or other toxic metabolics that contain hydrogen ions (the most common type of metabolic acidosis seen clinically);
2. a primary loss of bicarbonate; or
3. an increase in serum chloride level.

1. Increased Production of Acids. In a normal state of health, as acids are produced or introduced into the body, they are neutralized by the bicarbonate–carbonic acid buffering system and eventually excreted by the kidneys. With a sudden increase in acids in certain pathological states, the kidneys do not have enough time to excrete the acids or enough bicarbonate to neutralize them.

1. In diabetic acidosis, the acids produced are the ketone bodies.
2. In shock, the tissue hypoxia results in an excessive build-up of lactic acid.
3. In renal failure, or in severe dehydration, the kidneys can no longer excrete hydrogen ions or acids such as the phosphates and sulfates.
4. In cardiac arrest, there is an immediate build-up of lactic acid (as well as a high pCO_2, so the patient has both respiratory and metabolic acidosis).
5. Aspirin overdose floods the system with an acid. (Initially the ASA acts as a respiratory stimulant causing some respiratory alkalosis, but the end result is acidosis.)

Any situation that creates more acid (hydrogen ions) than can be handled by the body depletes the bicarbonate buffer system and results in acidosis.

The lactates, phosphates, ketone bodies, and other acids that can cause metabolic acidosis are negative ions (anions) in the bloodstream. So an increase in these acids increase the anion gap, which is the amount of unmeasured negative ions or anions in the bloodstream (see Chapter 5). It is determined by comparing the total amount of positive ions in the serum (primarily sodium and potassium) with the total amount of negative ions in the serum (primarily chloride and bicarbonate). When the total positive and the negative ions are compared in the bloodstream, there is a gap because one type of negative ions, namely the acids, are not measured. Yet the total numbers of positive and of negative ions must always balance in the bloodstream. Usually, since the unmeasured acids account for about 12 mEq of the total negative ions (Smithline 1977), the anion gap is considered to be no more than that 10 to 14 mEq.

In metabolic acidosis the increase in the negative ions of ketoacids, lactate, phosphate, sulfate, or other acids makes the anion gap larger because more unmeasured negative ions are present in the bloodstream. The anion gap is useful in distinguishing this first type of metabolic acidosis from the other two types because in them there is no increase in the acids that comprise the unmeasured negative ions and therefore no anion gap (Narins 1977).

2. Primary Loss of Bicarbonate. A primary loss of bicarbonate can occur with gastrointestinal losses below the pylorus because the intestinal tract and pancreatic secretions are rich in bicarbonate (Copeland 1977). (As a general rule, gastrointestinal losses above the pylorus, such as vomiting or gastric suctioning, tend to cause alkalosis due to the loss of hydrogen, potassium, and chloride ions. So alkalosis is related to vomiting and acidosis to diarrhea. However, dehydration from either vomiting or diarrhea is likely to result in acidosis due to the kidneys' inability to excrete acid byproducts.) The primary loss of bicarbonate (a negative ion) leads to an increased chloride level to keep the positive negative charges balanced in the serum. The anion gap does not increase.

3. An Increase in The Serum Chloride Level. A primary increase in the serum chloride level means that chloride, a negative ion is increased and that another negative ion, bicarbonate, must be proportionally decreased. The lowering of the serum bicarbonate level keeps the electrical charges of the serum electrolytes balanced, but it creates acidosis because the buffering ability of the serum is decreased.

This type of metabolic acidosis is a much less common clinical occurrence than the first two types. High doses of chlorides in intravenous therapy may raise the serum chloride level. Also, certain types of renal failure result in an inability to properly excrete chloride ions.

Possible Nursing Implications.

Assessing. Laboratory tests are meaningless without clinical assessments. The serum bicarbonate level must always be interpreted in relation to the pCO_2 and to electrolyte levels. The pathophysiological process may or may not be readily apparent given the patient's history, such as diabetes.

It is important for nurses to recognize early symptoms of acidosis, because severe acidosis can be life-threatening. When a patient has a lowered serum bicarbonate level that is creating metabolic acidosis, one of the key symptoms is hyperventilation. This deep and rapid respiration (Kussmaul's breathing) is an attempt to restore the 20:1 bicarbonate-carbonic acid ratio by decreasing the carbonic acid in the blood. (Recall that 3% of the pCO_2 is carried in the bloodstream as carbonic acid.) These fast and deep respirations may look like the patient has "air hunger," but they really reflect an attempt to blow off extra pCO_2. This increased respiratory rate may be one of the first clues that the pH is dropping. As the pH drops lower, the patient begins to exhibit signs of confusion, lethargy, and eventually coma. (A diabetic coma is a form of severe metabolic acidosis.) Newborn infants can develop severe metabolic acidosis if they are not kept warm and given sufficient calories. Acidosis can develop immediately, such as with a cardiac arrest, or very slowly, as in a patient with renal failure. Some diabetics who do not take their insulin may go into a coma within a day or so. A young child who is diabetic may go into acidosis very quickly, whereas an adult diabetic may take several days to develop ketoacidosis. The important thing is to know the type of situation that can lead to metabolic acidosis so any changes can be detected early.

Assisting with Medical Interventions. The major goal of treatment is to eliminate the cause of the acidosis. The cold-stressed newborn must be warmed and fed. The diabetic patient requires insulin so that glucose, rather than fats, can be used as the primary source of energy. Patients in shock must have increased oxygen perfusion at the cellular level so that there is no longer the anerobic metabolism that has caused a build-up of lactic acid.

Although the goal of treatment is to eliminate the cause of the acidosis, the patient may need sodium bicarbonate intravenously to bring the serum pH back to normal immediately. For example, in cardiac arrest sodium bicarbonate is usually the first drug administered to counteract the severe metabolic and respiratory acidosis. Adrenalin, and many other drugs, are maximally effective only when the pH of the blood is normal. Sodium bicarbonate may be given direct intravenous push or in a continuous intravenous solution. Other drugs should not be mixed with the bicarbonate solution because they may preciptate in an alkaline pH. For example, calcium precipitates in a strongly alkaline pH.

The respiratory rate is one objective assessment of the effectiveness of therapy. When acidotic patients are given sodium bicarbonate, the hyperventilation decreases as the pH of the blood returns to normal. Sometimes the patient may be given enough sodium bicarbonate to create a rebound metabolic alkalosis. Symptoms such as tingling can be signs that the pH of the blood is rising too much. However, in most situations where the physician orders massive doses of sodium bicarbonate, the acidotic state is a much more severe problem than the possibility of a rebound alkalosis. In an acute emergency, such as a cardiac arrest, it is essential that someone, usually the nurse, keep a detailed record of all the medications given the patient.

Very close monitoring of the intake and ouptut for patients in acidosis is essential to prevent severe dehydration and further electrolyte imbalances. (See Chapter 5 on the relationship of hyperkalemia and acidosis.) During acidotic states, more hydrogen ions go into the cells, and potassium ions are forced out. The potassium that leaves the cells is eventually excreted by the kidneys so that the aftermath of metabolic acidosis is a depletion of total body potassium. In connection with the anion gap, chloride levels may or may not be increased, depending on whether the metabolic acidosis is due to an increase of acids, which are negative ions. Sodium may also be depleted, particularly in diabetic acidosis where diuresis has been a prominent feature. The nurse caring for a patient who is recovering from metabolic acidosis must be aware of all the nursing implications for changes in each of these electrolytes, each of which was discussed separately in Chapter 5.

pO₂ (PARTIAL PRESSURE OF OXYGEN)

The pO_2 measures the amount of oxygen dissolved in the blood. The partial pressure is calculated by multiplying the amount of gas in a solution (%) by the total pressure (mm Hg or millimeters of mercury). Hence the laboratory reports the pO_2 as ''so many millimeters of mercury (mm Hg).'' In a healthy young person, arterial blood may have about 13% oxygen dissolved in the plasma. At sea level, the partial pressure of oxygen would be 13% times 760 mm Hg or 98.8 mm Hg. As can be seen by the reference values, breathing pure oxygen, moving to a high altitude, or just simply aging makes quite a difference in the partial pressure of oxygen in the bloodstream.

Reference Values

Adults	75-100 mm Hg while breathing room air. May be above 225 mm if breathing 40% oxygen (with normal lungs).
Newborns	60-70 mm Hg are usually given as maximum reference values, or 40-60 mm Hg in some laboratories.
Aged	The pO_2 drops about 3 to 5 mm Hg for each decade after 30. After age 60, a pO_2 of around 80 mm Hg is the maximum reference value (Engberg 1976).
Location	In high altitudes, such as Denver where the atmospheric pressure is 670 mm Hg, the maximum reference value for a person under 30 is around 81 mm Hg.

Increased pO₂

Clinical Significance. The only clinical situation that creates a high pO_2 is the administration of high doses of oxygen. 100% oxygen may increase the pO_2 to over 500 mm Hg. Whether high oxygen pressures in the blood can alter certain bodily conditions, such as aging, is a controversial subject that is being explored.

Possible Nursing Implications. It was discovered many years ago that high doses of oxygen can cause irreversible blindness in premature infants. The high oxygen level causes a condition called *retrolental fibroplasia.* Nurses must routinely check the oxygen content of incubators to make sure that the oxygen delivery is correct. More recently it has been discovered that the prolonged use of high concentrations of oxygen can cause airway irritation and eventually damage to the lungs in both children and adults (Nielson 1980).

Oxygen may also have a toxic effect on the central nervous system when oxygen is delivered under pressures greater than normal. The nurse should question any order for the prolonged use (over eight hours) of 100% oxygen. In severe and complicated cases of hypoxia, the patient may have to be on high concentrations of oxygen for an extended period of time. Frequent monitoring of blood gases is necessary to evaluate whether the oxygen therapy is satisfactory.

The key thing for the nurse to remember is that oxygen, like any other drug, can be misused to the detriment of the patient's well-being. (The danger of even normal concentrations of oxygen for the patient with carbon dioxide retention was discussed under the section on pCO_2.)

Decreased Arterial pO_2

Clinical Significance. Many different conditions can cause hypoxia, which is usually defined as a pO_2 of less than 70 mm Hg in the adult. With atelectasis or emphysema there may be ventilation to blood flow abnormalities so that oxygen does not reach the bloodstream. A lack of oxygen in the atmosphere, such as when a child is trapped in a refrigerator, leads to a severe drop in pO_2. Hypoventilation, such as in the patient who has taken a respiratory depressant, causes hypoxia. Anatomic defects, such as when arterial and venous blood intermix, cause hypoxia. In essence, any situation that interferes with the CO_2–O_2 exchange leads to a lowered pO_2.

Since the pCO_2 may be elevated, normal, or decreased with a decreased pO_2, it is important to look at the laboratory reports for both pCO_2 and pH when evaluating the clinical significance of a low pO_2. With many types of hypoxia, the pCO_2 may remain normal because carbon dioxide can diffuse much more readily than oxygen can across alveolar surfaces. If the hypoxia state is causing marked hyperventilation, the pCO_2 may actually drop below normal. For example, with pneumonia, both the pO_2 and pCO_2 may be lower than normal. The infection in the lungs interferes with oxygen exchange more than with carbon dioxide exchange. The hypoxia leads to hyperventilation in an attempt to increase oxygen. The hyperventilation causes more blowing off of carbon dioxide so the pCO_2 becomes lower than normal. In respiratory depression, such as that caused by general anesthesia, pO_2 levels cannot stimulate increased respirations, so the pCO_2 level rises. In chronic lung disease, there may first be only hypoxia, but eventually an increase in the pCO_2 level as the lung damage becomes worse. The clinical significance of hypoxia, compounded by hypercapnia (high pCO_2), is quite different from hypoxia alone.

Possible Nursing Implications.
Assessing for Hypoxia. The nurse may be instrumental in preventing serious complications from hypoxia by detecting it before cyanosis occurs, which is a late symptom of hypoxia. Peripheral cyanosis that occurs in the nailbeds reflects poor peripheral perfusion,

but not necessarily an extremely low pO$_2$. Central cyanosis is best assessed by looking at the tongue. In the adult the pO$_2$ is less than 50 mm Hg by the time central cyanosis occurs. The blue color of central cyanosis denotes at least 5 grams of unoxygenated hemoglobin in the arterial blood—or over one-third of the total hemoglobin in the blood. The nurse needs to look for early symptoms of hypoxia, such as tachycardia and restlessness. By the time this one-third or more of the hemoglobin is unsaturated, the patient may be in real distress.

Assessing for Cyanosis in Dark-Skinned People. Since cyanosis is difficult to assess in the dark-skinned person, nurses must become familiar with the patient's pre-cyanotic color. When cyanosis is suspected, nurses can press on the skin to create pallor. In cyanotic tissue the color returns slowly by spreading from the periphery to the center. Also the lips and tongue become ashen gray in a black person who is cyanotic (Bloch 1981: 26).

Assisting with Oxygen Therapy. When oxygen is ordered for the patient with hypoxia, nurses must make sure that the safety and comfort of the patient are maintained. Patients and family need clear instructions about the danger of smoking. Discontinuing oxygen for just a few minutes may cause a significant drop in the pO$_2$ of some patients, and it may take as much as twenty minutes to restore the previous level (Felton 1978). Since hypoxia can contribute to the development of severe cardiac arrhythmias, 100% oxygen may be given before and after suctioning a patient. The nurse should consult with the physician about whether oxygen therapy can be interrupted for oral temperatures, feedings, or other procedures. The most objective assessment of the need for continual oxygen therapy is the blood gas report. The patient on a ventilator may have blood gases drawn frequently to assess if the ventilator is properly adjusted.

The possible nursing implications for patients with a low pO$_2$ and a high pCO$_2$ were covered in the section on pCO$_2$. It is essential for the nurse to understand the potential danger of giving high concentrations of oxygen to patients who have hypoxia coupled with a chronically increased pCO$_2$. Recall that a patient with chronic emphysema who has an elevated pCO$_2$ and a "normal" pO$_2$ of 50–60 mm Hg is using the hypoxia as a stimulus for breathing.

Other Interventions to Decrease Hypoxia. Even with patients who have only hypoxia, and not an elevated pCO$_2$, oxygen may not be their primary need. For example, if the hypoxia is due to mucus plugs blocking some of the airways, then coughing, deep breathing, and maybe suctioning need to be instituted. When a patient is allowed to stay in one position, not all areas of the lungs are equally ventilated; so some unoxygenated blood goes back to the left atrium. This is called *physiologic shunting.* By changing the patient's position frequently, physiologic shunting does not add to the problem of hypoxia. However, if the hypoxia is due to a poor cardiac output, changing positions often may be tiring to the patient and not a top priority. It is very important to understand the basic reason for the hypoxic state so that nursing measures are geared to help the patient to utilize oxygen effectively and to conserve energy so that oxygen need is not increased.

OXYGEN SATURATION

Since the pO$_2$ measures the amount of dissolved oxygen in the blood, not the amount of oxygen carried by the hemoglobin, one must determine the oxygen saturation of the blood to evaluate its total carrying capacity. If hemoglobin is carrying the normal amount of oxygen, the oxygen saturation is close to 100%. The oxygen saturation of the hemoglobin is affected by the partial pressure of oxygen, by the temperature, by the pH, and by the chemical and physical structure of the hemoglobin itself. Unless there is a significant change in the last three factors, the oxyhemoglobin dissociation curve can be used to compute the oxygen-carrying capacity of the blood.

References Values

95–100% (arterial sample)

Comparison with pO_2 values (normal pH and temperature):
98% = pO_2 of 100 mm Hg
95% = pO_2 of 80 mm Hg
89% = pO_2 of 60 mm Hg
84% = pO_2 of 50 mm Hg
35% = pO_2 of 20 mm Hg

Decrease in the Oxygen Saturation

Clinical Significance. A decreased oxygen saturation of arterial blood occurs any time there is a decrease in the pO_2. So usually all one needs to do to assess the hypoxic state is simply to measure the pO_2 of the blood. The oxygen saturation is lowered with the lowered pH.

Besides a low pH, either abnormal hemoglobin or shunting blood from the venous to the arterial system causes decreased oxygen saturation. The oxygen saturation is also very low with carbon monoxide poisoning because CO combines with hemoglobin over 200 times faster than O_2 does.

Possible Nursing Implications. The key points about the care of the patient in a hypoxic state were covered in the discussion on pO_2. The additional information from the oxygen saturation test is usually part of the assessment of a patient who is having cardiac catherization studies. Surgical procedures may be done for various types of cardiac defects.

Questions

6–1. In addition to blood pH, the two other basic laboratory tests for assessing acid–base balance are which of the following?

    a. pO_2 and pCO_2.   **c.** HCO_3- and pO_2.

    b. pCO_2 and bicarbonate (HCO_3^-).   **d.** Na+ and K+.

6–2. In a patient who has no metabolic acid–base problems, hyperventilation will cause which of the following?

    a. ↓ pCO_2 ↓ pH of serum.   **c.** ↑ pCO_2 ↑ pH of serum.

    b. ↓ pCO_2 ↑ pH of serum.   **d.** ↑ pCO_2 ↓ pH of serum.

6-3. In the patient with no metabolic acid–base imbalances, hypoventilation will result in which of the following?

    a. ↓pCO₂ and ↓pH of serum.   **c.** ↑pCO₂ and ↑pH of serum.

    b. ↓pCO₂ and ↑pH of serum.   **d.** ↑ pCO₂ and ↓pH of serum.

6-4. In the patient with chronic lung disease, the kidneys can compensate for an elevated pCO₂ by which of the following?

    a. Retaining additional HCO₃⁻ (bicarb).

    b. Excreting more Na+ and K+ ions.

    c. Excreting carbonic acid.

    d. Retaining H+ ions to balance the pCO₂.

6-5. When a patient has blood drawn from the radial artery for arterial blood gases (ABG) the nurse should do all of the following *except* which?

    a. Pack the blood sample in ice for transport to the laboratory.

    b. Keep pressure on the puncture site for at least 5 minutes.

    c. Transfer the blood sample to a heparinized test tube.

    d. Record whether or not the patient was breathing room air when the ABG's were drawn.

6-6. Which of the following assessments by the nurse does *not* support the possibility that the patient is going into metabolic acidosis?

    a. Headache.   **b.** Drowsiness.   **c.** Confusion.   **d.** Muscle spasms.

6-7. Mrs. Candy is admitted in a diabetic coma. The aide reports to the nurse that, on admission, Mrs. Candy's respirations are rapid (38) and seem very deep. The nurse should do which of the following?

    a. Recheck the respirations since it is usual to have such a high rate since she is retaining CO₂.

    b. Check for signs of infection since this is probably causing the increased rate.

    c. Notify the doctor that the patient is having dyspnea.

    d. Know that none of the above actions show an understanding of acid–base balance.

6-8. Which of the following assessments by the nurse does not support the possibility that a patient is going into metabolic alkalosis?

    a. Twitching.   **c.** Slow, shallow breaths.

    b. Irritability.   **d.** Difficult to arouse.

6-9. Michael, a 7-lb newborn, has an Apgar score of 7 (the normal is 10). He lost points for heart rate, respiratory rate, and color. The meperidine (Demerol) given to his mother before delivery has resulted in the newborn having a slight:

a. metabolic alkalosis (bicarbonate excess).

b. respiratory alkalosis (low pCO_2).

c. metabolic acidosis (bicarbonate deficit).

d. respiratory acidosis (high pCO_2).

6-10. In a normal pregnancy blood gases are which of the following?

a. The same as in the nonpregnant state.

b. A lower pCO_2 and a lower HCO_3^-.

c. A higher pCO_2 and a higher HCO_3^-.

d. A lower pCO_2 and a higher HCO_3^-.

6-11. High concentrations of oxygen may be dangerous for the patient with a chronically elevated pCO_2 because the patient:

a. may develop respiratory distress due to oxygen toxicity.

b. will no longer have hypoxia as a stimulus for breathing.

c. depends on the pCO_2 as a stimulus for breathing.

d. has a high pCO_2, not a low pO_2.

6-12. Respiratory alkalosis (low pCO_2) could result from all of the following situations *except* which?

a. Hypoxia.   b. Fever.   c. Hysteria.   d. Narcotic overdose.

6-13. Which *one* of the following patients should be observed for possible signs of tetany if the calcium levels are borderline normal?

a. Mr. Vick who had a cardiac arrest yesterday.

b. Ms. Rona who tends to hyperventilate when she is anxious.

c. Mrs. Degas who was hypotensive after her delivery today.

d. Baby Fong who is in respiratory distress.

6-14. Deborah, age 18, is in the emergency room. She says she is having an ''anxiety'' attack. She complains of feeling light-headed and ''shaky'' all over. Which action by the nurse would *not* be appropriate in this situation?

a. Have Deborah practice taking rapid deep breaths.

b. Provide a calm, soothing environment.

c. Help her identify what has made her so anxious now.

d. Ask Deborah to breathe into a paper bag.

6-15. Which type of loss from the gastrointestinal tract contributes to the development of metabolic alkalosis (high serum bicarbonate)?

    a. Draining fistula from pancreatic cyst.   **c.** Diarrhea.

    b. Gastric suctioning.   **d.** Ileostomy drainage.

6-16. Which one of the following conditions does not cause a decrease in the serum bicarbonate (HCO_3^-) level?

    a. Prolonged decrease in the pCO_2.   **c.** Markedly increased serum ketones.

    b. Increased serum chloride level.   **d.** Decreased serum potassium level.

6-17. Jimmy, age 6, has lost an abnormal amount of chlorides because of vomiting. The loss of chlorides would contribute to which of the following?

    a. Respiratory alkalosis (low pCO_2).   **c.** Metabolic alkalosis (base excess).

    b. Respiratory acidosis (high pCO_2).   **d.** Metabolic acidosis (base deficit).

6-18. Betty Parker was admitted to the hospital with severe hyperemesis gravidarum. She has been unable to retain any meals or liquids. Her dehydrated and near-starvation state make her a candidate for which of the following?

    a. Metabolic acidosis (base deficit).   **c.** Respiratory acidosis (high pCO_2).

    b. Metabolic alkalosis (base excess).   **d.** Respiratory alkalosis (low pCO_2).

6-19. Rhonda, a 6-lb, 2-oz newborn, had a normal Apgar score. A half-hour after birth, her temperature is 96.8 R. She must burn extra calories because she is cold-stressed. Unless she is warmed and fed, she is likely to develop which of the following?

    a. Metabolic acidosis (base deficit).   **c.** Metabolis alkalosis (base excess).

    b. Respiratory acidosis (high pCO_2).   **d.** Respiratory alkalosis (low pCO_2).

6-20. The anion gap is increased (that is, the unmeasured negative ions are increased) in which of these types of metabolic acidosis?

    a. Primary loss of serum bicarbonate.   **c.** Increase of chlorides.

    b. Build-up of organic acids.   **d.** All of the above.

6-21. Mrs. Landino has been receiving sodium bicarbonate intravenously for an acidotic state. The nursing assessment that would indicate that the sodium bicarbonate has restored the blood pH to normal is which of the following?

    a. Blood pressure is in normal range.

    b. Urine output has increased.

    c. Irritability and muscle spasms are less.

    d. Respirations have returned to normal.

6-22. For a middle-aged adult, hypoxia is generally defined as a pO_2 less than:

   a. 90 mm Hg.   **b.** 80 mm Hg.   **c.** 70 mm Hg.   **d.** 60 mm Hg.

6-23. In the adult, central cyanosis is present as a symptom of hypoxia, when the pO_2 is below:

   a. 70 mm Hg.   **b.** 60 mm Hg.   **c.** 50 mm Hg.   **d.** 40 mm Hg.

6-24. For a patient with a low pO_2, regardless of the cause for the hypoxia, nursing interventions would *always* include which of the following?

   a. Assisting with correcting the underlying acid–base imbalance.

   b. Ensuring optimal oxygen utilization.

   c. Administering oxygen.

   d. Keeping the patient as quiet as possible.

6-25. Blood gases drawn on a patient reveal a normal pO_2, a slightly low pCO_2, and a slightly high pH. Which of the following situations would most likely produce these blood gas results?

   a. Mr. Emory who has chronic emphysema.

   b. Bobby Black who is in diabetic acidosis.

   c. Mrs. Calhoun who is recovering from anesthesia and has had a lot of muscle relaxants.

   d. Mrs. Delgado who has been using breathing exercises during her labor contractions.

6-26. Mr. Cope has been admitted with a diagnosis of respiratory acidosis due to a chronic lung condition. When looking at his lab data, which of the following would be indicative of his acid–base difficulty? (Assume some compensation has occurred.)

   a. High blood pH, low pCO_2, high HCO_3^-.

   b. Low blood pH, high pCO_2, high HCO_3^-.

   c. High blood pH, low pCO_2, low HCO_3^-.

   d. Low blood pH, high pCO_2, low HCO_3^-.

6-27. Bill Phillips is on a respirator due to a drug overdose. Which of the following set of blood gases would be an indication that the respirator needs to be set at a lower rate?

   a. pCO_2 60 mm Hg, pO_2 100 mm Hg, pH 7.32, HCO_3^- 28 mEq.

   b. pCO_2 40 mm Hg, pO_2 80 mm Hg, pH 7.42, HCO_3^- 25 mEq.

   c. pCO_2 30 mm Hg, pO_2 98 mm Hg, pH 7.56, HCO_3^- 26 mEq.

   d. pCO_2 45 mm Hg, pO_2 110 mm Hg, pH 7.42, HCO_3^- 29 mEq.

REFERENCES

Bloch, Bobbie and Hunter, Mary. "Teaching Physiological Assessment of Black Persons," *Nurse Educator* 6 (January–February 1981): 24–27.

Boyce, Barbara and King, Thomas. "Blood–Gas and Acid–Base Concepts in Respiratory Care," *American Journal of Nursing* 76 (June 1976): 963–992.

Chan, James. "Clinical Disorders of Sodium, Potassium, Chloride and Sulfur Metabolism. Diagnostic Approach to Children," *Urology* 12 (November 1978): 504–508.

Copeland, Lucia. "Chronic Diarrhea in Infancy," *American Journal of Nursing* 77 (March 1977): 461–463.

Dingle, Rebecca *et al*. "Continuous Transcutaneous O_2 Monitoring in the Neonate," *American Journal of Nursing* 80 (May 1980): 890–893.

Engberg, Sandra. "Blood Gases," *Journal of Emergency Nursing* 2 (November–December 1976): 9–13.

Felton, Cynthia. "Hypoxemia and Oral Temperatures," *American Journal of Nursing* 87 (January 1978): 56–57.

Holum, John. *Elements of General and Biological Chemistry,* 5th ed. New York: John Wiley & Sons, Inc., 1979.

Kaplan, Alex and Szabo, LaVerne. *Clinical Chemistry: Interpretation and Technique.* Philadelphia: Lea and Febiger, 1979.

Lee, Carla *et al*. "What to Do When Acid–Base Problems Hang in the Balance," *Nursing 75* 5 (August 1975): 32–37.

Miller, Marjorie and Sherman, Raymond. "Metabolic Acid–Base Disorders, Part I: Chemistry and Physiology," *American Journal of Nursing* 77 (October 1977): 1619–1650.

Miller, Marjorie and Sherman, Raymond. "Metabolic Acid–Base Disorders, Part II: Physiological Abnormalities and Nursing Actions," *American Journal of Nursing* 78 (January 1978): 87–108.

Miller, Marjorie and Sherman, Raymond. "Metabolic Acid–Base Disorders, Part III: Clinical and Laboratory Findings," *American Journal of Nursing* 78 (March 1978): 1–16.

Milne, J. A. "The Respiratory Response to Pregnancy," *Postgraduate Medical Journal* 55 (May 1979): 318–324.

Narins, Robert *et al*. "The Anion Gap (Letters to the Editor)." *Lancet* 11 (June 18, 1977): 1304.

Nielson, Lois. "Pulmonary Oxygen Toxicity and Other Hazards of Oxygen Therapy." *American Journal of Nursing* 81 (December 1980): 2213–2215.

Pavlin, Edward and Hornbein, Thomas. "The Control of Breathing," *Basics of Respiratory Disease* 7 (November 1978): 1–6.

Sandvik, Jacqueline. "The Emergency Management of Hyperventilation," *Journal of Emergency Nursing* 3 (July–August 1977): 17–20.

Shrake, Kevin. "The ABC's of ABG's or How to Interpret a Blood Gas Value," *Nursing 79* 9 (September 1979): 26–33.

Smithline, Neil and Gardner, Kenneth. "Gaps—Anionic and Osmolal," *JAMA* 236 (October 4, 1976): 1594–1597.

Sumner, Sara. "Refining Your Technique for Drawing Arterial Blood Gases," *Nursing 80* 10 (April 1980): 65–69.

Waites, Thad. "Hyperventilation—Chronic and Acute," *Archives International Medicine* 138 (November 1978): 1700–1701.

Worthington, Laura. "What Those Blood Gases Can Tell You," *RN* 42 (October 1979): 23–27.

CHAPTER SEVEN

Three Less Commonly Measured Electrolytes

Objectives

1. Explain the relationship of parathyroid hormone (parathormone) to serum and urine levels of calcium and phosphorus.
2. Identify nursing assessments useful in detecting hypercalcemia or hypocalcemia, including the Sulkowitch test for urine calcium.
3. Plan appropriate nursing interventions to decrease the harmful effects of hypercalcemia.
4. Analyze clinical situations to determine which patients are likely to have changes in serum phosphorus or calcium levels.
5. Describe the nursing implications of treatment and medications used for calcium/phosphorus imbalances.
6. Prepare a teaching plan for patients who must decrease or increase calcium and phosphorus intake.
7. Identify nursing assessments useful in detecting serum magnesium excess and deficiency.
8. Describe the nurse's role in treatments for magnesium excess and deficiency.

This chapter covers three electrolytes or minerals that appear in small amounts in the serum: calcium, phosphorus, and magnesium.

Both calcium and phosphorus serum levels are controlled by parathyroid hormone (parathormone or PTH), which also promotes the reabsorption of calcium and the excretion of phosphorus. The end results of an increased secretion of parathormone are an increased serum calcium and a decreased serum phosphorus level. Although the serum calcium level often varies inversely with the phosphorus level due to this hormonal control, both calcium and phosophorus may be increased or decreased together in other clinical situations. Calcium and phosphorus are discussed in separate sections, but the reader needs to be aware that both tests are useful in assessing an imbalance of either electrolyte. In addition, urinary tests for both may give additional information about their overall metabolism. Methods of testing for calcium and phosphorus in the urine are discussed after each section on the electrolytes.

Magnesium is less well understood than the other two electrolytes. It is known that a marked increase in serum magnesium has been shown to decrease the release of parathyroid hormone (Goodman 1975:970), and that aldosterone causes an increase of serum magnesium as it does of potassium. The section on magnesium discusses the interrelationship of magnesium to calcium and potassium in deficiency states.

Unlike the more commonly measured electrolytes discussed in Chapter 5 ($Na+$, $K+$, $Cl-$, HCO_3^-), the three electrolytes in this chapter are not always measured in milliequivalents (see Chapter 5 for a definition of milliequivalent). Since a particular laboratory may use either mg or mEq, reference values using both systems are presented. In addition, some laboratories may use the SI (Systeme International) discussed in Chapter 1. For Na, K, Cl and HCO_3, the SI and the mEq figures are the same. But with Ca, P, and Mg, the SI figures are different from the mEq. (See Appendix A for the SI equivalents.)

CALCIUM

Calcium is a positively charged ion ($Ca++$) that is in small concentrations in the bloodstream. Calcium circulates in the bloodstream both in the free or ionized state and bound to plasma proteins. The bound calcium, carried chiefly by albumin, is about half of the total calcium in the bloodstream. Since most laboratories measure the total calcium level, not just the ionized calcium, a change in the serum albumin level means a change in the total serum reference values. A decrease of 1 g of albumin means that the serum total calcium level is about 0.8 mg less. Since the free, or ionized, calcium affects neuromuscular function, a low calcium level due to a low albumin level does not make the patient symptomatic for hypocalcemia. When the serum albumin level is not normal, some laboratories measure the ionized part of the serum calcium to get a clearer picture of any calcium deficiency. Factors that cause decreased serum albumin levels are discussed in Chapter 10.

The amount of calcium in the serum is quite small compared to that present in the teeth and bones. The bones contain a tremendous reservoir of calcium that can be used if needed to keep the serum calcium level normal. Two hormones control serum calcium levels. Calcitonin, a hormone secreted by the thyroid gland, protects against a calcium excess in the serum. Parathormone (PTH), secreted by the parathyroid gland, functions to keep a sufficient level of calcium in the bloodstream; an increase in parathormone not only increases the serum calcium level, it also decreases phosphorus levels. Thus, for many types of serum calcium imbalance, it is important to evaluate the serum phosphorus level too. The relationship of phosphorus to calcium is discussed in detail in the next section on serum phosphorus levels.

Calcium is obtained in several food sources, of which milk products are the best: A cup of milk, for example, contains 236 mg of calcium. Other sources that contain a fairly large amount of calcium include vegetables, such as turnip greens, collard greens, white beans and lentils (Table 7-1). Intestinal cells also need vitamin D to absorb calcium. Vitamin D is a unique vitamin made entirely in the body from cholesterol and a photochemical reaction (Wood 1977). Thus sunlight and a diet adequate in fat are also impor-

TABLE 7-1. EXAMPLES OF FOODS HIGH IN CALCIUM
AND/OR PHOSPHORUS*

Food in 100-g Portions	Calcium in mg	Phosphorus in mg
Swiss cheese	925	563
Cheddar cheese	750	478
Brick cheese	730	455
American cheese	697	771
Turnip greens	246	58
Almonds	234	504
Collard greens	203	63
Beans, white	144	425
Milk (100 g = scant ½ cup)	118	93
Frankfurter	32	603
Bologna	32	581
Peanuts	69	401
Whole wheat flour	41	372
Liver	8	352

* Modified from Linkswiler (1979) with permission.

tant to ensure proper levels of vitamin D. Protein is also required for the proper utilization
of calcium. Chronic nutritional deficiencies of calcium, vitamin D, and protein eventually
result in lowered serum calcium levels. Yet, due to the vast reservoir of calcium in the
bones, dietary deficiencies do not immediately cause lowered serum calcium levels.

Infants require 360 to 540 mg of calcium, depending on age. Children and adults
require around 800 mg of calcium. Adolescents, as well as pregnant and lactating women,
have the greatest requirement for calcium, which is around 1,200 mg (American Academy
of Pediatrics, 1978). Excess calcium is excreted in the urine. The measurement of urinary
calcium is covered after the discussion on serum calcium levels.

Preparation of the Patient
And Collection of the Sample

Three ml of serum are needed. Some laboratories require a fasting state, although water is
allowed. BSP dye interferes with the test.

Reference Values

Adults	Calcium levels tend to be slightly higher in males. 8.5 to 10.5 mg/dl or 4.3 to 5.3 mEq/l.
Pregnancy	Falls gradually to a level at term about 10% below nonpregnant level. Consistent with the fall in albumin.
Newborns	7.4 to 14 mg/dl or 3.7 to 7 mEq*
Children	Slightly higher in children—may be up to 12 mg.

* Children's Hospital San Francisco considers below 8 abnormal for a 1,500 gm
infant and below 7.5 mg/dl abnormal for an infant below 1,500 g. Remember
that if the serum albumin level drops 1 g, the total serum calcium level drops
0.8 mg, even though the ionized calcium remains the same. Always interpret
calcium levels in relation to serum albumin levels.

Increased Serum Calcium Level (Hypercalcemia)

Clinical Significance. As with many other tests, dehydration gives a pseudo-high reading for the serum calcium level. An increased level of the parathyroid hormone, parathormone, causes a persistently elevated serum calcium level. Since adenomas of the parathyroid gland can cause the gland to produce additional amounts of parathormone, the physician may order several other tests, including an assay of parathormone levels (PTH) to rule out the possibility that a parathyroid tumor is responsible for hypercalcemia.

There are several more common reasons for the serum calcium level being higher than normal. The most common is the release of calcium in metastatic bone disease as bone is destroyed. Also, some of the hormonal changes in malignant states may contribute to raising the serum calcium level. Some tumors produce parathormone-like substances. (See Chapter 15 for a discussion on ectopic hormone production.) Long-term immobilization may result in increased serum calcium levels because the lack of normal bone stress causes the release of calcium from bone. Thiazide diuretics are another reason for hypercalcemia. Excessive milk intake (meaning at least three quarts of milk a day) is a less frequent cause of hypercalcemia. Vitamin D intoxication can also result in hypercalcemia.

Possible Nursing Implications.

Assisting with Follow-Up for Diagnosis. Often the patient may be asymptomatic even though the laboratory report shows a higher-than-normal serum calcium level. In borderline cases, the test may be repeated several times over a period of weeks or months, in addition to other diagnostic studies, such as the parathyroid hormone assay (discussed in Chapter 15). If the high serum calcium level is due to parathyroid dysfunction, the patient may eventually have to undergo surgery to remove part of the parathyroid gland.

TABLE 7-2.   COMMON CAUSES OF HYPERCALCEMIA AND HYPOCALCEMIA*
(Serum P = Serum Phosphorus Levels Which Help with Interpretation of Serum Ca)

Hypercalcemia (Serum Ca++ levels above 10.5 mg/dl or see values for specific laboratories.)
1. Pseudo-rise due to dehydration
2. Hyperparathyroidism (serum P decreased)
3. Malignancies
4. Immobilization
5. Thiazide diuretics
6. Vitamin D intoxication (serum P increased)

Hypocalcemia (Serum Ca++ levels below 8.5 mg/dl or see values for specific laboratory.)
Infants have lower values to 8 or 7.5 mg/dl.
1. Pseudo-decrease due to low albumin levels
2. Hypoparathyroidism (serum P increased)
3. Early neonatal hypocalcemia
4. Chronic renal disease (serum P increased)
5. Pancreatitis
6. Massive blood transfusions
7. Severe malnutrition (serum P decreased)
8. Symptoms of hypocalcemia when patient is alkalotic although total serum calcium is normal (see text).

* See text for explanation and Chan (1979), Tripp (1976), Canalis (1977), and Felver (1980).

Other types of hypercalcemia are not treated surgically. In some situations, such as the patient with a malignancy, since treating the elevated serum calcium levels may be very difficult, the patient continually has elevated serum calcium levels.

Preventing Pathologic Fractures. If the hypercalcemia is a result of loss of calcium from the bones, the patient becomes very susceptible to fractures. These types of fractures are referred to as *pathologic fractures* because the bone is made fragile by a pathological process. Patients who are prone to pathological fractures must be handled very gently. The nurse must be alert to any vague symptoms of bone pain. Sometimes just turning in bed can cause a fracture. If ambulation is possible, weight bearing can help to minimize loss of calcium from the weight-bearing bones. A walker or other supportive device is essential for safety.

Preventing Renal Calculi. An increased serum calcium level almost always means an increased calcium excretion by the kidneys. Thus, insofar as a high concentration of calcium in the urine may lead to the formation of renal stones (*calculi*), it is very important that a patient with hypercalcemia stay well hydrated. Some authorities suggest that the urine volume needs to be above 2,500 ml in 24 hours (Smith 1978). Health teaching for the patient at home should include information on how to make sure the urine is never concentrated; the person must be aware of the importance of drinking fluids at bedtime and also during the night. A visiting nurse can help make out a schedule for the patient or for a member of the family to follow.

Calcium is more likely to precipitate in an alkaline urine. Yet, since the urine pH is normally acid (around 6), precipitation may not be a threat unless the patient gets a urinary tract infection, which may make the urine alkaline. Measures, such as the intake of cranberry juice, to change an alkaline urine to acid are discussed in Chapter 3.

Assessing for Other Effects of Hypercalcemia. The patient with an increased serum calcium level may demonstrate some slowing of reflexes. Because increased serum calcium levels decrease the permeability of nerve cell membranes to sodium, the depolarization process is affected, and the nerve fibers have a decreased excitability. This condition may result in some lethargy or a general sluggish feeling. Other possible problems may be vague abdominal pains and constipation; confusion may develop. An elevated serum calcium level also tends to slow the heart. So if the patient is on digoxin, a high serum calcium level may be particularly dangerous because it potentiates the effect of the digoxin.

Assisting with Drug Therapy for Hypercalcemia. Although several drugs may be used to reduce high serum calcium levels, none of them are entirely satisfactory. So a search is continuing for more effective drugs (Canalis 1977). Currently used drugs include:

1. calcitonin,
2. phosphates,
3. mithramycin, and
4. glucorticosteroids.

Forcing fluids and diuretics may also be prescribed.

1. *Calcitonin* (Calcimar), a synthetic preparation of the hormone produced by the thyroid gland, is being investigated as a treatment for certain types of transitory hypercal-

cemia. Presently calcitonin is used mostly to lower serum calcium levels and to increase bone formation in the patient with Paget's disease who has considerable bone destruction. Patients with Paget's disease may take calcitonin injections daily over a long period of time. Often the nurse needs to teach the patient how to do the injections at home. The serum calcium levels needs to be evaluated periodically when the patient is on this drug.

2. *Phosphates* decrease serum calcium levels on the principle that an increased serum phosphate level causes a decreased serum calcium level. Presumably, the higher phosphate level promotes the deposition of calcium in the bone and decreases the reabsorption of bone (Goodman 1975:787). The disadvantage is that there may be some deposition of calcium in soft tissues as well. The use of phosphates is a slow process, and the patient must have good renal function.

3. *Mithramycin,* an antineoplastic drug, is also sometimes used to reduce high serum calcium levels in patients with malignancies. A single dose may reduce elevated serum calcium levels for three to fifteen days (Canalis 1977). However, a rebound hypercalcemia, along with many toxic side effects, may result from the use of this drug.

4. Of the *glucorticosteroids,* prednisone and some others reduce serum calcium levels, but they may take a week to ten days to do so. As with all the other drugs, the nurse must be aware of the potential side effects from the use of corticosteroids. (See Chapter 15 on hormones.)

Sometimes more than one type of drug therapy may be tried to see which one has the best effect on lowering the serum calcium level. With all these drugs, the patient must be well hydrated all the time, including during the night.

Teaching About Dietary Restrictions. Depending on the underlying pathophysiology, the dietary restriction of foods high in calcium may be used to control hypercalcemia. Restricting milk and milk products very dramatically reduces the calcium intake. Other sources of calcium—such as dried legumes, broccoli, and some other dark green leafy vegetables—probably do not need to be restricted if dairy products are reduced or eliminated (Mundy 1977). The nurse needs to consult with the doctor about what degree of diet restriction may help to alleviate the high serum calcium levels. Then any restrictions can be explained to the patient. Since hypercalcemia may be due to complex pathological processes, the value of diet restriction must be evaluated in relation to the particular medical problem that exists. Table 7–1 gives examples of foods high in calcium.

Decreased Serum Calcium Level (Hypocalcemia)

Clinical Significance. First of all, since much of the serum calcium is bound to albumin it is important to make sure that the lowered serum calcium level is not due to a lowered serum albumin level.

Just as *hyper*parathyroidism causes *hyper*calcemia, *hypo*parathyroidism causes *hypo*calcemia, because the parathyroid hormone, parathormone, controls serum calcium levels. Hypoparathyroidism, or a lack of parathormone, can be due to accidental damage to the parathyroids during thyroid surgery. The hypocalcemia may be more severe from surgical removal of the parathyroids than from the other various causes of hypoparathyroidism.

Early neonatal hypocalcemia is a clinical condition experienced by many pre-term infants in the first 24 to 48 hours of life. The exact reason for this kind of hypocalcemia is not known (Domenech 1978).

Hypocalcemia is also commonly seen in patients with renal failure when there is an impaired elimination of acid phosphates. The increase of phosphates in the serum causes a decreased calcium level due to the inverse relationship between these two levels. (See the beginning of the chapter for an explanation of this interrelationship due to parathormone control.) Also in chronic renal disease, since the kidney is unable to finish the process of making vitamin D chemically active, calcium absorption is impaired. The tubules of the kidney are responsible for the final active form of vitamin D, which functions as calcitriol, a hormone necessary for calcium absorption. Vitamin D is the only vitamin known to be converted to a hormonal form (DeLuca 1981:1). Children who have chronic renal disease may develop rickets because of the lowered serum calcium levels.

Serum calcium levels can also be lowered because calcium is being deposited in tissues. In pancreatitis, the fatty acids that are released can bind up calcium. The pancreas may actually become calcified in areas of necrotic tissue. In massive blood transfusions, the serum calcium level may drop because the calcium ions in the blood are bound by the citrate that the blood bank uses as the anticoagulant. The liver removes the citrate from the circulation, but it may not be able to do so fast enough when a large amount of blood is infused.

Severe malnutrition may eventually lead to hypocalcemia, but, due to the vast reserves of calcium in the bones, a calcium-deficient diet does not immediately cause a drop in serum calcium levels. Hence a pregnant or lactating woman who does not have enough calcium intake continues to have a normal serum calcium level as she loses calcium from the teeth and bones. Children and elderly people who have calcium-deficient diets usually retain normal serum calcium levels too. But the child develops rickets, and the older person develops osteomalacia or a softening of the bones. A very severe malnutrition that includes a lack of vitamin D and protein eventually causes a lowered serum calcium level when calcium cannot be released from the bones or teeth.

The nurse should bear in mind the effect of pH on calcium solubility. In alkalotic states, even though the total serum calcium does not change, the amount of ionized calcium is less because calcium is less soluble in an alkaline medium. A decrease in the ionized portion of serum calcium causes symptoms of hypocalcemia even though the laboratory test looks normal. (Recall that the serum calcium level measures both bound calcium and ionized calcium.)

When the patient is acidotic, the total serum calcium level may be low, but the patient has few symptoms as long as he or she is acidotic because more calcium is in the ionized state. When the pH returns to normal, there is less ionized calcium and the symptoms of hypocalcemia become apparent. Thus acidotic states may ''mask'' a true hypocalcemia state.

Possible Nursing Implications.

Assessing for Hypocalcemia. The symptoms of hypocalcemia vary depending on how low the level of serum calcium drops and on how abruptly it drops. Hypocalcemia causes muscle twitching and cramps, which may lead to generalized muscle spasms that are called *tetany*. These cramps in the muscles are due to the neuromuscular irritability from the lack of calcium ions. In the patient with a low serum calcium level, a tapping of the jaw causes a facial spasm (Chovstek's sign). Another assessment for low serum calcium levels is to look for carpopedal spasms or spasms in the hands. The carpopedal spasms may be elicited when the arm becomes a little ischemic. For example, when the nurse takes the blood pressure, the patient's hand may twitch when the cuff is left inflated for a couple of minutes (Trousseau's sign). Very subtle signs of neuromuscular irritability due to hypocalcemia, such as a twitching of the nose, may be overlooked unless the nurse is aware that any neuromuscular irritability should be watched for in a patient who is a candidate for hypocalcemia. In the newborn the symptoms may include twitching or convulsions. Treatment for newborns is advocated when levels drop below 7.0 mg/dl (Domenech 1978). The symptoms of hypocalcemia often coincide with hypoglycemia in the newborn. (See Chapter 8 for a discussion on hypoglycemia in the newborn.)

Since the patient with the potential for hypocalcemia may have a convulsive state, the nurse must be prepared for such a possibility. Calcium gluconate for intravenous administration should be on an emergency cart. After thyroid or parathyroid surgery, an ampule of calcium gluconate is usually kept at the bedside. Patients at risk for hypocalcemia usually have their serum calcium levels measured daily.

Assisting with Replacement of Calcium. The treatment for hypocalcemia depends on the underlying cause. To prevent tetany and convulsions, the serum calcium level must be raised quickly to normal. If the signs of tetany are severe, the physician orders calcium to be given intravenously. Several different salts of calcium are available, but usually calcium gluconate is given for fast replacement. Unlike potassium, calcium can be given directly by intravenous push. (In most clinical situations, the physician must give medications that are given by intravenous push.) The medication may give the patient a feeling of warmth due to the vasodilation that occurs, along with a drop in the blood pressure, for which the patient must be monitored.

In less acute situations—when the patient is having few symptoms—an ampule of calcium gluconate may be added to a bottle of intravenous fluid. Since calcium precipitates in an alkaline medium, calcium salts can never be added to intravenous fluids with an alkaline pH. Most dextrose and saline solutions are acid in pH, but this point must be carefully checked since an intravenous may also contain sodium bicarbonate.

Before the start of any type of calcium replacement, a blood sample must be drawn to determine the baseline serum calcium level. After or during calcium replacement therapy, other samples may be drawn to make sure that the serum calcium level is not becoming higher than normal. Because calcium has a profound effect on the heart, some physicians may choose to have the patient on a cardiac monitor all the while calcium is being replaced. This precaution is all the more likely if the patient is also on digoxin, since calcium increases the possibility of digitalis toxicity.

For mild hypocalcemia, and in chronic states, the patient may be given various oral preparations of calcium salts. Newborns may be given oral supplements, once feedings are tolerated. The nurse needs to find out whether the particular preparation being used should be taken on an empty stomach. With some preparations, alkaline foods and milk tend to decrease the absorption of calcium. The calcium of other preparations may have a bitter taste or cause gastrointestinal irritation, so that it is better tolerated with food. Patients on calcium supplements should not take tetracyclines since calcium interferes with the absorption of this type of antibiotic (Goodman 1975). Metabolites of vitamin D, such as calciferol, or calcitrol, are used to increase serum calcium levels. The use of vitamin D supplements requires careful monitoring of serum calcium levels because vitamin D has a cumulative effect.

Dietary Teaching. Calcium requirements are best met by having adequate calcium in the diet. So the nurse must assess the dietary habits of individuals to determine whether their calcium intake is adequate. If the patient does not like milk or cheese (which, as dairy products, are among the best sources for calcium), powdered milk can be added to many dishes without changing their taste. A tablespoon of powdered milk contains nearly 50 mg of calcium. Since elderly patients may have a decrease in gastric hydrochloric acid, for example, their calcium absorption is impaired; also a lack of protein decreases calcium utilization (Tripp 1976).

Another way to help raise the serum calcium level is to reduce the amount of phosphate intake. (The relationship of high phosphorus levels to low serum calcium levels is discussed next in the section on phosphorus.) Oral antacids that contain magnesium or aluminum (Aludrox) are sometimes ordered with meals to help bind up phosphates so that more calcium can be absorbed. If the low serum calcium level, related to a high serum phosphorus level, is due to renal failure, medications containing aluminum, not magnesium hydroxide, are prescribed to lower the serum phosphorous level. The reason is that magnesium is not excreted well in renal dysfunction (Goodman 1975).

Special Emphasis for Symptoms of Hypocalcemia in Alkalosis. If the patient is having symptoms of tetany because less calcium is in an ionized state, the patient is not given calcium as the treatment. In alkalosis, the symptoms arise from a lack of ionized calcium, not from a *true lack* of calcium. When the pH returns to normal, the calcium is once again ionized in the correct amount for neuromuscular functioning. (The possible nursing implications for the patient in alkalosis are covered in Chapter 6.)

URINARY CALCIUM LEVELS

Quantitative Method (24-Hour Urine Sample)

Preparation of Patient and Collection of Sample. All urine for 24 hours is collected in a special bottle that contains 10 ml of hydrochloric acid. The HCl is to keep the pH of the urine low (pH of 2 to 3) because calcium tends to precipitate in an alkaline medium. The patient stays on the usual diet. Any increased intake of protein by the patient should be noted since more calcium is excreted on a high-protein diet. (See Chapter 3 for general instructions about 24-hour urine collections.)

Reference Values

Adults	50–300 mg/d depending on dietary intake, usually less than 150 mg/d or 75 mEq.
Children	Range is around 5 mg per kg of body weight if on normal dietary intake of calcium (Chan 1978).

Clinical Significance of Results. Normally up to 99% of the calcium filtered by the kidneys is reabsorbed. An increased urinary calcium level is almost always due to an elevated serum calcium level (Chan 1979). The amount of calcium being excreted in the urine may differ for various types of hypercalcemia, so the 24-hour urine collection may give the physician extra diagnostic clues. For example, a highly elevated urine calcium does not usually accompany primary hyperparathyroidism because the increased amount of parathormone promotes additional reabsorption of calcium. In other types of hypercalcemia, such as with malignant tumors, the urine calcium level may be as high as 800 or 900 mg in 24 hours. In conditions where there is a low serum calcium level, the urinary excretion of calcium is very low.

Qualitative Method (Sulkowitch Test)

This is a test done on one specimen of urine to get a rough indication of the amount of calcium being excreted in the urine. The findings are reported as normal, increased, or decreased. Either the patient may be taught to do this test, or a visiting nurse can do it on a visit, since it is easy to perform.

Preparation of Patient and Collection of Sample. The patient should continue with the usual diet. If hypercalcemia is suspected, the urine should be collected before a meal. If hypocalcemia is suspected, the urine should be collected after a meal. A few drops of calcium oxalate solution are added to the urine specimen to see if precipitation occurs.

Reference Values

1. Heavy white precipitate indicates more-than-normal calcium in the urine.
2. Fine white cloud is considered to be within the normal range.
3. Clear specimen indicates less-than-normal calcium in the urine specimen.

Clinical Significance of Results. If hypercalcemia is suspected, the urine specimen should be collected in the morning before eating. An increased calcium in the urine in an early morning fasting specimen would be a strong indicator of persistent high serum calcium levels. If hypocalcemia is suspected, the urine specimen should be collected after meals. If the specimen remains clear even after meals, there is a strong possibility that the serum calcium level is always abnormally low. Patients may do these tests over a period of weeks to help assess the presence or absence of a problem. If they do, they must record not only the results but also the timing of the specimens in relation to meals.

SERUM PHOSPHORUS OR PHOSPHATES

Serum phosphorus levels are actually measured as phosphate ions. Laboratories may report phosphorus levels as phosphorus (P) or phosphate (PO_4) levels. Whereas potassium is the major intracellular *cation*, phosphorus is the major intracellular *anion*. So the majority of phosphorus is in bone tissue and skeletal muscle, and phosphates regulate many enzymatic actions that are critical for energy transformations. Since phosphorus has a very close relationship to calcium, the phosphorous level is usually more useful as a diagnostic tool when looked at in relation to the serum calcium level.

The phosphate electrolyte is the only electrolyte that is markedly different in values for children and adults. (The bicarbonate ion discussed in Chapter 5 does have slight variations with age.) The marked increase in phosphate ions in young children is partially explained by the increased amount of growth hormone that is present until puberty.

The recommended dietary allowances for phosphorus, except in infancy and lactation, is a one-to-one ratio to calcium. Thus an adult requires about 800 mg of phosphorus a day. In the infant and the lactating woman, the need for calcium exceeds the need for phosphorus. However, in most American diets, the intake of phosphorus is probably twice that of calcium: The average calcium intake may be around 700 mg, while the average phosphorus intake is about 1,500 mg (Linkswiler 1979). This higher phosphorus intake occurs for two reasons. First, phosphorus is abundant not only in dairy products but also in many natural foods. Second, many food additives contain a lot of phosphates. Linkswiler (1979), in a detailed discussion of the additional source of phosphorus from food processing, concludes that at the present time there are no data to suggest harm from the extra phosphates in the diet. Processed meat, cheese, and soft drinks are three sources that are quite high in phosphates. See Table 7–1 for a list of other foods that are high in calcium and/or phosphates.

Like calcium, phosphorus is controlled by the parathyroid hormone. Increases in the level of parathormone cause a decrease in the serum level of phosphorus and an increased secretion of phosphorus by the kidney.

Additional phosphates are excreted by the kidney. Some phosphate is also excreted in the feces. Drugs, such as aluminum hydroxide (Aludrox) can significantly increase the fecal excretion of phosphates.

Special Preparation of Patient
And Collection of Sample

Two ml of serum are needed. The patient should be in the fasting state, although water is allowed. Since increased carbohydrate metabolism lowers serum phosphorus levels, the patient should not have intravenous solutions of glucose running before the test. If an intravenous of glucose is being administered, note it on the laboratory slip. The serum needs to be sent to the lab as soon as possible since the laboratory must quickly separate the serum from the cells.

Reference Values

Adults	3.0–4.5 mg/dl or 1.8–2.6 mEq/l. Male values are slightly higher than female values.
Pregnancy	Slightly lower in pregnancy.
Newborns	5.7–9.5 mg/dl. May be higher ranges in prematures and for a few days after birth.
Infants and Children	4–7 mg. Levels decline with maturity.
Aged	May be slightly lower in the aged.

TABLE 7–3.   COMMON REASONS FOR CHANGES IN SERUM
PHOSPHATE LEVELS* (Serum Calcium Ca++ Helps in Interpretation)

Hyperphosphatemia (Serum phosphorus over 4.5 mg/dl in adult)
1. Hypoparathyroidism (serum Ca decreased)
2. Renal failure (serum Ca decreased)
3. Increased growth hormone
4. Vitamin D intoxication (serum Ca increased)

Hypophosphatemia (Serum phosphorus below 3 mg/dl in adult)
1. Hyperparathyroidism (serum Ca increased)
2. Diuresis
3. Malabsorption or malnutrition (serum Ca decreased)
4. Increased glucose metabolism—carbohydrate loading
5. Antacid abuse

* See text and Kreisberg (1977), Chan (1979), and Knochel (1977) for more details
and for less common medical conditions.

Increased Phosphate Level (Hyperphosphatemia)

Clinical Significance.   The clinical significance of an elevated phosphorus level is always
evaluated in relation to the serum calcium levels to get a clearer picture of what may be a
very complicated pathological process (see Table 7–3):

1. When the phosphorus level is elevated and the serum calcium level is low,
   hypoparathyroidism may be the reason. The lack of parathyroid hormone
   (parathormone) decreases the renal excretion of phosphates.
2. In some types of renal dysfunction, the kidneys cannot excrete phosphate ions. A
   high phosphate level in the serum then depresses the serum calcium level
   through several hormonal actions.
3. Diseases of childhood may sometimes involve an increase in the production of
   growth hormone. In such a case, the serum calcium level would not be elevated.
4. If the phosphates in the serum are·elevated due to vitamin D intoxication or to the
   excessive intake of milk, then the serum calcium is most likely elevated too.
5. In certain malignant conditions, the serum phosphate level may either remain
   normal or be somewhat elevated when the serum calcium is elevated.

Possible Nursing Implications.

Assessing for Other Pathology. There are no specific symptoms for an elevated
serum phosphorus level since it is but one aspect of one sort of complex pathophysiology
or another. Hence the related nursing implications depend on the underlying
pathophysiology. If the underlying problem is due to hypoparathyroidism, then replacement with calcium and vitamin D corrects the problem. If the phosphorus and calcium
levels are both elevated, the patient may be put on a moderately reduced calcium and
phosphorus diet by limiting dairy products.

Use of Medications and Dietary Restrictions. If the phosphorus level is high and the
calcium level is low, as often happens in renal failure, the patient may be put on medication to reduce the phosphate level. Aluminum hydroxide gels (AluCaps or Aludrox),

given by mouth, unite with the phosphates present in food to form insoluble aluminum phosphate. These insoluble phosphate compounds are then excreted in the feces. Magnesium hydroxide also binds phosphates, but the additional magnesium intake is contraindicated in renal failure. If the serum phosphorus level is increased and the serum calcium is normal or decreased, the restriction of dairy products must be countered by calcium supplements. It is hard to significantly reduce the serum phosphorus level by diet alone because phosphorus is abundant in many more foods than is calcium (Mundy 1977). Neither is it possible to reduce phosphorus levels by dialysis.

Decreased Serum Phosphorus Level (Hypophosphatemia)

Clinical Significance. Moderate hypophosphatemia can result from a variety of conditions (see Table 7–3):

1. Hyperparathyroidism results in a high serum calcium level and a low phosphorus level.
2. Diuretics may cause a low phosphorus level.
3. Phosphates can be lost in large amounts in some types of renal diseases, although phosphate retention is more common.
4. Drugs that bind up phosphate, such as aluminum or magnesium gels, can cause phosphate deficiency. However, diets are usually high in phosphates so this pharmacological binding of antacids is usually not a major concern.
5. Malabsorption syndromes may eventually lead to low serum phosphorus levels.

Other clinical conditions in which serum phosphorus concentrations may fall are alcoholic withdrawal, diabetes mellitus, the recovery diuretic phase after severe burns, hyperalimentation therapy, and nutritional recovery syndrome. Exactly why these clinical conditions cause hypophosphatemia is not completely understood. It is known that, when glucose metabolism is increased (carbohydrate loading), the phosphorus ions become tied up. Also a decrease in serum magnesium ions or a shift in potassium ions tends to create hypophosphatemia. Knochel (1977) has an extensive review of research done on hypophosphatemia over the past fifty years.

Possible Nursing Implications.
Assessing for Hypophosphatemia. Although severe hypophosphatemia has definite clinical consequences, the nurse may not be able to assess specific symptoms. A lack of serum phosphorus results in erythrocyte, leukocyte, and platelet dysfunction, but the effect clinically is still a subject of research (Knochel 1977). Also it is hypothesized that lowered serum phosphorus levels create central nervous system symptoms such as irritability and confusion. Hence nurses must be aware that patients with any altered electrolyte may not be able to function normally; so safety precautions become very important.
Assisting with Replacement. Therapy for low serum phosphate levels may include administration of phosphate salts in oral or intravenous form. In a patient with a severe metabolic problem, such as alcohol withdrawal or diabetic coma, numerous electrolyte disturbances must be corrected. Since patients likely to develop low phosphorus levels may also develop low potassium and low magnesium levels, the nurse must be familiar

with all the replacements being used. The greatest hazard of giving large amounts of phosphates is that hypocalcemia may result. If the patient can tolerate oral feedings, milk is a very good source of phosphorus. It is usually not necessary to do long-term health teaching about phosphorus intake because in a regular diet phosphates are abundant. The concern with the patient who has a low serum phosphorus level is to correct the often complex metabolic problem that has caused the deficiency in the serum. If the lowered serum phosphorus level is due to hyperparathyroidism, surgery is usually done.

URINARY PHOSPHORUS LEVELS

Preparation of Patient
And Collection of Sample
All urine is collected over a 24-hour period. There is no need for a preservative in the bottle, and the urine does not need to be iced. (Note that for urine calcium a preservative is needed. when both calcium and potassium are to be collected the preservative will not interfere with the test for phosphorus.)

Reference Values

All groups	0.4–1.3 g in 24 hours. Varies with intake. Average is 1 g in 24 hours.

Clinical Significance of Results. Urinary phosphorus levels usually reflect the amount of both organic and inorganic phosphates taken in the diet. Because parathormone causes a decreased renal reabsorption of phosphorus, hyperparathyroidism causes an increased urinary phosphorus level. This test may help to explain the alterations in serum calcium and phosphorus levels. In renal failure, the excretion of phosphates may be impaired so that the urinary phosphorus level is decreased. However, testing the urine in renal failure usually does not give any additional clinical help. The urinary phosphorus test is most often used when there is a complex metabolic problem, such as an endocrine disturbance or malnutrition problems, and when a very complete investigation of all electrolyte disturbances needs to be done to monitor the progress of the patient.

MAGNESIUM (Mg + +)

Primarily an intracellular ion, magnesium appears in the bloodstream only in very small amounts. The bulk of magnesium is combined with calcium and phosphorus in the bones. Magnesium is essential for neuromuscular function and for activation of certain enzymes in the body. Changes in serum magnesium levels affect other serum ions, too, such as potassium, calcium, and phosphorus. Thus magnesium deficiency is not usually seen alone. Evidently the body can store magnesium, because deficiencies usually develop in chronic conditions not in acute conditions.

Since magnesium is present in a variety of foods, a normal diet supplies the recommended daily allowances. Magnesium requirements for infants and children may range from 60 to 250 mg, depending on age, but optimum levels for children are not clearly established (Chan 1979). Adult males need around 350 mg and adult females around 300 mg. Pregnancy and lactation increase the need to around 450 mg. The average intake of magnesium in the adult diet is probably around 400 mg (Elbaum 1977).

Magnesium is excreted primarily by the kidney. The hormone aldosterone causes an increased excretion of magnesium as it does of potassium. Compared to the facts known about potassium, much is still to be learned about how magnesium functions in the body. (See Chapter 5 for a detailed discussion of the effect of aldosterone on potassium levels.)

Preparation of Patient
And Collection of Sample

The patient does not have to be fasting. One ml of serum is needed. Calcium gluconate may interfere with some test methods. Hemolysis of the specimen must be avoided because magnesium is primarily an intracellular ion.

Reference Values

Adults	1.5–2.0 mEq/l or 1.4–2.5 mg
Pregnancy	Gradual fall of about 10 to 20%
Children	1.54–1.86 mEq/l
Aged	No reported difference

Increased Serum Magnesium Level (Hypermagnesemia)

Clinical Significance. Renal failure is the most common reason for magnesium excess, because the kidneys are unable to excrete magnesium normally. If the renal output is not adequate, an increased magnesium level may result from the administration of medications containing magnesium, such as milk of magnesia. (See Table 7–4.)

TABLE 7–4. COMMON REASONS FOR CHANGES IN THE SERUM MAGNESIUM LEVEL*

Hypermagnesemia (Serum Mg++ level above 2 mEq/l)
1. Renal failure
2. IV administration of $MgSO_1$ for toxemia

Hypomagnesemia (Serum Mg++ level below 1.5 mEq/l)
1. Chronic malnutrition (i.e., alcoholism)
2. Diarrhea or draining gastrointestinal fistulas
3. Diuretics
4. Diabetes
5. Hypercalcemia or other complex metabolic disorders

*See text and Chan (1979), Elbaum (1977), Freeman (1977), and Felver (1980) for more details.

Obstretic patients who receive magnesium sulfate ($MgSO_4$) parenterally for treatment of preeclampsia or toxemia can develop extremely elevated serum magnesium levels if the intravenous rate and the urinary output are not carefully monitored. Therapeutic serum levels for patients receiving $MgSO_4$ are kept in a range of 2.5 to 7.5 mEq/l (Butts 1977).

Possible Nursing Implications.

Assessing for Hypermagnesemia. Higher-than-normal levels of serum magnesium produce sedation, depression of the neuromuscular system, and some reduction in the blood pressure. If the mother had $MgSO_4$, the newborn may have lethargy and respiratory depression. Whether the excess magnesium is due to renal failure or intravenous therapy treatment for toxemia, an excess of magnesium eventually leads from muscle weakness to muscle paralysis and from sedation to coma. Deep tendon reflexes are weak or absent. Severe hypotension occurs. The electrocardiogram (EKG) shows changes similar to those of potassium excess. Thus nursing assessments for the patient who is at risk for developing serum magnesium excess should include: (1) frequent blood pressure and pulse monitoring; (2) assessment of the patient's level of consciousness, and (3) the presence of normal reflexes, such as the knee jerk.

Assisting with Treatments. The patient with a magnesium excess is sedated and thus less aware of the surrounding environment. The nurse must take whatever measures are necessary to protect the patient from injury. If the magnesium excess is causing acute problems, the physician may order calcium gluconate to be given intravenously since calcium antagonizes the sedative effect of the magnesium. Calcium gluconate 10% should be available for emergency use (Felver 1980).

Patient Teaching. Patients with chronic renal failure should not be given any medications that contain magnesium. The nurse needs to do some patient teaching since several over-the-counter drugs contain magnesium. For example, antacids used should be those that contain aluminum hydroxide gels, not magnesium hydroxide. A popular cathartic, epsom salts, is a compound of magnesium sulfate. Many other laxatives contain magnesium too. The dietary restriction of magnesium intake is not a focus for teaching since most foods contain only a small amount of this trace mineral.

Decreased Serum Magnesium Level (Hypomagnesemia)

Clinical Significance. A decrease in serum magnesium is usually due to some type of chronic problem involving a low intake of dietary magnesium over a long period of time. For example, people who use alcohol as the primary source of calories may become deficient in magnesium. Deficiencies may also result from impaired absorption, such as that associated with a draining intestinal fistula. Various metabolic disorders, such as hypercalcemia, may contribute to magnesium deficiency. Recent research has suggested that there is a lowering of magnesium levels in long-term insulin-treated diabetics. Hypomagnesium appears to be an additional risk factor for the development of retinopathy in diabetics (McNair 1978). Patients with low magnesium levels may also have unexplained hypocalcemia and hypokalemia, which cause complex electrolyte imbalances.

Possible Nursing Implications

Assessing for Hypomagnesemia. Perhaps the public health nurse or a nurse in a nursing home first spots symptoms that could be related to magnesium deficiency. Usually this deficiency is found in chronic, not acute, conditions. Early symptoms of a lack of magnesium are related to neuromuscular irritability: The patient may have tremors, muscle cramps, and insomnia. The nurse should assess for any involuntary movements or twitching by the patient. See the section on hypocalcemia on how to check for a positive Chvostek's sign and a positive Trousseau's sign. The patient may eventually show symptoms that look very similar to the tetany of hypocalcemia. Often the patient may have several deficiencies so that the clinical picture is not so simple. Laboratory tests have to be done to identify exactly which electrolyte imbalances coexist. A low calcium or a low potassium that is unresponsive to treatment may be due to a coexisting low magnesium (Elbaum 1977).

Assisting with Magnesium Replacement. Magnesium deficits are corrected by the intravenous use of magnesium sulfate, which comes in concentrations of 10% and 50%. One gram of $MgSO_4$ is equal to 8.12 mEq or 4.06 millimoles. Usually 2 to 4 g (17 to 34 mEq) may be given daily in divided doses (Goodman 1975). The dosage for children is calculated on the basis of weight. If magnesium is being given intravenously, the nurse must assess carefully for the signs and symptoms of magnesium excess discussed in the section on hypermagnesium. The intravenous infusion should be stopped if there is a sharp decrease in blood pressure, extreme sedation, or weak reflexes. The importance of assessing for the patellar reflex (knee jerk) was already stressed.

Patient Teaching. An assessment for magnesium deficiency is appropriate for patients who have to be fed by artificial means or who are chronically malnourished. As long as a patient is able to take a regular diet, increasing foods that are high in magnesium has little practical significance; the trace mineral is sufficient in a regular diet. Recent studies have suggested that magnesium requirements may be increased during total parenteral nutrition. The average need for the patient on long-term hyperalimentation may be around 400 mg (Freeman 1977). Nurses should be aware of the need for replacement therapy of magnesium for any patient who has poor nutrition over an extended period of time. Serum magnesium level tests can determine whether dietary intake is adequate.

Questions

7-1. When the serum albumin level is low, the total serum calcium level is also low for which of the following reasons?

    a. about half of the serum calcium is bound to albumin.

    b. conditions that deplete albumin cause an increased metabolism of calcium.

    c. the oncotic pressure of the serum is decreased.

    d. albumin levels are controlled by the parathyroid hormone.

7-2. An increased level of the parathyroid hormone, parathormone, causes which of the following?

    a. Increased serum calcium and serum phosphate levels.

    b. Decreased serum calcium and serum phosphate levels.

    c. Increased serum calcium and decreased serum phosphate levels.

    d. Decreased serum calcium and increased serum phosphate levels.

7-3. A public health nurse is visiting Mrs. Johnson, an elderly woman who lives alone and who does her own cooking. She considers milk to be ''for babies.'' If she does not wish to drink milk or use it in cooking, which alternative foods would offer the highest calcium intake?

   a. Fresh greens, beans, whole wheat products.

   b. Rice, liver, and chicken.

   c. Apples, oranges, and other citrus fruits.

   d. Potatoes, shellfish, and cornmeal.

7-4. Hypercalcemia (high serum calcium levels) should be assessed as a potential problem for all of the following patients *except* which?

   a. Mr. Robbins, who is in acute renal failure.

   b. Mrs. Berry, who has been on bedrest for several weeks with multiple fractures.

   c. Mr. Clancy, who has metastatic bone disease.

   d. Mr. Berlin, who takes vitamin D capsules and drinks a lot of milk.

7-5. All of the following medications are sometimes used to reduce high serum calcium levels *except* which?

   a. Aluminum hydroxide.   **c.** Mithramycin.

   b. Corticosteroids.   **d.** Calcitonin.

7-6. Which nursing action is the most important to prevent complications for patients with a high serum calcium level?

   a. Keeping the pH of the urine alkaline.

   b. Checking for signs of tetany.

   c. Making sure the patient is well hydrated.

   d. Checking for tachycardia.

7-7. A lactating mother who drinks only one or two glasses of milk a day will most likely continue to have a normal serum calcium level for which of the following reasons?

   a. Two glasses of milk supply the minimum calcium requirements for lactation.

   b. Calcium is also available in most meat products and leafy green vegetables.

   c. Lactation causes a decrease in the parathyroid hormone.

   d. Calcium is being drawn from the reservoir in the bones and teeth.

7-8. Which of the following is a characteristic symptom of a low serum calcium level?

   a. Flank pain.   **c.** Bradycardia.

   b. Carpopedal spasms.   **d.** Constipation.

7-9. All of the following patients should be assessed for symptoms of hypocalcemia (low calcium levels) *except* which?

 a. Baby Lynn, a premature infant born this morning.

 b. Mrs. Thomas, who had a subtotal thyroidectomy today.

 c. Mrs. Rhoades, who has metastatic cancer of the liver.

 d. Jack Benson, who has acute pancreatitis.

7-10. Which of these patients is the most likely to have decreased serum calcium and serum phosphorus levels?

 a. Mr. Lamb, who takes a lot of antacids and milk.

 b. Mr. Babiloni, who is in renal failure.

 c. Baby Wong, who is on a low-fat diet and who is never taken outdoors.

 d. Mrs. Candy, who is in a diabetic coma and who is being treated with glucose and insulin.

7-11. Which of the following statements does not illustrate the principle that calcium is more soluble in an acid medium?

 a. Calcium gluconate should not be added to intravenous solutions containing sodium bicarbonate.

 b. Urine collected for a 24-hour test of calcium should have hydrochloric acid as a preservative.

 c. In respiratory alkalosis, the patient should be watched for signs of hypocalcemia, even though serum calcium is normal.

 d. A urine with a low pH contributes to the formation of renal stones in hypercalcemia.

7-12. When a qualitative method of testing for calcium in the urine (Sulkowitch test) is being done to assess the possibility of hypocalcemia, the patient should be taught to collect the urine specimen when?

 a. Before meals. **b.** After meals. **c.** Randomly. **d.** Upon arising.

7-13. Mr. Jacobs is on therapy to reduce his serum phosphorus level. Which of the following foods is not high in phosphorus content and would thus be allowed on his diet?

 a. Processed luncheon meat. **c.** Soft drinks.

 b. Skim milk. **d.** Apples.

7-14. In a patient with chronic renal failure, aluminum hydroxide may be useful in lowering serum phosphorus levels because the drug:

 a. causes precipitation of insoluble phosphates in the intestine.

 b. increases secretion of phosphorus in the urine.

   c. counteracts the effect of the parathyroid hormone.

   d. balances the pH of the serum.

7-15. As a general rule, an increase of glucose metabolism or "carbohydrate loading" has which effect on the serum phosphorus level?

   a. Transitory decrease.   **c.** Prolonged decrease.

   b. Transitory increase.   **d.** Prolonged increase.

7-16. The nurse should be assessing all of the following patients for symptoms of magnesium deficiency *except* which?

   a. Sally, age 5, who has had vomiting and diarrhea for 24 hours.

   b. Mrs. Leandro, who is on hyperalimentation therapy.

   c. Mr. White, who has a long history of alcohol abuse.

   d. Mrs. Warzenkiak, who has a chronic problem with a draining gastrointestinal fistula.

7-17. Mr. Olino is an elderly man who has had poor nutritional habits over an extended period of time. The public health nurse suspects that magnesium deficiency may be one of his problems. Which of the following symptoms would *not* be indicative of a low serum magnesium?

   a. Leg and foot cramps.   **c.** Irritability.

   b. Tremors.   **d.** Unusual amount of sleeping.

7-18. Mrs. Long is receiving magnesium sulfate ($MgSO_4$) intravenously as treatment for preeclampsia. Which of the following nursing assessments is an indication that Mrs. Long may be developing a serum magnesium excess?

   a. Rise in pulse and blood pressure.

   b. Exaggerated patellar reflex (knee jerk).

   c. Sedation.

   d. All of the above.

7-19. The antidote for high serum magnesium levels is the administration of which of the following?

   a. Potassium chloride.   **c.** Aluminum hydroxide.

   b. Calcium gluconate.   **d.** Calcitonin.

REFERENCES

American Academy of Pediatrics Committee on Nutrition. "Calcium Requirements in Infancy and Childhood," *Pediatrics* 62 (November 1978): 826–833.

Butts, Priscilla. "Magnesium Sulfate in the Treatment of Toxemia," *American Journal of Nursing* 77 (August 1977): 1294–1298.

Canalis, Ernest *et al*. "Hypercalcemia: Diagnosis and Therapy," *Connecticut Medicine* 41 (January 1977): 16-21.

Chan, James. "Clinical Disorders of Calcium, Phosphate, Magnesium and Hydrogen Ion Metabolism: Diagnostic Approach in Children," *Urology* 13 (February 1979): 122-128.

DeLuca, Hector. "Modern Views of Vitamin D," *Contemporary Nutrition* 6 (February 1981):1-2.

Domenech, E. and Maya, M. "Calcium Intake in the First Five Days of Life in the Low Birthweight Infant," *Archives of Disease in Childhood* 53 (October 1978): 784-787.

Elbaum, Nancy. "Detecting and Correcting Magnesium Imbalance," *Nursing* 77 7 (August 1977): 34-35.

Felver, Linda. "Understanding the Electrolyte Maze," *American Journal of Nursing* 80 (September 1980): 1591-1595.

Freeman, Joel and Wittine, Marion. "Mg Requirements are Increased During Total Parenteral Nutrition," *Surgical Forum* 28 (October 1977): 61-62.

Goodman, Louis and Gilman, Alfred. *The Parmacologic Basis of Therapeutics*, 5th ed. New York: Macmillan, Inc., 1975.

Knochel, James. "The Pathophysiology and Clinical Characteristics of Severe Hypophosphatemia," *Archives of Internal Medicine* 137 (February 1977): 203-225.

Kreisberg, Robert. "Phosphorus Deficiency and Hypophosphatemia," *Hospital Practice* 12 (March 1977): 121-128.

Linkswiler, Hellen and Zemel, Michael. "Calcium to Phosphorus Ratios," *Contemporary Nutrition* 4 (May 1979): 1-2.

McNair, P. *et al*. "Hypomagnesemia: A Risk Factor in Diabetic Retinopathy," *Diabetes* 27 (November 1978): 1075-1077.

Mundy, Gregory *et al*. "Calcium and the Kidney: Renal Osteodystrophy and Renal Calculi," *Connecticut Medicine* 41 (April 1977): 205-209.

Smith, Lynwood *et al*. "Current Concepts in Nutrition: Nutrition and Urolithiasis," *New England Journal of Medicine* 298 (January 12, 1978): 87-89.

Tripp, Alice. "Hyper and Hypocalcemia," *American Journal of Nursing* 76 (July 1976): 1142-1145.

Wood, Camilla. "Calcium Metabolism," *Nurse Practitioner* 2 (September 1977): 30-32.

CHAPTER EIGHT

Tests to Measure the Metabolism of Glucose and Other Sugars

Objectives

1. Describe the hormonal control of serum glucose levels.
2. Compare the patient preparation, usefulness, and limitations of the various tests of glucose to detect diabetes.
3. Describe the expected laboratory findings and related assessments in hyperglycemic hyperosmolar nonketotic coma (HHNK) and in ketoacidosis.
4. Identify appropriate nursing and medical interventions for patients with hyperglycemia of varying severity.
5. Compare and contrast the assessment of hypoglycemia in adults, children, newborns, and the elderly.
6. Determine the priority nursing and medical interventions for various types of hypoglycemia, including reactive hypoglycemia.
7. Identify nursing assessments that would indicate the possibility of a rebound effect from insulin (Somogyi effect).
8. Develop a teaching plan to inform patients about urine and serum glucose tests done at home.
9. Analyze the similarities and differences in galactose and lactose intolerances, along with the laboratory tests used to identify each abnormality.

FBS, PPSB, RBS, GTT, and S and A's—these abbreviations should all be familiar to the nurse because they represent very common measurements of the glucose in the blood and urine. Each test is discussed in this chapter. At the present time there is no general agreement over which is the best to use for detecting diabetes mellitus. Clinicians may use several of these tests both to diagnose and to evaluate the therapy for diabetes mellitus, as well as for other conditions involving an elevated blood sugar level (hyperglycemia) or a low blood sugar level (hypoglycemia).

Normally, all complex carbohydrates, including sugar and starches, are eventually broken down to glucose. In some metabolic abnormalities, such sugars as lactose and galactose are present in the serum and urine. The tests that may be done to detect these abnormal sugars are covered in the last part of this chapter.

BRIEF SUMMARY OF GLUCOSE METABOLISM

Although the majority of glucose comes from the dietary intake of carbohydrates, the liver can convert fats and protein into glucose when not enough glucose is available for the cells. The liver also stores extra glucose in the form of glycogen. With an excess of glucose intake, the glucose that is not stored as glycogen is converted into adipose (fat) tissue. Several hormones influence serum glucose levels:

1. *Insulin,* secreted by the beta cells of the pancreas, is essential for the transport of glucose (and potassium) into the cells. A lack of insulin causes an increase in the blood glucose level and a potassium imbalance because the glucose and potassium cannot get into the cells.

2. *Glucagon,* secreted by the alpha cells of the pancreas, elevates blood glucose levels by promoting the conversion of glycogen to glucose. The role of glycogen in the treatment of hypoglycemia is explained in the section on hypoglycemia.

3. Other hormones that cause an elevation of blood glucose levels are the *corticosteroids, adrenalin,* and *growth hormone.* The hyperglycemic effects of these hormones are discussed under the section on the clinical significance of hyperglycemia.

4. In pregnancy, *human placental lactogen* (HPL) promotes increased blood glucose levels. Other hormones in pregnancy, *progesterone* and *estrogen,* may also either have a "diabetogenic effect" or at least raise the blood glucose level.

The actual presence or absence of diabetes may be difficult to assess, both in pregnant and nonpregnant patients, due to the complex hormonal interactions that control glucose metabolism (Widmann 1979). Table 8–1 summarizes the effect of hormones on glucose metabolism.

TABLE 8–1.   EFFECTS OF HORMONES ON SERUM GLUCOSE LEVELS*

Hormones That May Promote Hyperglycemia
1. Growth hormone	5. Human placental lactogen (HPL)
2. Glucocorticoids	6. Estrogen
3. Epinephrine and norepinephrine	7. Progesterone
4. Glucagon	8. Thyroxin

Hormone That Promotes Hypoglycemia
1. Insulin

* See Chapter 15 for detailed discussion on the tests for hormones.

For most people, the renal threshold for glucose is around 160 to 190 mg/dl; that is, glucose is not spilled into the urine until the blood glucose level is above 160 to 190 mg/dl. For some people, however, the renal threshold may be higher or lower. For example, in the elderly with a high renal threshold, glucose may not be excreted by the kidney even though the blood glucose is elevated above normal limits (Hayter 1981). Urine sugar levels need to be compared to blood glucose levels to determine the specific renal threshold for an individual.

Besides some confusion about which values of urine and blood glucose levels indicate diabetes, there may also be additional confusion over the different testing methods used to determine the amount of glucose in the blood. Laboratories may use either the reducing method or an enzymatic method to measure glucose; the enzymatic methods are more often used since they are specific for glucose only. The differences between these two methods are discussed in Chapter 3 on urine testing for sugar because these two methods give different results in urine too. Usually a laboratory chooses to employ only an enzymatic or only the reducing method for serum or blood glucose levels.

As with other tests, these different methods will not be confusing for nurses as long as they always compare the results of a test to the reference values used by the laboratory. If a laboratory uses whole blood to test for blood glucose, for example, the values are about 10 to 15% lower than if plasma or serum is used, because the red blood cells are not as rich in glucose as is plasma (Widmann 1979:286). In this chapter, reference values for several methods are given so the reader is aware of the possible variations. When values are phrased only in general terms—"such as "over 140 mg" or "below 300 mg"—they must be considered practical only as general guidelines to the more precise reference values in a particular setting. In clinical practice, the more general term "blood *sugar* level" is often used interchangeably with the more precise term "blood *glucose* level."

FASTING BLOOD SUGAR (FBS)

Special Preparation of Patient

For a fasting blood sugar test, the patient may not eat for at least four hours, but water intake may continue. If the patient has an intravenous that contains dextrose, the test is not valid. If the patient is a diabetic being treated with insulin, both food and the insulin are withheld until the specimen is drawn.

The blood is collected in a tube with an EDTA-fluoride mixture as a glycolytic inhibitor. (Gray-topped Vacutainer is usually used, but check with the laboratory for the-specific method.) Three milliliters of serum or whole blood are needed.

Reference Values (Serum Values, Not Whole Blood Values)

Adults	(Average around 70–110 mg/dl, but check with laboratory concerning technique used).
	90–120 mg/dl Folin–Wu method (a reducing method)
	65–95 mg/dl Somogyi–Nelson (a reducing method)
	60–105 mg/dl Glucose Oxidase (an enzyme method)
Newborns	20–80 mg/dl

(*continued*)

Reference Values (*continued*)

Newborns (*continued*)	Full-term infants around 30 mg. Low-weight infants stabilize around 20 mg in 72 hours. Must consult specific orders in neonatal unit. May treat premature if less than 40 mg/dl (San Francisco Children's Hospital).
Pregnancy	Slightly higher values may be "normal."
Children	Basically same as adults.
Aged	Reference values may be slightly higher with aged, particularly with glucose tests other than FBS. The FBS increases only 1–2 mg per decade (Hayter 1981).

As a general rule, in an adult, a FBS over 140 mg for two to three times indicates probable diabetes.

POSTPRANDIAL BLOOD SUGAR (PPBS) OR TWO-HOUR P.C. BLOOD SUGAR

Purpose of Test And Preparation of Patient

''Postprandial'' means after a meal. Sometimes the patient is given a meal consisting of a standard amount of carbohydrate, but, more commonly, the laboratory draws the blood after a regular meal. The purpose of this test is to see how the body responds to the ingestion of carbohydrates in a meal.

So the person must eat the entire meal and may not be vomiting after the meal. The timing of the blood specimen drawing must be accurate. The laboratory technician usually draws the blood sample, but the nurse manages the time of the meal, observes what was eaten, and makes sure the patient is available for the blood sample within two hours. All the factors that affect the glucose tolerance test results may also affect the p.c. blood sugar levels.

Reference Values

"Normally" the 2-hour postprandial blood sugar will have returned to the pre-meal levels, but such may not always be the case. A value over 165 mg may suggest diabetes (Koepke 1979:226). Since the 2-hour value rises about 5 mg/dl for each decade of life, a person of 60 has a 2-hour p.c. blood sugar about 15 mg higher than a person at age 30 (Hayter 1981).

RANDOM BLOOD SUGAR (RBS)

Purpose of Test And Preparation of Patient

Since random blood sugars are not drawn in relation to a meal, there is no specific preparation of the patient. Blood sugars may be ordered to be drawn at 4 PM, at 8 PM, or at other times to assess the fluctuations of blood glucose levels during a 24-hour period. In addition, a random blood glucose may be drawn when the patient shows signs of hypo-glycemia. Because treatment for hypoglycemia should not be delayed, a nurse or available physician usually draws the blood as a stat procedure rather than waiting for a laboratory technician, if an immediate blood sugar is needed to assess the symptoms of a patient.

Reference Values

For the nondiabetic person or for a diabetic patient in good control, the random blood sugars should be within the normal ranges for fasting blood sugars or elevated only in direct relation to meal times. Values above 180 mg/dl are usually considered abnormal.

DEXTROSTIX TESTING BY THE NURSE OR PATIENT

Purpose of Test And Preparation of Patient

Dextrostix (Ames) permits clinicians and patients to determine the approximate blood glucose levels since it does not require a venipuncture to obtain a sample of blood. Venous blood may also be used, but fluoride must be avoided as a preservative. If a venous specimen has been refrigerated, it must reach room temperature before it is tested. Dex-trostix is not used with serum or plasma (Ames Product Profile). Since other companies may make serum glucose test strips, the explicit instructions for each brand must be heeded.

A drop of capillary blood is obtained by a finger stick, or in the case of an infant by a heel stick. The skin area must be warm so there is no stasis of the blood. (See Chapter 1 on the procedure for finger and heel sticks.) A drop of blood is placed on a strip of reagent paper and left for 60 seconds. The blood is then washed off and the paper is compared to a color chart.

Reference Values

Glucose:	0 mg	Yellow color
	25 mg 45 mg 90 mg 130 mg	Varying shades of bluegray indicate approximate value.
	175 mg	Dark blue.

Usefulness of Dextrostix

Testing for blood glucose with Dextrostix takes place often in the newborn nursery where infants may need to be tested frequently for hypoglycemia. Also in home situations, parents may be taught to test the blood sugar level of the child who begins showing behavioral changes that could be due to hypoglycemia. Older people may be taught to do the finger stick to themselves if they are having periods of insulin rebound. (The Somogyi effect or insulin rebound is discussed in the section on hypoglycemia.) In elderly patients or in other diabetics who have an abnormally high renal threshold for glucose, the

Dextrostix may be needed to demonstrate hyperglycemia since the urine tests remain negative even with high blood sugar levels.

Glucose Monitoring with a Photometer

The strips used to monitor blood glucose can also be put into photometers which give a digital readout. Dextrostix, for example, is used in the Dextrometer made by Ames, while Chemstrip B.G. is used in the Stat-Tek, manufactured by Bio-Dynamics Company. (Chapter 1 lists the addresses of the major companies that make laboratory testing kits.)

The meters require one drop of capillary blood placed on the paper strip. The strip is put into the photometer, which produces a digital readout from 0 to 350 mg/dl of glucose. (There will be some variations in the range depending on the brand used.) In general, the accuracy of the meters is within 10% of the obtained results from a blood sample tested in the laboratory.

Six types of patients may benefit from monitoring of blood sugar levels with a photometer:

1. patients with abnormal or unstable renal threshold,
2. patients in renal failure,
3. unstable-type juvenile diabetics,
4. patients with impaired color vision,
5. patients who have difficulty recognizing true hypoglycemia, and
6. pregnant diabetics (Christiansen 1980:13).

These patients can buy a small apparatus to do capillary sticks, which most surgical supply houses sell. The meters can be rented or purchased. Christiansen (1980) has done a survey of all the methods used for home blood glucose monitoring and has found the meter particularly useful for patients who cannot rely on urine sugars to monitor the blood glucose level at any given time. She also gives specific details on the accuracy and cost of various meters on the market.

GLUCOSE TOLERANCE TEST (GTT)

Purpose of Test

The oral glucose tolerance test used to be considered the best way to diagnose diabetes mellitus. Yet since so many factors can render the test invalid, the current trend is to rely more on fasting blood sugar levels and/or postprandial blood sugars (Siperstein 1975). Bedrest, infections, and trauma—as well as drugs, such as diuretics, birth control pills, or cortisone—all cause an abnormal glucose tolerance test. Even stress can alter the results. In fact, most clinicians feel that a glucose tolerance test is useless when a patient is in the hospital because the person is always under some type of stress that makes the test results questionable.

One objection to the GTT is that normally no one ever sits down and eats pure glucose. Hence the response to the oral glucose load may not reflect the normal response to carbohydrate in food. In puzzling conditions, clinicians may still use the GTT to document the individual's reaction to a measured amount of glucose. Since the glucose tolerance test may be of limited value in any setting, one option is to have the patient eat a high-carbohydrate diet for a few days and then draw a 2-hour p.c. blood sugar.

Preparation of Patient

The patient needs to be on a normal diet for several days before the GTT is done. The test is usually scheduled for early morning after the patient has been fasting all night. Water is not withheld so that urine samples can be collected at the proper times.

At the start of the test, blood is drawn for a fasting blood sugar, and urine is obtained for testing for glycosuria. The patient is then given 100 g of glucose dissolved in water. The glucose drink may be flavored with lemon juice to make it more palatable. (If the patient cannot swallow the glucose, the glucose is sometimes given intravenously; but the intravenous glucose may make the test reflect normal carbohydrate metabolism even less.)

Urine and blood samples of glucose are collected at 1-, 2-, and 3-hour intervals. (Some laboratories may collect in half-hour intervals, and others may continue the test for up to 5 hours.) It is essential that the nurse and the patient know the timing for each collection so that the blood and urine samples are all collected at the specified times. Although the patient may not eat anything during the test, he or she should continue to drink plenty of water so that all the urine samples can be obtained. Patients are not able to urinate every hour unless they have adequate fluid intake. Even if they cannot void on time, the blood sample should be taken because this is the more important part of the GTT.

The results of all the samples are plotted on a graph to see how long it takes the blood sugar to return to normal. Diabetics may either take longer to return to baseline readings or never return at all to fasting levels. Patients with reactive hypoglycemia may drop to subnormal blood sugar levels in response to the glucose load. The meaning of the curve must be carefully interpreted by the physician (Koepke 1979:227). The sample reference values that follow are based on information from several sources, and they show some of the differences that may be expected in GTT results.

Reference Values

	Range of Values Below Age 55	Average After 75	Average in Pregnancy
Fasting blood sugar	80–110 mg/dl	110 mg	90 mg
Blood sugar in 1 Hour	120–160 mg/dl	200 mg	165 mg
Blood sugar in 2 Hours	80–110 mg/dl	150 mg	145 mg
Blood sugar in 3 Hours	80–110 mg/dl	140 mg	125 mg

GLYCOSYLATED HEMOGLOBIN

With prolonged hyperglycemia, some of the hemoglobin remains saturated with glucose for the life of the red cell. So a test of glycosylated hemoglobin (HbA_{1c}) is a reflection of serum glucose over a period of weeks. Due to problems with standardization and cost, HB_{1AC} is not a routine test in most laboratories, but it is being used as an adjunct to therapy (Garofono 1981). Laboratory values must be verified by the laboratory.

Preparation of Patient
And Collection of Sample

Usual diet and medications are taken, including insulin or oral hypoglycemic agents. A 5-ml specimen of venous blood is collected in a lavendar-top Vacutainer.

Reference Values

Must be verified by the laboratory.

Clinical Significance

In the diabetic patient, continually high levels of glycosylated hemoglobin demonstrates a lack of effective treatment of hyperglycemia.

Elevated Blood Sugar Level (Hyperglycemia)

Clinical Significance. The most common reason for a persistently elevated blood sugar is diabetes mellitus, in which condition the relative lack of physiologically active insulin results in an increased blood sugar level. With extremely high serum glucose levels, diagnosis is easily confirmed, even though the exact level of blood sugar that is diagnostic of diabetes mellitus is controversial.

On the other hand, values that denote diabetic coma are fairly standard:

1. In mild diabetic coma, the blood glucose is usually around 300 to 450 mg/dl.
2. In moderate diabetic acidosis, the blood sugar is around 450 mg to 600 mg/dl.
3. In severe diabetic coma, the blood sugar is usually over 600 mg/dl.

Hyperglycemia from other causes is not as pronounced as the hyperglycemia in diabetic acidosis. In addition, the test for plasma acetone (covered next) will be positive in diabetic acidosis and not in other types of hyperglycemia. Sometimes acute pancreatitis may cause a diabetic state because the beta cells cannot function properly. More often the exact cause of the diabetic state is not known, since much is still to be learned about the disease labeled "diabetes" and about the other conditions that cause hyperglycemia.

In clinical conditions when certain hormones are elevated, hyperglycemia may be present.

1. The *glucocorticords,* for example, tend to raise blood sugar levels due to the breaking down of protein to form new glucose (neoglucogenesis). Patients with Cushing's syndrome or patients on high doses of cortisone may have higher-than-normal blood sugar levels.
2. Since *adrenalin* increases serum glucose levels, any stress such as shock, burns, or trauma may create an elevated blood sugar level.
3. The *growth hormone,* secreted by the pituitary gland, creates an elevated blood sugar by making the cells more resistant to insulin. Tumors or other factors may cause abnormal functioning of the pituitary gland. (See Chapter 15.)
4. During pregnancy, several hormones tend to cause some hyperglycemia. The placenta secretes *human placental lactogen* (HPL) or *human chorionic*

somatomotropin, which tends to raise the blood sugar level. In addition, the increased levels of *estrogen* and *progesterone* may cause some increase in blood sugar level.

Pregnant patients are classified A through F, according to the severity of the diabetes and of the potential problems that may occur during pregnancy. McAteer (1979) describes in detail the use of White's classification system, along with the diagnostic testing done in pregnancy and in the newborn. As a general rule, women who become diabetic only during pregnancy (Class A) are not diabetic when the stress of pregnancy is over. Also, diabetics who require additional insulin during the last two trimesters of pregnancy usually return to a lower need or to no need at all for insulin when pregnancy is over.

Juvenile onset diabetes (before age 15) differs in many ways from adult or maturity onset diabetes. In children, the lack of insulin is usually severe so that diabetic coma or ketoacidosis is much more likely to occur (Waechter 1976:703).

Possible Nursing Implications.

Supporting the Patient During a Diagnostic Work-Up (Patient Teaching). An elevated fasting blood sugar level is an indication for a medical work-up to determine whether the patient is diabetic. The next step may be a two-hour postprandial blood sugar or, more rarely, a glucose tolerance test. Some clinicians prefer to order several fasting blood sugars. In all these situations, the patient also needs to be tested for sugar and acetone in the urine to see the pattern of glucose spillage over a 24-hour period. Nurses need to be aware of the particular diagnostic work-up planned for the patient so that they can answer the patient's questions correctly when the urine testing is begun. (Nursing implications for doing sugar and acetone tests are covered in Chapter 3.) Urine testing may also be done as part of a screening program to detect diabetes in adult populations at risk. Nurses can be valuable resource persons to answer questions about diabetes when mass screening programs are conducted.

Patients with elevated blood sugars may be very anxious while further testing is being done. The possibility of diabetes may be particularly frightening if they have known someone who had numerous complications from the disease. Assessments may indicate the need for some health teaching while they are undergoing a diabetic work-up.

1. Excess glucose in the blood can be deposited in the lenses of the eyes, causing blurred vision. It may be several weeks before the sugar deposits are cleared from the lenses (Hayter 1981:35). Thus eye examinations for fitting glasses should not be done until the hyperglycemia is controlled.
2. Of course, talking about a specific diabetic diet during testing would be premature. But if the person is overweight, diet counseling may be very appropriate if aimed at motivating the person to shed extra pounds.
3. The importance of exercise in helping the body utilize glucose could also be discussed.
4. Since an elevated blood sugar makes the person more susceptible to infections, cleanliness becomes very important.

If the patient is eventually diagnosed as diabetic, the nurse is instrumental in helping the patient learn to manage the disease. The American Diabetic Association provides excellent resource material for both health professionals and patients. A handy guide for teaching adult diabetics is included in the reference by Guthrie (1979). The articles by Rancilia, Schuler, and Wimberly (1978) contain excellent tips for the nursing care of the diabetic patient, through pregnancy, labor, and delivery.

Assessing and Preventing Complications. Two of the most important nursing impli- cations for patients with elevated blood sugars are (1) to keep them from becoming dehydrated and (2) to assess for electrolyte imbalances. Glucose in high concentrations in the bloodstream functions as an osmotic diuretic because it makes the plasma hypertonic. Extra water is pulled into the vascular system from the interstitial spaces and even from the cells if the hyperglycemia is severe and long-lasting. As excess glucose is excreted by the kidneys, so are enormous amounts of water. Thus the key symptoms of hyperglycemia are thirst (polydipsia) and increased urination (polyuria).

As long as the patient can drink large amounts of water, dehydration may not occur, but the continued diuresis causes a loss of potassium and sodium. The loss of these electrolytes leads to some of the specific problems discussed in Chapter 5.

If the hyperglycemia is due to a lack of insulin, then the other two cardinal signs of diabetes, polyphagia and weight loss, eventullay occur, because the cells are literally starving for glucose.

When dehydration becomes pronounced, the person has the characteristic signs and symptoms such as the loss of skin turgor, flushed warm skin, and soft eyeballs. The soft eyeballs are due to the lack of fluid in the interstitial tissue of the eyeball.

Interventions for Hyperosmolar Hyperglycemia Non-Ketotic Coma. The progression of these symptoms is called *hyperosmolar hyperglycemia nonketotic coma* (HHNK). A hyperglycemic coma can occur as a result not only of diabetes but of any pathological condition entailing a persistently high blood sugar that causes severe dehydration and electrolyte imbalance. The coma is called "nonketotic" because ketones are not part of the pathological problem; the serum ketones (see the test on plasma acetone) do not increase. Therapy is geared to reducing the blood sugar level by replacing fluids and perhaps by giving some insulin to help the body utilize the excess sugar. Since throm- boembolic episodes can occur due to the increased viscosity of the blood, nurses should institute measures to decrease the chance of venous thrombi. HHNK can be a complication of hyperalimentation therapy if glucose levels are not closely monitored. (See Chapter 3 on urine sugar levels in hyperalimentation therapy.)

Interventions for Diabetic Coma Due to Ketoacidosis. In diabetes, the three levels of glucose intolerance are hyperglycemia, ketosis, and ketoacidosis. Diabetic coma is caused by severe dehydration and by the acidosis resulting from the build-up of ketone bodies. When glucose is not available for the cells due to the lack of insulin, fats and sometimes protein are converted to glucose and used as the source for energy. The incomplete oxidation of fats and proteins leads to the build-up of ketones in the bloodstream (ketosis). Eventually the ketones, which are acid, exhaust the buffering capacity of the blood and ketoacidosis occurs. The serum bicarbonate level is decreased. Ketoacidosis, as one type of metabolic acidosis, is discussed in Chapter 6 in the section on decreased serum bicar- bonate levels. (Note also that the pCO_2 level decreases in an attempt to compensate for an overwhelming acidotic state.) See Table 8–2 for a summary of some of the symptoms of

TABLE 8–2.   OUTSTANDING SIGNS AND SYMPTOMS OF HYPERGLYCEMIA AND
HYPOGLYCEMIA
(Including HHNK as One Type of Hyperglycemia)*

Hyperglycemia (Note most of symptoms are due to dehydration, occurs gradually)
 1. Frequent urination (positive for sugar)
 2. Thirst, dry mouth, and skin
 3. Soft eyeballs
 4. Nausea, vomiting, abdominal pain
 5. Weakness, confusion, blurred vision
 6. Severe dehydration and electrolyte imbalance
 7. Possible coma
 8. Urine positive for ketones**
 9. Kussmaul's respiration**
10. Actone breath**
11. See Table 8–3 for other laboratory tests in diabetic ketoacidosis.

Hypoglycemia (Many of symptoms due to release of epinephrine, also due to lack of sugar
for CNS, happens quickly.)
1. Diaphoresis (see exceptions for newborns and elderly)
2. Tachycardia, anxiety
3. Weakness, hunger
4. Irritability, confusion, behavioral changes
5. Tremors to convulsions
6. Coma
7. Urine negative for sugar
8. Dextrostix or blood sugar low

* See text and Slater (1978) for more details.
**Present only if ketosis and ketoacidosis develop.

hyperglycemia and of hypoglycemia, along with Table 8–3 for the laboratory reports used
for diabetic ketoacidosis.

Nursing interventions for ketoacidosis include the careful regulation of intravenous
fluid and electrolyte replacements, as for HHNK. Electrolytes must be carefully
monitored during the acute stages of diabetic coma. Potassium levels are high in the serum
because insulin is needed for optimal transportation of potassium into the cells. Potassium
also leaves the cell as more hydrogen ions go into it. (See Chapter 5 on the effect of
acidosis on the potassium level.) When the acidosis is corrected, hypokalemia may occur
if adequate replacement is not given, and hyponatremia may result from the loss of sodium
by diuresis. Since dehydration may cause a pseudo-elevation of serum sodium levels,
osmolality test of serum and urine (Chapter 4) are useful to assess the magnitude of the
dehydration.

Administering Insulin. Regular insulin is the only type of insulin used in treating
elevated serum glucose levels that may fluctuate every few hours. It is also used to control
glucose blood levels during labor and delivery or during surgery when the unusual stress
causes unpredictable levels of hyperglycemia (Wimberley 1979). The intermediate insulins (NPH and Lente) are begun when the severe hyperglycemia in ketoacidosis has been
corrected and the person is in a more stabilized condition. Both urine and blood glucose
levels are used to monitor the return of the blood sugar to a lower stable level. The nurse
must carefully monitor urine sugar and acetone levels because additional units of regular
insulin are usually ordered on the sliding scale format discussed in Chapter 3. (Chapter 3

TABLE 8-3. LABORATORY TESTS USED IN DIABETIC KETOACIDOSIS*

	Ketoacidosis		
	"Mild"	"Moderate"	"Severe"
Serum glucose	300–450 mg/dl	450–600 mg/dl	600 mg/dl +
Plasma ketones	4+ in undiluted sample	4+ in 1:1 diluted sample	4+ in 1:2 diluted sample
Serum bicarbonate (see Chapter 6)	More than 15 mEq/l	10–15 mEq/l	Less than 10 mEq/l
pH (see Chapter 6)	More than 7.3	7.2–7.3	Less than 7.2
BUN (see Chapter 4)	Less than 25 mg/dl	25–40 mg/dl	40–100 mg/dl
Urine glucose (see Chapter 3)	2%	2%	2%
Urine acetone (see Chapter 3)	Small	Moderate	Large

* See text, other chapters in this book, and Walesky (1978) for more details.

contains not only specific instructions on different methods of urine testing for sugar and acetone, but also charts to illustrate the effect of drugs on Clinitest and Tes-Tape.) The disappearance of ketones from the urine is one way to evaluate that ketoacidosis no longer exists. The usefulness of the serum acetone level in comparison to urine testing is discussed in the next section.

SERUM ACETONE OR KETONE LEVELS

When glucose is not available to the cells and the body mobilizes fat and protein as sources of energy, the ketone bodies (acetoacetic acid, acetone, and beta-hydroxybutyric acid) are the byproducts. The acidity of these ketone bodies causes the ketoacidosis that results from uncontrolled diabetes mellitus or starvation.

When ketoacidosis is suspected, the laboratory can quickly test a blood sample to determine the relative amount of ketones in the blood. Some laboratories may test acetoacetic acid and acetone rather than just ketones. Normally the levels of ketone bodies should be negative. Various laboratories use slightly different techniques to estimate the presence of ketone bodies, and consequently they report serum ketone or acetone levels in different ways.

Preparation of Patient And Collection of Sample

The laboratory usually needs about 2 ml of blood to do any form of these tests, and there is no special preparation of the patient. The tablets used for urine testing of ketones can also be used to test ketones in serum or blood (Acetest, Ames Company 1980). For serum testing, the color of the tablet is compared two minutes after a drop of serum is placed on it. If whole blood is put on the tablet, the clot is removed after 10 minutes and the tablet is compared to the chart. Except when laboratory facilities are not readily available, such as during a home visit or in a camp setting, it is better to let the laboratory do the measurement of serum acetone under more controlled conditions where serum can be separated from whole blood and properly diluted.

Reference Values

Acetoacetate plus acetone levels	0.3 to 2.0 mg/dl
Serum ketone levels:	
Undiluted sample	4+ is considered mild ketoacidosis
1:1 diluted sample	4+ is considered moderate ketoacidosis.
1:2 diluted sample	4+ is considered severe ketoacidosis.

Some laboratories may just report abnormal results as small, moderate, or large amounts of ketones.

A Positive Test for Ketones in Serum

Clinical Significance. The presence of large amounts of ketones in the serum is diagnostic of ketoacidosis. More often, the presence of ketones is assessed by frequent urine testing since ketones are excreted by the kidney. (The specific procedure for testing urine for ketones is covered in Chapter 3.) As ketones enter the bloodstream, the excess is excreted by the kidneys so that the urine test is positive before the build-up in the serum is excessive. However, in severe ketoacidosis, the dehydrated state may cause oliguria so that obtaining urine for testing is difficult. Also, when the acidosis is coming under control by therapy, the serum level is more reflective of the current status of the patient because the serum levels begin to drop while the urine level remains high. The serum acetone level is thus the more useful as an immediate indicator of the amount of ketones in the bloodstream. When patients have a continuing positive serum acetone level, the nurse may note a fruity odor to their breath, which is similar to nailpolish remover, and which is due to the excretion of some acetone by the lungs.

A Low Blood Glucose Level (Hypoglycemia)

Clinical Significance.
    Hypoglycemia in the Diabetic Patient. Hypoglycemia in the diabetic patient is caused by:

1. too much insulin, or less frequently, by too high a dose of oral hypoglycemia agents,
2. too little food, or
3. increased exercise without additional food intake.

Less insulin is needed for the utilization of glucose when the body's activity is increased by work or exercise. Recall also that, in the case of stressful events, such as infection or trauma, more insulin is needed to control hyperglycemia. Hence, if bouts of hyperglycemia and hypoglycemia are to be prevented, the well controlled diabetic must have a balance between diet, medication, and exercise, plus a lack of stress.

In the pregnant woman, hypoglycemia is most likely to occur at two times during the pregnancy: During the first three months, since the growing fetus requires additional glucose, the mother may experience some periods of low blood sugar. Again during labor, the extra exertion may also make the woman more prone to hypoglycemia (Schuler 1979).

Hypoglycemia is always a potential problem in infants whose mothers are diabetic. During uterine life, the infant's pancreas secretes large amounts of insulin due to the high blood glucose levels in the mother. Glucose crosses the placental barrier but insulin does not. After birth, the infant's pancreas may continue to secrete large amounts of insulin even though the blood glucose levels are much less than in utero. Usually glucose levels drop the lowest an hour or two after birth, reach a plateau in 2 to 4 hours, and then gradually increase (Vogel 1979:459). Infants that are premature or that have a low birth weight are also prone to hypoglycemia due to a lack of glycogen reserves in the immature liver.

Hypoglycemia in Nondiabetic Patients. Hypoglycemia in nondiabetic patients is not well understood. In a few patients, a low blood sugar level can be traced to a tumor of the pancreas, to a lack of cortisone (Addison's disease), to extensive liver disease, or to pituitary hypofunction. Alcohol-induced fasting hypoglycemia can cause death if not identified and corrected (Dipp 1978).

Most cases of hypoglycemia, however, are termed ''functional'' because their exact cause cannot be attributed to organic pathology. Sometimes this type of hypoglycemia is termed ''reactive'' because the hypoglycemic attack may follow a meal of high carbohydrates, particularly one with a lot of sugar. Sometimes the functional hypoglycemia may be related to anxiety and stress.

Glucose tolerance tests may be used to determine the response of the person to a load of sugar. Yet most authorities feel that even a blood sugar as low as 40 mg should not be considered hypoglycemia if the patient has no symptoms (Siperstein 1975). The diagnosis of ''hypoglycemia'' usually refers to the presence of hypoglycemic symptoms rather than to a certain blood glucose level.

Possible Nursing Implications.

Assessing for Hypoglycemia in the Adult and Older Child. For patients who are likely to develop hypoglycemia due to too much insulin, the key nursing implication is to assess for early symptoms of hypoglycemia so that treatment is given quickly. Hypoglycemia occurs rapidly and can lead to coma if it is not treated. In contrast, the coma that may develop from hyperglycemia usually takes much longer to develop as the person gets progressively more dehydrated and as the ketones build up in the bloodstream.

One of the most outstanding symptoms of hypoglycemia in many adults and children is diaphoresis (excessive sweating). Since infants do not perspire, however, this clinical sign is not useful in the newborn nursery. The diaphoresis, along with weakness, dizziness, and tremors is the result of an increased surge of adrenalin (epinephrine) to raise the blood sugar level.

Symptoms of hypoglycemia are also due to a lack of glucose for normal cellular function. If the brain is deprived of glucose for more than a few minutes, the person begins to experience irritability, confusion, and severe behavioral outbursts that may make it impossible to get the person to take some juice. In an adult, a low blood sugar causes convulsions and coma. Permanent brain damage can result from severe hypoglycemia. The onset of hypoglycemia in the elderly may not show the signs and symptoms of increased epinephrine usually seen in the young. As a result, the episodes of confusion or other cerebral dysfunctions may be wrongly attributed to cerebral arteriosclerosis. Eliopoulos (1978) and Hayter (1981) describe the unique reactions of the elderly person with diabetes.

Interventions to Raise the Blood Sugar Level. Anytime that hypoglycemia is suspected, don't wait for a progression of symptoms; have the person drink a glass of orange juice or eat some candy. If the symptoms are not due to hypoglycemia, the extra sugar does not significantly affect other conditions. But if the symptoms *are* due to hypoglycemia, the concentrated sugar quickly restores the blood sugar level and the symptoms disappear. If a patient is brought to an emergency room in an unconscious state from an unknown cause, a diagnostic procedure is to draw laboratory blood for a serum glucose level and then immediately give 50 cc of 50% glucose. If the unconscious state is due to hypoglycemia, the patient immediately becomes more responsive as the blood sugar returns to normal (Koepke 1979:295). Nurses should be aware that alcohol intoxication can cause severe hypoglycemia, for which the mortality rate is 25% in children (Dipp 1978:651).

Assessing and Treating Hypoglycemia in the Newborn. In the newborn infant, the symptoms of hypoglycemia are tremors, listlessness, apnea, cyanosis, a shrill cry, changes in muscular tone, and an unstable temperature. When the infant is hypoglycemic, the resultant release of glucagon stimulates the secretion of calcitonin from the thyroid (Vogel 1979:460), which may cause a rapid fall of serum calcium, which in turn causes the symptoms of tetany. (See Chapter 7 for a discussion of hypocalcemia.) Usually the newborn of a diabetic mother is fed early with 10 to 20% glucose by a bottle, by gavage, or by intravenous infusion if necessary. The infant is also frequently tested for blood glucose levels (see the Dextrostix procedure discussed earlier in this chapter). Any infant prone to hypoglycemia is usually kept in a special care nursery for close observation.

Assessing for Hypoglycemia When Clinical Symptoms Are Not Obvious. Patients who have experienced hypoglycemia are usually aware of the beginning of symptoms and take some orange juice or candy to offset the reaction. For some people the early symptoms of hypoglycemia may not be so obvious or the hypoglycemia may occur during sleep. For example, with the intermediate acting insulins (NPH and Lente), the peak action is 8 to 12 hours after administration and the duration is around 24 hours. Headache and weakness may be the only symptoms.

Two signs of hypoglycemia can be objectively measured by nurses: (1) a fall in temperature and (2) a rise in the systolic blood pressure of about 4 to 6 mm Hg, with a larger drop in the diastolic blood pressure (Hite 1979:44). With objective documentation of these two measurements, nurses can assess drops in blood sugar that might not be otherwise detected.

Use of Glucagon as Treatment for Hypoglycemia. Some physicians may order the hormone glucagon as treatment for an insulin reaction when it is not feasible to give intravenous glucose immediately. The hormone, available in 1 mg ampules, is injected the same as insulin, and it should be effective in raising the blood sugar in 15 to 20 minutes (Goodman 1975:1,528). Glucagon, secreted by the alpha cells of the pancreas, stimulates the formation of glucose from glycogen stores. So it is not effective for the person who is malnourished and who thus has little stored glycogen. The physician must make the decision as to whether the drug may be useful for a patient in a home situation. A member of the family needs to be instructed on how to give glucagon when the patient has an insulin reaction that does not respond to oral sugar.

Patient Teaching to Prevent Hypoglycemia in Diabetic Patients. The nurse and patient need to be aware that unusual exercise increases the chance of hypoglycemia. Because active muscular exercise increases the utilization of carbohydrates, the person requires more food intake or less insulin. When a person is in the hospital, the stress of the hospitalization and the lack of normal muscular activity both contribute to increasing the blood sugar level. When the person is discharged, the stress is less and normal muscular activities are resumed. So the insulin requirement may be decreased. Sometimes in pediatric units, children are taken to a park or playground for a few times before they are actually discharged from the hospital so that insulin maintenance dose matches the food intake and exercise level of the child. This may be very helpful in preventing hypoglycemic attacks after the child is at home.

Preventing Hypoglycemia in Nondiabetic Patients (Patient Teaching). In contrast to the patient who has hypoglycemia due to an insulin reaction, the patient with functional hypoglycemia does not have symptoms that progress to a coma. The light-headedness, sweating, and palpitations may be relieved by the intake of some carbohydrate. For the long-term management of hypoglycemic attacks, the person is usually advised not to eat concentrated sugars at all since they may cause a surge of insulin in the bloodstream. The diet usually consists of a high-protein, low-carbohydrate diet with frequent feedings. For example, the person should eat cottage cheese and maybe some fruit for a mid-morning snack rather than pastry or a doughnut and coffee. Stimulants such as caffeine should be avoided because the caffeine may cause a sudden rise in blood sugar that stimulates insulin production.

The relationship of diet, stress, and anxiety to functional hypoglycemia still is not well understood. The nurse needs to evaluate the potential stress in the environment since this may be a contributing factor for the development of the hypoglycemic symptoms. Emphasis is placed not on the symptoms, but rather on eradicating the stimulus for the symptoms—be it food indiscretions, anxiety, or some yet undetected organic abnormality. Blood glucose levels drawn during a hypoglycemic attack may be helpful in documenting the physiological nature of the symptoms.

Assessing for Insulin Rebound in the Diabetic Patient. With so many variables affecting it, the blood glucose level may fluctuate a lot during a 24-hour period. The Somogyi effect, named after the man who first described the phenomenon (Kaiser 1980), is the occurrence of insulin rebound. After a period of hypoglycemia, several hormones (epinephrine and the glucocorticosteroids) are released to raise serum glucose levels. So repeated episodes of slight hypoglycemia may have the end result of making the person hyperglycemic, which may partially explain why some patients on insulin still have wide fluctuations of blood sugar levels that are not directly related to food intake. Based on this theory, a plan for reducing the insulin dose may bring about a more stable blood sugar because there is no longer the rebound effect from the periods of slight hypoglycemia.

The nurse can be useful in detecting this pattern of slight hypoglycemia reactions followed by hyperglycemia. For example, a patient may suddenly have a lot of sugar in the urine after being negative only a few hours before. Perhaps the person feels a little weak or hungry during the time the urine is negative, but eats something and soon feels better. Yet patients may not think that such small symptoms are important enough to report. The nurse may also note that one random blood sugar was unusually low while the next one was unusually high. The patient at home may be taught to do blood glucose testing with tape (see Dextrostix discussion) a few times before meals and at bedtime to make sure that slight hypoglycemia is not occurring. The importance of clearly establishing the presence of any slight hypoglycemic attacks is that the patient has better control when the insulin is slightly decreased. Having more stable blood sugar levels when the insulin is slightly reduced is considered proof that the Somogyi effect or insulin rebound was creating the problem (Hite 1979).

URINE TESTING FOR SUGAR AND ACETONE

The techniques for both the enzyme method (TesTape) and the reducing method (Clinitest) are discussed in Chapter 3. Also discussed in that chapter are the differences between the two methods and the nursing implications for urine testing in general. When a diabetic patient is on insulin, the urine is tested before meals and at bedtime. If the patient is being controlled on oral hypoglycemic agents, the urine testing is typically done once a day after the largest meal. The patient is taught to call the physician or clinic if the sugar is 1 to 2% for one or two days. In children, one day of spilling 1 or 2% sugar would be reason to notify the physician or clinic. Guthrie (1980) includes a pictorial summary of how to teach a patient to do urine self-testing at home, along with other tips to foster self-care.

TESTING FOR SUGARS
OTHER THAN GLUCOSE IN THE URINE

As discussed in Chapter 3, using the copper-reduction technique (Clinitest), rather than the enzyme method (TesTape), is important if an assessment is to be done for the presence of sugars other than glucose. Lactose, fructose, and galactose can be detected only by the reduction method. In the newborn, metabolic abnormalities due to genetic defects can cause various sugars to be present in the urine. The excretion of abnormal sugars begins after the baby is begun on a milk diet. Thus the testing for abnormal sugars must not be done when the baby is still taking just glucose and water. Most of the sugars, such as lactose (discussed next), are fairly benign. The most important other sugar to detect in the urine is galactose, since its presence is a potentially dangerous condition.

Lactose Tolerance Test
(Testing for Lactase Deficiency)
Lactase, an enzyme found only in the small intestine, usually diminishes by early childhood. Due to both genetic and other factors, some people have less of this enzyme than others. Black and Oriental people are more likely to have a deficiency of it.

A lack of this enzyme leads to an intolerance for milk because the lactose in the milk cannot be converted to a simple sugar. (One glass of milk contains 12 g of lactose.) The stools are sour and have a low pH, rather than an alkaline pH, due to the presence of undigested milk. The test for lactose tolerance is to give a measured amount of lactose and then test the blood *glucose* level at various intervals. An increase of less than 20 mg of glucose, associated with gastrointestinal symptoms (bloating or diarrhea) is strongly suggestive of lactase deficiency. The treatment is to use lactose hydrolyzed milk or milk fermented products. Newcomer (1980) gives a detailed description of this disorder and the testing done.

Serum Test for
Galactose-1-Phosphate-Uridyl Transferase

Galactosemia is an inherited disorder in which galactose cannot be converted to glucose due to a lack of the enzyme galactose-1-phosphate-uridyl transferase. The galactose is wasted in the urine. Once galactose has been detected in the urine, the test for this enzyme verifies that there is a genetic defect in metabolizing galactose. To prevent mental retardation and other complications, a diet containing no milk products should be instituted within the newborn period. If milk is not eliminated from the diet, cataracts may appear within one month and any neurological defects may be permanent (Waechter, 1976:638).

All parents, especially those who have home deliveries, need to be aware of the importance of early detection of the presence of any sugar in the urine or any intolerance to milk. Galactosemia is one of the three tests done on all newborns in California. (see Chapter 18 on genetic screening tests).

Questions

8-1. All of the following hormones cause an increase in serum glucose levels *except* which?

    a. Growth hormone.   **c.** Testosterone.

    b. Cortisone.   **d.** Epinephrine.

8-2. In comparing the tests for fasting blood sugar (FBS), postprandial blood sugar (PPBS), and random blood sugar (RBS), which statement is the most accurate?

    a. The patient must be NPO before all three tests are done.

    b. An abnormality of any two of the tests indicates diabetes mellitus.

    c. RBS gives the most accurate picture of carbohydrate metabolism.

    d. The exact timing of the drawing of the specimen is most critical for the PPBS.

8-3. Which of the following would not be considered a reason to postpone a glucose tolerance test? The fact that the person:

    a. is on bedrest.   **c.** is on a reducing diet.

    b. has a fever.   **d.** had hypoglycemic symptoms yesterday.

8–4. Which of the following statements is correct about glucose tests in the elderly patient (over 65)?

    a. The curve for a glucose tolerance test for the elderly should return to baseline as soon as the curve for a person under 50.

    b. The renal threshold for glucose is usually decreased in the elderly.

    c. The postprandial blood sugar level in the elderly tends to be higher than p.c. blood sugar levels for younger adults.

    d. Normals for fasting blood sugar tests tend to border on hypoglycemia in the elderly.

8–5. The plasma acetone level is:

    a. Increased in both diabetic coma and hyperosmolar hyperglycemic nonketotic coma (HHNK).

    b. Decreased in both diabetic coma and HHNK.

    c. Unchanged in either diabetic coma or HHNK.

    d. Increased in diabetic coma and not changed in HHNK.

8–6. Mrs. Forini is a diabetic patient in labor. She is on sliding scale insulin coverage for 1 or 2% glycosuria. Which type of insulin is used to control hyperglycemia in acute situations such as labor and delivery?

    a. Regular insulin.   **c.** NPH insulin.

    b. Lente insulin.   **d.** Combinations of all three.

8–7. Which of the following nursing actions would be *inappropriate* for the patient with an elevated blood sugar level of 300 mg/dl?

    a. Testing the urine periodically for sugar and acetone.

    b. Restricting all fluid intake to prevent nausea and vomiting.

    c. Observing for any signs of infection.

    d. Assessing for possible signs of acidosis such as faster-than-normal breathing.

8–8. All of the following patients should be watched carefully for hypoglycemic symptoms *except* which?

    a. Baby Tell, born 4 hours ago to a diabetic mother who is on sliding scale coverage.

    b. Ms. Fannin, who is in her first trimester of pregnancy and is insulin-dependent (Lente 20 units).

    c. Mr. Lord, who has been controlled on NPH 40 units, but who now is on bedrest with an infected toe.

    d. Mr. Sloan, with a possible diagnosis of functional hypoglycemia, who has just eaten two candy bars to ''tide him over'' until meal time.

8-9. A characteristic symptom of hypoglycemia in *both* the adult and newborn is which of the following?

  a. Diaphoresis. **b.** Tremors. **c.** Shrill cry. **d.** Confusion.

8-10. The night nurse discovers Mr. Riley, a newly diagnosed diabetic patient, wandering about in his room. He says he has a headache. He appears flushed and warm. The nurse knows that Mr. Riley had 20 units of Lente insulin in the AM and 10 units of regular insulin at bedtime to cover a 2% sugar. Which action would be the most appropriate for the nurse to do first?

  a. Get Mr. Riley back to bed and check to see if he has an order for pain relief for the headache.

  b. Call the intern to check Mr. Riley for possible diabetic acidosis.

  c. Obtain a blood sample for a blood sugar and give Mr. Riley a glass of orange juice.

  d. Assess his vital signs, particularly the temperature and blood pressure and wait to see if he is becoming diaphoretic.

8-11. Glucagon, a hormone from the alpha cells of the pancreas, is sometimes used to do which of the following?

  a. Treat mild cases of diabetes.

  b. Counteract the effect of epinephrine.

  c. Help promote conversion of glycogen to glucose.

  d. Reduce the blood sugar level in newborns.

8-12. The patient who has functional or reactive hypoglycemia needs to be taught to maintain a diet that includes all *but* which of the following?

  a. High carbohydrates.   **c.** Low carbohydrates.

  b. High protein.   **d.** Frequent small feedings.

8-13. Which of the following is *not* characteristic of a patient who may be experiencing insulin rebound (Somogyi effect)?

  a. Urine and blood sugars that are higher after meals.

  b. High urine sugars a few hours after negative urine tests.

  c. Headaches, tremors, and diaphoresis before a meal.

  d. Wide fluctuations in blood sugars that are not related to meals.

8-14. Mrs. Hobdey, age 54, is being discharged from the hospital. She is on an oral hypoglycemic agent. Which of the following should be taught Mrs. Hobdey about testing her urine?

    a. She can use either Clinitest tablets or TesTape since the tests are the same and give the same results.

    b. She should test her urine at least once a day after her largest meal of the day and do so more often only if the test is positive.

    c. She should test her urine before meals and at the hour of sleep, and report any positive signs immediately.

    d. She does not need to test her urine since she is not taking insulin.

8-15. Sarah is a 5-year-old with diabetes. Which of these points would *not* be correct to teach Sarah's parent about testing in diabetes?

    a. Dextrostix may be useful to assess for hypoglycemia if Sarah has unexplained behavioral outbursts.

    b. Regular exercise is important in keeping blood sugar levels more stable.

    c. If the urine sugar is positive, an acetone should always be done.

    d. If the sugar and acetone remain positive after more than two days, the clinic or physician should be notified.

8-16. Which of the following conclusions is *incorrect* in comparing galactose and lactose intolerances and the tests done for each?

    a. Both galactose and lactose can be detected in the urine by Clinitest tablets.

    b. Galactose intolerance is a more serious defect than lactose intolerance.

    c. A nonmilk diet in the infant eliminates the symptoms of both lactose intolerance and galactose intolerance.

    d. The blood glucose level will be abnormally elevated in both conditions.

REFERENCES

Ames Product Profiles, *Acetest, Dextrostix, Clinitest* and *KetoDiastix*. Elkhart, Indiana: Ames Company, Division of Miles Laboratories, 1980.

Dipp, Stephen. "Metabolic Effects of Alcohol," *Arizona Medicine* 35 (October 1978): 651–652.

Christiansen, Constance and Sachse, Marti. "Home Blood Glucose Monitoring," *The Diabetes Educator* 6 (Fall 1980): 13–21.

Eliopoulos, Charlotte. "Diagnosis and Management of Diabetes in the Elderly," *American Journal of Nursing* 78 (May 1978): 884–887.

Garofono, Catherine. "A Simpler Test for Diabetes?" *RN* 44 (September 1981): 155.

Goodman, Louis and Gilman, Alfred. *The Pharmacologic Basis of Therapeutics,* 5th ed. New York: Macmillan, Inc., 1975.

Guthrie, Diana. "Helping the Diabetic Manage Self-Care," *Nursing 80* 10 (February 1980): 57–65.

Hayter, Jean. "Diabetes and the Older Person," *Geriatric Nursing* (January/February 1981): 32–36.

Hite, Anna and Humphrey, James. "How to Spot the Vicious Cycle of Insulin Rebound," *RN* 42 (July 1979): 44–47.

Kiser, Debra. "The Somogyi Effect," *American Journal of Nursing* 80 (February 1980): 236–238.

Koepke, John. *Guide to Diagnostic Tests,* 2nd ed. New York: Appleton-Century-Crofts, 1979.

McAteer, Jane. "Clinical Implications of Laboratory Studies: Diabetic Pregnancy and Neonatal Outcome," *Critical Care Quarterly* 2 (December 1979): 61–72.

Newcomer, Albert. "Lactose Deficiency," *Contemporary Nutrition* 4 (August 1979): 1–2.

Rancilia, Nancy. "When a Pregnant Woman is Diabetic: Postpartal Care," *American Journal of Nursing* 79 (March 1979): 453–456.

Schuler, Katherine. "When a Pregnant Woman is Diabetic: Antepartal Care," *American Journal of Nursing* 79 (March 1979): 448–450.

Siperstein, Marvin. "The Glucose Tolerance Test," *Advances in Internal Medicine* 20 (1975): 279–323.

Slater, Norma. "Insulin Reactions vs. Ketoacidosis: Guidelines for Diagnosis and Intervention," *American Journal of Nursing* 78 (May 1978): 875–877.

Vogel, Margery. "When a Pregnant Woman is Diabetic: Care of the Newborn," *American Journal of Nursing* 79 (March 1979): 458–460.

Walesky, Mary. "Adult Diabetes: Diabetic Ketoacidosis," *American Journal of Nursing* 78 (May 1978): 872–874.

Waechter, Eugenia et al. *Nursing Care of Children.* Philadelphia: J.B. Lippincott Co., 1976.

Widmann, Frances. *Clinical Interpretation of Laboratory Tests,* 8th ed. Philadelphia: F.A. Davis Co., 1979.

Wimberly, Dian. "When a Pregnant Woman is Diabetic: Intrapartal Care," *American Journal of Nursing* 79 (March 1979): 451–452.

CHAPTER NINE

Tests to Measure Lipid Metabolism

Objectives

1. Define hyperlipidemia and discuss the factors that seem to contribute to its development.
2. Describe the patient preparation necessary for tests of serum cholesterol and serum triglyceride levels.
3. Discuss the controversial aspects about the relationship of serum cholesterol and serum triglyceride levels to the development of cardiovascular disease.
4. Plan a diet low in cholesterol and saturated fats.
5. Identify nursing interventions, other than diet teaching, that may be useful for the patient with elevated serum cholesterol levels.
6. Identify nursing assessments that might indicate a lack of essential fatty acids in the diet.
7. Give examples of how serum triglyceride levels are used as an evaluation tool.
8. Describe lipoprotein electrophoresis and explain how the research findings from this test have been applied to clinical situations.

Hyperlipidemia is a broad term that means high plasma concentrations of cholesterol, triglycerides, or the complex lipoproteins. Although cholesterol is the lipid that seems to get the most publicity, it is just one that can be measured in the serum. Other lipids found in the serum include the triglycerides and the phospholipids, such as lecithin and sphingomyelin. Lecithin and sphingomyelin comprise the basis of the L/S ratio, a test done on amniotic fluid to evaluate the maturity of the fetus.

Serum cholesterol levels and, less frequently, triglyceride levels are two tests done to evaluate the risk potential for the development of atherosclerosis. Based on current knowledge, the serum cholesterol level is the more important laboratory test to assess for hyperlipidemia that may be helped by therapy.

In addition to the use of these two tests to evaluate hyperlipidemia, lipoprotein electrophoresis may be done to evaluate rarer types of lipid abnormalities. Lipoproteins are complex protein molecules that contain several proteins and lipid components. Lipoprotein molecules can be separated into four different bands on a strip of paper by using an electric current to cause migration of the molecules. Identification of abnormal patterns for the four bands on the electrophoresis strip has resulted in a classification system of various types of hyperlipidemia, the six types of which are briefly discussed in this chapter. For an in-depth knowledge about the present use of this classification system, however, the reader must consult recent literature since its usefulness is controversial at the present time. Researchers are trying to discover whether some types of lipoproteins, such as the high-density lipoproteins, may actually be protective against the development of atherosclerosis. A test called *HDL-cholesterol* (*high-density lipoprotein*) is currently being used to assess the potential for developing coronary vascular disease. This is the last test covered in this chapter.

SERUM CHOLESTEROL LEVELS

Cholesterol, a natural constituent of the serum, is essential for the production of bile salts, for the manufacture of many of the steroid hormones, and for the composition of cell membranes. The liver esterfies cholesterol by combining it with a fatty acid. Most of the cholesterol is present in the bloodstream in the esterfied form. Usually only the total cholesterol is measured, unless there is possible liver dysfunction. Because cholesterol has been so closely linked to the development of atherosclerosis, there is great concern about how much of this natural constituent should be in the serum. At the present time, there is no general agreement about which levels of serum cholesterol are "normal." Only about one-third of the adult population in America has cholesterol levels below 200 mg. In other countries, the adult population may have considerably lower values. Cholesterol levels seem to differ greatly depending on such variables as age, diet, geographic location, and genetic influences. Values in the United States are considered normal up to around 335 mg, depending on age. Many authorities question whether these "normal" values of cholesterol are ideal for optimal health (Kannel 1976). Because a high cholesterol level has not been proven as a cause of vascular disease, cholesterol as an assessment tool is used in conjunction with an assessment of other known risk factors for the development of atherosclerotic vascular diseases.

Preparation of Patient
And Collection of Sample
Serum cholesterol requires 2 ml of serum. The patient needs to have fasted for a minimum of four hours. Because there may be significant variations from day to day in the same individual, the test may be repeated more than once to determine which variations are occurring. The patient should be on a regular diet until the fasting period. Some laboratories may require overnight fasting. Water is allowed. Certain drugs, such as vitamin E, phenytoin, or steroids, may cause false elevations, while other drugs, such as some antibiotics, may cause falsely low readings.

Reference Values

Adults by age*	Less than 30	120–255 mg/dl
	30 to 40	140–295 mg/dl
	41 to 60	155–330 mg/dl

These figures are only averages for different age groups. The "ideal" level is not known (Kaplan 1979).

Women tend to have lower cholesterol levels than men of the same age until after menopause.

Pregnancy Cholesterol levels increase in pregnancy to around 240–300 mg/dl. Values return to pre-pregnancy values within one month (Hytten 1975).

Newborns 90 mg at birth, increases to around 120 mg by third day.

Children From one year, around 130 mg to around 175 mg by age 19. A cutoff point of 205 mg is used for some studies (Morrison 1979).

Aged Most authorities consider an increase of cholesterol to be proportional to age increases, so that a cholesterol of 260 mg would be acceptable for a 60-year-old, but questionable for a 30-year-old. Range after 60: 160 –335 mg/dl. Cholesterol levels may decline in persons over age 70.

* Values are for total cholesterol: In liver disease when liver can not esterfy cholesterol, the laboratory may measure "esterfied" cholesterol since this value decreases. Normally 65 to 75% of total cholesterol will be esterfied.

Increased Serum Cholesterol Level

Clinical Significance. For the majority of patients, the reason for a high cholesterol level is not known. Much research is being done to try to discover to what extent genetic, dietary, or other environmental factors contribute to high cholesterol levels. Three recognized genetic disorders lead to hyperlipidemia: (1) familial hypercholesterolemia, (2) familial combined hyperlipidemia, and (3) familial hypertriglyceridemia. Although these three disorders affect 0.5 to 1% of the population and are the most common genetic diseases (Breslow 1978:514), they do not cause the vast majority of high cholesterol levels seen in adults.

There is an association between high cholesterol levels and the development of atherosclerosis, but the cause and effect relationship is not known. In some clinical situations, however, the cause of the increased serum cholesterol level can be identified. For example, liver disease with biliary obstruction, hypothyroidism, and pancreatic dysfunction all cause increased cholesterol levels. Certain drugs, such as corticosteroids, may cause an increased cholesterol level, but the significance of this is not known. Although cholesterol levels are normally high in pregnancy, they rise even higher in preeclampsia (Hytten 1975). Also in nephrotic syndromes, the cholesterol levels may increase.

Possible Nursing Implications. Depending on the clinical situation, the patient may undergo other tests, such as serum triglycerides or high-density lipoprotein analysis (HDL), to further investigate the characteristics of the hyperlipidemia. The nurse working with patients with hyperlipidemia needs to be aware of the most recent developments in the area of diet and drugs.

Patient Teaching on Diets. Once a patient has been definitely identified as having hyperlipidemia, the usual recommendation is to decrease the amount of fat in the diet and to replace saturated fats with polyunsaturated fats. Vegetable oils tend to be high in polyunsaturated fats, while animal fats are high in saturated fats, which contain high amounts of cholesterol. Meat, egg yolks, and dairy products are the major source of cholesterol in the American diet (see Table 9-1). (See the section on lipoprotein electrophoresis for more details on diet regimens.) Some physicians may recommend a ratio of twice as much polyunsaturated fats as saturated, with a total amount of fat being not more than 30 to 35% of the total caloric intake. A diet plan may limit cholesterol intake to 200 to 300 mg per day.

The specific dietary recommendations published by the American Heart Association (1978:3) are as follows:

1. Caloric intake should be adjusted to achieve and maintain ideal body weight.
2. Reduction in total fat calories should be achieved by a substantial reduction in dietary saturated fatty acids. Saturated fats should be no more than 10%, polyunsaturated fats should be no more than 10%, and the rest of the fat should come from monounsaturated sources. (Not all dietary plans follow these figures exactly.)
3. Substantial reductions in dietary cholesterol are in order. The average daily intake for adults should be less than 300 mg. If hypercholesterolemia is present, even greater reduction may be warranted.
4. A slight increase in carbohydrate intake can make up the caloric difference resulting from less fats in the diet. This may lower the postprandial serum triglyceride level.
5. Avoid excessive dietary sodium. The level of sodium restriction must be determined by the physician based on signs of hypertension and other conditions (see Chapter 5 on low-sodium diets).
6. Other dietary factors, such as alcohol, should be limited because of the increased calories and possible hyperlipidemia effect.

Despite the advertising world's use of "low-cholesterol" labeling to sell food, the need for the strict dietary restriction of cholesterol is controversial. At the present time, dietary restrictions do not seem to be the perfect treatment for high serum cholesterol levels because so many factors seem to influence the metabolism of cholesterol (Sodhi 1977). Some authorities maintain that it is not necessary to restrict cholesterol in the diet, because most studies have failed to demonstrate a consistent relationship between changes in serum cholesterol (Reiser 1980). In healthy men, eating two eggs a day for three months made no change in their cholesterol levels as compared to a diet with no eggs (Flynn 1979). However, other studies have shown a reduction in serum cholesterol levels if the change in diet continues for as long as 17 months (Mallison 1978). Because high

TABLE 9–1. FIVE MAIN SOURCES OF
CHOLESTEROL IN THE DIET

	Approximate Amount of Cholesterol
Liver, one serving	90 mg
Egg, one	275 mg
Whole milk, one glass	24 mg
Cheese, 1 ounce	30 mg
Butter, 1 tablespoon	35 mg

serum cholesterol levels do seem to indicate a state of less than optimal health, most physicians put their patients on some type of restricted fat diet.

When a patient has a high serum cholesterol level, the nurse's role in diet teaching may be crucial. Rather than emphasizing a diet that is based on restrictions (no eggs, no steak, no ice cream, no butter), it may be better to take a more positive approach and stress the foods to choose. Thus the person can be encouraged to choose fish and chicken rather than beef, which is high in fat, polyunsaturated margarine rather than butter, and more fresh fruit for dessert. Patients should also be made aware of the food served in "fast food" places, which specialize in selling food that contains high amounts of fats and calories. Most of the deep-fried chicken parts or donuts are cooked in melted lard. On the other hand, the patient at home can use corn oil, a polyunsaturated fat, to prepare food. The person who is following a diet very restricted in saturated fats faces the possibility of some vitamin E deficiency since this vitamin is found mainly in saturated and animal fat.

Any plan for diet restrictions must be looked at in relation to the total nutritional needs of the person. The American Heart Association has excellent material for teaching patients about low-fat diets. Diet modification for children is especially controversial. Some pediatricians have suggested that as early as the second year of life, American children should be on the modified low-fat diet described for adults (Breslow 1978).

Assisting with Drug Therapy. If dietary changes are not sufficient to lower cholesterol levels, the physician may order certain medications, such as cholestyramine, clofibrate (Atromid-S), and nicotine acid. Cholestyramine (Questran, Cuemid) is also used for patients with elevated direct bilirubins because it binds up bile salts. (See Chapter 11 on direct bilirubin.) Other drugs are being investigated as possible aids in reducing serum cholesterol levels. Yeshurum (1976) has an excellent review of the variety of medications that have been used in the past for the treatment of hyperlipidemia.

Nurses must be aware of the information for the specific drug chosen for the patient. The patient has serum cholesterol, and maybe serum triglyceride levels, checked every few weeks for the first few months. Some drugs, such as clofibrate (Atromid-S) may have more effect on the triglyceride levels than on cholesterol levels. With most of the drugs, the serum level of cholesterol may not drop for about two months (Yeshurum 1976). The patient needs encouragement to continue whatever diet has been prescribed and to report any side effects of the drug. If the drug is ineffective or if there are undesirable side effects, the patient is switched to other drugs.

Treatment of hyperlipidemia in children is somewhat the same as adults. As a general rule intensive dietary therapy for 6 months to a year is done before drugs or other interventions are tried.

Helping the Patient Adopt Healthier Lifestyle. The nursing implications for the patient with a high serum cholesterol level are broader than just teaching about diet and drug therapies because cholesterol seems to be only one of the risk factors for the development of cardiovascular disease. Thus, it is important to identify the other risk factors that may be present, such as lack of exercise, obesity, hypertension, stressful environments, and cigarette smoking. All these risk factors seem to be interrelated, along with other factors such as glucose levels. For example, hypertension may be a critical factor in the development of atherosclerosis since low pressure areas of the circulation, although bathed in the same lipid-laden blood, do not develop atherotic placques as do the arteries in the body that have the highest pressures (Kannel 1976:274). Obesity and stress both contribute to the development of hypertension. For each 5 lbs of extra weight, the diastolic pressure rises about 1 mm Hg. It is not enough to tackle just one of the risk factors, because all are part of a still *poorly understood* pathophysiology. Exactly why lipid deposition occurs is under intense investigation (Ross 1976).

Hence a nurse, skilled in health teaching and counseling, can help the person with a high serum cholesterol level to find ways to achieve a healthier lifestyle. It is essential that patients know both what is known, and what is still not known, about the role of serum cholesterol and other risk factors in the development of vascular disease. The patient can then make choices about what can be changed in his or her style of living to reduce some or all of the risk factors.

Family Follow-Ups. Although the influence of genetics cannot be controlled by the person, it is important to consider genetic implications in counseling a patient with an elevated serum cholesterol level. Since severe hyperlipidemia may sometimes be partly genetically based, the family members of patients with diagnosed hyperlipidemia need to be screened for the same condition. It is usually considered advisable to screen close relatives when a person has a coronary event before the age of 60. If a familial hyperlipidemia is suspected and a child's lipid levels are normal, rescreening every three to five years is recommended (Breslow 1978:510). Most authorities feel the early treatment of hyperlipidemia, particularly in young people, is warranted. However, it has not yet been *proven* that the control of hyperlipidemia reduces the risk of cardiovascular disease in either the young or the old.

Decreased Serum Cholesterol Level

Clinical Significance. Common conditions that cause low serum cholesterol levels include:

1. *hyperthyroidism,* in which the increased metabolism accounts for an increased utilization of fat;
2. *severe liver damage*, after which the liver can no longer manufacture cholesterol; and
3. *malnutrition,* which eventually leads to a deficiency of cholesterol due to the lack of fats in the diet.

Possible Nursing Implications. If the low serum cholesterol level is the result of one of these three disease processes, nursing care is geared toward the particular pathphysiology. The low serum cholesterol level, by itself, is not of specific concern. Remember that, since the "normals" for cholesterol levels are arbitrary, low cholesterol levels are unlikely to cause any symptoms in the patient.

If the patient is on a diet or on drugs to reduce the cholesterol levels, a gradual lowering of the serum cholesterol levels is an indication of the effectiveness of therapy. Even with drugs, the cholesterol does not usually drop below the lower end of the reference values.

TRIGLYCERIDES

Triglycerides, like cholesterol and the phospholipids, are lipids that are normally present in the serum. The more precise chemical term for this group of lipids is *tricylglycerols,* but the laboratory test is called triglycerides (Widmann 1979). The triglycerides, the most abundant group of lipids, are neutral fat and oils that come from both animal fat and vegetable oils. A heavy meal or alcohol causes a transient increase in the serum triglyceride level. Excess intake of triglycerides, which are useful for energy, is stored in the body as adipose tissue. The triglyceride test is useful in identifying some types of hyperlipidemia.

Preparation of Patient
And Collection of Sample
The test should be done in the fasting state, but the patient should be on a regular diet before the fasting begins. The laboratory needs 2 ml of serum. Since there is much variation in what is considered "normal," the patient usually has the test done more than once if it is elevated.

Reference Values

Adults	40–150 mg/dl. Age- and diet-related.
Pregnancy	Level rises progressively during pregnancy. Note oral contraceptives also cause an increase (see Appendix D).
Newborn	Lower than 40 mg at birth but in adult range by third day.
Children	Same reference values as adults. Some authorities use 125 mg as upper limit in children (Morrison 1979).
Aged	Most authorities may consider levels higher than 150 mg "normal" as the person ages.

Increased Serum Triglyceride Levels

Clinical Significance. Many of the clinical conditions that cause an increase in serum cholesterol levels also cause increases in triglyceride levels. Thus patients with nephrotic syndrome, pancreatic dysfunction, diabetes, toxemia of pregnancy, and hypothyroidism have elevated triglyceride levels. Pancreatitis may cause a very high elevation of tri-glycerides. Fatty meals and alcohol always raise the triglyceride level for a while. The serum triglyceride level peaks about five hours after a fatty meal. An increase of serum triglycerides is sometimes associated with certain abnormal patterns of lipid metabolism that are probably genetic in origin (Kaplan 1979).

Possible Nursing Implications. The serum triglyceride level is usually measured in con-junction with the serum cholesterol level to get a clearer picture of the type of hyper-lipidemia present. In the discussion on lipoprotein electrophoresis, the marked changes in cholesterol and/or in serum triglyceride levels are discussed briefly in relation to the six types of hyperlipidemia.

Treatment modalities depend on which lipids are elevated. Often weight reduction and a low-fat diet can significantly lower the serum triglyceride level, and some of the drugs used to lower cholesterol also lower triglyceride levels.

Once again, the reduction of hyperlipidemia needs to be done in conjunction with other measures to improve the total health of the individual. The American Heart Associa-tion considers cigarette smoking, hypertension, and cholesterol as the three major risk factors for cardiovascular disease. The elevated serum triglyceride level is not as firmly established as cholesterol as a risk factor.

Since alcohol is a major cause of secondary hyperlipidemia, the possibility of alcohol abuse should be investigated when there is unexplained high levels of triglycerides (Dipp 1978).

Decreased Serum Triglyceride Levels

Clinical Significance. A decreased triglyceride level is rarely seen as a clinical problem. Some rare genetic defects may cause low serum triglycerides, and severe malnutrition may lead to low levels. Although hypothyroidism may cause an abnormally high tri-glyceride level, hyperthyroidism does not contribute to a low level.

Possible Nursing Implications. If the low serum triglyceride level is due to an exhaustion of the body's store of essential fatty acids, the patient may have sparse hair growth, scaly and dry skin, poor wound healing, and a decrease in blood platelets, which may lead to some bleeding. The nurse should look for these signs when patients are not getting enough fat in their diet.

Patients who are deficient in fatty acids can be given fat emulsions intravenously. Since the usual hyperalimentation fluids contain only glucose and amino acids, the fat is given as a separate solution. The fat used for intravenous replacement is composed of soybean oil emulsions and purified egg phosphatides in glycerol and water. This lipid emulsion (Intralipid, Liposyn) can be given via a peripheral vein. Maintaining the emul-sion's stability before and during infusion as well as watching for untoward reactions, are the major responsibilities of the nurse. Specific instructions about how to set up the emulsion are included with the bottle of solution. The patient's ability to use lipid emul-sions is evaluated by testing the serum triglyceride levels. Within 18 hours after the lipid infusion, the serum triglycerides should return to the baseline. Jacobson (1979) covers some of the important points about giving fat emulsions. If the serum triglyceride level remains elevated beyond 18 hours, the patient should not be given more fat emulsions.

LIPOPROTEIN ELECTROPHORESIS

Lipoproteins are complex molecules that contain lipids, such as cholesterol and tri-glycerides, in combination with various proteins. Researchers have been able to make some broad classifications of these lipoproteins based on the varying density of their molecules: high-density lipoproteins (HDL), which weigh the most, low-density lipoproteins (LDL), and very low-density lipoproteins (VLDL). Electrophoresis can separate these types by using an electric current to cause migration of the molecules. The direction of the different protein molecules is based on size and electrical charge. After the lipoproteins have separated into distinct layers, the paper is stained to show the relative distribution of four bands of lipoproteins:

1. chylomicrons (particles representing dietary fat in transport),
2. pre-beta lipoproteins (very low-density lipoproteins),
3. beta lipoproteins (low-density lipoproteins), and
4. alpha lipoproteins (high-density lipoproteins).

Reference Values

A change from the typical pattern in one or more bands on the electrophoretic pattern would be considered abnormal. Several atypical patterns of electrophoresis have been observed and classified as different types of hyperlipidemia. The following brief summary of the six types of patterns are based on several references. The classification system was developed in the late sixties (Fredrickson 1967).

Type I	Lipoprotein pattern of increased chylomicrons. Serum cholesterol may be normal. Triglycerides are markedly elevated. This is the rarest type of hyperlipidemia. May be treated with just low-fat diet and restriction of all alcohol.
Type II, A	Lipoprotein pattern of increased beta (low-density) lipoproteins. Increased serum cholesterol levels and normal serum triglyceride levels. Therapy would include a restricted cholesterol diet. This is a relatively common pattern of hyperlipidemia and is the most resistant to diet therapy.
Type II, B	Lipoprotein pattern of increased pre-beta and beta lipoproteins. Cholesterol and serum triglyceride levels are both elevated. This is a relatively common type of hyperlipidemia.
Type III	Lipoprotein pattern shows abnormal type of beta lipoproteins and increased beta lipoproteins. Cholesterol level moderately elevated and triglycerides moderately elevated. Relatively uncommon.
Type IV	This is the most common type of hyperlipidemia. Lipoprotein pattern shows an increase of pre-beta (very low-density) lipoproteins. Serum cholesterol is normal or slightly elevated, with serum triglycerides markedly elevated. Diabetics often show this type of hyperlipidemia. Treatment usually includes control of carbohydrate intake.

(continued)

Reference Values (*continued*)

Type V	This is an uncommon type of hyperlipidemia. The lipoprotein pattern shows an increase of chylomicrons and of the pre-beta lipoproteins, along with serum cholesterol that is either normal or slightly elevated. Serum triglycerides are elevated.
	Types II, III, and IV are particularly associated with the develop ment of coronary artery disease.

Abnormal Lipoprotein Patterns

Clinical Significance. It has been hypothesized that these six different patterns are due to genetic differences while other secondary changes may be induced by high carbohydrate and/or fat intake or by disease states such as diabetes. Some clinicians may feel that identifying the type of hyperlipidemia is important in choosing the correct diet and/or drug therapy. Other clinicians may prefer to designate the hyperlipidemia simply as primary

TABLE 9-2.   SAMPLES OF DIETARY REGIMEN AS PART OF TREATMENT FOR VARIOUS TYPES OF HYPERLIPOPROTEINEMIAS*

Type I	Limit fat intake (25-35 g/day) No alcohol.
Type IIA	Increase polyunsaturated fat. Reduce cholesterol. Limit alcohol.
Type IIB	Maintain ideal weight. Limit carbohydrate (40% of calories). Normal fat (40% of calories). Increase polyunsaturated fat. Reduce cholesterol. Limit alcohol.
Type III	As in Type IIB.
Type IV	Maintain ideal weight. Limit carbohydrates (35–40% of calories). Increase polyunsaturated fat. Normal cholesterol (up to 500 mg/day). Limit alcohol.
Type V	Maintain ideal weight. Normal carbohydrate (48–53% of calories). Reduce fat (25–30% of calories). High protein (21–24% of calories). Limit cholesterol (300–500 mg/day). No alcohol.

* Summary from Kritchevsky (1980:2), reprinted with permission. See text for discussion on types and Fredrickson (1967) for original description of types of hyperlipoproteinemia.

hypercholesterolemia, as primary hypertriglyceridemia, or as a combination of both (Havel 1977).

Since these six categories were developed, much research has been done to establish possible causes for the different types of hyperlipidemia (Ross 1976). Still not known is whether these various types of hyperlipidemia are really separate categories or not. Much of the data from lipoprotein electrophoresis is more appropriate for research purposes than for specific diagnoses. Different authorities have different opinions about the usefulness of this drug or that for different types of hyperlipidemia. However, almost all authorities do agree that the treatment of any primary hyperlipidemia begins with diet changes. The usual diet recommendations for each of the six types of hyperlipidemia are summarized in Table 9-2. As research progresses, more light may be shed on specific treatments for specific types of hyperlipidemia, and each classification may become a more precise category with a more definite treatment.

Newer research is focusing more on the high-density lipoproteins. In all the abnormal patterns that have been implicated with hyperlipidemia, none contain increased amounts of the high-density lipoproteins. About 20% of cholesterol is carried via the high-density lipoproteins. Thus the speculation is that the high-density lipoproteins (HDL) may actually protect against the development of coronary artery disease.

HIGH-DENSITY LIPOPROTEIN (HDL CHOLESTEROL)

The cholesterol component of the high-density (alpha) lipoproteins is measured for this test. Normally about 20% of cholesterol is HDL cholesterol. Data from the Framingham study, a longitudinal study of the cardiovascular risk for a population in Massachusetts, has supported the theory that low levels of HDL are associated with an increased incidence of coronary vascular disease. Persons with high levels of HDL cholesterol had less vascular disease. Gordon (1977) presents the statistical evidence for the benefit of higher levels of HDL cholesterol. Levels above 45 mg/dl are considered to be beneficial in that the patient may be less likely to develop atherosclerosis. Levels below 45 mg/dl indicate a higher risk for the development of coronary disease.

Preparation of Patient

Patient should be fasting overnight. Water is allowed. The patient should not have had weight changes in the last few weeks. Since many drugs may affect the pattern, drugs should be withheld for 24–48 hours, if possible. Radiological contrast dye interferes with the test.

Reference Values

At all ages, women have higher levels than men. Values in newborns, children, and pregnancy are still being researched.

Average adult female	55 mg/dl
Average adult male	44 mg/dl

Clinical Significance. There is a *theoretical* risk of cardiovascular disease when the HDL is below 45 mg/dl. However, since laboratory techniques may cause a variation of 5–10 mg, the test is more for research than for clinical screening. The results of the HDL must be interpreted with caution since much is still to be learned about HDL. Furthermore, the HDL can be subfractionated into HDL_2 and HDL_3 which may have implications for future studies (Kritchevsky 1980).

Possible Nursing Implications. Some of the recommendations to increase HDL cholesterol have included eating less meat, consuming fewer calories, drinking 5–6 oz of alcohol each week, and eating 1–2 tablespoons of lecithin a day. Studies have shown that long distance runners have higher levels of HDL (Smith 1979). Several studies have also suggested that some alcohol may be protective against coronary heart disease; still, the other negative aspects about alcohol must be considered. Most authorities stress that the best way to increase the amount of HDL cholesterol is to lose excess weight and then to maintain the proper weight, because high-density lipoprotein cholesterol concentration decreases with increasing weight (Bradley 1978). The nurse can stress to patients that they should talk to the physician and also read the latest information about HDL. In summary, being at risk for developing atheroscleroic vascular disease can be a strong motivation for patients to evaluate the effect of their total lifestyle on their health and to make changes in other risk factors as discussed throughout this chapter.

Questions

9–1. Hyperlipidemia is defined as increased serum:

    a. cholesterol levels.   **c.** lipoproteins.

    b. triglyceride levels.   **d.** any or all of the above.

9–2. In a female, a rise in the serum cholesterol level is an expected occurrence at all these times *except* when?

    a. About three days after her birth.   **c.** During pregnancy.

    b. At onset of menses.   **d.** After menopause.

9 3 Guidelines for patient preparation for tests of serum cholesterol or serum triglycerides include which of the following?

    a. The patient should be in the fasting state.

    b. A usual diet for at least two weeks before the test.

    c. Test done more than once to confirm.

    d. All of the above.

9–4. At the present time, whether serum cholesterol levels can be significantly lowered by diet is controversial due to which of the following reasons?

    a. The liver continues to make cholesterol even though food intake contains little cholesterol.

    b. In the majority of cases of high cholesterol levels, the actual cause of high serum cholesterol has not been proven yet.

    c. Most patients with high cholesterol levels do not have diets unusually high in cholesterol.

    d. Serum cholesterol levels are genetically determined.

9-5. Which one of the following meals contains the least amount of cholesterol?

    a. Steak, baked potato with sour cream, roll and butter, tossed salad with French dressing and coffee.

    b. Lobster, rice, salad with Thousand Island dressing, milk, apple pie with cheese slice.

    c. Chicken, mashed potatos, green beans, salad with Blue Cheese dressing, wine and strawberries with powdered sugar.

    d. Liver, rice, peas, cole slaw, tea, and ice cream.

9-6. For patients with hyperlipidemia, the nurse needs to help patients assess whether their lifestyles contain other high risk factors for the development of a cardiovascular disease. All of the following are considered high risk factors for development of cardiovascular disease except which?

    a. Alcoholic beverages.   c. Hypertension.

    b. Cigarette smoking.   d. Obesity.

9-7. Mr. Riley, age 44, has been started on drug therapy for a high serum cholesterol level that did not respond to diet and weight control. Which of the following information about hyperlipidemia and drug therapy is appropriate to use to teach Mr. Riley about his disease and drug therapy?

    a. Serum cholesterol levels should show a significant drop in a week or two after drugs are begun.

    b. Drug therapy eliminates the need for dietary restrictions.

    c. Drug therapy reduces the chance of a heart attack.

    d. Family members of Mr. Riley should be screened for abnormal lipid levels since they might need treatment.

9-8. Assessment of a patient who has a decrease in essential fatty acids may include all these findings *except* which?

    a. Sparse hair growth.   c. Increased serum triglyceride levels.

    b. Dry and scaly skin.   d. Decreased serum cholesterol levels.

9-9. Serum triglyceride levels are useful in all the following conditions *except* which?

    a. Evaluating the effect of intravenous fat emulsions.

   b. Assessing the presence of hyperthyroidism.

   c. Evaluating the effectiveness of some drugs used to control hyperlipidemia.

   d. Assessing the type of hyperlipidemia that may be present.

9-10. Lipoprotein electrophoresis is a laboratory test that reports which of the following?

   a. Pattern for four different types of lipoproteins (chylomicrons, pre-beta, beta, and alpha).

   b. Numerical values for these four types of lipoproteins.

   c. Ratio of triglycerides to cholesterol levels.

   d. All of the above.

9-11. According to data from the Framingham study, the type of lipoproteins that may offer some protection against the development of cardiovascular disease is which of the following?

   a. Chylomicrons.

   b. Pre-beta (very low-density) proteins, VLDL.

   c. Beta (low-density) lipoproteins, LDL.

   d. Alpha (high-density) lipoproteins, HDL.

9-12. A factor that tends to increase the level of HDL cholesterol is which of the following?

   a. Losing weight if obese.   **c.** Eliminating alcohol from the diet.

   b. Eating meat.   **d.** Lack of exercise.

REFERENCES

American Heart Association. *Diet and Coronary Heart Disease: Statement for Physicians and Other Health Professionals.* New York: American Heart Association, 1978.

Bradley, Douglas *et al.* "Serum High Density Lipoprotein Cholesterol in Women Using Oral Contraceptives, Estrogens and Progestrins," *New England Journal of Medicine* 299 (1978): 17-21.

Breslow, Jan. "Pediatric Aspects of Hyperlipidemia," *Pediatrics* 62:4 (October 1978): 510-551.

Dipp, Stephen. "Metabolic Effects of Alcohol," *Arizona Medicine* 35 (October 1978): 651-652.

Flynn, M. A. *et al.* "Effect of Dietary Egg on Human Serum Cholesterol and Triglycerides," *American Journal of Clinical Nutrition* 32 (May 1979): 1051-1057.

Fredrickson, D. S. *et al.* "Fat Transport in Lipoproteins—An Integrated Approach to Mechanisms and Disorders," *New England Journal of Medicine* 276 (1967): 215.

Gordon, Tavia. "High Density Lipoprotein as a Protective Factor Against Coronary Heart Disease," *American Journal of Medicine* (May 1977): 707-714.

Havel, Richard. "Classification of the Hyperlipidemias," *Annual Review of Medicine* 28 (1977): 195-209.

Hytten, Frank and Lind, Tom. *Diagnostic Indices in Pregnancy.* New Jersey: Ciba-Geigy Corporation, 1975.

Jacobson, Nancy. "How to Administer Those Tricky Lipid Emulsions," *RN* 42 (June 1979): 63–64.

Kannel, William. "Some Lessons in Cardiovascular Epiderminology from Framingham," *American Journal of Cardiology* 37 (February 1976): 269–282.

Kaplan, Alex and Szabo, LaVerne. *Clinical Chemistry Interpretation and Techniques*. Philadelphia: Lea & Febiger, 1979.

Kritchevsky, David and Czarnecki, Suzanne. "Lipoproteins," *Contemporary Nutrition* 5 (May 1980): 1–2.

Mallison, Mary. "Updating the Cholesterol Controversy Verdict—Diet Does Count," *American Journal of Nursing* 78 (October 1978): 1681.

Morrison, John *et al.* "Diagnostic Ramifications of Repeated Plasma Cholesterol and Triglyceride Measurements in Children: Regression Toward the Mean in a Pediatric Population," *Pediatrics* 64:2 (August 1979): 197–201.

Reiser, Raymond. "Diet and Blood Lipids: An Overview," *Food and Nutrition News* 51 (January 1980): 104.

Ross, R. and Glomset, J. A. "Pathogenesis of Atherosclerosis," *New England Journal of Medicine* 295 (August 12, 1976): 364–377.

Sodhi, Harbhajon and Mason, Dean. "New Insights into the Homeostasis of Plasma Cholesterol," *American Journal of Medicine* 63 (September 1977): 325–327.

Smith, Tim. "Medical Advice," *Nor-Cal Running Review* 75 (Winter 1979): 18.

Widmann, Francis. *Clinical Interpretation of Laboratory Tests*, 8th ed. Philadelphia: F. A. Davis Co., 1979.

Yeshurum, D. and Golto, A. M. "Drug Treatment of Hyperlipidemia," *American Journal of Medicine* 60 (March 1976): 379–392.

CHAPTER TEN

Tests Related to Serum Protein Levels

Objectives

1. Identify the serum proteins measured by electrophoresis and immunoelectrophoresis.

2. Illustrate how cellular and humoral immunity are assessed by specific laboratory tests.

3. Identify nursing implications for patients with low serum albumin levels (hypoalbuminemia).

4. Explain the general clinical significance of various aclonal, monoclonal, and polyclonal patterns of immunoglobulins in serum and urine.

5. Identify basic nursing interventions for any patients who has an abnormal pattern or deficiency of IgG, IgA, IgM, or IgD.

6. Describe how the RAST test is used in the assessment of allergies.

7. Identify the types of medications and food that must be withheld when a patient has an elevated serum ammonia level.

8. Describe the clinical usefulness of serum alpha-1 antitrypsin levels and alpha fetoprotein (AFP) levels.

This chapter focuses on the most common tests used to measure proteins in the serum. The difference between serum and plasma proteins is that plasma proteins include those involved in the clotting of the plasma. (The plasma proteins, fibrinogen and prothrombin, are discussed in Chapter 13.)

The two serum proteins measured in the test for "total proteins" are albumin and globulin. Albumin is a singular type of protein that is either in the serum in sufficient amounts or not. The tests for globulins are more complex because there are five types of globulins (Alpha-1 and -2, beta-1 and -2, and gamma globulins). In addition, there are many singular types of proteins in each of these major classes.

The exact amounts of albumin and of the five major globulin types are determined by a procedure called *electrophoresis*. If certain of the gamma globulins are shown to be

TABLE 10-1.   TESTS OF SERUM PROTEINS*

Measured as Total Proteins (T/P)	Measured by Protein Electrophoresis		Measured by Immunoelectrophoresis
Serum proteins (6-8.4 g/dl)	Albumin (3.5-5 g/dl) (52-68%)		
		Alpha-1 globulins (4.2-7.2%)	
		Alpha-2 globulins (6.8-12%)	
Globulins** (2.3-3.5 g/dl)		Beta-1 globulins (3-10%)	
		Beta-2 globulins (1-9%)	IgG 75%
			IgA 10 to 15%
		Gamma globulins (13-23%)	IgM 7 to 10%
			IgD Less than 1%
			IgE Less than 1%

* Values are approximate values for adults. See text for variations.
** Note that many of the alpha and beta globulins can be measured by individual tests for alpha-1 anti-trypsin, alpha feto-protein, and so on.

abnormal, a further test, *immunoelectrophoresis,* is done to separate out the five major types of gamma globulins. Electrophoresis uses an electrical current to separate the six protein fractions, while *immuno*electrophoresis involves, as an added step, the use of antiserum to cause precipitation of the five gamma globulins. The proteins that are identified by these tests are shown in Table 10-1.

These tests can be done not only for the serum but also for urine and spinal fluid. Cawley (1978) gives explicit details on the technical aspects of each of these tests, including the medical interpretation of results. This chapter includes a brief summary about electrophoresis and immunoelectrophoresis of urine; serum ammonia levels are discussed in this chapter because they have a direct relationship with protein metabolism. One serum protein, alpha fetoprotein, normal in pregnancy and very abnormal otherwise, is discussed at the end of the chapter.

FUNCTIONS OF ALBUMIN IN THE SERUM

Albumin, produced only by the liver, is essential in maintaining the oncotic pressure in the vascular system. A lack of albumin in the serum allows fluid to leak out into the interstitial spaces and into the peritoneal cavity. Albumin is also very important in the transportation of many substances in the bloodstream. For example, when the serum albumin level is less than normal, the total serum calcium level is depressed. (See Chapter 7 on how albumin affects the interpretation of serum calcium levels.) Many drugs, lipids, hormones, and toxins are bound to albumin while they are circulating in the bloodstream.

Once the drug or other substance reaches the liver, it is detached from the albumin and made less toxic by conversion to a water soluble form that can be excreted. (See Chapter 11 for further discussion about the role of albumin in the conjugation process of bilirubin.) Albumin is also one of the buffers that functions to maintain acid–base balance in the bloodstream, as discussed in Chapter 6.

FUNCTIONS OF GLOBULINS IN THE SERUM

As can be seen in Table 10–1, the globulins are a very complex and diversified group of serum proteins, for which both the alpha and the beta types are synthesized in the liver:

1. *Alpha-1 globulin* is composed of various lipoproteins, glycoproteins, antitrypsin, and other proteins such as thyroid-binding globulin.
2. *Alpha-2 globulin* contains macroglobulins, haptoglobulin, ceroloplasmin, and hormones such as erythropoietin.
3. *Beta-1 globulins* contain hormones, fat soluble vitamins, transferrin, and plasmingen, in addition to other lipoproteins.
4. *Beta-2 globulins* contain most of the various components of the complement system and other proteins.

For more than this short summary of the alpha and beta globulins, see Arguembourg (1975), who gives a very detailed explanation on how these globulins are identified in electrophoresis.

Nurses need not necessarily remember which specific proteins go under which type of alpha or beta globulin. The point is that the globulins are comprised of many types of proteins. Liver dysfunction is the usual reason for overall changes in alpha and beta globulins. Disease conditions that change an individual alpha or beta globulin, such as the lack of erythropoietin in renal disease, do not cause a major change in the whole broad grouping of serum globulins. (Some of the individual tests for the various components of the complement system, as well as other serological tests involving protein reactions, are covered in Chapter 14.) The lipoprotein electrophoresis, which measures specific alpha and beta globulins involved in fat (lipid) transport, is used to detect certain types of hyperlipidemia. (Lipoprotein electrophoresis is covered in Chapter 9.)

Unlike the alpha and beta globulins, gamma globulins, now called immunoglobulins, are not synthesized by the liver. They are made by B lymphocytes in response to a stimulus from an antigen. Classified as five main types that are designated by the letters IgG, IgA, IgM, IgD, and IgE, these five immunoglobulins are changed considerably in different types of immunological responses. To understand the clinical significance of testing for the immunoglobulins, one must recall some basic facts about the concepts of cellular and humoral immunity.

The Immune System
Nysather (1976) contains a detailed review of the development and functions of the immune system. Optimal immunological defense probably depends on interactions be-

tween cellular and humoral immunity, but much is still to be learned about the interaction of these two systems.

Cellular Immunity. Cellular immunity, or delayed hypersensitivity, is a function of the T lymphocytes that are controlled by the thymus. The presence of adequate cellular immunity can be demonstrated by a positive response to various skin tests. Cellular immunity is not identified by tests on plasma because T lymphocytes do not produce antibodies, although they may help mediate this function of the B lymphocytes.

Humoral Immunity. Because the immunoglobulins secreted by the B lymphocytes are found in the bloodstream and in other secretions such as saliva, tears, and colostrum, this type of immunity is called *humoral*. Humoral immunity is the type directly measured by assessment of the circulating antibodies in serum and in other body fluids, since the antibodies or immunoglobulins are produced by the B lymphocyte system. The "B" stands not for blood but for bursa, because earlier research discovered this type of lymphocyte in the bursa of chickens. In man, the B lymphocytes are thought to be produced in the lymphoid tissue of the gastrointestinal tract. The distinctions between the five types of gamma globulin are discussed under the section on the test of immunoelectrophoresis.

The complement system contains several proteins that are classified by the letter C and a number (such as C2, C4, and the like). The complement system enhances the antibody–antigen reaction of the humoral system. The tests involving the complement system are discussed in Chapter 14.

ALBUMIN/GLOBULIN RATIO

Older nursing texts may still refer to the albumin/globulin ratio as a test done for liver function. Characteristically, the albumin level drops and the globulins rise in liver dysfunction. The exact percentages of albumin and the globulins, however, is much more useful than just a ratio. Since the total protein measures the actual amount of albumin and globulin, this is a much more useful test. In addition, the electrophoresis gives much more information about all the types of globulins.

SERUM TOTAL PROTEIN AND PROTEIN ELECTROPHORESIS

In this test, the laboratory uses an electrical current to separate normal human serum into six distinct protein fractions, through a migration of protein molecules. Various protein molecules, after separating out in a gel mixture or on a coated film, are fixed on a sheet of paper. Albumin, the largest component, has the greatest mobility, so it moves the farthest away from the point of the electrical current. The alpha globulins line up next, then the beta globulins (Cawley 1978). Since the gamma globulins migrate the least from the electrical point, this group makes the last big distinct band on the paper. Once the six protein fractions have been separated out on the strip of paper, the sheet is stained to identify the pattern.

This pictorial representation of the amounts of each protein type is useful as a screening device because significant changes in the patterns can be noted and further testing done if deemed necessary by the clinician. The pathologist is usually the one to compare the pattern to known abnormal patterns that are seen in various disease states. The strip of paper, or electrophorectogram, can be put into a machine that quantifies the six serum protein fractions and reports the amount in percentages. This report in percentages can be read by the nurse since the percentages can be compared to reference values for each type of protein fraction.

Preparation of Patient and Collection of Sample

The patient should be fasting but can have water. One milliliter of whole blood is ample for total protein and electrophoresis. Fresh samples are ideal, but older samples can be used. The dye used for a BSP test makes the results falsely elevated for a couple of days.

Reference Values

Essentially, the same for all people. Variations noted for electrophoresis results are as follows:

Total serum protein   6–8.4 g/100 ml
Serum albumin   3.5–5.0 g/100 ml
Serum globulins   2.3–3.5 g/100 ml

Electrophoresis (reported as a percentage of total protein):

Adults	Albumin	52–68%
	Globulins	
	Alpha-1	4.2–7.2%
	Alpha-2	6.8–12%
	Beta-1	3–10%
	Beta-2	1–9%
	Gamma	13–23%

Newborns   Essentially fall in the same distribution with a little lowering of Beta-1. See details about gamma globulins in text.

Pregnancy   Albumin falls quickly the first few months and then more slowly during rest of pregnancy. Overall fall is about 1 g/100 ml. The alpha and beta globulins show slight increases while the gamma globulins may decrease slightly (Hytten 1975).

Note that oral contraceptives may cause a slight decrease (see Appendix D).

Children	Tend to have slightly greater amounts of alpha-2. Types and amounts of gamma globulins depend on age. See text.	
Ages 4–11	Total protein	6.6–7.9 g
Ages 12–20	Total protein	6.8–8.4 g

Aged   The gamma globulins, or at least the immunological response, decreases with age (Dharan 1976).

Elevated Serum Albumin Level

Clinical Significance. No pathological conditions cause the liver to produce extra amounts of albumin. So an increased value of albumin on a laboratory report is a reflection of dehydration. (Recall that many tests can be falsely elevated by dehydration.) The inclusion of excess amounts of protein in the diet does not raise the serum albumin level since protein is first broken down into amino acids and then used for various purposes, including storage as adipose (fat) tissue.

Dilution by Excess IV admin. ↓Total protein - Assoc. c ↓alb. + sm. change in globulin resulting in Low A/G ratio. ↑ loss albumin in urine ↓ protein intake - Neph. Synd.

Decreased Serum Albumin Level

Clinical Significance (Hypoalbuminemia). Since albumin is totally synthesized by the liver, liver dysfunction is a common reason for a decreased serum albumin level. Reduced albumin levels are not seen in acute liver failure because it takes several weeks of non-production before the albumin level drops. The most common reason for a lowered level is chronic liver dysfunction due to cirrhosis. A loss of albumin in the urine due to renal dysfunction (nephrotic syndrome) can also cause a decrease of albumin in the serum. Although a drop of about 1 g/100 ml is normal in pregnancy, there is even more of a drop in preeclampsia. (Albuminuria, or albumin in the urine, is a key sign of both renal pathology and eclampsia. See Chapter 3.) Severe burns, with the related damage to capillaries and blood vessels, result in a large loss of serum proteins, including albumin. The increased capillary permeability due to the burn damage may cause a continual leak of serum proteins out of the vascular system. Also, the long-term depression of protein synthesis after a burn may last for a couple of months.

If there is inadequate intake of protein, the body begins the breakdown of muscles and of other protein tissue (catabolism) to obtain enough amino acids for the continuing synthesis of serum albumin. Thus albumin levels do not drop in fasting states or in malnutrition until the condition is severe. Protein requirements may be greatly increased during stress, infection, or injury. The patient is in a negative nitrogen balance when the catabolic process is greater than the anabolic process and when the protein deficiency is longstanding. A combination of illness with prolonged protein deprivation is eventually reflected in a reduced serum albumin level.

In the United States, a true protein deficiency (kwashiorkor) is a rare condition. Certain elderly groups, particularly black and Spanish-American women, may contain people who have lower than the recommended daily allowance of protein (Palombo 1980). However, this low-protein diet does not affect serum albumin levels directly unless illness increases the need for more protein. On rare occasions, when children, who require more protein than adults, are placed on an inadequate cult-type vegetarian diet, they may become so depleted in protein that this causes a lowered serum albumin level. Vegetarians who choose a diet with a sufficient variety of grains, nuts, fruits and vegetables maintain adequate protein synthesis.

↓T.S. protein is assoc. c edema + ↓ Transport function such as hypocalcemia, caused by ↓ iron intake - Excessive administration of IV glucose in water

Possible Nursing Implications.

Assessing for Edema. Because albumin is responsible for the oncotic pressure in the vascular system, a reduction in serum albumin causes edema. Without adequate albumin in the bloodstream, fluid leaks out into the interstitial spaces and into the peritoneal cavity. Unlike the edema due to too much volume in the vascular space, this type of edema is not found primarily in dependent areas. For example, patients with an increased volume due to congestive heart failure have edema in the feet if they are sitting up or in the sacral area if in bed. In contrast, patients with edema due to a lack of albumin may also have puffy eyelids or hands and a swollen abdomen due to the leakage of fluid into the peritoneal cavity. (The cirrhotic patient who has hypoalbuminemia is also likely to have portal hypertension that intensifies the collection of fluid in the peritoneal cavity.) In addition to weighing these patients and checking their ankles and sacral area for edema, the nurse should also measure the abdominal girth to check the progression of edema. Since skin breakdown is also a problem with edema, these patients need good skin care.

Assisting with Interventions to Decrease Edema. A collection of fluid in the peritoneal cavity may make it impossible for the patient to breathe comfortably in a reclining position. Sometimes a paracentesis must be done to take the pressure off the diaphragm. The disadvantage of a paracentesis is that proteins are lost in the peritoneal fluid. Diuretics, along with some restrictions of fluids and of sodium, may be ordered because an increased amount of aldosterone may also be contributing to the formation of edema. (See Chapter 5 on hypernatremia.)

Diet Teaching on Protein Foods. The primary treatment for edema caused by a lack of serum albumin is to increase the albumin level. If the liver can still synthesize albumin, a diet with adequate protein is appropriate for long-term therapy. The recommended daily allowance for protein for healthy adults is around 44 to 56 g a day depending on age and weight. These general figures are set higher than what may be the minimum needed. Palombo (1980) suggests that many Americans eat as much as 90 g of protein while the minimum needed may be as little as 35 to 50 g.

Often the patients who need the protein the most can tolerate it the least because their livers are unable to handle the ammonia that results from protein breakdown. (See the test for serum ammonia at the end of this chapter.) If protein is well tolerated, however, then eggs, cheese, fish, and meat are excellent sources, along with a correct mixture of nuts, grains, and vegetables. If protein needs to be increased in the diet, one egg or an ounce of cheese supplies about 7 g of protein. A glass of milk made from dried milk powder supplies 8 grams of protein without increasing the cholesterol intake. (See Chapter 9 for the cholesterol controversy.) Also, dried milk is economical and can be added to many foods and beverages. Commercially made protein supplements can be used, although they tend to be expensive. If the patient is also deficient in minerals and vitamins, these liquid diets may ensure a higher level of many necessary nutrients. The patient must have plenty of calories from carbohydrates so that protein is not used as an expensive energy source. See Table 10-2 for a comparison of the protein content in various foods.

Assisting with Albumin Replacement Intravenously. For the patient who needs albumin replacement immediately, albumin can be given intravenously. Brand names for albumin include Albumisol, Albuspan, Burminate, Albuminar, Albuteen, and Proserum. Some albumin, which is collected from human donors, is obtained from placental blood, which is a significant fact since the infusion of some albumins causes a rise in the alkaline phosphatase level. (See Chapter 12 for this enzyme test.) Albumin does not need to be refrigerated as does whole blood. It does not have any preservatives added so it must be used soon after it is opened.

Albumin comes in a 5% and a 25% concentration. The 25% solution is salt poor. The removal of the salt from the solution makes the albumin more therapeutic if the edema is due to sodium retention as well as to a lack of albumin. The 25% solution is usually given at a rate no faster than 1 ml a minute. The 5% solution can be given at a rate of around 2 ml to 4 ml a minute (Govoni 1978:11). The intravenous infusion must be given slowly due to the danger of circulatory overload. Otherwise the safety of albumin is very high.

As the oncotic pressure returns to normal, edematous fluid is pulled back into the

TABLE 10-2.   FOODS HIGH IN PROTEIN*

Food Item	Grams of Protein
Complete proteins	
1 egg	7
1 oz meat or fish	7–8
1 oz cheese	6–7
8 oz milk	8.5
1 Tbsp dried milk	1.6
Incomplete proteins**	
1 Tbsp peanut butter	4
2 slices wheat bread	4
1 cup nuts	7–8
3 oz lentils	7
¼ cup garbanzo beans	10

* Estimates are from various food labels and nutritional pamphlets.
** Consult a nutrition text on how incomplete vegetable proteins can be balanced to supply all needed amino acids.

vascular system. The mobilization of edema from the tissues causes an increased urine output. The albumin remains in the bloodstream for several days, but with a severe albumin deficiency, the patient may need repeated infusions over time. Serum albumin levels are assessed every few days, or even daily, to determine how much replacement is needed. Giving albumin intravenously is not only costly, but also recent studies suggest that protein by oral feedings helps to raise albumin levels even when protein synthesis seems questionable (Tullis 1977).

Change in the Alpha and Beta Globulins

Clinical Significance. Many of the individual proteins of which the alpha and beta globulins are comprised can be measured specifically, since most of them do not make major changes in overall pattern of the globulins. In general, the usual causes for significant changes in the alpha and beta globulins are due to liver dysfunction and, if any other abnormalities are suspected, more specific testing must be done. For example, if there is a lack of alpha-1, further testing would be done to see if there is a lack of the specific antitrypsin.

Possible Nursing Implications. Since the most common reason for a change in the alpha and beta globulins is liver dysfunction, the nursing care depends on the exact pathological state, which may be cirrhosis or hepatitis. The nurse needs to see if there is a change in the patient's gamma globulins, as well as in other globulins, since the implication for nursing is much more specific for gamma globulin changes.

ALPHA-1 ANTITRYPSIN

The role of antitrypsin is to inhibit the damaging effects from proteolytic enzymes released by bacteria and phagocytes in the lung. The relationship of antitrypsin to the liver is not well understood, but a lack of this protein is found in young children with cirrhosis (Widmann 1979:389). Children with lung or liver dysfunctions are screened for a lack of this alpha protein.

Preparation of Patient
And Collection of Sample

No special preparation of patient is necessary. Laboratory needs 10 ml of blood.

Reference Values

200–400 mg/100 ml

Decreased Alpha-1 Antitrypsin

Clinical Significance. The lack of this type of protein is due to a genetic defect. People with a lack of antitrypsin tend to have fibrotic changes in the lung and liver.

Possible Nursing Implications. The key nursing implication for the patient with a lack of antitrypsin is to protect the patient against respiratory infections. The reader is referred to more advanced texts for current treatment on abnormalities of specific globulins.

Change in Gamma Globulins

Clinical Significance. There is usually more diagnostic significance in the patterns of gamma globulins than in the alpha and beta globulins. There may be an increase either of various types (polyclonal) or of only one type (monoclonal), or there may be an absence (aclonal) of gamma globulins. The use of the term "clonal" refers to the origin of the globulins from a particular *clone* of plasma cells. All these patterns can be detected by electrophoresis. Cawley (1978) and Dharan (1976) are recommended for more detailed explanations of these patterns' clinical significance, which can range from a slight infection to a terminal disease, such as multiple myeloma.

   Polyclonal Pattern. This pattern is a reflection of an overproduction of almost all the immunoglobulins in response to antigens. Several different clones of plasma cells are producing increased amounts of various immunoglobulins. The end result is a general hypergammaglobulinemia, a characteristic response to infections (the inflammatory response). Autoimmune diseases and certain liver diseases cause a generalized increase too.

   Monoclonal Patterns. In this pattern, only one type of gamma globulin is increased. Patterns of this sort may be more specifically diagnostic because they involve a spike of a single globulin, which can be closely examined by immunoelectrophoresis to detect

paraproteins or abnormal varients of an immunoglobulin. Monoclonal patterns are found
in a number of situations:

1. A majority of patients with multiple myeloma have a peak of a paraprotein or
abnormal globulin. (The discussion on immunoelectrophoresis explores paraproteins.)
2. Sometimes the elderly have a monoclonal pattern that appears to be more the
result of the aging process than of a specific disease. However, for patients that
show a monoclonal pattern, half may eventually develop multiple myeloma
(Dharan 1976:1677).
3. Macroglobulinemia, an increase in the IgM, is characterized by an increase in
just one type of immunoglobulin.
4. Malignant lymphomas and acute infections are other conditions that may cause
an increase of only one type of immunoglobulin.

Aclonal Patterns. In aclonal patterns, or hypogammopathies, the gamma globulins
are absent or markedly decreased.

1. The lack of gamma globulins may be congenital. Infants with an aclonal pattern
may appear normal at birth due to the presence of immunoglobulins from the
mother. But then frequent and severe infections begin to occur when the passive
immunity from the mother no longer exists.
2. Acquired hypogammaglobulinemia is most often seen with chronic lymphocytic
leukemia, malignant lymphomas, or other diseases affecting the bone marrow.
3. Drugs, such as corticosteroids and cytotoxic drugs used for treatment of malignancies, may reduce gamma globulin levels or at least make the gamma
globulins ineffective.
4. Radiation therapy and toxins in the environment can also produce an acquired
lack of gamma globulins.

Possible Nursing Implications.

Protecting the Patient from Infection. The person with either less gamma globulins
or abnormal gamma globulins is very susceptible to opportunistic pathogens. High levels
of abnormal immunoglobulins are always accompanied by lower levels of normal immunoglobulins. So the single most important nursing implication for a patient who has an
abnormal gamma globulin pattern is to protect the patient from infection. Since bacterial
pneumonia is often the cause of death, for example, the patient must be protected from
others who have upper respiratory infections. Sometimes it may be necessary to initiate
reverse isolation to protect the patient, particularly with infants who have a severe immunodeficiency disorder. With the older person, meticulous hand washing is probably the key
point, since reverse isolation, with its extra cost, still does not protect persons from the
bacteria on their own skin or from the bacteria in food. A concentrated effort should be
made to keep the environment relatively free of pathogens; Donley (1976) gives many
tips on how to make the environment as germ-free as possible. Since the main defense
against invading organisms is intact skin and mucus membranes, the nurse must promote
good skin care. Proper nutrition with adequate protein is also important for the production

of immunoglobulins. (See the discussion on albumin for ways to ensure adequate protein intake.) The premature infant and the aged person are particularly vulnerable to infections due to their more severe lack of enough antibodies to offer resistance to pathogens.

Assisting with Therapy to Replace or Remove Gamma Globulins. Gamma globulin may be administered to patients to increase immunoglobulin levels temporarily. Immune serum globulin (Gamastan by Cutter) may prevent serious infection if circulatory levels of IgG (discussed next) are kept at about 200 mgm/dl. However, Gamastan may not prevent chronic infections of the secretory tissues such as the respiratory tract. The gamma globulin may be needed every three to four weeks. Since now and then serum globulin injections can cause anaphylaxis, the person should be observed for 20 to 30 minutes after the injection (Cutter 1979). Plasma therapy may also be used if larger doses of passive immunity are needed.

In addition to the replacement of normal gamma globulins there may also be an attempt to remove abnormal proteins from the bloodstream by pheresis. *Pheresis* is the process whereby a specific plasma constituent is separated from other blood constituents and removed from the patient's plasma. (Pheresis can also be used to obtain platelets for transfusion.) If the patient has an excessive amount of abnormal IgM (see the discussion on macroglobulinemia), this protein can be filtered out of the blood by the pheresis machine. Rossman (1977) discusses the nursing care of two patients undergoing pheresis therapy for monoclonal gamma globulin patterns.

Since the specific therapy for abnormal gamma globulin patterns depends on which gamma globulins are affected, the test for immunoglobulins is discussed next.

IMMUNOELECTROPHORESIS OF SERUM PROTEINS (IgG, IgA, IgM, IgD, AND IgE)

When a protein electrophoresis demonstrates abnormalities in the gamma globulins, it may be useful to find out exactly which of the gamma globulins are changed. Before 1960, the term "gamma globulins" was used to include those known to give the body immunity against antigens or foreign proteins. According to the World Health Organization, *immunoglobulins* are defined as proteins of animal origin that are endowed with known antibody activity (Arguembourg 1975:9). Certain other proteins that do not have antibody activity are also called immunoglobulins. These paraproteins are the type seen elevated in the monoclonal patterns of multiple myeloma and in other abnormal productions of plasma cells. Although there are only five main groups of immunoglobulins (IgG, IgA, IgM, IgD, and IgE), forty or more fractions can be distinguished by researchers. This discussion is limited to some general knowledge about the five major types of immunoglobulins.

The laboratory uses antiserum preparations to cause a precipitation of each of the five major types of immunoglobulins. The precipitations may be done in a gel or on a glass slide and then transferred to a sheet of paper. The final result is a pattern of bands that have a certain curvature, position, and intensity of color. Abnormalities in any of the immunoglobulins cause the band for that precipitation to be displaced, bowed, lighter in color, thicker than normal, or absent. The laboratory can also quantify each type of immunoglobulin. Some laboratories may report in milligrams and some in grams. Thus the results may be, for example, 0.8 to 1.5 g/dl or 800 to 1,500 mg/dl. The reference values used here are in milligrams.

Preparation of Patient
And Collection of Sample

The patient should not eat for eight hours before the test. A fresh sample is the sample of choice, but aged serum or plasma can be used. Depending on the technique, only 1 ml of blood may be needed. Other techniques require 10 ml. Any blood transfusions or blood component therapy within the last 6 weeks, as well as any immunizations or vaccines within the last 6 months, should be noted on the laboratory requisition (Byrne 1981).

Reference Values

	IgG	IgA	IgM	IgD	IgE
Adult	540–1.663 mg/dl (usually about 75% of total)	66–344 mg/dl (10–15%)	39–290 mg/dl (7–10%)	0.5–3 mg/dl (less than 1%)	0.01–0.04 mg/dl (less than 1%)

Newborns	IgG 640–1.250 mg/dl IgD —
	IgA 0–11 mg/dl IgE —
	IgM 5–30 mg/dl

Children	Depends on age. By age 6 months to a year. levels begin gradual increase. Adult values may be reached by late teens.
Pregnancy	Evidently IgE falls somewhat during pregnancy. while the others show no significant change.
Aged	Even healthy older people may show abnormal patterns with increase of paraproteins. (Dharan 1976). In response to a challenge, such as an infection. immunoglobulin production is likely to be reduced.

Changes in Immunoglobulins

Clinical Significance. The exact significance of changes in immunoglobulins may be determined only in conjunction with other tests such as urine immunoelectrophoresis and perhaps bone marrow studies. Following is a brief summary of the general characteristics of changes in each component of the immunoglobulins. One way to rememer which one is the most abundant and which is the least is to say "*G A M D E,*" since G is the most abundant and E the least abundant in the adult. Kyle (1978) contains an extensive review of the studies done on the immunoglobulins.

IgG. This immunoglobulin, which makes up about three-fourths of the total immunoglobulins, is the only one that crosses the placenta. Hence the infant has a high level, which shows some decrease until about 6 months to a year when the infant begins ample production of IgG.

IgG protects against virus, bacteria, and toxins. It is more for a secondary response. IgG, IgM, and IgA are all elevated in the inflammatory response. A lack of IgG causes severe immunodeficiency. IgG increases when the person is desensitized to antigens, and it apparently blocks IgE actions (Voignier 1978:618). Note that injections of immune serum globulin (Gamastan by Cutter) contain primarily IgG.

IgA. The second most common immunoglobulin in the bloodstream, IgA is also present in watery fluids and in surface secretions, such as saliva, tears, and colostrum. These immunoglobulins are thought to be the first line of defense against organisms invading the respiratory, gastrointestinal, or urinary tracts. The infant begins producing IgA after a few months. Deficiencies of IgA may be combined with other deficiencies or be alone. The antinuclear antibodies (ANA), febrile agglutinins, and cold agglutinins (Chapter 14) belong to this class of immunoglobulins.

IgM. In the bloodstream in slightly lower levels than IgA, IgM does not cross the placenta, but the infant may begin synthesizing IgM sooner than IgA. IgM is particularly important for resistance to gram negative bacteria (Heagarty 1980:204). IgM is the major component in a primary immune response. The rheumatoid factor and heterophile antibodies are also in this group. IgM activates the complement system, its level remaining high as long as the antigen is present. The antibodies to blood group antigens are in the group of IgM immunoglobulins. (See Chapter 14 for the specific tests for ABO incompatibility, Rh factor, rheumatic factor (RF), heterophile antibody test (HAT), and the complement system.)

Since IgM has a high molecular weight, abnormal increases in it are called *macroglobulinemia*. There immunoglobulins tend to make the blood highly viscous. Normal viscosity of blood is 1.4 to 1.8 as compared to the viscosity of water. The increase of macroglobulins also makes the person very sensitive to cold (Dharan 1976:1628). As discussed earlier, pheresis therapy may be used to remove abnormal immunoglobulins (Rossmann 1977).

IgD. This immunoglobulin is in the bloodstream in very small amounts. The exact functions of IgD are unclear at the present time.

IgE and the RAST (Radioallergosorbent Test for IgE Antibodies). IgE, which is in the bloodstream in very small amounts, increases in allergic states and in the event of parasitic infestation. Evidently IgE is responsible for severe hypersensitive reactions. A measurement of specific IgE antibodies in the serum helps to establish the diagnosis of allergic disease by identifying which allergens are causing clinical symptoms such as hay fever, asthma, or skin rashes (Hamburger 1978).

The radioallergosorbent test (RAST) measures the quantity and the increase of antigen-specific IgE present in the serum. Hence the exact quantities of antibodies to a variety of pollens, such as animal dander or food, can be tested. Although more expensive than conventional skin testing, the RAST gives precise information without causing any hypersensitivity reactions. The test has become the most reliable for the diagnosis of food allergy of the immediate type. No satisfactory laboratory test is available to aid in the diagnosis of delayed (up to 5 days) food allergy (Breneman 1979:2). Voignier (1978) explains the nurse's role in testing and treating for allergies in children.

URINE PROTEIN ELECTROPHORESIS
AND IMMUNOELECTROPHORESIS

The techniques for doing electrophoresis and immunoelectrophoresis of urine are similar to those for serum testing. If an abnormal amount of protein is discovered in the urine, these tests can identify exactly which kinds of proteins are being excreted. (See Chapter 3 for the screening technique for proteinuria.) Normally, a 24-hour urine has a protein content of around 40 to 150 mg with no more than 10 mg in a random specimen. The dipstick used for screening registers 1+ when there are about 30 mg in the specimen; less than 30 mg causes a trace showing.

The dipstick method of screening for proteinuria tests primarily for albumin. The dipstick for protein is not reliable as a screening test for proteins other than albumin. The laboratory uses other methods to screen for abnormal proteins, such as Bence-Jones protein which may occur with multiple myeloma. The electrophoresis and, if necessary, an immunoelectorphoresis are used to follow up a quantitative or qualitative report of abnormal protein in the urine.

Protein in the urine may not always be pathological. Glomerular permeability increases in some people when they are in the upright position (orthostatic proteinuria). Another nonpathological reason for protein in the urine is vigorous exercise.

Reference Values

Three main types of pathological patterns may be identified by separating out the protein fractions in urine (Cawley 1978:74):

1. There may be a marked increase in the albumin fraction and some increase in alpha and beta globulins. This signifies increase glomerular permability such as that seen in some renal disease and in eclampsia.

2. There may be a marked elevation in alpha and beta globulins with a decrease in albumin. This most likely signifies tubular damage.

3. There may be various abnormal proteins or paraproteins, such as those found in multiple myeloma or in other disorders of the gamma globulins. This is considered a prerenal pattern. Just as in the serum, immunoelectrophoresis can then be used to identify exactly which globulins are present.

SERUM AMMONIA LEVELS

The liver normally converts ammonia, a byproduct of protein metabolism, into urea, which is excreted by the kidneys. When the liver is unable to convert ammonia to urea, toxic levels of ammonia accumulate in the bloodstream. In severe liver failure, the blood urea nitrogen (BUN) drops as the ammonia level rises. (See Chapter 4 on the use of the BUN as a test for renal function.)

Preparation of Patient And Collection of Sample

Although the patient should be in the fasting state, water is allowed. Either venous or arterial blood can be used. The blood is put into a heparinized tube (green top Vacutainer) and packed in ice for transport to the laboratory. If the patient is on antibiotics (such as neomycin) for treatment of hepatic coma, write this fact on the laboratory slip.

Reference Values

Adults	35–65 mcg/dl	(tested by enzymatic method,
Newborns	90–150 mcg/dl	Children's Hospital San Francisco, California)
Children	45–80 mcg/dl	

Values may vary considerably from laboratory to laboratory. See Appendix A for another set of values.

Increased Ammonia Level

Clinical Significance. Increased ammonia levels, which occur in liver dysfunction, may be due either to blood not circulating through the liver well or to actual hepatic failure. For example, in Reyes syndrome, an increasing ammonia level signifies major liver damage. In terminal cirrhosis, the patient has an elevated ammonia level. Cirrhotic patients who have portal-caval shunts done to relieve portal hypertension may have increased ammonia levels after surgery because blood is shunted away from the liver.

Possible Nursing Implications.

Assessing for Asterixis. Although high levels of ammonia occur in hepatic coma (hepatic encephalopathy), the ammonia may not be what actually causes the neurological symptoms. Most likely, many toxins in hepatic failure cause the symptoms of disorientation and tremors seen in hepatic encephalopathy. The patient should be checked for a certain kind of tremor of the hand called liver flap or *asterixis* (which can also be caused by high levels of uremia or other central nervous system toxins). Ask the patient to extend his or her arms out in front of the body, spread the fingers, and hold the hands in a dorsiflexed position. Patients who have a high level of ammonia in their blood and who are developing hepatic encephalopathy cannot hold their palms up in a steady manner. The hands will flap. Asking the patient to write his or her name or to draw a star are other ways to assess the neurological dysfunction. The nurse may often be the first one to notice subtle changes in the patient's ability to perform simple tasks that require coordination and mental alertness. The lack of mental alertness and coordination may progress to a coma unless treatment is begun.

Reducing All Sources of Ammonia from Protein Breakdown. Since a rising serum ammonia level indicates an inability of the liver to handle the breakdown of protein, the patient should have *no* protein intake until the ammonia level returns to normal. If the patient in hepatic failure has a gastrointestinal bleed, this makes the progression to hepatic coma faster because ammonia is produced when the blood proteins in the intestine are broken down. Enemas and gastric lavage may be needed to get as much of the blood out of the gastrointestinal tract as possible. Since intestinal bacteria produce ammonia by breaking down protein, the amount of bacteria may also be reduced by giving neomycin, a nonsystemic antibiotic, which may be given orally or by enemas (Phipps 1979).

Resuming Protein Intake. When the ammonia level returns to normal, protein is cautiously put back into the diet in increasing amounts. The diet may be limited to only 20 g of protein per day for awhile. (See Table 10–2 for a list of the protein content of foods.) As the protein level in the diet is increased, the nurse must watch carefully for any signs of hepatic encephalopathy. Serum ammonia levels are useful in evaluating the ability of the liver to once again handle protein.

Recognizing the Potential Danger of Sedatives and Diuretics. In addition to the amount of protein in the diet, other factors that contribute to the development of hepatic coma include hypokalemia and the use of sedatives and narcotics. The body is less able to handle ammonia when the potassium level is low or when alkalosis is present (Phipps 1979). Thus diuretic therapy (which often causes potassium loss) may be contraindicated when the patient has an increased ammonia level. In addition, the failing liver is unable to detoxify many drugs, including sedatives and narcotics. When a patient has a rising ammonia level, all previous drug orders need to be reevaluated to see if they are still appropriate in respect to the change in the patient's condition.

ALPHA-FETOPROTEIN

Normally this globulin, formed only in the yolk sac and liver of the fetus, disappears from the bloodstream after birth, except for trace amounts which may be detected by radioimmunoassay. (See Chapter 15 for a description of RIA.) The test for alpha-fetoprotein is done on amniotic fluid to detect certain congenital defects, as well as in the serum of pregnant women and other adults to detect a specific pathology.

Preparation of Patient
And Collection of Sample

There is no special preparation of the patient for a serum sample. The laboratory needs 5 ml of clotted blood.

Reference Values

After infancy	Abnormal if present.
Pregnancy	Serum levels increase during pregnancy to levels of 53–350 μg/l.

Elevated Alpha-Fetoprotein Level in
Serum or Amniotic Fluid

Clinical Significance. The serum alpha-fetoprotein has the distinction of being the first maternal serum test to screen for a genetic defect in the fetus. In the fetus, if the neural tube fails to close properly, enormous amounts of fetal protein leak out into the amniotic fluid all during the pregnancy. Hence this test is useful to detect closure defects of the neural tube. In the pregnant woman, levels above the usual reference values for a particular gestational age may also indicate a neural tube defect in the fetus. (See Chapter 18 for a detailed discussion of this test.) The alpha-fetoprotein level is also usually increased in the serum of the mother when the infant has died in utero (Hytten 1975:43).

In the nonpregnant adult, a markedly increased alpha-fetoprotein level is associated with primary carcinoma (hepatoma) of the liver, since metastatic cancer to the liver does not cause such a rise. Very small amounts are present in some nonmalignant liver diseases in children and adults. The appearance of a fetal protein in an adult malignancy gives support to the theory that cancer somehow arises from very primitive cells. Other fetal proteins may also be present in some types of malignancies. As a group, these antigens are called oncofetal antigens (OFA) (Phipps 1980:201). For some time, it has been known that a change in the immunological makeup of a person seems to increase one's susceptibility to cancer (Donley 1976:1622). Cancer immunology is still more in the research stage than in general use. So the reader is encouraged to consult current literature for the newest developments in testing for oncofetal antigens.

Questions

10-1. Which of the following proteins in the blood is a plasma protein rather than a serum protein?

    a. Fibrinogen.
    c. Gamma globulins.

    b. Alpha and beta globulins.
    d. Albumin.

10-2. The test for gamma globulins (immunoglobulins) measures which of the following?

    a. Both cellular and humoral immunity.

    b. Antibodies produced by antigenic stimulation of T lymphocytes.

    c. Antibodies produced by antigenic stimulation of B lymphocytes.

    d. Reactions of delayed hypersensitivity.

10-3. Protein electrophoresis is a more useful test than the albumin/globulin ratio for the measurement of serum proteins because electrophoresis does what?

    a. Identifies specific proteins other than albumin and globulin.

    b. Reports the percentages of both albumin and the five globulins.

    c. Measures two types of albumin as well as the various types of globulins.

    d. Requires less sophisticated technical equipment.

10-4. The only clinical condition that creates an elevated serum albumin level is which of the following?

    a. Early liver dysfunction.
    c. Dehydration.

    b. Increased protein intake over a long period.
    d. Kwashiorkor.

10-5. A lowered serum albumin level (hypoalbuminemia) is likely to be a clinical problem for all these patients *except* which?

    a. Mrs. Lehman who is in her last trimester of pregnancy and has been admitted for preeclampsia.

    b. Tommy, age 6, who has severe nephrosis.

  c. Mr. Buber, who has advanced cirrhosis.

  d. Shirley, age 17, who has been on a very restricted diet (only juices) for the past 8 days.

10-6. The major clinical manifestation of the patient with a lowered serum albumin level is which of the following?

  a. Increased susceptibility to infection.   **c.** Loss of weight.

  b. Edema.   **d.** Tendency to bleed.

10-7. Mr. Buber is receiving a 5% solution of albumin intravenously because his serum albumin level was 2 g/100ml. Which of the following nursing actions in *inappropriate?*

  a. Run the solution no faster than 2 to 4 ml a minute.

  b. Observe the patient frequently for possible circulatory overload.

  c. Tell Mr. Buber he will probably have increased urination over the next several hours.

  d. Keep the albumin refrigerated until 30 minutes before it is hung.

10-8. For the patient who can tolerate oral feedings, the most efficient and economical way to increase protein intake is to do which of the following?

  a. Use commercially prepared protein mixtures or powders.

  b. Add extra tablespoons of powdered milk to foods and beverages.

  c. Increase meat consumption.

  d. Reduce carbohydrate intake so the person can eat more protein.

10-9. The most common reason for a significant change in the alpha and beta globulins would be what?

  a. Lack of one specific protein such as erythopoietin.

  b. Liver dysfunction.

  c. Inherited deficiency of antitrypsin or other alpha proteins.

  d. Immunologic responses to antigens.

10-10. The major nursing implication for the patient who is deficient in alpha-1 antitrypsin is which of the following?

  a. Protect the patient from upper respiratory infections.

  b. Increase protein in the diet.

  c. Limit protein in the diet.

  d. Assess for edema.

10-11. The disease multiple myeloma causes an overproduction of immunoglobulins in a pattern classified as which of the following?

    a. Monoclonal.   **c.** Aclonal.

    b. Polyclonal.   **d.** Any of the above.

10-12. Which of these patients is the least likely to have lowered or absent immunoglobulins?

    a. Baby Federini, a premature infant born yesterday.

    b. Mrs. Patch, who is a month pregnant and diabetic.

    c. Mr. Regoni, who is on corticosteroid therapy for chronic emphysema.

    d. Mrs. Adams, who is 85 years old and has been admitted for a hernia repair.

10-13. The single most important nursing implication in caring for any patient with an abnormal gamma globulin pattern is which of the following?

    a. Prevent dehydration.   **c.** Increase protein in diet.

    b. Minimize potential for infection.   **d.** Observe for edema.

10-14. Which immunoglobulin crosses the placenta and provides immunity for the newborn for several months?

    a. IgG   **b.** IgA   **c.** IgM   **d.** IgD

10-15. Which type of immunoglobulin is elevated in response to incompatible blood?

    a. IgG   **b.** IgA   **c.** IgM   **d.** IgE

10-16. The radioallergenosorbent test (RAST) is useful to do which of the following?

    a. Measure all the various types of immunoglobulins in the serum.

    b. Distinguish between cellular and humoral immunity.

    c. Measure the quantity of antigen specific IgE antibodies in the serum that increase in immediate allergic reactions.

    d. Discriminate the globulins of high molecular weight (macroglobulinemias) from other globulins.

10-17. What is urine immunoelectrophoresis used to do?

    a. Quantify the total protein in the urine.

    b. Identify the ratio of albumin to globulin in the urine.

    c. Diagnose orthostatic proteinuria.

    d. Detect specific immunoglobulins and paraproteins in the urine.

10-18. Mr. Buber is a patient with cirrhosis who has an ammonia level of over 100 mcg/100 ml. He states he wants ''something to eat.'' Which diet would be appropriate for Mr. Buber this morning?

    a. Eggs, toast, jelly, and coffee.

    b. Grapefruit juice, cereal, and a glass of milk.

    c. Orange juice and sliced banana.

    d. Pancakes, syrup, butter, and coffee.

10–19. In a nonpregnant state, what might the presence of large amounts of alpha-fetoprotein in the serum indicate?

    a. Metastatic cancer of the liver.   **c.** Congenital enzymatic defect.

    b. Lack of adult proteins.   **d.** Primary cancer of the liver.

REFERENCES

Arguembourg, Pierre. *Immunoelectrophoresis,* 2nd ed. Basel, Switzerland: S. Karger, 1975.

Breneman, James. "Food Allergy," *Contemporary Nutrition* 4 (March 1979): 3.

Byrne, Judith *et al. Laboratory Tests: Implications for Nurses and Allied Health Professionals.* Menlo Park, Cal.: Addison-Wesley Publishing Co., Inc., 1981.

Cawley, Leo *et al. Electrophoresis and Immunochemical Reactions in Gels,* 2nd ed. Educational Products Division, American Society of Clinical Pathologists, 1978.

Cutter Product Information, *Immune Serum Globulin—Gamastan,* Berkeley, Cal.: Cutter Biological Laboratories, 1979.

Dharan, Murali. "Immunoglobulin Abnormalities," *American Journal of Nursing* 76 (October 1976): 1626–1628.

Donley, Diana. "Nursing the Patient Who is Immunosuppressed," *American Journal of Nursing* 76 (October 1976): 1619–1625.

Govoni, Laura and Hayes, Janice. *Drugs and Nursing Implications,* 3rd ed. New York: Appleton-Century-Crofts, 1978.

Hamburger, Henry. "Diagnostic Usefulness of Specific IgE Antibody Measurements," *Mayo Clinic Proceedings* 53 (July 1978): 459–462.

Heagarty, Margaret *et al. Child Health: Basics for Primary Care.* New York: Appleton-Century-Crofts, 1980.

Hytten, Frank and Lind, Tom. *Diagnostic Indices in Pregnancy.* Ciba-Geigy Corporation, Summitt, New Jersey, 1975.

Kyle, Robert and Greipp, Philip. "Laboratory Investigation of Monocloncal Gammopathics," *Mayo Clinic Proceedings* 53 (November 1978): 719–739.

Nysather, John *et al.* "The Immune System: Its Development and Functions," *American Journal of Nursing* 76 (October 1976): 1614–1616.

Palombo, John and Blackburn, George. "Human Protein Requirements," *Contemporary Nutrition* 5:1 (January 1980): 1–2.

Phipps, Wilma, ed. *Medical–Surgical Nursing: Concepts and Clinical Practice.* St. Louis: The C. V. Mosby Company, 1979.

Rossmann, Maureen *et al.* "Pheresis Therapy: Patient Care," *American Journal of Nursing* 77 (July 1977): 1135–1141.

Tullis, James. "Albumin," *Journal of the American Medical Association* 237 (January 1977): 355–360.

Voignier, Ruth and Bridgewater, Sharon. "Allergies in Children: Testing, Treating and Teaching," *American Journal of Nursing* 78 (April 1978): 617–621.

Widmann, Frances. *Clinical Interpretation of Laboratory Tests,* 8th ed. Philadelphia: F. A. Davis Co., 1979.

CHAPTER ELEVEN

Tests to Measure the Metabolism of Bilirubin And Liver Function

---

Objectives

1. Diagram the normal pathway for bilirubin excretion and explain the five laboratory tests used as assessment tools.
2. Distinguish between prehepatic, intrahepatic, and post-hepatic jaundice in regards to etiologies, symptoms, and changes in laboratory values.
3. Compare and contrast the nursing assessments and interventions appropriate for increased indirect and/or direct serum bilirubin levels in the infant and the adult.
4. Describe the role of the nurse in assisting with medical interventions for newborns with markedly elevated serum indirect bilirubins.
5. Describe the nurse's role in assisting with medical interventions for patients with elevated serum direct bilirubin.
6. Discuss the psychological impact of jaundice on the patient and on significant others.
7. Explain the clinical significance of measuring the bilirubin content in amniotic fluid.
8. Describe the purpose of the BSP test and the necessary preparation of the patient.

The tests for bilirubin were first used over forty years ago, but they are still useful in assessing the patient who has jaundice. Because the tests clearly pinpoint any changes in the breakdown of the metabolism of bilirubin, there is no controversy about the meaning of the results. This chapter begins with a discussion about the normal pathway of bilirubin excretion. Then, to understand the different types of jaundice, it is essential to know the differences between the two types of bilirubin, direct and indirect. The clinical symptom of any elevated bilirubin is jaundice, but the nursing implications are somewhat different depending on whether the jaundice is prehepatic, post-hepatic, or hepatic in origin. The chapter ends with a discussion about general nursing implications for any patient with an elevated bilirubin (jaundice), along with some more specific implications depending on the origin of the jaundice. Understanding the various laboratory tests is the first step in understanding which pathophysiological process is creating the jaundice.

PATHWAY OF NORMAL BILIRUBIN EXCRETION

Bilirubin is a normal component of red blood cells (erythrocytes). When the reticuloen-dothelial system breaks down old or nonuseful red blood cells, bilirubin is one of the waste products. This "free" bilirubin, which is not water-soluble, is a lipid-soluble waste product that needs to be made water-soluble to be excreted. So it is carried by albumin to the liver, where it is conjugated by the liver and made water-soluble. Only water-soluble conjugated bilirubin can be excreted in the urine.

The liver handles bilirubin in a similar way to other poorly water-soluble compounds such as steroids, drugs, and toxins (Schmid 1972). In general, such substances are carried by the plasma proteins (see Chapter 10) to the liver, where they are detached from the protein and made less toxic by conversion to a form that can be excreted.

An enzyme, glucuronyl transferase, is necessary for the transformation or conjuga-tion of bilirubin. Either a lack of glucuronyl transferase or the presence of drugs that interfere with this enzyme renders the liver unable to conjugate bilirubin.

Urine, however, is not the major pathway of excretion for conjugated bilirubin, almost all of which is excreted as one of the components of bile salts. In fact, bilirubin, a vivid pigment, gives bile the characteristic bright greenish-yellow color. When the bile salts reach the intestine via the common bile duct, the bilirubin is acted upon by bacteria to form chemical compounds called *urobilinogens*. Technically, the breakdown of conju-

TABLE 11-1.   RELATIONSHIP OF NORMAL BILIRUBIN EXCRETION TO THE FIVE TESTS USED TO MEASURE BILIRUBIN METABOLISM

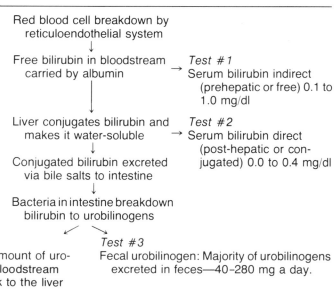

Red blood cell breakdown by
reticuloendothelial system
↓
Free bilirubin in bloodstream   *Test #1*
    carried by albumin   →   Serum bilirubin indirect
                                    (prehepatic or free) 0.1 to
                                    1.0 mg/dl
↓
Liver conjugates bilirubin and   *Test #2*
    makes it water-soluble   →   Serum bilirubin direct
↓   (post-hepatic or con-
Conjugated bilirubin excreted   jugated) 0.0 to 0.4 mg/dl
via bile salts to intestine
↓
Bacteria in intestine breakdown
bilirubin to urobilinogens
↙   ↘

Test #4   *Test #3*
Urine urobilinogen: Small amount of uro-   Fecal urobilinogen: Majority of urobilinogens
    bilinogen absorbed into bloodstream   excreted in feces—40–280 mg a day.
    and goes to urine or back to the liver
    to be excreted again.

Test #5
Note: No *bilirubin* is normally in urine. It
    can be detected by Icotest tablets in
    pathological conditions.

TABLE 11-2. CHANGES IN SERUM, URINE, AND FECES IN THREE TYPES OF JAUNDICE*

	Indirect Serum Bilirubin	Direct Serum Bilirubin	Urine Bilirubin	Urine Urobilinogen	Fecal Urobilinogen
Reference values	Average 0.5 mg/dl	Average 0.1 mg/dl	None	0.4 to 1 mg/day	40 to 280 mg/day
Prehepatic jaundice (hemolytic)	Elevated usually not more than 5 mgm in adults. May be above 20 mgm in newborns	Normal	None	Up to 10 mg	Up to 1,400 mg
Hepatic jaundice	Elevated. May be 15 to 20 mg in severe liver failure.	Slight elevations depending on amount of stasis of bile.	Elevated if obstruction present.	Normal or increased (see text).	Normal or little decreased (see text).
Post-hepatic jaundice (obstruction)	Normal in beginning.	Elevated—May be 30 to 40 mg if obstruction complete.	Elevated—Urine dark orange and foams.	Slight decrease or normal.	Absent—clay-colored stools.

* See text for explanation of each test.

gated bilirubin in the intestine creates several other compounds, but the end product that is measured in both urine and feces is labeled as urobilinogen. These breakdown products give feces their dark color; hence an absence of bilirubin in the intestine causes clay-colored stools. Most of the urobilinogen is excreted in the feces, while some is reabsorbed and goes through the liver again and still another small amount is excreted in the urine. Thus tests for fecal and urine urobilinogens can detect abnormalities in bilirubin excretion.

Because the bilirubin is chemically different after it goes through the conjugation process in the liver, laboratory tests of the serum can differentiate between the bilirubin that is free (prehepatic) and the bilirubin that is conjugated (post-hepatic). The laboratory therefore reports the test results either as total bilirubin or as "direct" or "indirect" bilirubin, terms that refer to the way the two types react to certain dyes (sometimes referred to as the Van de Bergh reaction):

1. The conjugated water-soluble (post-hepatic) bilirubin reacts *directly* when dyes are added to the blood specimen.
2. The nonwater-soluble, free (prehepatic) bilirubin does not react to the reagents used for the test until alcohol is added to the solution; hence their measurement is *indirect* (Mukher 1979).

The exact technical procedure for the test is not of major concern for nurses. They should know, however, enough about how the tests are done so that the words "direct" and "indirect" make some sense when they are interpreting laboratory reports. To understand the clinical significance of changes in one or both types, nurses must clearly understand the origin and route for each type of bilirubin. Table 11–1 can be used as a quick summary of how each of the bilirubin tests are related to the normal pathway of bilirubin excretion. Table 11–2 summarizes how each of the five tests of bilirubin are changed in the three types of jaundice (prehepatic, intrahepatic, and post-hepatic).

SERUM BILIRUBINS
(VAN DE BERGH REACTION)

Preparation of Patient
And Collection of Sample

Most laboratories require the patient to fast for eight hours before the test because a large intake of fat interferes with the chemical testing. The test requires 3 ml of serum. The specimen should be protected from bright light because bilirubin is broken down by exposure to sunlight or to high-intensity artificial light. The test should not be done for 24 hours after a dye has been used for X-ray studies.

Reference Values

Most laboratories report only the figures for the total and the direct. The indirect is calculated by subtracting the direct from the total.

Adults and children past
newborn stage
   Indirect bilirubin   0.1–1.0 mg/dl   This is the prehepatic, free, or
                                Mean 0.5 mg   unconjugated bilirubin.

(continued)

Reference Values (*continued*)

Direct bilirubin	0.0–0.4 mg/dl Mean 0.1 mg	Post-hepatic, conjugated bilirubin.
Total bilirubin	0.1–1.4 mg/dl	Includes both types of bilirubin.
Newborns	See text for explanation of physiological jaundice in new- borns. Examples used here, from Jensen (1981), reflect *total* bilirubins.	
Term infants	First 24 hours Up to 48 hours 3 to 5 days	2–6 mg 6–7 mg 4–12 mg
Premature infants	First 24 hours Up to 48 hours 3 to 5 days	1–6 mg 6–8 mg 10–15 mg
Pregnancy	Bilirubin levels usually remain in normal ranges, but several studies have shown that about 15% of normal pregnancies may have total bilirubins as high as 10 mg (Hytten 1975: 16).	

Increased Indirect Bilirubin

Clinical Significance. An increase in the indirect portion of bilirubin can be caused in two different ways:

First, the breakdown of red blood cells can increase, thus causing an excess of free bilirubin in the bloodstream. Many conditions cause an increased destruction (hemolysis) of red blood cells:

1. sickle cell disease,
2. autoimmune diseases,
3. hemorrhage into a body cavity when the red blood cells are broken down,
4. drug toxicity,
5. any physical or physiological stress (a slight increase),
6. a transfusion reaction due to incompatible blood (see Chapter 14 on transfusion reactions),
7. similarly, Rh or ABO incompatibility in an infant.

The indirect bilirubin of a newborn with Rh incompatibility (erythroblastosis fetalis) is often above 20 mg. Usually the indirect bilirubin, in an adult, does not go much above 5 mg due to hemolysis.

Second, the indirect portion of bilirubin can be elevated when the liver's ability to conjugate the free bilirubin that circulates in the bloodstream is decreased. Liver dysfunction causes high elevations of the indirect bilirubin in both adult and newborns. In severe liver disease, the indirect bilirubin may be over 20 mg (Koepke 1979:78). Although the most common reason for severe liver dysfunction in the adult is cirrhosis, hepatitis may also make the liver less capable of conjugating bilirubin. As a rare example, some people have a lack of the enzyme glucuronyl transferase (Gilbert's syndrome), which is necessary for the conjugation of bilirubin in the liver. The lack of this specific enzyme results in an increased amount of indirect bilirubin. Drugs, viral diseases, and other toxins may also injure the liver or interfere with enzymatic actions, so that the liver cannot conjugate bilirubin efficiently.

The newborn is particularly susceptible to environmental contaminants because the epidermis is thinner and percutaneous absorption is thus greater. The faster respiratory rate also increases the intake of any environmental contaminant. For example, two epidemics of neonatal hyperbilirubinemia were linked to the use of a phenol disinfectant detergent (Wysowski 1978). Several infants had very high indirect bilirubins after a new detergent was used to clean bassinets.

Liver diseases often involve not only some inability to conjugate bilirubin, but also some obstruction to drainage from the liver. With obstruction, the direct bilirubin increases. While the impact of liver disease on the direct bilirubin is covered in the next section, suffice it to say here that several pathological processes may be causing elevations of both the indirect and direct bilirubins.

Physiological Jaundice in the Newborn. An increase in the indirect bilirubin is a physiological occurence in the newborn that is due both to an increased hemolysis and to a slower conjugation by the liver. The infant is born with a large number of fetal red blood cells that have a short lifespan. So the hemolysis that occurs after birth is a normal adaptation to the new environment. Yet, since the newborn's liver has inadequate glucuronyl transferase, the liver takes longer to conjugate and to remove bilirubin from the bloodstream. Then the synthesis of the enzyme occurs a few days after birth in a full-term infant and a little longer in a premature. Due to these events, about 50% of newborns have some physiological jaundice that disappears in a few days.

Distinguishing this physiological jaundice from any other kind is important. If the indirect bilirubin rise is elevated the first day, or if it does not begin to drop after three to five days, the jaundice may be pathological rather than physiological. For example, the infant with Rh incompatibility has a high indirect bilirubin immediately after birth. (See Chapter 14 for other tests done for Rh babies.) Lowered serum albumin levels, hypoxia, cold, stress, drugs, and other metabolic factors may also cause abnormal rises in the indirect bilirubin by interfering with the transportation or conjugation of bilirubin. Thaler (1977) explains all the causes for elevations of both indirect (unconjugated) bilirubin and direct (conjugated) bilirubin, as well as how to distinguish these from the physiological jaundice of the newborn.

In a few instances, breast feeding may intensify the physiological jaundice because an enzyme present in some women's milk inhibits the action of glucuronyl transferase. Gartner, one of the original researchers into neonatal jaundice and breastfeeding, does not consider an elevated bilirubin to be significant if the bilirubin is below 20 mg for the first week and if the infant is otherwise healthy (White 1979). The potential danger of a high level of indirect bilirubin in the newborn is covered in the section on nursing implications of patients with elevated bilirubin levels.

Increased Direct Bilirubin Level

Clinical Significance. Normally the amount of conjugated bilirubin circulating in the bloodstream is very small because the larger portion of this type of bilirubin is excreted via the bile salts into the intestine. Thus a marked increase in the direct bilirubin is an indication of an obstruction in the normal flow of bile. Jaundice due to an elevation in direct bilirubin is called *obstructive jaundice*. The obstruction may be in the collecting channels in the liver, in the hepatic ducts, or in the common bile duct. For example, a gallstone lodged in the common bile duct prevents the normal excretion of bile salts (which contain the conjugated bilirubin) into the intestine. The conjugated bilirubin is thus absorbed into the bloodstream in much larger amounts than normal. In complete biliary obstruction, the direct bilirubin may be as high as 30 to 40 mg. Another example of an obstruction would be cancer of the head of the pancreas, for which jaundice is often the first symptom. Newborns with a congenital malformation in the biliary tree (biliary atresia) also have high direct bilirubins.

Sometimes the direct bilirubin may be elevated even though biliary obstruction is not apparent. Certain drugs, notably contraceptive steroids and some of the phenothiazines such as chlorpromazine (Thorazine), may cause a stasis of bile in the liver (intrahepatic cholestasis). The bile tends to be viscous, and the small bile ducts in the liver become dilated. The direct bilirubin is elevated due to this partial obstruction to the normal outflow of bile. A similar condition of stasis occurs in what is called the ''benign jaundice'' of pregnancy. The rise in bilirubin is an occasional occurence in pregnancy, and the bilirubin returns to normal after delivery (Seymour 1979). Inflammation of the liver as in hepatitis, or scarring as in cirrhosis, may also cause partial obstruction to the flow of bile out of the liver and thereby cause an elevation of the direct bilirubin.

Although the discussion has attempted to make a clear distinction between elevations of direct and of indirect bilirubin, clinical situations often entail elevations of both. Any clinical condition, any drug, or any toxic condition that causes obstruction to the flow of bile may eventually cause some increase in the indirect bilirubin too, because the stasis of bile in the collecting ducts eventually impairs the normal functioning of the liver. Intrahepatic disease, such as cirrhosis or hepatitis, and drug toxicity may cause elevations in both the direct and indirect bilirubins. Urine bilirubin, urine urobilinogen, and, less frequently, fecal urobilinogen tests may give additional information about the nature of the jaundice. Table 11–2 summarizes the usual findings in jaundice that is prehepatic (hemolytic) intrahepatic (liver dysfunction), or post-hepatic (obstruction). Ostrow (1975) is an excellent overview for the reader who is interested in more detail about the differential diagnosis in older children and adults.

For clinical jaundice, tests other than those for bilirubin and urobilinogen may also be needed. For example, alkaline phosphatase, an enzyme normally excreted in the bile, is elevated in biliary obstruction. The transaminases are also elevated in most types of liver disease. (See Chapter 12 on using these enzymes in detecting liver and biliary disease.)

URINE BILIRUBIN (ICOTEST)

Since only the water-soluble conjugated (direct) bilirubin can cross the glomerular filter, it is the only type of bilirubin even found in the urine. Normally even this type of bilirubin is not in the urine in detectable amounts because it has been converted to urobilinogen in the intestine. Bilirubin becomes apparent in the urine when there is an obstruction to the normal pathway of conjugated bilirubin. This test is therefore used to detect obstructive jaundice, and it is sometimes said incorrectly to be a test for ''bile'' in the urine.

Preparation of Patient
And Collection of Sample

A few milliliters of freshly voided urine are needed. The urine must be fresh since oxidation affects the results, and exposure to strong lights also changes the chemical composition of the bilirubin.

Sometimes the nurse or patient may test urine for bilirubin by using either a tablet or a dipstick. For the Icotest (Ames), five drops of urine are placed on a special test mat. A tablet is then placed on the mat and 2 drops of water are added. If the mat turns blue or purple within 30 seconds, the test is positive for bilirubin. With the dipstick method, the positive reaction is a tan to purple color. The dipstick method is two to four times less sensitive than the tablet method (Ames Product Information 1980). Drugs that change the color of the urine may mask the color change on the tablet or strip of paper. (See Chapter 3 for a list of drugs that cause color changes in urine, as well as for a dipstick method to check for ascorbic acid since this may interfere with the bilirubin tests.)

Reference Values

All groups	Normally bilirubin is present in such small quantities in the urine that it is not detected by routine screening procedures.

Bilirubin in the Urine (Bilirubinemia)

Clinical Significance. Bilirubin in the urine indicates the beginning of obstructive jaundice, and its presence is detected before there are any clinical signs of jaundice. (No bilirubin is in the urine if the jaundice is due to an elevated indirect bilirubin.) Since this test is likely to be positive for bilirubin before the person has signs of clinical hepatitis, it may be a screening procedure done on populations that were known to be exposed to hepatitis. It may also be useful to screen out potential blood donors, food handlers, and the like, when controlling the spread of subclinical cases of hepatitis is imperative.

Bilirubin makes urine a dark orange color, and it also makes urine foam when it is shaken (shake test). Urine does not foam or become dark if it contains only urobilinogen. Since the nurse or patient may be the first to notice that the urine color is abnormal, the color of urine and stools should always be a priority assessment when an obstruction of the common bile duct is suspected.

URINE UROBILINOGEN

Urobilinogen is formed in the intestine from the conjugated bilirubin normally present in bile salts. Most of the urobilinogen is excreted in the feces, but a small amount that finds its way into the bloodstream either goes through the liver again or is excreted in the urine. This test may be used to detect hemolytic jaundice or early liver dysfunction.

Preparation of Patient
And Collection of Sample

If a 24-hour specimen is needed, a preservative must be used. (See Chapter 3 for tips on 24-hour urine collection.) The more common procedure is to collect a 2-hour urine sample in the afternoon, because the excretion of urobilinogen is at a maximum from mid-afternoon to evening when food is being digested. The urine should be taken to the laboratory immediately after collection. Strongly acid urine may make the results inaccurate; so if a patient is on drugs, such as high doses of salicylates, note this fact on the laboratory slip. Drugs that color the urine also interfere with the test. Laboratories may report in milligrams or in units.

The nurse can also check for urobilinogen by using a dipstick, which shows 0.1–1 Ehrlich units as normal. For amounts from 2 to over 12 Ehrlich units, the color goes from dark yellow to orange when read after 45 seconds (Ames 1980).

Reference Values

All groups	0.3–1.0 Ehrlich units in a 2-hour sample (1–3 PM).
	0.5–4.0 Ehrlich units in a 24-hour sample (ask lab about preservative).
	0.4–1 mg a day. Note specific color chart if doing by dipstick method.

Changes in Urinary Urobilinogen
(Urobilinogenuria)

Clinical Significance. An increase in urine urobilinogen follows an increased breakdown of red blood cells, with the increase in fecal urobilinogen even more pronounced than that in urinary urobilinogen. Since some of the urobilinogen that is in the feces is picked up by the portal circulation and carried to the liver again, and since urinary urobilinogen excretion is increased when the liver cannot excrete the recycled urobilinogen, urinary urobilinogen can also be used to detect early liver dysfunction. The inability of the liver to handle urobilinogen occurs before bilirubin excretion is affected (Widmann 1979: 579).

In obstructive jaundice, the lack of bilirubin excreted into the intestine causes a decrease in the amount of urobilinogen to the urine, which is not important to measure since it is very small even in normal health. The amount of urinary urobilinogen also decreases when there is a lack of intestinal flora to convert bilirubin to urobilinogen; this effect, however, is more of academic interest than of clinical usefulness.

FECAL UROBILINOGEN

The amount of urobilinogen in the feces depends on the amount of conjugated bilirubin that is excreted via the bile salts into the intestine. Since urobilinogen is the end-product of conjugated bilirubin, a lack of bacteria to break down the bilirubin may reduce the urobilinogen in the intestine, and thus the feces become lighter in color. The test for fecal urobilinogen is not done often because urine and serum tests may give enough information about the cause of the impaired bilirubin excretion.

Preparation of Patient
And Collection of Sample

The laboratory gives specific instructions if a specimen of feces is to be saved for 24 hours or for several days. Usually patients can collect the specimen if they are given the correct container. Having patients do so is desirable both to avoid their embarrassment and to protect the nurse from possible contamination in transferring feces. Special waxed containers are used for stool collections.

Reference Values

75–350 mg/100 g of stool

40–280 mg in a 24-hour period

Changes in Fecal Urobilinogen

Clinical Significance. The fecal urobilinogen is significantly increased when there is an increased breakdown of red blood cells (hemolytic jaundice) because much more bilirubin is conjugated by the liver and excreted into the intestine. A lack of fecal urobilinogen occurs in obstructive jaundice because the conjugated bilirubin cannot be excreted into the intestine. A lack of conjugated bilirubin in the intestine is apparent to the eye because the feces are clay-colored. In the infant, this condition may not be apparent because the stools are normally light-colored.

Bilirubin Level
(Hyperbilirubinemia)

Possible Nursing Implications.

Assessing for Clinical Signs of Jaundice. Although the serum tests are used to monitor the exact level of the bilirubin from day to day, the nurse should also record color changes on a daily basis. An excess of serum bilirubin, either the direct or indirect type, gives a yellowish coloration to the sclera of the eyes, skin, and mucus membranes. The symptoms of jaundice begin to appear when the total bilirubin is around 2 to 4 mg in the adult or older child. In the infant, jaundice may not be apparent until the total bilirubin is around 5 to 7 mg (Heagerty 1980). Often the yellow color is noted first in the sclera of fair-skinned people. In dark-skinned people, the inner canthus of the eye may show more change. In dark-skinned or Oriental people, the yellowish tinge also becomes apparent in the mucous membranes of the hard palate (Roach 1977). Blanching the skin of newborns by pressing on the sternum makes the jaundice of the skin more apparent. With proper lighting, one can see jaundice in the abdomen nearly as easily as in the sclera. Also observations for jaundice should be done in natural daylight, if possible.

In a community health setting or clinic, the nurse may be the first one to notice the beginning of jaundice. In high-risk populations composed of alcohol or other drug abusers, inspections of the eyes and skins would be especially important to detect liver damage. Actually, since patients may be the best judges of day-to-day changes in their own skin color, this source of data should never be overlooked.

Nurses must also know whether the direct or indirect bilirubin is elevated because the nursing implications vary for each type of elevation. Some of the implications, such as changes in body image or ways to assess for jaundice, are the same for both types. However, the potential danger to the central nervous system, itching, discomfort, and bleeding are problems associated more with one type than the other. The treatment of each of these problems must be considered in relationship to the type of bilirubin elevated. Therapeutic interventions to reduce each type of bilirubin are also included in the following section.

Preventing Central Nervous System Damage in the Newborn. In older children and adults, an increase in the indirect (unconjugated) bilirubin is not in itself dangerous or uncomfortable for the patient. After infancy, a blood-brain barrier prevents the indirect bilirubin from affecting the central nervous system. (Very rarely, an extremely high indirect bilirubin in an adult may affect the brain.) High indirect bilirubins in newborns, however, are of grave concern. In infants, indirect bilirubin does leak through the vascular walls and can damage the central nervous system. *Kernicterus* (kern = kernel + icterus = yellow) is the term used to describe the central nervous system damage that results from high indirect bilirubins (usually over 20 mg) in newborns.

No one figure—such as "over 20 mg"—defines the upper limits of indirect bilirubin that necessitate interventions in the newborn. The physician must consider many factors, such as whether the bilirubin level is rising rapidly or not falling after the first few days. In an individual case, the physician may determine that the bilirubin should not be more than 15 or 18 mg.

New parents, on the other hand, usually need a figure to hold on to so that they can make sense of the laboratory report that is given. A mother may be anxiously awaiting the laboratory report of the bilirubin each day because a bilirubin that exceeds the limit for the newborn may mean that the baby will have to stay in the hospital a few days longer. This news can be devastating to the new parents. Nurses may be able to alleviate some anxiety by a brief explanation about how elevated bilirubins are usually treated in their hospital. The mother and father may prefer not to see the heel sticks done to obtain blood.

Assisting with Treatments to Decrease the Indirect Bilirubin in Newborns. Three different methods are used in the newborn to reduce indirect bilirubin:

1. *Exchange transfusions* are used primarily for severe cases of blood type incompatibility. Jensen (1981:866) describes in detail the procedure for exchange transfusions.

2. *Phototherapy,* more commonly used for other causes of jaundice with a high indirect bilirubin, is the use of a high-intensity light to help break down the indirect bilirubin to a nontoxic substance. Phototherapy converts bilirubin to derivatives that apparently can be excreted in the bile and urine without being conjugated by the liver. It is important that the baby's eyes be protected under the lights, since they can damage the eyes. It is also crucial to monitor the temperature to prevent hypo- or hyperthermia. Extra fluids need to be given to prevent dehydration. The skin becomes lighter in the areas under the light. Evidently, turning the baby so that no areas are shaded is not important since the rapidity of the bilirubin level drop is due to the dose of light, not to the amount of skin illuminated (Tan 1975).

3. *Drugs* constitute another method of treating high levels of indirect bilirubin. Phenobarbital is given to help promote the hepatic clearance of bilirubin, and it may be given to a woman during pregnancy as well as to the newborn.

Assisting with Treatments to Decrease Indirect Bilirubins in Older Children and Adults. The therapeutic interventions used to reduce the indirect bilirubin level in older children and adults depend on the underlying pathophysiology. For hemolytic anemias or liver dysfunction, refer to nursing texts for discussions on nursing care and treatment. Since the indirect bilirubin itself is not of danger to the older child or adult, little effort is made to decrease the level itself. Theoretically, sitting in the sun would be beneficial to the child or adult who has a high indirect bilirubin, but it is more important to correct the pathophysiologic process causing the elevation. When the indirect bilirubin is elevated, the urinary and fecal urobilinogen is increased too, due to the extra bilirubin excreted into the intestine.

When the elevated bilirubin is due to an elevation of the direct (conjugated) bilirubin, the nursing implications are different because patients have a tendency to bleed and to itch. They may also experience pain, intolerance to fatty foods, and a general lack of appetite. All these problems are related to the fact that the normal flow of bile is obstructed.

Relieving Pruritis. It is presumed that the severe itching (pruritis) that often accompanies an elevated direct (conjugated) bilirubin is due to something toxic in the ''bile salts'' deposited in the skin. Keeping the environment cool is useful since perspiring may accentuate the pruritis. Soothing baths and lotions may also give some relief. Aveeno, a colloidal oatmeal bath for irritated skin contains no soaps or synthetics that can harm the skin. The bath soothes and cleanses naturally because of its unique adsorption action. Oatmeal baths can be used for infants as well as adults who have pruritis. Children may need to be restrained from scratching.

Although there is not direct evidence that the pruritis is directly attributed to bile salts, the use of medication that binds the bile salts may relieve the itching. Cholestyramine (Cuemid, Questran) is a resin that is taken orally to bind bile salts in the intestine so that there is a larger increase in the feces (Goodman 1975:972). This treatment may be helpful when the obstruction is not complete. To prevent constipation, the person taking cholestyramine needs a large intake of fluids and a diet high in roughage. Since the drug may bind up other drugs, it should be given at least one hour before or four hours after other drugs. Supplements of fat-soluble vitamins may be needed if the patient is on long-term therapy with the drug. (Cholestyramine is also used as a drug to lower cholesterol levels. See Chapter 9.)

Preventing Bleeding. For fats and fat-soluble vitamins to be emulsified and absorbed from the intestine, there must be adequate bile salts. For this reason, a patient with an elevated direct bilirubin may develop a tendency to bleed. Without bile salts, fat-soluble vitamins, including vitamin K, are not absorbed from the small intestine. If vitamin K is not absorbed into the bloodstream, the liver cannot make enough prothrombin and other factors needed for normal blood clotting. Patients with obstructive jaundice thus often have increased prothrombin time. Patients with elevated prothrombin times due to obstructive jaundice are given parenteral injections of vitamin K. Parenteral vitamin K can reach the liver because the bile salts were not needed to get the vitamin from the intestine into the bloodstream. Specific actions on how to prevent bleeding when the patient has an increased prothrombin time are covered in Chapter 13 on clotting tests.

Relieving Pain. Although jaundice due to an elevation of indirect bilirubin is painless, pain, other than that associated with pruritis, may or may not be associated with jaundice due to an elevation of the direct bilirubin. Since obstruction of the biliary tree by a pancreatic tumor may be painless for quite awhile, the first indications of biliary obstruction would be jaundice and a tendency to bleed. On the other hand, jaundice due to a gallstone in the common bile duct tends to cause severe abdominal pain in the right upper outer quadrant. In such a case, the patient may need narcotics to relieve the pain. Characteristically, the pain tends to radiate to the right shoulder, and it may be intensified by an attempt to eat fatty foods.

Providing Adequate Food and Fluids. Since patients with an elevated direct bilirubin usually have some intolerance to fatty foods, their nutritional status must be carefully assessed so that their caloric needs are met. If indicated, surgery is done to relieve the obstruction. Before surgery, the patient may need intravenous feedings to maintain hydration and caloric intake. Fat-soluble vitamins can be added to intravenous fluids. Even with just a partial or clearing obstruction, the patient may have little appetite for food, so the nurse must plan meals carefully. (As a general rule, an increase in the indirect bilirubin does not seriously interfere with appetite unless the liver is involved.)

Hepatitis which causes cholestasis, is accompanied by anorexia. Even if foods are not desired, the patient should be encouraged to drink fruit juices. These provide some calories and help flush out the water-soluble direct bilirubin into the urine. As the patient's appetite returns, food is needed to supply adequate calories and protein for liver regeneration. Fats can be allowed as tolerated.

Recognizing Other Problems Associated with Jaundice. Not all cases of jaundice can be as neatly classified as "nonobstructive" and "obstructive". Patients with liver disease, such as hepatitis or cirrhosis, usually have elevations of both types of bilirubin. In addition, patients with liver dysfunction have many other problems besides jaundice. Some of these problems, such as a lack in plasma proteins (Chapter 10), a reduction in prothrombin (Chapter 13), and an inability to detoxify drugs (Chapter 17) are covered elsewhere in this book. Refer to a medical–surgical nursing text for a more comprehensive view of the patient with cirrhosis who has jaundice, since the nursing care for these patients is quite complex and they usually have a poor prognosis.

Meeting the Psychological Needs of the Patient with Jaundice. A concentration on the physical aspects of care for patients with an elevated bilirubin must not overshadow their psychological needs. Nurses need to be aware that jaundice is a definite change in the body image of the person. Jaundice may be very upsetting not only to patients but to their families as well. Some patients are afraid to look in a mirror, and others may prefer not to have any visitors. If these patients must come to a clinic, they may not want others to stare at them. (In addition, other patients may be afraid that the jaundice is catching.) Soft, subdued lights make the jaundice less apparent while treatments are begun to reduce the bilirubin level.

Patients' reactions, of course, can also be unexpected. A young man was once admitted to the hospital with severe jaundice due to cirrhosis. Blue dye for a lymphogram turned the man's sclera and skin from yellow to green. One might jump to the conclusion that the patient would not want anyone to see him and that he would be upset by the parade of nursing students, residents, and interns who came to examine the "green man." On the contrary, the patient enjoyed all the extra attention from being unique and seemed a little disappointed when his color began to return to normal. So, as with all generalizations about nursing implications, nurses must choose which ones are applicable for a certain patient in a certain setting. Usually, since jaundice is upsetting to patients and to their families, nurses must be sensitive to this aspect when caring for patients who are jaundiced. They should also recognize that a change in body image due to a specific *external* source (such as the dye) may be quite a different experience from a longer-term and less specific *internal source (the elevated bilirubin)*.

Bilirubin in the Amniotic Fluid

It is not known for sure how bilirubin reaches the amniotic fluid; some of it may diffuse across the skin. Since it is the indirect, nonwater-soluble type, it cannot be excreted in the urine of the fetus. The bilirubin content of amniotic fluid is often high during early pregnancy, but it should fall progressively after mid-pregnancy. The importance of measuring the bilirubin content in amniotic fluid is to determine whether the normal downward progression of bilirubin concentration in the last half of pregnancy is continuing. If the bilirubin content is not dropping, or if it begins to rise for the fetus of a Rh negative mother, medical interventions may be necessary to save the fetus. Laboratories may use either light or chemical methods to determine the amount of bilirubin in the amniotic fluid. (See Chapter 14 for Rh antibody titers and the Coomb's test.)

BROMSULPHALEIN (BSP)

Bromsulphalein (BSP), a dye used to evaluate liver function, is given intravenously and a blood sample is taken 45 minutes later. The liver should remove the dye from the blood, conjugate it, and excrete it into the bile. The conjugation of the dye is similar to the conjugation of bilirubin described in the beginning of this chapter. More than 5% of the dye in the 45-minute blood sample is an indication that the liver cannot excrete substances normally.

Although rare, BSP dye can cause allergic reactions. Indocyanine green (Cardio-Green) is another dye that is metabolized by the liver cells in a manner similar to BSP. Cardio-Green is more expensive and not widely used (Ravel 1978).

Preparation of Patient
And Collection of Sample

The patient should not have had other dyes for X-ray studies within the last 48 hours. Many drugs may interfere with the test too. Also, since BSP dye interferes with other tests, any other blood work should be done before the BSP is given. The patient fasts overnight.

Because 5 mg of dye is given for each kilogram (2.2 lbs) of body weight, the patient is weighed. The physician then injects the dye. Adrenalin and any equipment necessary for emergency resuscitation should be available to treat severe allergic reaction. Three ml of blood are withdrawn 45 minutes after the dye is injected. The timing must be precise if the results are to be meaningful. The dye should be withdrawn from the arm opposite to the one that received the dye.

Reference Values

Less than 5% retention of dye in the 45-minute blood sample.

In pregnancy, BSP retention is increased (Seymour 1979).

Increased Retention of BSP Dye

Clinical Significance. The inability of the liver to excrete the dye normally indicates liver dysfunction. Dye excretion tests, however, do not give as much information as the newer techniques that use radioisotopes (liver scans) or ultrasound (sonograms) to assess liver pathology.

Questions

11–1. When the body is utilizing the normal pathway of bilirubin excretion, which laboratory test will be negative?

   a. Serum bilirubin level (indirect portion).   **c.** Urine urobilinogen.

   b. Fecal urobilinogen.   **d.** Urine bilirubin.

11–2. Which of the following terms is not a synonym for direct bilirubin?

   a. Conjugated bilirubin.   **c.** Post-hepatic bilirubin.

   b. Water-soluble bilirubin.   **d.** Free bilirubin.

11–3. The laboratory slip on Mrs. Fong's chart shows a total bilirubin of 3.0 mg and a direct bilirubin of 0.3 mg. Her indirect bilirubin is which of the following?

   a. Unknown at the present time.   **c.** 2.7 mg/dl.

   b. 3.3 mg/dl.   **d.** 3.0 mg/dl.

11–4. Baby Toler has a very elevated indirect bilirubin due to physiological jaundice. What would be the effect on the fecal and urine urobilongens?

   a. Both decreased.   **c.** Increase only in fecal urobilongen.

   b. Both increased.   **d.** Increase only in urinary urobilongen.

11–5. Which of the following assessments is not found in a patient with an elevated direct bilirubin?

   a. Urine will be dark and will foam when shaken.

   b. Stools will be clay-colored.

    c. Urine test for bilirubin will be negative.

    d. Urine test for urobilongen will be decreased.

11–6. In an infant, clinical jaundice becomes apparent when the total bilirubin level is around which of the following levels?

    a. 2–4 mg/dl. **b.** 5–7 mg/dl. **c.** 7–9 mg/dl. **d.** Over 9 mg/dl.

11–7. In an adult, clinical jaundice becomes apparent when the serum bilirubin (total) is about which of the following levels?

    a. 2–4 mg. **b.** 5–7 mg. **c.** 7–9 mg. **d.** Over 9 mg.

11–8. The indirect part of the serum bilirubin is increased in all these clinical situations *except* which?

    a. Mrs. Rhoades, age 31, who has anemia due to a lack of iron in her diet.

    b. Baby Holmes, 2 days old, on breastfeeding and slightly jaundiced.

    c. Shirley, age 7, who has been admitted to the pediatric unit in a sickle cell crisis.

    d. Mr. Smith, age 42, who has terminal cirrhosis.

11–9. An increase in the direct part of the serum bilirubin would be an expected assessment finding in all these patient care situations except which of the following?

    a. Mrs. Fonolini, who has gallstones in the common bile duct.

    b. Mr. Petersen, who is undergoing surgery (Whipple procedure) for cancer of the head of the pancreas.

    c. Baby Jones, who has a malformation in the biliary tree (biliary atresia).

    d. Reggie, age 7, who had a transfusion reaction due to incompatible blood.

11–10. In a patient who has moderate hepatic dysfunction and some stasis of bile in the hepatic ducts, the laboratory test for serum bilirubin will most likely show which of the following?

    a. An increase in the indirect portion of bilirubin.

    b. A decrease in the direct portion of bilirubin.

    c. Increases in both the indirect and direct bilirubins.

    d. An increase in the direct portion of bilirubin.

11–11. Key nursing implications for the patient with an elevated bilirubin (indirect and/or direct) would include all *except* which of the following?

    a. Evaluating the effect of jaundice on the body image of the person.

    b. Assessing in natural daylight, the color of the sclera, mucous membrane, and skin.

    c. Charting the color of both urine and stools.

    d. Encouraging foods that are high in fat-soluble vitamins.

11–12. When jaundice is due to a high elevation of the direct bilirubin, rather than of the indirect bilirubin, the nursing actions may include all of the following *except* which?

    a. Use of soothing baths to relieve pruritis.

    b. Special attention to safety measures due to the tendancy to bleed.

    c. Making sure that foods high in fat are not served to the patient.

    d. Assessing for effects of central nervous system damage, especially in the newborn.

11–13. The current methods used to treat high levels of indirect bilirubin in the newborn include all of the following *except* which?

    a. Complete elimination of breast milk to reduce the factors that interfere with glucuronyl transferase in the liver.

    b. Exchange transfusions to remove toxic products from the bloodstream.

    c. Phototherapy with high-intensity lights to help break down the bilirubin.

    d. Drug therapy with phenobarbital to promote the hepatic clearance of bilirubin.

11–14. All of the following therapeutic interventions may be used for the person who has jaundice due to an elevated direct bilirubin *except* which?

    a. Vitamin K by injection to return the prothrombin time to normal.

    b. Cholestyramine (Cuemid, Questran) to bind up bile salts in the intestine.

    c. Surgical intervention to remove the obstruction.

    d. Use of phototherapy to break down the bilirubin.

11–15. The clinical significance of measuring the bilirubin content in amniotic fluid is that:

    a. the presence of any bilirubin denotes pathology because there should be no bilirubin in the amniotic fluid after the first trimester of pregnancy.

    b. a rise in bilirubin during the later part of pregnancy signifies that the liver of the fetus is functioning normally, so no treatment is needed.

    c. a rise or a cessation of a downward trend in the bilirubin during the last part of pregnancy means a poorer prognosis for the fetus unless medical interventions are begun.

    d. an increase in both the indirect and direct levels of bilirubin signifies both liver dysfunction and hemolysis, so both must be treated.

11–16. Which of the following nursing actions is *not* needed for the patient who is to have a BSP test?

    a. Weighing the patient.

    b. Making sure that adrenalin is available.

    c. Saving all urine voided during the test.

    d. Withholding food until the test is completed.

REFERENCES

Ames Product Information on *Icotest*. Elkhart, Indiana: Ames Division, Miles Laboratories, 1980.

Goodman, Louis and Gilman, Alfred. *The Pharmacologic Basis of Therapeutics,* 5th ed. New York: Macmillan, Inc., 1975.

Heagarty, Margaret *et al. Child Health: Basics for Primary Care.* New York: Appleton-Century-Crofts, 1980.

Hytten, Frank and Tom Lind. *Diagnostic Indices in Pregnancy.* Summit, N.J.: Ciba-Geigy Corporation, 1975.

Jensen, Margaret *et al. Maternity Care: The Nurse and the Family,* 2nd ed. St. Louis: C. V. Mosby Co., 1981.

Koepke, John. "Chapter 7: Jaundice," *Guide to Clinical Laboratory Diagnosis.* New York: Appleton-Century-Crofts, 1979.

Mukher, Kanai. *Review of Clinical Laboratory Methods.* St. Louis: C. V. Mosby Co., 1979.

Ostrow, Donald. "Jaundice in Older Children and Adults: Algorithms for Diagnosis," *Journal of the American Medical Association* 234 (5) (November 3, 1975): 522–526.

Ravel, Richard. *Clinical Laboratory Medicine,* 3rd ed. Chicago: Year Book Medical Publishers, 1978.

Roach, Loya, "Color Changes in Dark Skin," *Nursing '77* 7 (January 1977): 48–51.

Seymour, Carol and Chadwick, V. S. "Liver and Gastrointestinal Function in Pregnancy," *Postgraduate Medical Journal* 55: (May 1979): 343–351.

Schmid, Rudi. "Bilirubin Metabolism in Man," *New England Journal of Medicine* 287 (October 5, 1972): 703–709.

Tan, K. L. "Comparison of the Effectiveness of Single Direction and Double Direction Phototherapy for Neo-Natal Jaundice," *Pediatrics* 56 (4) (October 1975): 550–553.

Thaler, M. M. "Jaundice in the Newborn: Algorithmic Diagnosis of Conjugated and Unconjugated Hyperbilirubinemia," *Journal of the American Medical Association* 237 (January 3, 1977): 58–62.

White, Mary. "Information Please on Jaundice," *LaLeche League News* 21 (July–August 1979): 71–72.

Widmann, Frances. *Clinical Interpretation of Laboratory Tests,* 8th ed. Philadelphia: F. A. Davis Co., 1979.

Wysowski, Diane *et al.* "Epidemic Neo-Natal Hyperbilirubinemia and Use of a Phenolic Disinfectant Detergent," *Pediatrics* 61 (2) (February 1978): 165–170.

CHAPTER TWELVE

Tests to Measure Enzyme And Isoenzyme Levels

Objectives

1. Identify factors, other than pathological processes, that tend to cause elevations in the majority of the serum enzyme tests.
2. Explain the usual clinical significance for a patient with an elevated serum alkaline phosphatase level (ALP).
3. Explain the primary purpose of the serum acid phosphatase level as an assessment for a malignancy.
4. Describe the nursing assessments and interventions required when a patient has marked elevations of the transaminases, ALT (formerly SGPT), and AST (formerly SGOT).
5. Discriminate between four cardiac enzymes—CPK, AST (SGOT), LDH, and HBD—in relation to the onset, peak, and duration of elevation after a myocardial infarction.
6. Explain why isoenzymes of CPK and LDH are often more valuable than the measurement of the total amounts of the enzymes.
7. Identify the most important nursing implication for the cardiac patient who has unexpected normal levels of cardiac enzymes.
8. Plan an appropriate activity schedule for a patient who has an elevated serum aldorase level due to a muscular disorder.
9. Explain how serum amylase and lipase and how urinary amylase are used as assessment tools for pancreatitis.
10. Describe the nursing implications for patients who have marked elevations of serum amylase and lipase levels.

This chapter covers the most common enzymes measured in the serum. As an additional assessment, only one of the enzymes, amylase, is also measured in the urine. Almost all cells contain these major enzymes, although some types of tissue contain larger concentrations of particular enzymes. So when tissue cells are damaged, the enzymes leak out into the serum.

Although the enzymes are not tissue-specific, various types of tissue have isoenzymes with different chemical and physical properties. Isoenzymes of a particular enzyme all control the same specific metabolic function even though their molecular forms vary slightly from one to another. The enzyme lactic dehydrogenase (LDH), for example, which is abundant in most tissues, can be separated into five distinct types of isoenzymes. LDH_1 is abundant in heart tissues, while LDH_5 is abundant in liver tissue. Each of the five LDH isoenzymes are still not organ-specific, however, since the heart or liver may have more than one type of isoenzyme and isoenzymes may come from several different tissues. Nonetheless, the use of isoenzymes narrows the possibilities of the origin of the elevated enzyme in the serum. (The various isoenzymes are separated by the electrophoresis method, explained in Chapter 10 for protein electrophoresis.)

Enzyme names are generally easy to understand and recognize. Particular enzymes are often named for the reaction that they catalyze. For example, lipase is an enzyme used for the reaction of a lipid or fat, and transaminases transfer amino groups in energy production. Enzymes are easy to recognize because their names almost always end in -*ase* (Holum 1979). However, since many of the serum enzyme tests are known by initials rather than by names, there is no way to know that CPK is an enzyme test unless one sees it written out as creatine phosphokin*ase*.

To make matters more confusing, the transaminases, which until recently were called SGPT and SGOT, are now called ALT and AST because the new names are more correct in a chemical sense. The enzyme that used to be called serum glutamic-pyruvic transaminase (SGPT) is now called alanine aminotransferase (ALT). The transaminase serum glutamic-oxalacetic transaminase (SGOT) is now called asparate aminotransferase (AST). Laboratory reports may use both the old and new names, or only the new names. Older reference books will, of course, use the terms SGPT and SGOT. To lessen the confusion during this transition time, both abbreviations for the transaminases are used in this chapter.

There is a movement to have all enzyme tests reported in a standard way by the use of international units. By convention, the IU is expressed as so many ''International units per liter.'' However, various laboratories may still use different methods to measure enzymes. Results are reported as Bodansky units, Somagyi units, or other units, which usually bear the names of the originators of the method. In this chapter, the IU system for reference values is emphasized, but examples of other values are given too. *Caution:* The only reliable reference values are those determined by the laboratory doing the testing. For example, even two laboratories using Bodansky units may have slightly modified the testing method for their respective laboratories.

Table 12–1 summarizes the most important enzyme elevations for several common pathological conditions. With a quick glance at the table, the reader sees that none of the enzyme tests is totally specific and that many are changed by several pathological conditions. Also, various nonpathological factors, such as exercise, cause elevated serum enzymes. Certain treatments, such as intramuscular injections and the administration of opiates, cause serum elevations of some enzymes. Improper handling of the specimens also bring about elevations due to hemolysis.

In this chapter, each of the factors that affects a particular enzyme is discussed with the specific test. Since only one of the enzymes (alkaline phosphatase) is affected by food,

TABLE 12-1. ENZYME ELEVATIONS IN COMMON PATHOLOGICAL CONDITIONS

↑ = Significant Elevation: Note that any tissue injury causes *slight* increase in many of these enzymes.
(↑) = Used as Major Diagnostic Tool: See text for elaborations.

Serum Enzymes	Eclampsia	Cancer of Prostate	Obstructive Jaundice	Bone Metastasis	Liver Metastasis	Hepatitis	Cirrhosis	Myocardial Infarction	Infectious Mononucleosis	Hemolytic Disease	Pulmonary Infarction	Muscular Necrosis or Inflammation	Pancreatitis	Brain Tissue Injury
1. Alkaline phosphatase	↑	↑	(↑)	(↑)	(↑)	↑	↑		↑				↑	
2. Acid phosphatase	↑	(↑)			↑					(↑)				
3. ALT or SGPT	↑	↑	↑	(↑)	(↑)	(↑)	↑	↑	(↑)	↑	↑	↑	↑	↑
4. AST or SGOT	↑	↑	↑	(↑)	(↑)	(↑)	↑	(↑)	(↑)	↑	↑	↑	↑	↑
5. CPK total								(↑)			↑	(↑)		↑
CPK I (BB)														
CPK II (MB)								(↑)						
CPK III (MM)												(↑)		
6. LDH Total	↑	↑	↑	↑	↑			↑	↑	(↑)	↑	↑	↑	↑
LDH_1								(↑)		↑				
LDH_2								(↑)		↑				
LDH_3											(↑)		↑	
LDH_4													↑	
LDH_5					↑	↑	↑		↑			↑	↑	
7. HBDH								(↑)		↑		↑	↑	
8. Aldorase		↑				↑		↑	↑		↑	(↑)		
9. Amylase			↑										(↑)	
10. Lipase			↑										(↑)	

251

none of the other tests discussed in this chapter requires fasting. The exact timing of each specimen must be documented since several of these enzymes peak quickly and are of short duration, while others do now show up in the bloodstream for a couple of days after tissue injury. For most of the enzyme tests, only elevations of the enzymes or isoenzymes are clinically significant. However, decreasd alkaline phosphatase levels and, very rarely, decreased transaminase levels may be clinically significant.

ALKALINE PHOSPHATASE (ALP)

Two types of phosphatases are measured in the bloodstream: alkaline and acid. These two types of phosphatases are so termed because their activity is best measured in a pH around either 10 (alkaline) or 5 (acid).

The alkaline phosphatase (ALP) is the much more common clinical test. Alkaline phosphatase is found in the tissues of the liver, bone, intestine, kidney, and placenta. Its three isoenzymes can be identified by electrophoresis:

1. *Band I:* liver, vascular endothelium, and lung.
2. *Band II:* bone, kidney, and placenta.
3. *Band III:* intestinal mucosa.

However, unlike the other isoenzymes, the isoenzymes of alkaline phosphatase are not commonly used in clinical evaluations of pathology.

Except in pregnancy, most of the serum alkaline phosphatase is made up of liver and bone isoenzymes. Since alkaline phosphatase is increased with new bone formation (osteoblastic activity), children have much higher levels than adults. Since the placenta is a rich source of alkaline phosphatases, a high level of this enzyme is also normal in pregnancy. The alkaline phosphatase from liver tissue is normally excreted into the bile, so biliary obstruction causes an increase of alkaline phosphatase. The ingestion of a fatty meal also causes a temporary increase of serum alkaline phosphatase.

Preparation of Patient
And Collection of Sample
The patient should be fasting but can have water. (This is the only enzyme test where food interferes with the results.) BSP dye causes an elevation in results. If the patient is on oral contraceptives, phenothiazines, or morphine, note the use of the drug on the laboratory slip, since elevations in the enzyme level may be related to the drug. The laboratory needs 1 ml of serum.

Reference Values

Adults	13–39 IU (international units)
	1.4–4.4 Bodansky units
	4–13 King-Armstrong Units
Pregnancy	Levels increase due to production by placenta. Levels may be as high as 107 IU by late pregnancy. Levels return to normal about three weeks after delivery (Hytten 1975).

(continued)

Reference Values (*continued*)

Infants and children	Up to 104 IU
	5–14 Bodansky units
	15–30 King-Armstrong units
	Levels remain elevated until puberty when the epiphyses close.
Aged	After age 60, values tend to be slightly lower than in younger adults.

Increased Alkaline Phosphatase (ALP) Level

Clinical Significance. A markedly increased alkaline phosphatase level in a nonpregnant adult is a general warning of a bone or liver abnormality. An elevation several times normal is usually the case with liver or bone pathology (Burke 1978).

In Paget's disease, with considerable bone destruction and bone rebuilding, the alkaline phosphatase level is higher than normal. Metastatic cancer to the bone also often causes an elevated alkaline phosphatase if the body attempts to continue to form new bone. If bone is only being broken down (osteolytic process), alkaline phosphatase is not elevated. However, most types of osteolytic processes are accompanied by some osteoblastic activity. A healing fracture causes a modest rise in the alkaline phosphatase level. Conditions, such as hyperparathyroidism and vitamin D or calcium deficiencies, cause an increased amount of alkaline phosphatase, even though bone growth may be abnormal.

Liver dysfunction is the other main reason for increased alkaline phosphatase levels. The elevation may be due either to actual liver tissue damage or, since alkaline phosphatase is excreted in the bile, to an obstruction of bile flow. Morphine sulfate may cause some spasm of the sphincter of Oddi, and thus it may elevate the alkaline phosphatase level (Koepke 1978). Conditions that cause obstructive jaundice, such as a stone in the common bile duct or cancer of the head of the pancreas, cause a markedly elevated alkaline phosphatase.

Certain drugs, such as the estrogens and phenothiazines, may cause a stasis of bile (cholestatic effect), thus elevating the alkaline phosphatase in the serum. It has also been postulated that some drugs may induce a synthesis of increased amounts of alkaline phosphatase and other liver enzymes (Rock 1980). The elevation of the alkaline phosphatase may be the first indication of an adverse reaction to a drug and indicates the drug should be stopped.

In eclampsia, the alkaline phosphatase levels are increased above the normally high levels of pregnancy, probably due to a liver dysfunction.

Often patients with liver problems, such as cirrhosis, receive albumin intravenously. (See Chapter 10 for a discussion on albumin deficiency.) In such cases, the fact that the placenta is normally a rich source of alkaline phosphatase is important to remember. Administration of albumin derived from placentas causes an elevation of the serum alkaline phosphatase level.

Possible Nursing Implications.

Preventing Injury to Fragile Bones. One of the most common uses of the alkaline phosphatase test is to screen for the possibility of bone metastasis in patients with malignancies. Whether the alkaline phosphatase is elevated, the possibility of bone metastasis is an indication that the patient may be prone to pathological fractures and thus should be handled very carefully and protected from injury. Remember that the metastatic destruction of bone causes an increase of alkaline phosphatase only if osteoblastic activity is occurring along with bone destruction. So not all bone metastasis causes elevated alkaline phosphatase levels. In metastatic disease, any elevated alkaline phosphatase is usually followed with a bone scan to determine the exact points of bone destruction.

Assessing for Jaundice. If the elevated alkaline phosphatase is due to any type of obstruction in the common bile duct, specific nursing implications are related to the presence of obstructive jaundice. (The problems associated with obstructive jaundice are discussed in Chapter 11 in the section on direct bilirubin levels.)

Recognizing the Influence of Drugs. If the patient has an elevated alkaline phosphatase due to the administration of albumin, this condition is not pathological but rather just the result of the product used. So no particular nursing implications are warranted. Also, since some patients may have increased alkaline phosphatase levels without any apparent disease process, these patients may have no special needs related to the laboratory test. However, if the patient is on drugs that can cause cholestasis, such as estrogens or phenothiazines, even a small increase in the alkaline phosphatase level may be an indication that the patient should not continue on the drug (Burke 1978). The patient who is on oral contraceptives that contain estrogen needs information about other forms of birth control.

Decreased Alkaline Phosphatase (ALP) Level

Clinical Significance. In the child before the onset of puberty, a decrease of alkaline phosphatase to adult levels indicates a lack of normal bone formation. This condition may be due to pathological conditions, such as hypothyroidism, celiac disease, cystis fibrosis, or chronic nephritis. Very low levels of alkaline phosphatase are seen in scurvy. Adults with a lack of bone formation due to malnutrition or excessive vitamin D intake may have lowered alkaline phosphatase levels.

Possible Nursing Implications. The exact nursing implications depend on the reason for a lack of normal bone formation. Usually a dietary plan is needed to ensure an adequate intake of protein, vitamins, and minerals for optimal bone growth.

ACID PHOSPHATASE

Acid phosphatase is found in high concentrations in the prostate gland, erythrocytes, and platelets. Since this enzyme is excreted in the seminal fluid, a test for acid phosphatase is sometimes done on vaginal secretions as supportive evidence for alleged rape (Byrne 1981). Because the prostatic portion of the enzyme is in such small amounts in the serum, the laboratory may use radioimmunoassay to measure the prostatic isoenzyme. The test is primarily used to assess prostatic cancer.

Preparation of Patient
And Collection of Sample
There is no special preparation of the patient. It is important, however, that the specimen not be hemolyzed since the erythrocytes are rich in acid phosphatase. The specimen should be examined within one hour. The laboratory needs 1 ml of serum.

Reference Values

Adults	Total: 0–3 IU (international units/l)
Female	Total: 0.01–0.56 Sigma units/ml
Male	Total: 0.13–0.63 Sigma units/ml Prostatic isoenzyme: 0.0–0.7 Fisherman-Lerner units/100 ml
Newborns	Increased levels due to the hemolysis of newborn period.
Pregnancy	Very little change, if any.

Increased Serum Acid Phosphatase Level

Clinical Significance. Operative trauma or instrumentation of the prostate gland, such as a cystoscopy, can cause a transient increase in the acid phosphatase level. However, the major reason for a marked elevation of the prostatic portion of this enzyme is cancer of the prostate that has invaded the capsule surrounding the gland. Conditions that cause an increased destruction of red blood cells, such as the various hemolytic anemias, also cause an increase of the nonprostatic portion of acid phosphatase. Acute renal impairment, liver dysfunction, and some diseases of the bone may also cause an increase in the total acid phosphatase level, but this test is not used to evaluate these conditions.

Possible Nursing Implications.

Assisting with Cancer Therapy. The major use of the serum acid phosphatase level is to evaluate carcinoma of the prostate gland. Since usually the man is elderly when this test is ordered, he may have other physical problems besides the malignancy. The patient needs help in coping with what may be a terminal illness. If the tumor is successfully treated by surgery, the acid phosphatase levels decrease in a few days. If estrogen therapy is used as the treatment for the prostatic cancer, the levels of acid phosphatase may not return to normal for several weeks (Widmann 1979:365). An increasing acid phosphatase level may signal a much worse prognosis for the patient.

ALANINE AMINOTRANSFERASE (ALT)
(OR FORMERLY SGPT)

Formerly known as serum glutamic-pyruvic transaminase (SGPT), this transaminase is found in the largest concentration in liver tissue, but it is also present in kidney, heart, and skeletal muscle tissue. Like the other transaminase (AST or SGOT), ALT is increased in various types of tissue damage, and so it is not very specific. ALT (or SGPT) may be used if there is a specific need to evaluate the possibility of liver tissue necrosis, but AST (or SGOT) is elevated more dramatically in most types of tissue injury and thus stays in the serum longer. The ratio of the two enzymes, ASAT (SGOT) to ALAT (SGPT), can also help to evaluate liver diseases.

Preparation of Patient
And Collection of Specimen

The patient does not need to fast. The specimen can be refrigerated after it is clotted, but it is important that the blood not be hemolyzed. The exact time that the specimen was drawn should be noted since serial measurements give useful information about the progression or lessening of liver necrosis. The laboratory needs 1 ml of blood. Various antibiotics, narcotics, and salicylates may cause false elevations of liver enzymes.

Reference Values

All groups	1–35 IU (International Units/l)
	5–35 Sigma-Frankel units

Labor and delivery or other active exercise may cause slight elevations. Newborns have higher levels.

A comparison of the ratio of ASAT (SGOT) to ALAT (SGPT) can help to evaluate liver disease. ASAT (SGOT) levels are greater than ALAT (SGPT) in cirrhosis and metastatic carcinoma of the liver. In acute hepatitis and nonmaligninant hepatic obstruction, the ASAT (SGOT) is usually lower than the ALAT (SGPT) (Rock 1980:69).

Increased ALT or SGPT

Clinical Significance. In severe hepatitis the ALT is often over 1,000 IU and may rise to 4,000 IU (Byrne 1978). In chronic hepatitis and cirrhosis, the levels are not so markedly elevated. Infectious mononucleosis, which often involves the liver, causes a significant rise in the ALT. (See Chapter 14 for tests for infectious mononucleosis.) Shock, congestive heart failure, and eclampsia all cause an increased ALT due to some liver tissue damage. Hydatidiform moles also cause elevations of the ALT. (Chapter 15 discusses the diagnosis of hydatidiform moles by hormone assay.)

Possible Nursing Implications.

Assessing for Liver Insufficiency. Since a markedly elevated ALT or SGPT may be indicative of severe liver tissue damage, nurses must carefully assess for any signs of liver insufficiency. (See Chapter 10 for the test of ammonia levels as a sign of liver dysfunction and for details on the symptoms that may be present. Chapter 11 discusses the special needs of the jaundiced patient.)

Promoting Rest and Nutrition. The basic ingredients for the encouragement of liver tissue regeneration are the promotion of rest, the avoidance of drugs toxic to the liver, and the provision of a nutritious diet that is high in calories, protein, and vitamins. Nurses may need to do some teaching to help patients learn how to conserve energy. For patients at home, someone should be available to see that they do indeed rest. Rest is not a luxury here; it is often *the* basic therapy. Enzyme levels, tested over a period of weeks, may be used to gauge the amount of activity allowed. Boredom and depression can occur due to a long convalescent period with prolonged restrictions on usual activities.

ASPARATE AMINOTRANSFERASE (AST)
(OR FORMERLY SGOT)

Formerly called serum glutamic-oxalacetic transaminase (SGOT), AST is found predominantly in heart, liver, and muscle tissue, although all tissues contain some of the enzyme. Since the transaminases are very important in energy transformation, the highest amounts of them are found in high-energy cells such as the heart, liver, and skeletal muscles. As discussed in the previous section, the highest concentration of ALT or SGPT is in the liver, and it is used primarily to detect liver necrosis. AST or SGOT can also be used to detect liver necrosis, since both transaminases rise before there are any signs of jaundice. Neither the ALT or AST are used to evaluate skeletal muscle necrosis because two other enzymes (CPK and aldorase) are more specific for muscle tissue necrosis. The AST or SGOT is most often used as one of the cardiac enzymes to detect the occurrence of a myocardial infarction. (ALT or SGPT is not elevated significantly in cardiac damage.) However, if isoenzymes of the other two cardiac enzymes (LDH and CPK) are available, the AST or SGOT may not give any additional information. A summary about the use of all the cardiac enzymes follows the discussion about each separate cardiac enzyme.

Special Preparation of Patient
And Collection of Specimen
The patient is prepared and the specimen collected in the same way and under the same conditions as for the other transaminase, ALT or SGPT. Note that various drugs may interfere with the test.

Reference Values

	10–40 IU (International Units/l)
	5–40 Sigma-Frankel units
All groups	Female values tend to be slightly lower than males but only marked increases are significant.
Pregnancy	Labor and delivery cause slight increases. Vigorous exercise also tends to increase transaminase levels.
Newborns	Higher values—check specific laboratory values.

Increased AST or SGOT Level

Clinical Significance. With the necrosis of tissue that accompanies myocardial infarction, AST is released from the damaged cardiac cells. If the patient experiences chest pain for other reasons, such as angina or pericarditis, the AST level is not markedly elevated because there is no actual cell death. The amount of enzymes released depends on the severity of the inflammation. After an acute infarction, the serum level of AST begins to rise in about 6 to 12 hours. A peak of 100 to 150 IU is reached in a couple of days, and the enzyme returns to normal in another two or three days. (See Table 12-2 for a comparison of the onset, peak, and duration of AST with the time frames for CPK, LDH, and HBD.)

TABLE 12–2.   TIME FRAME FOR CHANGES IN SERUM ENZYME LEVELS AFTER AN
ACUTE MYOCARDIAL INFARCTION*

	Appears in Serum (Hours)	Peaks (Days)	Duration (Days)
CPK (Isoenzyme II-B) *most significant	4–8	0.5–1.5	About 3
AST (Formerly known as SGOT)	6–12	1.5–2	4–6
LDH (Isoenzyme LDH₁ and LDH₂) **most significant, a "flipped" LDH.	12–24	2–6	8–14
HBDH	12	2–3	12–21

* These time frames are general approximations based on several references. Not all patients fall exactly into these patterns.
**See text for elaboration on relative efficiency of different tests. Also see Gann (1978) for discussion
on combination of tests.

In hepatitis, the AST or SGOT may reach levels as high as 1,000 to 2,000 IU (Ravel 1978), and it is elevated in the bloodstream even before jaundice appears. The return to normal may take weeks to months after hepatitis. Other types of liver involvement, such as that with shock, trauma, or cirrhosis, may cause lesser elevations of the AST. Muscular damage or pulmonary infarction are other causes of an elevated AST. Again, the ratio of AST (SGOT) to ALT (SGPT) is useful in distinguishing various types of liver pathology.

Possible Nursing Implications. Since the AST or SGOT can be elevated from many different causes, nursing care must be based on the underlying pathophysiology. If the AST is due to hepatic damage, the nursing implications for ALT or SGPT elevations would be useful as general guidelines. If the AST or SGOT is being used to rule out the possibility of a myocardial infarction, the enzymes must be carefully interpreted in relation to other clinical assessments of the patient. Some general nursing implications about the use of all the cardiac enzymes follows the discussion on the CPK and LDH tests.

Decrease in Transaminases ALT and AST (Or SGOT and SGPT)

Clinical Significance. Since the levels of transaminases are normally very low, a decrease is unlikely. In *rare* instances, both transaminases ALT (SGPT) and AST (SGOT) are decreased or nonexistent due to severe liver dysfunction because the liver can no longer make the enzymes.

CREATINE PHOSPHOKINASE (CPK) AND THE CPK ISOENZYMES

CPK, which is very important in energy utilization, is involved in the reaction that changes creatine to creatinine. (See Chapter 4 for the serum tests of creatine and creatinine.) Since almost all of the circulating CPK comes normally from muscular tissue, muscular activity and intramuscular injections are two common ways that CPK values are elevated. CPK can be measured as one total enzyme in the serum, or it can be separated into three different isoenzymes. The three types of CPK isoenzymes are:

1. CPK-I   (BB)   produced primarily by brain tissue.
2. CPK-II (MB)   produced primarily by heart tissue.
3. CPK-III (MM)   produced primarily by muscle tissue.

The isoenzymes of CPK are particularly useful in detecting myocardial infarction and progressive muscular diseases that cause muscle necrosis.

Preparation of Patient And Collection of Specimen

Because physical activity causes a transient increase in CPK, patients should not engage in vigorous activity before the blood sample is drawn. Since intramuscular injections may triple the amount of CPK in the serum, such injections should be delayed until the test is drawn if doing so is feasible. Otherwise, the fact that the patient has received IM injections should be noted on the laboratory slip. The timing of the drawing for the CPK is crucial since the enzyme may disappear from the bloodstream in less than 24 hours after a myocardial infarction. The laboratory needs 1 ml of serum of blood, which should be refrigerated if it cannot be sent to the laboratory immediately.

Reference Values

All groups:
  Females
  Males
	Total: 5–35 mU/ml
	Total: 5–55 mU/ml

	Values for black males are double those for white males, while female black and white values are nearly equal (Ravel 1978: 227).
Isoenzymes	CPK-I (BB) Brain 0% CPK-II (MB) Heart 0–3% CPK-III (MM) Muscle 97–100%
Pregnancy	Levels are reduced in first half of pregnancy but rise in second half of pregnancy. Slight increase during labor and delivery. Surgical procedures, such as an episiotomy, cause more increase. Also, intramuscular injections and vigorous exercise elevate the CPK.

Increased Serum CPK

Clinical Significance.
   Elevation of CPK-II. The CPK, the first enzyme to be elevated after a myocardial infarction, begins to rise in 3 to 6 hours and may peak in the first 24 hours (Table 12–2). In

some patients the CPK returns to normal within 16 hours after the chest pain. (Gann (1978) gives evidence that one CPK-II (MB) on admission and another after 12 hours are usually enough to diagnose or to exclude myocardial infarction occurring within 24 hours of admission. It is generally agreed that the CPK-II (MB) is very useful in the initial detection of an infarction, but it is not useful if the patient has had chest pain for a day or two before coming to seek medical help. For some patients, the duration of CPK may continue for about 3 days but the peak is missed; in such cases, other cardiac enzymes are more helpful.

Elevation of CPK. III CPK-III (MM) elevations are never diagnostic of a specific muscular disease, but high levels are an indication for further specific testing of muscular function. In the early stages of muscular dystrophy, CPK is as high as 3,000 IU/l. As the disease progresses, the CPK levels drop, and, by the time the person is bedridden, they may be normal. Healthy female carriers of X-linked Duchenne muscular dystrophy have raised levels of CPK. Once these women are pregnant, however, the lowering of the CPK in the first half of pregnancy may mask the elevation (Hytten 1974:45).

Elevation of CPK-I. The third type of isoenzyme, CPK-I (BB) may be elevated in the case of extreme shock, of brain tumors, or of severe cerebral accidents. However, this test is not of clinical value at the present time.

Possible Nursing Implications.

Assessing for Symptoms of A Myocardial Infarction. Since this CPK is the first cardiac enzyme to be increased and has a short duration in the serum, it should not be elevated after the first few days of an infarction. A sudden increase in the CPK after a day or two should be reported to the physician immediately and the patient assessed for the possibility of an extension of the infarction. In this respect, however, the nurse must remember the effect of intramuscular injections on the total CPK. The isoenzyme II is the one to note for the patient who has had a myocardial infarction. A general summary of key points in planning nursing care for the patient with elevated cardiac enzymes follows the discussion on the LDH test.

Assisting with Diagnostic Procedures for Muscle Necrosis. If the elevated CPK is related to muscle necrosis, the patient may need to undergo a battery of tests to discover the exact problem. Women who are found to be carriers of the sex-linked gene for muscular dystrophy may need to be referred to genetic counseling if they desire pregnancy. The enzyme aldorase is another test for muscular inflammatory diseases. Some general nursing implications for patients with myositis are covered in the section on aldorase later in this chapter.

LACTIC DEHYDROGENASE (LDH) AND THE FIVE LDH ISOENZYMES

Lactic dehydrogenase is an enzyme that helps remove a water molecule from lactic acid. LDH is found in large amounts in the heart, liver, muscles, and erythrocytes. It is also present in other organs such as the kidney, pancrease, spleen, brain, and lungs. Like the enzyme CPK, LDH can be separated into various isoenzymes:

1. LDH_1 is primarily from the heart and erythrocytes.
2. LDH_2 probably comes mostly from the reticuloendothelial system (Widmann 1979:359).
3. LDH_3 is from the lungs and other tissue.
4. LDH_4 comes from the placenta, kidney, and pancreas.
5. LDH_5 is largely from liver and muscle tissue.

Total LDH, as well as LDH_1 and LDH_2, are most often used in detecting a myocardial infarction. LDH is not typically used to assess liver function or muscle function, since other enzymes are more specific. (See Table 12-1 for elevations of LDH isoenzymes in various pathological states.)

Preparation of Patient
And Collection of Specimen

The sample must be handled carefully since any hemolysis of the red blood cells elevates falsely the results. Even if the hemolysis is not enough to turn the serum pink, there is still an increased LDH. The patient does not need to be fasting. The laboratory needs 2 ml of serum.

Reference Values

Adults	60–120 u/ml
Pregnancy	Normal in pregnancy but increases slightly during labor and delivery, as with other vigorous exercise.
Newborn	First week of life: 308–2,540 units due to increased breakdown of red blood cells.
Children	Decrease to adult levels by age 14.
Isoenzymes	LDH_1 (erythrocytes, heart tissue) 25% LDH_2 (reticuloendothial tissue, kidney) 40% LDH_3 (lungs, lymph nodes, spleen, and various other tissues) 25% LDH_4 (kidney, placenta, liver tissue) 5% LDH_5 (liver tissue, skeletal tissue, kidney 5%

(Values from Cawley 1978.)

Increased Serum LDH

Clinical Significance. In myocardial infarction, the LDH begins to rise about 12 to 24 hours after the cardiac damage. The peak, usually around 300 to 800 IU/l is in two to six days, and the enzyme remains in the bloodstream for up to two weeks. (See Table 12-2 for a comparison of this time frame with the other cardiac enzymes.) The measurement of the isoenzymes 1 and 2 gives an even more specific indication that damaged cardiac tissue is causing the elevation. As noted in the reference values, LDH_2 is usually higher in concentration than LDH_1. Since in a myocardial infarction the greatest rise is in the LDH_1 isoenzyme, it becomes more concentrated than LDH_2. This change in the percentage ratio between LDH_1 and LDH_2, called a *flipped LDH,* is considered to be highly suggestive of a myocardial infarction. A flipped LDH, or the reversal of the ratio of LDH_1 to LDH_2, is apparent sooner than the rise in the total LDH. It also remains evident for three to four days after the total LDH returns to normal after a myocardial infarction (Widmann 1979:359).

Other possible causes of LDH elevations are as follows:

1. Hemolytic and macrocytic anemias tend to cause elevations in LDH_1 and LDH_2.
2. In pulmonary infarction and infectious mononucleosis, LDH_2 and LDH_3 are elevated.
3. Leukemia and malignancies, in general, cause large increases in LDH_3.
4. Liver damage increases the last two isoenzymes, LDH_4 and LDH_5. Since the last two isoenzymes make up but a small portion (10%) of the total LDH, such an increase may not change the total drastically.
5. Shock and trauma may cause an elevation of all the isoenzymes, as does heart surgery. If the heart-lung machine is used, the LDH will be four to six times the normal reference values.
6. In pregnancy, placental disturbances, such as abruptio placenta, effects an elevation in the isoenzymes.
7. Hepatitis causes a more modest increase in the total than that accompanying myocardial infarction.
8. An LDH of 2,000 IU or more is almost always due to either megaloblastic anemia or cancer (Burke 1978:78).

The actual interpretation of the LDH isoenzymes can be very complicated because of the many variations possible. Cawley (1978) offers pictures and examples of how subtle differences in the overall pattern can be diagnostically significant. More commonly, the total amounts are used as guidelines in conjunction with the clinical symptoms of the patient.

Increased LDH

Possible Nursing Implications.

Assessing for Chest Pain. Although almost any type of tissue damage can change the LDH, the major use of this test is to determine the presence of a myocardial infarction. (The use of isoenzymes is even more definitive, of course.) Since LDH may remain elevated for a couple of weeks after a myocardial infarction, it is useful in monitoring the patient who is convalescing from an infarction. If the LDH begins to rise again after the first week, the physician should be notified immediately, since this rise may signal an extension of the infarction. Sometimes a second infarction is "silent," since the patient experiences no symptoms of chest pain, or it may be unnoticeable because the patient has been heavily medicated with morphine sulfate.

The sudden increase in LDH does not always mean a worsening of the infarction since other things may cause a rise. For example, pulmonary infarctions can occur as a complication of the bedrest. To pinpoint the exact reason for an increasing LDH in a patient recovering from a myocardial infarction, a thorough medical assessment and other tests, such as repeat electrocardiograms and lung scans, are needed. Some general nursing implications for the patient with a change in the cardiac enzymes are summarized after the discussion on the HBD test.

Assessing Other Needs of the Patient. If the elevated LDH is due to a malignancy, the nursing implications are based on the stage of the disease and on the therapeutic interventions needed for the individual case. If the highly elevated LDH is due to a type of megaloblastic anemia, some of the nursing implications discussed in Chapter 2 for anemias may be appropriate. For example, the patient may need teaching about diet and drug therapy.

HYDROXYBUTYRIC DEHYGROGENASE (HBD OR HBDH)

Some laboratories may do an HBD test, which is an indirect measure of LDH_1 and LDH_2, when isoenzymes for LDH cannot be done. The HBD is more specific than either the AST (SGOT) or the total LDH, but it is less specific than either the CPK isoenzymes or the LDH isoenzymes for detecting myocardial infarctions (Galen 1975). Since HBD is also easier and cheaper than isoenzymes, it may be used to follow a myocardial infarction over a period of time (Ravel 1978:226).

Preparation of Patient
And Collection of Sample
The same precautions apply to the HBD that apply to the LDH.

Reference Values
110–230 IU/l

Increased HBD or HBDH

Clinical Significance. Although malignancies, muscle disease, and megaloblastic anemias also cause elevations, the most common reason for an elevated HBD is a myocardial infarction. See the previous discussion on LDH_1 and LDH_2. Note that HBD may remain elevated for over two weeks after an infarction.

CHANGES IN THE CARDIAC ENZYMES
(AST OR SGOT, CPK, LDH, AND HBD)

General Nursing Implications.

Understanding the Limitations of Enzymes as Assessment Tools. The real patient in the clinical area is never quite as predictable as the one indicated by the textbook tables. So, although the diagnostic interpretation of cardiac enzymes is the responsibility of the attending physician, the nurse caring for cardiac patients needs some general knowledge about standard practices when enzyme levels are puzzling. Usually, in a patient with a myocardial infarction, the changes in the cardiac enzymes roughly follow the time frames given in Table 12–2. If all the enzymes, including the isoenzymes, are normal for a couple of days, then the patient most likely has not had a myocardial infarction (DeHoff 1976). If the cardiac isoenzyme of CPK-II (MB) is elevated and the LDH remains normal, the diagnosis is in question. The patient may have had myocardial ischemia rather than an actual infarction. However, angina does not usually cause elevations, and the LDH may not always be positive (Gann 1978). As a general rule, the flipped LDH is considered highly suggestive of a myocardial infarction. The routine use of AST (SGOT) and HBD may not be necessary when the CPK isoenzymes and LDH isoenzymes are available. Galen (1975:47) has suggested that the four most important criteria for the diagnosis of a myocardial infarction are:

1. a positive new Q wave in the electrocardiogram,
2. a classical acute clinical history,
3. the presence of CPK-II (MB) over 3%, and
4. a flipped LDH (LDH$_1$ greater than LDH$_2$).

The important point for nurses to remember is that they must always interpret the enzyme levels in the context of the patient's overall clinical picture.

Recognizing Clinical Situations That Cause Pseudo-Elevations of Myocardial Enzymes. When isoenzymes are not available, the enzyme tests may be even more likely to give a pseudo-myocardial pattern. For example, if the patient has any disease of the biliary tract, then the use of opiates, such as morphine or codeine, can cause a spasm of the sphincter of Oddi. This temporary narrowing or obstruction of the common bile duct can cause an increase in the LDH, and it may make the AST or SGOT markedly increased (Koepke 1978). Nurses must also remember that intramuscular injections significantly increase the total CPK level.

Strenuous exercise can significantly elevate the CPK, the AST or SGOT, and the LDH. Evidently the amount of increase of these enzymes is related directly to the vigor of the exercise and inversely to the level of training before the exercise (Statland 1979). So a man in poor physical condition from a lack of training may have chest pain after a vigorous run or a handball game. The cardiac enzymes may be elevated even though he has not had an infarction. Again the point is that the enzymes are never diagnostic when used alone.

Recognizing the Importance of Timing of Enzymes. Just as an elevation of serum enzymes is not always proof positive of an infarction, a lack of enzyme elevations does not always mean that an infarction can be ruled out. Table 12–2, in showing the importance of timing in relation to the serum levels of the enzymes, also demonstrates that missing the peak of the enzyme in the serum is possible. According to Wenger (1980:286), it takes at least a gram of necrotic myocardial tissue to release enough enzymes to cause elevated serum levels. Fatal arrhythmias can result from a very small infarct or from ischemic heart tissue. Thus normal cardiac enzymes must not give nurses a false sense of security.

Planning Interventions for the Patient with a Possible Infarction. When the presence of an infarction is open to question, it is prudent to continue to treat the patient as a possible myocardial infarction until the condition is definitely ruled out. The key nursing actions are to promote physical and mental relaxation and to watch the vital signs carefully. Ideally, such patients should be in a coronary care unit so that they can be monitored very closely. The use of the cardiac monitor does not take the place of the nurse. The nurse must be able to recognize that the patient is having a potentially dangerous arrhythmia so that early treatment can be initiated. The nurse can also detect distended neck veins or slight dyspnea as signals of a potential fluid overload. Even a slight change in vital signs may indicate impending cardiogenic shock (Wenger 1980). This very careful watching of the patient is essential any time there is a question of myocardial infarction. Refer to a nursing textbook for the general care of the patient who has definitely been diagnosed as having a myocardial infarction.

ALDORASE

Like most of the other enzymes in this chapter, aldorase is present in all cells. Its highest concentrations are found in skeletal muscles, heart, and liver tissue. Since damage to muscular tissue causes marked elevations of aldorase, it is a diagnostic test for certain types of muscle damage. Aldorase is not used as a diagnostic test in cardiac or liver disease because other enzyme tests are sufficient.

Preparation of Patient
And Collection of Sample
Fasting is not necessary. Aldorase is in erythrocytes, so the specimen must not be hemolyzed. The laboratory needs 2 ml of fresh serum.

Reference Values

All groups 1.3–8.2 m U/ml
Newborns and children have higher values than adults.

Increased Aldorase Serum Level

Clinical Significance. Muscular disorders that cause inflammation of the muscles (myositis) cause an elevation of aldorase. In the event of muscular wasting due to a muscular disease of the central nervous system, such as myasthenia gravis or multiple sclerosis, the aldorase level is not elevated. In progressive muscular dystrophy, the level may be ten to fifteen times normal in the early stages of the disease, but the level sudsides as muscle wasting continues (Widmann 1979:351). In some types of acute myositis the levels of aldorase return to normal when corticosteroid treatment is effective. Aldorase may be used in conjunction with more specific diagnostic measures to identify the exact reason for muscle necrosis.

Possible Nursing Implications.
  Assisting the Patient During Acute Episodes. The key nursing implication for the patient with a skeletal muscular problem is to help the person to be as independent as possible while conserving muscle strength. The person is comforted to know that the lack of muscle strength is temporary. If the muscular disorder is due to an acute condition, the

return of muscle strength occurs after the enzymes return to normal. Nursing care during the acute phase may center most on preventing any complications from the disuse of muscles. (The other enzymes that become elevated in acute muscular myositis are the transaminases, CPK, and LDH.) The effectiveness of treatment is indicated by a continual monitoring of alderose and, less likely, some of the other enzymes.

Helping the Patient Cope with a Chronic Muscular Disease. If the muscular disorder is a chronic problem, such as muscular dystrophy, the patient is faced with learning how to cope with a progressively debilitating disease. Since each case of muscle disease differs from all others, the nursing care plan must be individualized to the severity of the disease and to its effects on the person. The community health nurse may be very involved in helping patients adapt to a crippling disease. Januel (1977) gives such patients many helpful hints on ways to be independent in doing personal care and housekeeping, while using their limited energy wisely. The nurse needs to emphasize to patients that a schedule that allows frequent and short rest periods is much better than one with a long rest period. Patients may be able to do much more if they are not hurrying to accomplish several activities in a limited time. In addition to emphasizing a planned exercise and rest schedule, the nurse may also need to do some health teaching about the expected effects of the prescribed medications and the necessity for follow-up diagnostic tests.

SERUM AMYLASE

Amylase is an enzyme that helps with the digestion of starch. It is found in high concentrations in the salivary glands and in the pancreas, each of which contains a different isoenzyme. These two isoenzymes can be separated, but doing so is not clinically useful since any disease of the parotid gland (mumps) is evident from the swelling of the gland. So although an infection of the parotid gland (mumps) causes an elevated serum amylase level, the test is not used for this condition. Even though various types of trauma to the pancreas can cause elevated amylase levels, the major use of the amylase test is to detect the presence of pancreatitis.

Amylase is the only enzyme that is measured in both serum and urine as a routine test. The serum amylase is often done as a stat procedure in patients with acute abdominal pain to distinguish pancreatitis from other acute abdominal problems that would require surgery. Since amylase is excreted in the urine, urine amylase is increased in pancreatitis too.

Preparation of Patient
And Collection of Sample
Since the amylase test is often done as a stat procedure, the timing of the specimen is very important. The enzyme begins to rise in the bloodstream within three to six hours after an attack of pancreatitis. Drugs that cause spasm of the sphincter of Oddi, such as the opiates, may cause an elevation of the serum amylase. The increase is at a maximum five hours after drug administration (Koepke 1978:66). So, if possible, the stat amylase should be drawn prior to the use of opiate drugs. Thiazide diuretics and diagnostic dyes may also cause false elevations.

The patient does not need to be fasting. Hemolysis does not affect the results of this test. The laboratory needs 3 ml of serum.

Reference Values

Adults	4–25 U/ml 60–150 Somogyi units
Women	If taking oral contraceptives, will have slightly increased amylase levels.
Newborns	May have very low levels.

Increased Serum Amylase Level

Clinical Significance. Pancreatitis is the most common reason for marked elevations of serum amylase, which begins to increase about three to six hours after an attack of this disease. (See Table 12-3 for a comparison with serum lipase, the other pancreatic enzyme.) The severity of the disease is not directly related to the levels of the enzyme. In fact, about 10% of patients with fatal pancreatitis have normal serum amylase levels (Wallach 1974:196).

In the adult, the two most common reasons for pancreatitis are alcohol abuse and gallstones. Evidently, the obstruction of the pancreatic ducts or pancreatic ischemia triggers an acute inflammatory response and autodigestion of the pancreas begins. Oral contraceptives, hyperlipidemia, and hyperthyroidism are less common reasons for such response. Ruptured ectopic pregnancies, perforated ulcers, and other acute abdominal conditions may cause some elevation of the serum amylase level due to trauma to the pancreas. In children, pancreatitis is rare and often of an unknown cause. Sometimes it appears to have a hereditary base. In a study done by Sibert (1979), obesity and the beginning of puberty were related to the incidence of pancreatitis in female children.

Possible Nursing Implications.

Assessing for Fluid Loss. Since a markedly elevated amylase level is indicative of acute pancreatitis, which may be life-threatening, the nursing care is geared to this pathology. If the patient has massive hemorrhagic necrosis, the mortality rate may be as

TABLE 12-3. PANCREATIC ENZYMES USED TO DIAGNOSE ACUTE PANCREATITIS

	Begins Elevation	Peaks	Duration
Serum amylase	3–6 hours	20–30 hours	2–3 days
Urine amylase	6–10 hours after serum levels	Varies	1–2 weeks
Serum lipase	Increases after amylase	Varies	Up to 14 days longer than amylase

Time frames are general approximations based on several references.

high as 50 to 80% (Price 1978:280). If the pancreatitis is not hemorrhagic, the prognosis is much better, but fluid loss can still lead to shock. Thus one key nursing implication for the patient with an elevated serum amylase level is to observe for any change in vital signs that may indicate hypovolemia from the loss of pancreatic fluids or blood.

Relieving Pain. Since patients with pancreatitis usually have severe abdominal pain, comfort measures and pain relief are important. Often meperidine (Demerol) is used to relieve pain rather than morphine because opiates may cause spasms of the sphincter of Oddi. (Recall that the potential effect of opiates on the sphincter of Oddi can cause the elevation of the pancreatic enzymes, as well as of liver enzymes such as the transaminases and alkaline phosphatase.)

Decreasing Pancreatic Stimulation. Stimulation of the pancreas needs to be minimized as much as possible. So the patient must be NPO. Atropine, an anticholinergic drug, may be ordered to decrease gastrointestinal activity. A nasogastric tube may be used to decompress the bowel until the acute inflammation has subsided. Bowel sound may be hypoactive or absent if the inflammation is severe.

Preventing Infection. Antibiotics are used to prevent a secondary infection of the necrotic tissue in the pancreas. (See Chapter 2 on WBC differentials to assess infections.)

Assessing for Possible Hypocalcemia, Hypokalemia, Hyperglycemia, and Jaundice. When the patient has pancreatitis, four laboratory tests, besides lipase (discussed next), influence nursing care:

1. *Calcium levels:* Serum calcium may be lowered because calcium is deposited in the pancreas due to fat necrosis. The hypocalcemia may be severe enough to cause tetany. (See Chapter 7 for possible nursing implications for patients with a decreased serum calcium level.)
2. *Potassium levels:* Hypokalemia may result from a lack of intake and a loss of body fluids. (See Chapter 5 for the implications of a lowered potassium level.)
3. *Glucose levels:* Hyperglycemia may be brought about because the damaged pancreatic cells may not be able to produce sufficient insulin. (See Chapter 8 for serum glucose levels.)
4. *Bilirubin levels:* Direct bilirubin may increase if the pancreatic inflammation is due to obstruction of the common bile duct. (See Chapter 11 for the implications when the patient has obstructive jaundice.)

Assessing for Chronic Complications. Once the patient is over the acute stage of pancreatitis, the most common complications are abcess formation in the pancreas or pseudocysts, which are collections of fluids in sacs outside the pancreas. Gallium scans may be used to detect abcesses, while sonograms may show the presence of the pseudo-cysts.

Patient Teaching to Prevent Recurrent Attacks. Patients who have had an elevated serum amylase level may benefit from discharge planning that focuses on the ways that recurrent attacks can be reduced. Alcohol in all forms should be avoided for several months. If alcohol abuse was the precipitating factor, the patient may need to seek professional help to deal with a chronic problem. If gallstones are present and a cholecystectomy is to be done later, dietary modifications may be needed.

URINARY AMYLASE

Amylase is the enzyme that is elevated in the serum in acute pancreatitis and that can also be measured in the urine. Since the amylase may be elevated in the urine for as long as two weeks after an acute episode of pancreatitis, monitoring the amylase levels in urine may be useful after the acute peak in the serum has diminished. (See Table 12–3 for a comparison of the time frames for serum and urine amylases.)

Preparation of Patient And Collection of Sample

Usually the test is done on a collection of urine for a 2-hour time period, but sometimes a 24-hour specimen is used. The 24-hour specimen needs to be iced. See Chapter 3 for tips on collecting 24-hour urine specimens.

Reference Values

24–76 units/ml
260–950 Somogyi units in 24 hours

SERUM LIPASE

Lipase is a pancreatic enzyme that breaks down fat into glycerol and fatty acids. Since urine lipase levels are not clinically useful, this section deals exclusively with serum lipase. In acute pancreatitis (see Table 12–3, lipase rises later in the serum than amylase. So lipase may be used as a secondary test for pancreatitis when the diagnosis is questionable (Koepke 1979). Other types of pancreatic pathothogy, such as carcinoma or trauma, cause some release of the enzyme into the serum.

Preparation of Patient
And Collection of Sample

The precautions are the same as those for amylase. The laboratory needs 3 ml of serum.

Reference Values

All groups	2 U/ml or less Cherry and Crandall method: 1–1.5 U Maclay method: less than 0.3 U
Pregnancy	Increase in late pregnancy to around 15 IU (may be related to high levels of circulating lipids).

Increased Serum Lipase Level

Clinical Significance. Elevated lipase levels are a confirmation test of acute pancreatitis. See the discussion of amylase for the nursing implications when a patient has pancreatitis.

Questions

12–1. The measurement of isoenzymes is often more valuable than the measurement of a total enzyme in the serum for which of the following reasons?

  a. The units for measurement are standardized for the isoenzymes.

  b. A specific isoenzyme is formed by only one organ.

  c. Isoenzymes are more tissue-specific.

  d. Each type of isoenzyme controls different metabolic functions.

12–2. Which one of the following factors is the *least* likely to cause elevations in most of the common serum enzymes?

  a. Eating food four hours before the test.

  b. Vigorous physical activity.

  c. Administration of intramuscular injections of morphine sulfate.

  d. Hemolysis of the serum sample.

12–3. The physiological process in puberty that causes alkaline phosphatase levels to decrease to adult levels is which of the following?

  a. Increased production of sex hormones. **c.** Maturity of the liver.

  b. Loss of adipose tissue of childhood. **d.** Closure of the epiphyses.

12–4. A markedly elevated alkaline phosphatase level is a general warning of either:

  a. increased bone formation *or* obstruction to bile flow.

  b. mycardial infarction *or* angina.

  c. cancer of the prostate *or* of the liver.

  d. increased bone destruction or liver dysfunction.

12–5. Administration of intravenous albumin solutions may cause an elevated serum alkaline phosphatase level for which of the following reasons.?

  a. Albumin obtained from placentas is rich in this enzyme.

  b. Alkaline phosphatase is transported by albumin.

  c. The oncotic pressure is increased in the serum.

  d. The method used to purify albumin causes the release of the enzyme.

12–6. The main use of serum acid phosphatase levels is to diagnose and to evaluate malignancies of which of the following?

  a. Liver.   **c.** Prostate gland.

  b. Ovaries.   **d.** Bone.

12-7. When a patient has a marked elevation of the transaminases ALT (formerly SGPT) and AST (formerly SGOT), the key nursing implication is observation for signs and symptoms of which of the following?

    a. Liver dysfunction.

    b. Muscle weakness.

    c. Dehydration.

    d. Angina or other cardiovascular problems.

12-8. In myocardial damage, all these enzymes will probably be increased. Which one of the enzymes is most useful for detecting myocardial damage in the first 24 hours after an episode of chest pain?

    a. CPK.   **b.** AST or SGOT.   **c.** LDH.   **d.** HBD.

12-9. The three isoenzymes of CPK are useful in detecting all the following types of tissue damage except which?

    a. Brain.   **b.** Pancreatic.   **c.** Skeletal muscle.   **d.** Cardiac.

12-10. A flipped LDH is one of the characteristic signs of an acute myocardial infarction. A flipped LDH means that LDH_1 is which of the following?

    a. Greater than LDH_2.

    b. Less than LDH_2.

    c. In an abnormal form.

    d. Greater than LDH_4 and LDH_5.

12-11. HBD is not usually used as one of the cardiac enzymes, if:

    a. isoenzymes are done for LDH and CPK.

    b. AST (formerly SGOT) is ordered.

    c. the acute chest pain was more than 24 hours before admission.

    d. the patient is in a convalescent phase.

12-12. Mr. Marx is a 50-year-old businessman who was admitted to the coronary care unit with severe chest pain yesterday. His enzyme levels (CPK, LDH, and AST or SGOT) done on admission were normal. Since he wants to make several business calls, he has asked where he can find a phone. Which nursing action is appropriate?

    a. Allow him to go via wheelchair to a phone since his enzyme levels are normal.

    b. Tell him he has had a heart attack so he must stay on complete bedrest.

    c. Make sure that Mr. Marx understands the need for further assessment of EKG readings, serial enzyme levels, and a medical exam to rule out a possible myocardial infarction.

  d. Tell him that phone calls are not allowed and continue to observe him for arrhythmias, hypotension, or distended neck veins.

12–13. Mrs. Jackson is a 44-year-old mother with two teenaged girls. She has increased aldorase levels due to a still-undiagnosed muscular disease. Which advice by a community health nurse would be the most appropriate?

  a. "Schedule most of your activities for the morning when you have the most strength."

  b. "Ask your teenagers to take care of your personal needs such as baths and shampoos."

  c. "Why not hire someone to do all your housework?"

  d. "Try to alternate each small activity with a short period of rest."

12–14. In acute pancreatitis, the serum lipase level:

  a. is a more useful test than the serum amylase because the lipase rises quickly.

  b. remains in the serum longer than the amylase after an acute attack so it may be used as a secondary test.

  c. can be measured in the urine as well as in the serum to aid diagnosis.

  d. closely parallels the rise and fall of the serum amylase level, so it gives no additional information.

12–15. Mr. Bigelow is a 35-year-old artist who has been admitted with reoccurring pancreatitis. Both his serum and urine levels of amylase are markedly increased. The nurse should assess for any signs of which of the following?

  a. Hypocalcemia.   **c.** Circulatory overload.

  b. Hypoglycemia.   **d.** Hyperkalemia.

12–16. Mr. Bigelow's amylase levels have returned to normal, and he is being discharged. When he returns to the clinic next week, it would be *most important* to reemphasize a diet plan that includes which of the following?

  a. Decreased intake of starches and other carbohydrates.

  b. Total restriction of alcoholic beverages.

  c. Foods high in fat-soluble vitamins.

  d. Frequent small feedings with an emphasis on high-caloric foods.

REFERENCES

Byrne, Judith. "Using Enzyme Levels to Assess Liver Function," *Nursing* 78 (January 1978): 50–52.

Byrne, Judith *et al. Laboratory Tests: Implications for Nurses and Allied Health Professionals.* Menlo Park, Cal.: Addison-Wesley, 1981.

Burke, Desmond *et al.* "Laboratory Studies: When to Act on Unexpected Test Results," *Patient Care* 12 (January 30, 1978): 14–87.

Cawley, Leo. *Electrophoresis and Immunochemical Reactions in Gel.* Chicago: American Society of Clinical Pathologists, 1978.

DeHoff, Janet. "What You Should Know About Interpreting Cardiac Enzyme Studies," *Nursing '76* 6 (September 1976): 69–70.

Galen, R. S. *et al.* "Diagnosis of Acute Myocardial Infarction: Relative Efficiency of Serum Enzyme and Isoenzyme Measurements," *Journal of American Medical Association* 232 (April 14, 1975): 145–147.

Gann, Dietmar, *et al.* "Optimal Enzyme Test Combination for Diagnosis of Acute Myocardial Infarction," *Southern Medical Journal* 71 (12) (December 1978): 1459–1462.

Holum, John. *Elements of General and Biological Chemistry,* 5th ed. New York: John Wiley & Sons, Inc., 1979.

Hytten, Frank and Lind, Tom. *Diagnostic Indices in Pregnancy.* Summit, N.J.: Ciba-Geigy Corp., 1975.

Koepke, John. *Guide to Clinical Laboratory Diagnosis,* 2nd ed. New York: Appleton-Century-Crofts, 1979.

Janul, Linda. "Polymyositis—Dermamyositis: A Perplexing Disorder," *American Journal of Nursing* 77 (July 1977): 1184–1186.

Price, Sylvia and Wilson, Lorraine. *Pathophysiology: Clinical Concepts of Disease Processes.* New York: McGraw-Hill Book Co., 1978.

Ravel, Richard. *Clinical Laboratory Medicine,* 3rd ed. Chicago: Year Book Publishers, 1978.

Rock, Robert. "Recent Advances in the Diagnostic Enzymology of Liver Disease," *Continuing Education for Family Physicians* 13 (July 1980): 64–69.

Sibert, J. R., "Pancreatitis in Childhood," *Postgraduate Medical Journal* 55 (March 1979): 171–175.

Statland, Bernard. "Strenuous Activity and Serum Enzyme Values," *Journal of the American Medical Association* 241 (January 26, 1979): 404.

Wallach, Jacques. *Interpretation of Diagnostic Tests,* 2nd ed. Boston: Little, Brown and Co., 1974.

Wenger, Nanette *et al.* *Cardiology for Nurses.* New York: McGraw-Hill Book Co., 1980.

Widmann, Frances. *Clinical Interpretation of Laboratory Tests,* 8th ed. Philadelphia: F. A. Davis Co., 1979.

CHAPTER THIRTEEN

Coagulation Tests And Tests to Detect Occult Blood

Objectives

1. Describe the four major stages of the coagulation process, as well as the difference between the intrinsic and extrinsic system of clotting as a basis for laboratory tests.
2. Describe clinical situations where vitamin K is useful for returning the prothrombin time (PT) to normal.
3. Describe important nursing implications for the patient who has a bleeding tendency due to a lack of clotting factors.
4. Devise a teaching plan for a patient who is discharged on long-term coumarin therapy.
5. Compare and contrast the two most common coagulation tests, prothrombin time (PT) and partial thromboplastin time (PTT).
6. Explain the possible nursing implications when a patient has an abnormally decreased PT and/or PTT.
7. Explain the screening tests and confirmatory test for classical hemophilia (hemophilia A).
8. Identify appropriate nursing actions in caring for patients with increased and decreased platelet counts.
9. Identify the changes in fibrinogen levels, along with the changes in the PT, PTT, and platelet counts, that are clues that disseminated intravascular clotting (DIC) or consumption coagulopathy may be occurring.
10. Describe the important facts a nurse should know about guaiac tests (Hemoccult), used to detect occult blood in the feces or other specimens.

The delicate balance of the coagulation process makes it possible for a healthy person to experience neither hemorrhage nor thrombus formation. Tests such as the PT, PTT, and platelet counts are routine tests for the clotting ability of the blood. Tests of individual factors are needed to detect specific diseases, such as hemophilia A (test for Factor VIII).

Other tests, such as fibrinogen assays, help to assess severe coagulation problems, such as disseminated intravascular coagulation disease (DIC).

Besides the common tests for clotting ability, this chapter also includes information on guaiac and other tests, which are used to detect hidden or occult blood. Occult blood tests are used not only to detect bleeding tendencies, but also to screen for rectal cancer.

Laboratory tests both for clotting functions and for bleeding tendencies are of use to the nurse in three primary ways. First, these tests may alert the nurse to the possibility that the patient is vulnerable due to an increased bleeding tendency. Second, some of these tests may indicate that the patient is vulnerable due to an increased risk of thrombus formation. Third, three of these tests are specifically used to monitor the effects of anticoagulant drugs. The role of the nurse in anticoagulant therapy is stressed. No "magic number" determines when a patient will bleed or become subject to thrombus formation. At the very best, these laboratory tests are only guidelines for helping the nurse assess potential patient problems.

THE COAGULATION PROCESS

Twelve factors are involved in the clotting process. Remembering all the factors is not necessary, but knowing which test measures which factors is useful. A list of the twelve factors, along with the tests that show the deficiencies and the relation of vitamin K, is included in Table 13–1. Vitamin K was named K because it is the "Koagulation" factor. If the liver cannot obtain vitamin K, four coagulation factors cannot be manufactured: Factors II, VII, IX, and X (Koepke 1979). Note that the table contains thirteen numbers,

TABLE 13–1. COAGULATION FACTORS TESTED BY SPECIFIC TESTS AND RELATIONSHIP TO VITAMIN K

Name of Factor	Test of Deficiency	Vitamin K Needed for Production by Liver
I (fibrinogen)	Fibrinogen level,* PT, PTT	
II (prothrombin)	PT, PTT	Yes
III (thromboplastin)		
IV (calcium)		
V (labile or proaccelerin)	PT, PTT	
VI (unassigned at present time)		
VII (stable factor or proconvertin)	PT	Yes
VIII (antihemophilic globulin)	PTT	
IX (partial thromboplastin component, Christmas factor, PTC)	PTT	Yes
X (Stuart Prower factor)	PT, PTT	Yes
XI (plasma thromboplastin antecedent)	PTT	
XII (Hageman factor)	PTT	
XIII (fibrin stabilizing factor)		

* Specific assays can be done to test for each factor (see the reference values in Appendix A– Table 4).

since one factor (VI) was found to really be part of another factor. The factors were numbered, instead of named, in the order of their discovery, so there could be a universal understanding of which factor was being discussed.

Table 13-1 illustrates that both the prothrombin time (PT) and partial thromboplastin time (PTT) test several factors, but not always the same ones. Although the PTT is a broader screening test, certain deficiencies can be assessed by using both the PT and PTT. Also the laboratory can add one factor at a time to see which factor is missing.

The coagulation process can be initiated two ways. With the *extrinsic system,* the clotting is triggered by the release of tissue thromboplastin. With the *intrinsic system,* the coagulation process requires only the factors that are present in the plasma.

Regardless of how the process initiated, the coagulation process occurs in four stages. Stage I involves the release of platelet factors that begin the clotting process. Stage II is the generation of thromboplastin, as calcium and other factors interact. Stage III is the conversion of prothrombin to thrombin, and Stage IV is the formation of fibrin from fibrinogen. Some sources list three stages of coagulation because Stage I and II are combined as parts of Stage I. Table 13-2 outlines the stages of clotting.

The importance of calcium in the clotting process should be noted. Usually a defect in calcium is not a problem due to the tremendous reservoir of calcium in the bones and teeth (see Chapter 7 on calcium). About 90% of all clotting defects occur in Stage II, the thromboplastin generation stage (Price 1977). Thus the PTT is a useful screening tool for many bleeding disorders.

TABLE 13-2. STAGES OF CLOTTING AND COMMON LABORATORY TESTS

Time of Stage	Stage	Factors Involved	Major Tests for Stage
	Stage I	Platelets initiate clotting	Platelets clot retraction
Takes 3–5 minutes	Stage II	Thromboplastin (Factor III) is generated by reaction of Factors VIII, IX, X, XI, and XII. Factor IV Ca++ also needed.	PTT very sensitive Lee-White less sensitive Factor VIII
Takes 8–16 minutes	Stage III	Factor II (prothrombin) is converted to thrombin. Accelerator Factors V, VII, and X are involved.	PT very sensitive
Almost instantly	Stage IV	Factor II (fibrinogen) is converted to fibrin. Factor XIII, the fibrin stabilizing factor, is needed.	Fibrinogen levels

Note that some references combine Stages I and II so that:
  Stage I: Formation of thromboplastin or activation of Factor X
  Stage II: Prothrombin to thrombin
  Stage III: Fibrinogen to fibrin
See Ravel (1978), Price (1977), or Koepke (1979) for more details on the stages of clotting and tests used for differential diagnosing.

PROTHROMBIN TIME (PT, OR PRO TIME)

Prothrombin, or Factor II, is a plasma protein that is produced by the liver. The confusing thing about the test is that, although it is called prothrombin time (PT), it does not measure just prothrombin, but also Factor I (fibrinogen), Factor V (labile factor), Factor VII (stable factor) and Factor X (Stuart factor). (See Table 13-1.) Remembering the specific names of these other factors is not necessary. The point to remember is that a change in any, or all, of these factors causes an abnormal PT. Just like prothrombin, these other factors are manufactured in the liver and most of the factors require vitamin K for their manufacture. (See earlier discussion on vitamin K.)

The PT is used to test for a pathological lack of clotting factors due either to liver dysfunction or to an absence of vitamin K. While the absence of vitamin K may be due to an absolute lack in the body, more often it occurs because the body is unable to absorb the vitamin due to an obstruction in the common bile duct. The PT is also the specific, and the only, laboratory test used to measure the effectiveness of the coumarin type of anticoagulant drugs, such as warfarin sodium (Coumadin). Although heparin, a different type of anticoagulant, in large doses may change the PT level, two other tests are used to monitor heparin therapy. These are the partial thromboplastin time (PTT) and Lee-White Coagulation Time, both of which are discussed later in this chapter. Although the abbreviations, PT and PTT, are very similar and thus often confusing to the novice, the tests are very different and used for two very different anticoagulants (see Table 13-3).

Measurement in Seconds and Percentages

Prothrombin results may be reported (1) as time in seconds and (2) as a percentage of normal activity. The seconds reflect how long the blood sample takes to clot when certain chemicals are added. To obtain a control value, the laboratory also tests a known "normal" sample of blood by the same technique. It is important for each laboratory to establish control values since many environmental variables may change the PT results by several seconds. If the patient's blood sample is deficient either in prothrombin or in one of the other clotting factors that affect the test, the patient's PT in seconds will be higher than the control PT in seconds.

While many laboratories report the PT only in seconds, others report the percentage too. The percentage figure is a little harder to understand than the one in seconds. The percentage is a way of expressing the patient's clotting ability as compared to the normal or control activity. In other words, the activity of the factors being tested is considered to be 100% in a control or normal blood sample. With no straight-line relationship between time and percentage, a graph has to be plotted to convert seconds to a percentage. The laboratory dilutes the normal sample to various concentrations. These various dilutions, or percentages of concentrations, are then measured to see how long each takes to clot. A graph is made that plots how percentage equals time. If a patient's blood sample clots in, say, 19 seconds, then the laboratory can look at the curve and see where 19 seconds intersects with a certain percentage. The time of 19 seconds may reflect 50% of normal clotting ability.

Percentages may vary somewhat because each laboratory must make its own graph for correlating times and percentages. Since the percentages must be based on dilution curves, their use may lead to inaccuracy (Ravel 1978:72). It is important to realize that 19

TABLE 13-3.   COMPARISONS OF PT AND PTT*

	PT	PTT (Activated)
Drugs monitored	Coumarin-type drugs i.e., bishydro-xycoumarin (Dicumarol), sodium warfarin (Coumadin), phen-procoumon (Liquamar).	Heparin
Reference Values (control)	60–140% activity 12–15 sec	No report in percentage 25–37 sec
Desirable therapeutic levels	1.5–2.5 × control	1.5–2.5 × control
Time of drug to affect lab test	Oral coumarin takes several *days* to achieve therapeutic level.	Intravenous heparin acts immedi-ately. (Sub cu not usually used except for prophylaxis.)
Usual timing of lab test	On daily basis until stabilized. Then 2–3 times per week, and even-tually once every 3–4 weeks for long-term control.	Once daily if continuous intravenous or ½–1 hour before the next inter-mittent dose. (PTT not changed if mini doses of heparin used as prophylaxis.)
Measures used to return lab test to normal	a. Reduction of dosage b. Whole blood c. Vitamin K_1 parenterally (Aqua Mephyton)	a. Reduction of dosage b. Whole blood c. Protamine sulfate parenterally
Time of reversability	a. Varies with dosage reduction b. Immediate with transfusion c. Several hours for vitamin K	a. Varies with dosage reduction b. Immediate with transfusion c. Immediate with Protamine
Examples of common drugs affecting results of test	Increase PT time: 　Alcohol 　Anabolic steroids 　Antibiotics 　Cimitidine (Tagamet) 　Salicylates 　Sulfonamides 　Thyroxine 　Quinidine (plus many others)	Increase PTT time: 　Salicylates 　Dipyridamate (Persantin)
	Decrease PT time: 　Barbituates 　Ethchlorovynol (Placidyl) 　Glutethimide (Doriden) 　Griseofulvin 　Oral contraceptives 　Vitamin K in nutritional 　　supplements, such as Ensure	May decrease PTT time: 　Digitalis 　Tetracyclines 　Antihistamines 　Nicotine

* See text for explanation and references for more details.

seconds may be translated into two different percentages by two different laboratories. In a general sense, the percentage is useful in illustrating how the patient's clotting ability compares to the control. For example, a patient with a PT of only 20% has only about one-fifth of the clotting ability of the "normal" person used as the control. One might suppose that the most clotting factor ability that a patient could have would be 100%. Yet remember that, for a percentage of normal activity, there is a range in "normal." So a figure over 100% can result for the patient who has a clotting time that is faster than the control picked by the laboratory. Thus percentages of 60 to 140% are considered normal individual variations. See Appendix A for percentage values for all the other factors that may be measured. Note that some have as wide a variation as 50 to 200%.

Relationship of Time to Percentage

An increase in time always means a decrease in percentage of activity, and vice versa, because as the clotting activity of the blood decreases, the blood takes longer to clot. If the percentage of activity is below 60%, the patient's prothrombin time in seconds is increased to more than the control time. On the other hand, if the patient's PT in seconds decreases from, say, 20 to 12 seconds, then the percentage of clotting activity has increased or risen to somewhere near the 100% normal activity. PT results in textbooks or on charts are sometimes reported just as an "increased PT." This notation means an increase in *time*, not in activity. An increase in the PT time means the percentage of activity is less than normal.

Special Preparation of Patient

There is no special preparation of the patient for the prothrombin time (PT). Note that many drugs can affect the PT (see Table 13-3). Make a note on the lab slip of any heparin dosage, since the PT may be affected at the peak of heparin activity. The test is done on 4.5 cc of plasma, obtained by venipuncture. The blood is collected in plastic tubes with 3.8% sodium citrate. (Blue top Vacutainer).

Reference Values

Adults	Control 11–16 sec (+ or − 2 seconds). Percentage of normal activity should be close to 100%, but most sources consider a range of 60–140% to be normal variations in percentages.
Newborns	Certain clotting factors are lower than adults, so reference values may be around 12–21 seconds. Prematures may have even higher reference values in seconds.
Pregnancy	In late pregnancy, certain clotting factors are increased, so reference values may be slightly decreased for time in seconds (Howie 1979). Oral contraceptives also cause increase in clotting factors (see Appendix D).

Increased PT (Increase in Time and Consequent Decrease in Percentage)

Clinical Significance. A variety of pathological conditions cause an increased PT. (Remember that an ''increased'' PT means an *increase* in the seconds and a *decrease* in the percentage. It is just easier to speak of an increased PT, rather than spelling it out.)

A patient may have an increased PT because the liver is unable to make prothrombin and the other factors measured by the PT test. An increased PT is very characteristic of advanced cirrhosis of the liver. In cirrhosis, a lot of scar tissue takes the place of functioning liver cells, and these nonfunctioning liver cells can no longer make prothrombin. PT is a very valuable tool in assessing the amount of liver damage in the patient with liver disease. Unlike other situations where the PT is increased, vitamin K injections usually do not help much with advanced liver disease. The inability of the liver to respond to vitamin K, as evidenced by little change in the PT after the vitamin K injection, demonstrates that the liver is so damaged that it cannot produce more prothrombin and other factors, even with abundant vitamin K.

Another clinical reason for an increased PT is the body's inability to absorb vitamin K from the gastrointestinal tract. Since vitamin K is a fat-soluble vitamin, absorption depends on the presence of bile salts. With an obstruction of the common bile duct, bile salts cannot be released into the duodenum. So a patient who has obstructive jaundice, which is caused by an obstruction in the common bile duct, has an increased PT since the liver cannot get vitamin K.

Much rarer is a true deficiency of vitamin K in the body, because humans do not depend much on dietary sources for vitamin K. This vitamin is manufactured by the bacteria that normally reside in the intestinal tract. So if a patient is on long-term antibiotic therapy that wipes out the normal bacteria in the gastrointestinal tract, the patient may have an increased PT due to an absolute deficiency of vitamin K. Unlike the patient with a failing liver, the patient with a vitamin K deficiency or malabsorption problem has an increased PT that can be returned to normal by the administration of vitamin K. When the vitamin is given parenterally, it is absorbed into the bloodstream and bypasses the digestive step that requires bile salts. (See Chapter 11 for more discussion on obstructive jaundice in relation to the test of direct bilirubin.)

The newborn's prothrombin time is slightly prolonged because infants do not have the same quantity of some of the clotting factors as adults. Newborns also do not have a store of vitamin K, and they have not yet acquired the normal intestinal bacteria to produce the vitamin (Jensen 1981). Newborn infants of mothers who are deficient in vitamin K are thus susceptible to a disease called *hemorrhagic disease of the newborn*. A dose of vitamin K, given prophylatically to all newborns, guards against the possibility of hemorrhage in the first few days.

Another hemorrhagic situation with an increased PT is in the complex bleeding disorder called *disseminated intravascular clotting* (DIC). This clinical situation is discussed in detail at the end of this chapter, along with fibrinogen levels.

Effect of Coumarin on PT. In all the situations discussed, an increased PT time of 24 seconds, with a corresponding percentage of normal activity of around 20–25%, would be indicative of a severe pathological state. For a patient who is anticoagulated with one of the coumarin-type drugs, such as warfarin sodium (Coumadin), the therapeutic goal is usually to have the PT time about 1.5 to 2.5 time the control. Coumarin-type drugs cause a decrease in the production of prothrombin and of other factors because these drugs interfere with the liver's use of vitamin K. Since the coumarin-type drugs work in this indirect way, by depressing liver function, the change in the PT does not occur for a day or longer. It usually takes several days to get the PT time 1.5 to 2.5 times the control. Vitamin K, taken orally or parenterally, reverses the effects of these drugs, returning the PT to normal within several hours. Obviously, a PT in the normal range may be dangerous for the patient who needs to be anticoagulated in the first place. Refer to Table 13-3 for a summary about coumarin drugs and PT monitoring.

Possible Nursing Implications.

Collecting Data About the Chronic Nature of the Problem. The nurse caring for a patient with an increased PT needs a clear understanding of whether this person is likely to be vulnerable to bleeding for a long time or if this abnormal PT is of short duration. For example, if the patient has an increased PT due to obstructive jaundice, vitamin K brings the PT back to normal within a few hours or at most within a day or so. In this case, one should not need to burden the patient and family with a long list of all the possible ways to protect the person from bleeding. On the other hand, the patient who is being discharged on a coumarin-type drug needs to know that a PT of 24 seconds and 20–25% normal clotting activity makes a person vulnerable to bleeding. These patients and their families need detailed instructions on how to treat bleeding episodes. Vitamin K is one antidote for coumarin overdosage (whole blood is the other), but many physicians do not want patients to carry this drug if they are close to a medical facility. Patients with severe liver disease may also be functioning with an increased PT that is of a chronic nature. They need to be taught how to protect themselves from bleeding episodes. As mentioned earlier, probably vitamin K will not help this PT very much. Patients with liver disease are very likely to eventually have severe bleeding episodes.

Assessing and Preventing Bleeding Episodes. Nurses must always be looking for symptoms that could indicate that a patient might be bleeding, since a bleeding episode is the possible consequence of any patient with an increased PT. Nurses must also be aware of the ways to prevent bleeding. They must use their own judgment about which parts of the following assessment and interventions are needed for an individual patient. The degree of patient involvement in protecting him- or herself from bleeding depends on the level of illness and the setting of home or hospital. Nurses must assess the patient's level of understanding, readiness for information about the condition or treatment, and willingness and ability to participate in health care.

When caring for a patient who has a bleeding tendency due to an abnormal PT and other factors, nurses need to be aware of all the subtle clues that can be a symptom of bleeding. As the persons who probably spend the most time with the patient, nurses have the opportunity and responsibility to detect these subtle change before a bleeding episode becomes a major catastrophe. So a complete assessment and prevention of bleeding would include the following:

1. Headaches or changes in the neurological status could indicate bleeding into the cranium. A headache would be of particular concern if the patient has had a head injury.

2. Patients with increased PT must be protected from falls. Sports or other activities that could lead to head blows are risky.

3. Shaving should be done with an electric razor to prevent bleeding from accidental cuts.

4. Epistaxis (nose bleeding) and gum bleeding may occur too. So too vigorous tooth brushing, hard coughing, or blowing the nose may trigger a bleeding episode. Nose bleeding in these patients can be a serious matter.

5. Nurses must be particularly careful when suctioning a patient who has a bleeding tendency.

6. Vomiting or coughing up blood can be quite serious. The physician should be notified immediately, even if the vomitus contains only a small amount of blood. Often the small amount of blood that is vomited first is just the tip of the iceberg. Fresh blood looks like blood. Older blood, which has been acted upon by the gastric juices, has a characteristic dark brown color that is called "coffee-ground."

7. In a patient with a nasogastric tube, the drainage may be coffeeground color rather than the yellowish to pale green color of normal stomach contents. Not all coffee ground drainage from nasogastric tubes means the patient is having a lot of bleeding. Sometimes just the presence of the nasogastric tube causes enough irritation to have minimal and nonsignificant bleeding. Yet for a patient with an *increased PT,* any bleeding may be serious.

Tests can be done to detect occult bleeding in gastric secretions. Yet, obviously, if there is frank blood, doing a guaiac test is a waste. The nurse must also be very careful about the irrigations of a nasogastric tube for a patient with bleeding tendencies. Iced saline lavage may be used to control gastric bleeding. Antacids and cimitidine (Tagamet) may be ordered to decrease gastric hyperacidity. (See the section on guaiac and other tests at the end of this chapter.)

8. The patient with severe liver disease may also have esophageal varices (varicosities) that can be the source of a massive bleed. The patient with suspected varices may have diet restrictions so that only soft foods are served.

9. Abdominal or flank pain may indicate slow internal bleeding. Internal bleeding can be very subtle in the beginning, with few symptoms, since the bleeding usually takes place at a slow rate. A patient may complain of a backache that cannot be relieved with back rubs, a change of position, or the administration of a mild analgesic. No one may think about a possible connection to the anticoagulant the patient is receiving until the patient faints when he or she tries to get out of bed. Then it is discovered that the patient had been slowly bleeding into the retroperitoneal area.

Internal bleeding can cause pain due to the increasing pressure as blood collects. If the bleeding is into the gastrointestinal tract, however, there will probably not be any associated pain because the blood does not cause undue pressure. The blood eventually passes into the stool, but it may be occult or hidden.

So patients with a bleeding tendency should periodically test the stools for occult blood. Hematocrits will be useful to assess the exact amount of blood loss (see Chapter 2). The tests for occult blood, described at the end of this chapter, are simple enough that patients can be taught to do a test at home if the situation warrants doing so. If the bleeding is fairly copious and high enough in the gastrointestinal tract to be in contact with the digestive juices, the stools take on a dark black color that is described as "tarry". Straining at stool may cause bleeding, especially if the patient has hemorrhoids, so the nurse needs to help the patient find ways to avoid constipation.

10. Dark or smokey-looking urine may indicate blood in the urine. Hematuria is often the first indication of overdosage with anticoagulants. Sometimes the blood is bright red if it is fresh. Some physicians may order daily urine tests to check for the presence of red blood cells in the urine. While the laboratory can check for red cells by a microscopic examination, which is more sensitive for intact erythrocytes, nurses may do dipstick tests for blood in the urine too. (See Chapter 3 on hematuria.) Patients who have catheters may bleed from the irritation of the catheter. Nurses should make sure the catheter is securely anchored with tape so it does not slide up and down the meatus. Female patients with bleeding tendencies due to an abnormal PT will probably have heavy menses, and they should be aware of this possibility.

11. Pain in or immobility of a joint can indicate bleeding into the joint. Nurses must think of all the things necessary to protect the patient from falls and trauma. With active children as patients, doing so may be a real challenge to the mother and to the nurse. Specific points about bleeding due to classic hemophilia (hemophilia A) are discussed under the test for Factor VIII.

12. Taking blood pressure and the pulse are two other ways to detect bleeding. A slight but steady increase in the pulse rate may be a subtle sign of bleeding, long before the blood pressure drops.

13. Some hospitals have a policy of avoiding intramuscular injections, if at all possible, for patients with bleeding tendencies. One institution has a policy that encourages nurses to inform patients who are on anticoagulant therapy not to accept IM injections unless the physician is actually in the room (Shapiro 1974:442). If an intramuscular injection must be given, choose the smallest gauge needle possible and apply pressure for ten minutes after the injection.

Also alert laboratory personnel to the patient's bleeding tendency. Place a note on the Kardex so everyone is aware of the patient's bleeding tendency. When laboratory personnel come to draw blood, a nurse needs to remind them of the potential bleeding problem. The fingerstick method to obtain blood should be used whenever possible if the bleeding tendency is severe. (See Chapter 1 for the fingerstick procedure.) Laboratory personnel do not usually look at the Kardex, so another good idea is to make a notation about bleeding on the laboratory requisition. Some hospitals put a sign on the patient's door to alert all personnel to the bleeding tendency. The nurse can be inventive in particular settings to make sure everyone who will be doing things with the patient knows about the bleeding tendency.

Special Needs for the Surgery Patient. If a patient with an increased PT must go to surgery, it is imperative that the PT be medically corrected before the operation. To get the PT back to a safe level for surgery, vitamin K injections may be ordered. For example, patients who have had valve replacements are usually on long-term anticoagulation therapy to prevent thrombus formation around the valve. If the patient needs an emergency appendectomy, the conversion to a normal PT is done in conjunction with heparin replacement as an anticoagulant. When anticoagulant therapy is necessary during a surgical procedure, the patient will be switched to heparin because this short-term anticoagulent can be more easily controlled (see PTT next) and quickly reversed with protamine. Whole blood should always be available for the patient with an abnormal PT who must have surgery since whole blood supplies the missing clotting factors. A type and cross match are done as part of the preoperative preparation. (See Chapter 14 on type and cross match.)

Special Teaching Points in Relation to PT and Coumarin Therapy. Patients on coumarin therapy are usually on this anticoagulant for a long time. No matter how long they are taking the drug, they must continue to have prothrombin tests (PT) done periodically. It is critical that patients understand the importance of continuing the PTs because the balance between maintaining the needed anticoagulation and preventing bleeding episodes is always precarious. The PT should remain within the predetermined range considered therapeutic for that patient. It can be very dangerous for patients to take anticoagulants if they are not followed well with frequent assessments of the PT. Once a patient is on a maintenance dose of the drug, the PT may be drawn weekly or less often.

Patients also need explicit *written* instructions about the anticoagulation medicine and the date to return to the clinic office. Some patients may also need to be referred to a public health nurse for a follow-up visit, to more fully assess their health needs if they do not return to have their PT drawn at the clinic. Laboratories all over the world can check PTs. For example, if a person travels to Europe, arrangements can be made to get PTs done at various labs.

When the patient is on coumarin-type drugs, a wide variety of other drugs may interact with them so as to cause changes in the PT, either to increase or to decrease the PT time. Some of the more common drugs are listed in Table 13–3. Certainly the patient needs to be instructed not to take any medication without consulting the physician who is prescribing the anticoagulant. The coumarin-type drugs are responsible for more adverse drug reactions than any other group. Loebel (1977:203) describes in detail the interactive effect of over seventy drugs with coumarin anticoagulants.

Aspirin and other salicylates potentiate the effect of coumarin, thus increasing the PT time. Often the patient is not aware that many pain medications, such as cold remedies, contain aspirin. Brand drugs, such as Percodan, Empirin, or Darvon Compound, all contain aspirin. In fact, more than five hundred aspirin-containing compounds are available commercially (Shapiro 1974). For patients with bleeding tendencies, such as the patient on anticoagulants, it is usually advisable that acetaminophen (Tylenol, Datril, and the like) be used in place of the aspirin.

Other drugs—such as antihistamines, oral contraceptives, and barbituates—inhibit the action of coumarin drugs in various ways and thus tend to decrease the PT time. If a patient on coumarin drugs needs a sleeping medication, flurazpam (Dalmane) is usually ordered, since this hypnotic does not interfere with anticoagulant therapy.

Decreased Prothrombin Time

Clinical Significance. Sometimes patients may have a PT time of 8 or 9 seconds, compared to a control of 11 or 12 seconds, or their percentage of activity may be greater than 100%. The reduced prothrombin time may be associated with medications such as oral contraceptives, barbituates, digitalis, diuretics, or vitamin K. It may also reflect pathology, such as thrombophlebitis or certain malignancies (Byrne 1977). The reduced pro-thrombin time, however, is not of clinical significance as a diagnostic tool.

Possible Nursing Implications. A reduced prothrombin time may indicate hypercoagula-bility of the blood. Hypercoagulability of the blood, venous stasis, and injury to the venous wall are the three conditions that contribute to the formation of *venous* thrombi. Prolonged bedrest and surgery also increase the possibility of thrombus formation. (Note that the condition associated with *arterial* thrombosis is atherosclerosis. See Chapter 9 on lipid metabolism.) It is thought that at least two of the three conditions (Virchow's triad) must be present to have thrombosis formation in the veins (Luckmann 1980:1127). Ven-ous thrombi are found most often in the deep veins of the legs or in pelvic veins.

When a patient has known hypercoagulability of the blood, the primary goal of the nurse is to decrease the possibility of venous thrombi formation by such measures as leg exercises, adequate hydration, and no venous constrictions such as crossing the legs. (See the discussion under PTT on the effectiveness of low doses of heparin to prevent deep vein thrombosis.)

PARTIAL THROMBOPLASTIN TIME (PTT)

The partial thromboplastin time (PTT), a nonspecific test, can demonstrate a lack of any of the various clotting factors, except Factor VII (stable factor), that function in the intrinsic clotting system (see Table 13-1). Recall that, while the intrinsic system uses only the elements present in the plasma, the extrinsic clotting system is initiated by the clot-promoting abilities of tissue thromboplastin. So if the PTT tests for intrinsic factors, then it tests for those factors circulating in the plasma (with the one exception of Factor VII). Since some clotting tests, such as the prothrombin time, bypass the intrinsic clotting system, they are not useful to screen for general plasma deficiencies. On the contrary, the PTT is very useful in detecting the presence of many types of bleeding disorders due to defective or deficient circulating factors that compose the intrinsic system. If the PTT is abnormal, further tests are needed to pinpoint exactly which factor is defective or defi-cient, such as the lack of Factor VIII in classic hemophilia.

The other purpose for the PTT is to monitor heparin therapy because heparin, a short-acting anticoagulant that circulates in the plasma, increases the PTT. Table 13-3 summarizes the use of the PTT for monitoring heparin.

Essentially, the laboratory technique for measuring the PTT involves adding certain chemicals to the patient's blood sample and timing, in seconds, the formation of a clot. Deficiencies in any of the factors increase the time for clot formation. The patient's results in seconds is compared to a control that was tested using the same method. Like the prothrombin time, a control is done on "normal" blood since so many environmental variables can affect each individual situation. Unlike the PT, there is no percentage report.

The specific techniques may vary from laboratory to laboratory. If chemicals are also added to accelerate the clotting time, the result is reported as an "activated" PTT. The actual techniques are the concern of the laboratory and of the laboratory technician who does the test. The important thing for nurses to know is that the laboratory always notes if the PTT is the activated type.

Special Preparation of Patient
And Collection of the Sample

There is no special preparation of the patient. To do the test, the laboratory needs 4.5 cc of blood, which is obtained by venipuncture. Collect the blood in a tube containing 3.8% sodium citrate (Blue Vacutainer). If the patient is being anticoagulated, note the time and route of the last heparin dosage.

Reference Values

Adults	25–37 sec for activated PTT or 60–90 sec if not activated.
Pregnancy	May be normally decreased by a few seconds. Also may be decreased with oral contraceptives. (see Appendix D).
Newborn	Range is increased above adult level.

Increased PTT

Clinical Significance. An increased PTT, when the patient is not on heparin, signifies a bleeding disorder. Further tests must be done to determine which factor is deficient. The abnormality, or the lack of a factor, may be either acquired or hereditary.

The most common hereditary disorder is lack of Factor VIII (antihemophilic globulin), which results in the classical hemophilia or hemophilia A. An inherited deficiency in Factor IX (plasma thromboplastin component or Christmas factor) results in the condition known as Christmas disease or hemophilia B. Often the patient's history gives clues that the increased PTT is due to a familial condition. (See the tests for Factors VIII and IX). Specific assays for different factors in the plasma definitively establish the diagnosis.

Acquired deficiencies may be more subtle and difficult to connect to any specific cause. The PTT becomes elevated in a complex bleeding disorder where the clotting factors are used up at an abnormal rate. This disorder, called disseminated intravascular clotting (DIC), is discussed in detail at the end of this chapter, along with fibrinogen levels.

If the patient is on heparin, an increase in the PTT is the result of the effects of the circulating anticoagulant in the plasma. Usually the PTT is kept about 1.5 to 2.5 times the control value. So if the control is 36 seconds, a range of 54 to 90 seconds would be desirable for the patient. A report of 110 seconds would indicate more-than-adequate anticoagulation for that moment when the blood was drawn. A report of 45 seconds would indicate inadequate anticoagulation for the moment the blood was drawn. (At the very best, the PTT reflects only heparin activity at the moment the sample was taken, since heparin activity in the blood varies from moment to moment.)

Elevated PTT

Possible Nursing Implications.

Assessments Before Surgical Procedures. An abnormal PTT would necessitate postponement of the surgery unless it is an emergency. If the PTT is being used as routine check before surgery, such as a tonsillectomy, the test must be done early enough so that the reports are on the chart before the patient goes to surgery. A nonroutine PTT for other types of surgery is ordered if there is any reason to suspect that the patient might have a bleeding disorder. In talking to a patient before surgery, a nurse might discover that the patient has a history of bleeding in the family, easy bruisability, frequent nosebleeds, or some such characteristic. It is amazing how often patients forget to mention such details during a medical work-up and then later, in a conversation with a nurse, remember the information. Easy bruisability does not always mean a bleeding disorder, but any evidence of past bleeding difficulties needs to be medically assessed before operative or other invasive procedures, such as a liver biopsy, are done.

Protecting from Bleeding. If the PTT is elevated, several tests may be needed to evaluate the clotting ability of the patient. Nurses may also be helpful in allowing the patient and the family to express their concerns and anxieties about an unknown medical diagnosis. Any patient with an elevated PTT has an increased tendency to bleed. The incidence of hemorrhage from heparinization is increased in elderly patients and in patients with hypertension, obesity, or ulcer disease. The nursing implications for the patient who has a tendency to bleed are covered in detail under the prothrombin time (PT). The same principles apply to the patient with an increased PTT.

Use of PTT for Monitoring Heparin. Heparin may be given subcutaneously, intravenously q4h or q6h, or continuously by intravenous drip. The various techniques for giving heparin vary widely from hospital to hospital and from location to location, but for most situations, the nurse does have the responsibility of administering the heparin by one of these methods. Sohn (1981) describes proper nursing actions for administration of heparin subcutaneously and intravenously. Before each dose of heparin is given, the nurse should check to see the results of the latest PTT. To maximize the usefulness of the PTT, nurses must know the time that the PTT was drawn in relation to the last heparin dose. Usually PTTs are ordered to be done one-half to one hour before the next heparin dose (DeMeester 1978). The medical decision to give or not to give the antidote for heparin, protamine sulfate, depends partially on being able to establish how long ago the PTT was abnormally high. An abnormally high PTT should always be reported immediately before the next dose of heparin is administered.

The nurse must also note if the PTT is *below* the therapeutic range. For example, the nurse may note that the PTT drawn at 7 AM today was 46 seconds, compared to a control of 33 seconds. The nurse checks the medication sheet to make sure that the patient did have the heparin at 6 AM. It is charted. This patient appears not to be adequately anticoagulated. The PTT report should be called to the attention of the doctor now, so he or she can reevaluate the situation and readjust the dosage accordingly. It can be as dangerous for the patient to remain *under*-anticoagulated as over-anticoagulated.

Since heparin activity may vary from moment to moment, it would be mistake to think that all one needs to adjust the dosage is one PTT. Seeing the range of the PTT gives guidelines to the physician in adjusting the dosage for each individual. Some hospitals use flow sheets so that the PTT can be charted with each dosage of heparin and compared over an extended period. This chart makes it easier to get a clearer picture of the ongoing status of the anticoagulant therapy.

During the monitoring process, any factors that may invalidate the PTT must be assessed. For example, if the PTT was drawn when the intravenous was not running properly, the low PTT may be wrongly interpreted to mean that the patient needs more heparin added to the intravenous. The nurse can supply the information that the PTT may have been drawn when the intravenous was not dripping on schedule. Better still, when the laboratory technician is getting ready to draw the PTT, the nurse could explain that the intravenous is not on time, so a PTT would be useless for now.

Checking for Drug Interferences. Drugs that interfere with the action of heparin are not as numerous as those that interfere with the coumarin-type drugs, but certain drugs do affect the PTT. The use of digitalis, tetracyclines, nicotine, and histamines may partially counteract the effect of heparin. The potential interaction of these drugs may be significant if they are added or deleted during the time the patient is on heparin therapy. Since drugs containing aspirin increase the bleeding time, they should be avoided when the patient is on heparin. The reason is that, when a patient is anticoagulated, platelet aggregation is the main defense against bleeding, and aspirin decreases the adhesiveness of platelets, thus potentiating the bleeding tendency from any type of anticoagulation (Loebl 1977:209).

Patient Teaching. Because heparin must be given parenterally and requires close medical supervision, patients do not usually go home on heparin therapy. Patient teaching—about drugs to avoid, when to return for tests, and the like—is not a necessity as it is with long-term anticoagulants. If long-term anticoagulants are necessary to prevent other thromboembolic episodes, the usual pattern is to begin with a coumarin-type drug after five to six days of heparin therapy and continue both types of anticoagulants until the PT is within the desired range (DeMeester 1978). During this switch from heparin to long-term oral anticoagulants, both the PT and PTT need to be monitored.

Use of Heparin in "Mini-Doses." There is one type of clinical situation in which the PTT (or Lee-White coagulation time) need not be checked, even though the patient is on heparin. This is when heparin is given in low doses of usually about 5,000 units sub-cutaneously every eight or 12 hours. The purpose of the "mini-dose" is to prevent the possible occurrence of thromboembolic episodes in patients who are high risk due to certain surgical procedures or to prolonged bedrest. Studies have shown that the prophylactic use of heparin in small doses can significantly decrease the risk of pulmonary embolus in high risk patients (Sherry 1976). These doses of heparin are small enough so that they do not significantly affect the PTT. Nurses do not need to check PTT results before giving small prophylactic doses of heparin.

DECREASED PTT

Clinical Significance. A PTT that is lower than the control sample is not diagnostically significant, but it may be a clue reflecting hypercoagulability. (See the discussion under PT for the conditions that may cause increased clotting and how nursing care can help to prevent venous thrombus formation.) Some degree of hypercoagulability is normal in pregnancy (Howie 1979).

LEE-WHITE COAGULATION TIME

Although the partial thromboplastin time (PTT) is usually used to monitor heparin therapy, the Lee-White coagulation or clotting time can also be used. The Lee-White takes longer to do than the PTT, and it is harder to standardize. Also, the Lee-White is not sensitive enough to be used to detect other bleeding disorders. Since it may detect very severe bleeding disorders, but not mild ones, it is never used as a screening test. The Lee-White clotting time is reported in minutes, not seconds, as are the PT and PTT. Also, no control number is reported with Lee-White Clotting results, as with the other two tests.

Preparation of Patient and Collection of Sample

No special preparation of the patient is necessary. The laboratory collects blood by venipuncture and immediately transfers it to three tubes. Note the time, dosage, and route of heparin dosages.

Reference Values

Adults	Ranges are usually around 9–12 min. Some sources say 6–17 min. No significant differences reported for different age groups or for gender.

Increased Lee-White Coagulation Time

Clinical Significance. An increased value indicates the amount of anticoagulation achieved with heparin. Usually the desired therapeutic range is about 2.5 times the normal value established by the laboratory. For example, if a particular laboratory considered a value of 9 to 12 minutes as normal, a patient on heparin whose Lee-White time was above 30 minutes would probably be over-anticoagulated.

Possible Nursing Implications. As with the PTT, the interpretation of the Lee-White needs to be correlated with the time of the last heparin dosage. Since test results may vary quite a bit, the results are not significant unless the timing is correlated with drug administration. For a clearer picture of the true anticoagulated state of the patient, clinicians need to use a flow sheet that lists all the test results with the time and route of dosages given. The nurse giving the heparin needs to be aware of the results of the Lee-White. If the Lee-White coagulation time is not in the desired therapeutic range, the nurse has the responsibility to notify the physician before another does of heparin is given.

Some related aspects of monitoring the patient on heparin have been covered under the section on PTT. The nursing implications for a patient with bleeding tendencies are covered under the discussion on PT. The nurse must always keep in mind that a patient on any anticoagulation therapy can bleed, even if laboratory results indicate a satisfactory condition. Laboratory results can give a false sense of security.

HEMOPHILIA TESTING: FACTORS VIII AND IX

The two main types of hemophilia are called A (classical hemophilia) and B (Christmas disease). Classical hemophilia has been the curse of several royal families in Europe. Christmas disease was named for the family who was studied with the genetic defect of Factor IX. The specific diagnosis of classical hemophilia is made by assay of Factor VIII and for Christmas disease (hemophilia B) by assay of Factor IX. The cause of over 80% of all hemophiliacs is a deficiency of Factor VIII (Dressler 1980). Since the PTT is prolonged in hemophilia, it is a screening test for bleeding disorders. The patient has normal prothrombin time (PT) and platelet counts.

Preparation of Patient
And Collection of Sample

No special preparation of patient is necessary. The Test requires 4.5 ml of plasma. The blood is collected in plastic tubes with 3.8% sodium citrate (Blue Vacutainer).

Reference Values

Factor VIII (antihemophilic globulin)	50–200%
Factor IX (plasma thromboplastic cofactor)	60–140%

See Appendix A for reference values for other factors.

Deficiency in Factors

Clinical Significance. Both A and B are inherited as X-linked recessive traits. In other words, female carriers transmit the gene to half their daughters and to half their sons. The females who receive the defective gene do not have the disease because they also have another "healthy" X. On the contrary, any male who receives the defective X shows symptoms because he does not have a healthy X to balance the effect. Hemophilia may be mild, moderate, or severe, depending on how much of the factor is produced.

Nursing Implications. The general nursing implications for a patient with bleeding tendencies were discussed in the section on PT. Because factor replacement therapy is available, many bleeding episodes can be prevented or treated before damage occurs to joints or to other vital areas. Older children and their parents are also taught to mix the factor concentrate and to do the intravenous infusion. Pediatric textbooks give more specific instructions for the care of the patient with hemophilia. Dressler (1980) gives a good example of patient teaching aids, and Boulanger (1977) describes a national camp for children with hemophilia. (See Chapter 18 for a discussion on genetic counseling.)

PLATELET COUNT

Sometimes platelets are considered as a third type of blood cell in the plasma. (See Chapter 2 for RBC and WBC). Actually, platelets are not intact cells but only fragments of cytoplasm whose only role seems to be in the blood coagulation process. As platelets adhere to the wall of an injured vessel, they clump together (or aggregate) and release a substance that begins the coagulation process. Platelets are formed by the bone marrow and removed by the reticuloendothelial system when they are old. The spleen is a major component of the reticuloendothelial system. Because platelet counts are often done for disorders of the bone marrow and the spleen, nurses must understand their relationship to platelets.

Special Preparation of Patient
And Collection of Sample

No special preparation is necessary. The laboratory uses 0.5 cc of blood. EDTA is used as the anticoagulant (Lavender vacutainer). The count is usually done by a machine, but, if the count is low, it is confirmed by a hand count. Smears can also be done to estimate the number of platelets.

Reference Values

Adults 150,000–350,000/mm^3
  Females have a significantly decreased platelet count for the first few days of menses. Platelets are increased after labor and delivery.

Increased Platelet Count (Thrombocytosis)

Clinical Significance. Malignancies, especially advanced or metastatic cases, may cause an elevated platelet count or thrombocytosis. Many patients with an ''unexpected'' high platelet count are found to have a malignancy. Patients with polycythemia very often have high platelet counts too. (Polycythemia is discussed in Chapter 2 under the section on red blood cells.) Another reason for an increased platelet count is the removal of the spleen, or splenectomy, which causes a temporary increase in the platelet count.

Possible Nursing Implications.

  Preventing Thrombosis. A logical assumption is that an increased amount of platelets tends to make the blood more coagulable. As discussed in the section on decreased PT and hypercoagulability, dehydration could be dangerous for a patient with a high platelet count. Venous stasis may be of particular concern. Depending on the reason for the thrombocytosis, thrombus formation may or may not be a possibility. For example, the increased platelet count after a splenectomy does not seem to cause any problems.

  Teaching about the Use of Aspirin. If thrombus formation is considered a possibility, aspirin, which is used as a mild anticoagulant in certain situations, is sometimes ordered to decrease the adhesiveness of platelets. Recall that, due to the effect of aspirin on platelets, aspirin is not given with anticoagulants. To prevent gastric irritation, the patient needs to be taught either to take aspirin with milk or to dilute it with water.

  Assessing for Bleeding. Surprisingly, an increased number of platelets does not always mean an increased tendency to clot. In fact, it may mean an increased tendency to bleed. This paradox can be partially explained by the fact that sometimes the increased number of platelets are abnormal ones that cannot function properly in the coagulation process. Thus a patient with thrombocytosis may need to be watched for bleeding tendencies.

Low Platelet Count (Thrombocytopenia)

Clinical Significance. Since the cause of the low platelet count, or thrombocytopenia, is often unknown, this condition is called ''idiopathic'' (unknown cause) thrombocytopenia purpura. "Purpura" refers to bruising. Children who have idiopathic thrombocytopenia purpura often have spontaneous remissions. A low platelet count, or thrombcytopenia, can result from a number of causes. A low count can be associated with some types of anemias or other hemolytic disorders. Substances that depress bone marrow function, such as chemotherapeutic drugs or radiation, also depress the platelet count. Finally, an overactive spleen (hypersplenism) or an enlarged spleen (splenomegaly) destroys platelets at too fast a rate.

Possible Nursing Implications.

Preventing Bleeding. When caring for a patient with a low platelet count, the major nursing concern is protecting the person from bruising and bleeding. Petechiae are the most common manifestations of thrombocytopenia because the many microscopic injuries that occur continuously in the capillaries are not immediately sealed off due to the lack of platelets (Wroblewski 1981). A decrease in the platelet count to 50,000 or less/mm^3 usually puts patients at risk for spontaneous hemorrhage. Yet some patients do not bleed even with a count as low as 10,000/mm^3. Certain activities may need to be curtailed until the platelet count is returned to normal. In the case of an active child, protection from trauma requires a lot of ingenuity on the part of the nurse and the parents. Symptoms that indicate bleeding are described in detail in the section on nursing implications for a decreased PT. Patients may be embarrassed by the bruises on their arms and legs, and so they appreciate clothing to conceal the bruises from curious onlookers.

Assessing for Leukopenia and Anemia as Related Problems. If the thrombocytopenia is a result of general bone marrow depression, the implications about leukopenia (low white cell count) and anemia (low red cell count) must also be considered. These nursing implications are covered in Chapter 2.

Assisting with Medical Interventions. Adult patients, and sometimes children, with a low platelet count may be put on corticosteroid therapy, which is given to raise the platelet count to normal. There are several critical nursing implications when the patient is on one of the cortisone-type drugs. (See Chapter 15 on cortisone therapy.)

In idiopathic thrombocytopenia purpura, sometimes the removal of the spleen is necessary to get the platelet count back to normal. If such surgery is scheduled, the nurse can help to prepare the patient for the surgical experience. Adult patients usually have few problems after the spleen is removed because the role of the spleen can be taken over by other parts of the reticuloendothial system. For children, a splenectomy is usually not done because the spleen is important for antibody production (Luckmann 1980:1072).

If thrombocytopenia results from a malignancy or from treatment with chemotherapy drugs, platelet transfusions may be given. Patient with counts of less than 10,000/mm^3 usually require platelet transfusions, while those with more may receive transfusions only if hemorrhage begins (Wroblewski 1981). Since patients may become sensitized to the platelet concentrates, transfusions are reserved for those who are at great risk. When platelets are collected and transfused, Hernandez (1980) describes the nurse's role. Three of the major problems in platelet transfusions are allergic reactions, hyper-volemia, and bacterial sepsis. (See Chapter 14 for the laboratory tests done for transfusion reactions.)

CLOT RETRACTION TEST

Platelets have a major role in clot formation and in making it become very firm by causing retraction. If the platelets are lacking or defective, the clot does not shrink or retract but stays soft and watery. Also, if fibrinolysins are present in the serum, no clot retraction takes place (Koepke 1979). Fibrinolysis is discussed next under the section on decreased levels of fibrinogen.

Reference Values

50–100% in 2 hours

FIBRINOGEN LEVEL

Fibrinogen (Factor I) is a plasma protein that is manufactured by the liver. Vitamin K is *not* necessary for the formation of this factor, as it is for many of the others manufactured by the liver (see Table 13-1). The sole purpose of fibrinogen seems to be the formation of fibrin as the end-product (Stage IV) of blood coagulation (See Table 13-2). Fibrinogen deficiencies, which may be acquired or genetic, are most commonly associated with a complex bleeding disorder that is called disseminated intravascular clotting (DIC).

Preparation of the Patient
And Collection of Sample

No special preparation is necessary. The test requires 4.5 ml of plasma collected in a tube with sodium citrate (Blue Vacutainer).

Reference Values

Adults	0.15–0.35 g/dl Women tend to have slightly higher levels.
Pregnancy	Values may be as high as 0.60 g/dl Note that oral contraceptives may cause an increase in fibrinogen levels (see Appendix D).

Decreased Levels of Fibrinogen

Clinical Significance. Low fibrinogen levels can result from rare genetic disorders or from severe liver disease, either of which might first be detected with the partial thromboplastin test (PTT). More commonly, however, the decrease of fibrinogen is due to disseminated intravascular coagulation (DIC). DIC is a pathological overstimulation of the coagulation process. It is also called consumption coagulopathy or the defibrination syndrome.

Not a primary disorder, DIC is secondary to other severe illnesses. The theory is that widespread tissue injury somehow triggers the clotting mechanism so that a pathological formation of small thrombi occurs in the microcirculation. Paradoxically, the patient begins to bleed because the clotting factors are eventually depleted. Besides the low fibrinogen level, the prothrombin time (PT) is usually increased, the partial thromboplastin test (PTT) is increased, and the platelet count is lowered (O'Brien 1978). Since the placenta is a rich source of tissue thromboplastin, such abnormalities as abruptio placenta and fetal death can trigger massive clotting problems (Price 1978). Other patients that are the most likely to develop this abnormal clotting process are patients with toxemia of pregnancy, metastatic cancer, shock, sepsis, or burns. Respiratory distress syndrome, malaria, snake bite, and extracorporeal bypass may also contribute to DIC.

If some of the PT, PTT, or platelet count tests are positive for DIC, additional tests to check for fibrinolysis and fibrin degradation products may be ordered. (See Appendix A for values for these tests, Table A–4). Which additional tests should be ordered depends on the sophistication of the laboratory. In certain areas, tests of fibrin metabolism are also used to evaluate the clot formation that occurs after pulmonary embolism (Bynum 1979). Pregnant women have a reduced activity of the fibrolytic system. The increase of clotting factors and the decrease in fibrolysis protect against major hemorrhage, but these changes can also contribute to coagulation problems in pregnancy (Howie 1979).

Nursing Implications.

Assessing for DIC. Since a low fibrinogen level is often part of a complex pathological situation, the patients who are the most likely to develop DIC are usually those who are already in an intensive unit with a primary illness. Shock is often present. In the obstetrical area, women with toxemia or with any pathology of the placenta should be observed for DIC. The nurse giving direct care may be first to notice signs of bleeding, such as bruise marks or the appearance of blood in drainage tubes or on dressings. (Refer to the section on prothrombin time to review all the ways a nurse can make objective assessments for occult or hidden bleeding.) If thrombi have developed in the microcirculation, the patient may have unexplained pain or symptoms of poor circulation to specific areas, such as cyanosis of the fingers or toes.

Assisting with Medical Interventions. Whole blood or blood components may be given intravenously to replace the clotting factors. Nurses must understand the correct rate of flow for the particular blood component used, as well as the complications that may occur. Because blood components are obtained from a pool of donors, hepatitis is something that may happen later. (See Chapter 14 for tests used to screen blood products.) Not only is bleeding occurring, but thrombus formation may be taking place too. So heparin may be part of the therapy for this complex situation (O'Brien 1978). Either the Lee-White clotting time or the partial thromboplastin time (PTT) is used to monitor herapin therapy. Since for the patient with DIC these values are already prolonged, other assessments are used to evaluate whether an anticoagulant is needed. Consult current literature for the newest research about the treatment of DIC. Redman (1979) discusses in detail the coagulation problems in pregnancy and the specialized care needed when a patient has toxemia.

Increased Fibrinogen Levels

Clinical Significance. Although fibrinogen levels tend to increase with inflammatory conditions, such as pneumonia or rheumatic fever, the fibrinogen level is not a diagnostic test in these conditions. Note that, in pregnancy, women normally have increased fibrinogen levels.

Possible Nursing Implications. Increased fibrinogen levels could indicate some hypercoagulability of the blood. See the discussion under decreased PT for nursing measures to prevent venous thrombi.

OCCULT BLOOD:
HEMATEST, HEMOCCULT, AND OTHER GUAIAC TESTS

Occult (hidden) blood can be detected by simple tests that cause color changes in the presence of blood. Although all tests for blood in stool, urine, or other secretions are sometimes called ''guaiac tests,'' not all of them use the chemical guaiac. Some tests, Hematest being the common one, use another chemical, orthotolidin. Although tests, such as Hematest and Hemostix (Ames), can be used to detect occult blood in urine, a microscopic examination is needed to detect intact erythrocytes. (see Chapter 3 on tests for hematuria). The various tests for occult blood can also be done on emesis, but note that cimitidine may make the emesis falsely positive (Mar 1981).

Many studies have been done to see which test is the most sensitive for feces. At the present time, Hemoccult, which uses a guaiac-impregnated paper, seems to be the best screening test for stools (Glouberman 1978). The most important use of such tests as Hemoccult is to screen patients for cancer of the bowel, since bleeding is one of the very early symptoms (Miller 1977). A screening for blood in the stool is much easier and less expensive than a sigmoidoscopy.

Preparation of Patient
And Collection of Sample

The patient may be instructed to avoid meat and to eat a high roughage diet for one to three days before a screening test of the feces. The reason is that meat, especially red meat, may make a false positive. Some places may restrict the patient's diet only after an initial screening test is positive. More than one stool specimen may be needed to detect intermittent bleeding. Only a small amount of stool (or emesis) is needed for any of the tests. (For urine samples, see Chapter 3 for the dipstick method.) Stool specimens should be tested within 48 hours after collection, and they must be protected from sunlight.

Nurses should be aware of potential influences on these tests. Vitamin C in large doses may produce false negative results, whereas iron pills may give false positive results. Turnips, horseradish, and aspirin, all of which contain perioxidase, may also make a false positive; so these foods are to be avoided during the test.

Patient Teaching

The collection of stool can be done at home by the patient, who is given a commercially prepared filter paper in a protective cover (Hemoccult by Smith, Kline Diagnotics). The written instructions tell the patient to collect a small specimen of stool on an applicator and smear the stool on Part A of the paper. A second specimen from a different part of the stool is put on Part B of the paper. After the sample is collected and brought to the clinic or laboratory, two drops of a commercially prepared developing solution are placed on each smear, and the color change is noted after 30 seconds.

A newer technique involves the use of a filter paper as toilet paper. The stool is then tested for blood by spraying the paper. The use of newer techniques, which involve the use of a filter paper as toilet paper, may become more widespread in the future, because patients do not have to handle their feces, and thus may be more willing to do the test.

Reference Value

Appearance of a blue color indicates the presence of blood. A second test may be done to confirm a positive report.

Presence of Blood

Nursing Implications. Nurses may use the Hemoccult Test for on-the-spot assessments of patients who have bleeding tendencies. Enough stool for a guaiac test can often be obtained by a digital exam, and only a drop of emesis is needed. Nurses may also be involved in instructing patients on how to do the test as a screening measure at home. For example, the San Francisco Public Health Department offers a program of colorectal screening to all people. The screening, which includes the Hemoccult test done at home, is provided free to any senior citizen. Nurses can educate the public about the importance of the resources available in their communities. As discussed in Chapter 1, screening for occult blood in the feces is one of only four tests that are generally recommended routinely for even apparently healthy people over age 40. The community health nurse or the family nurse practitioner can offer this screening test to clients.

Questions

13–1. Which of the following is a description of Stage II in the *four* stages of the coagulation process?

   a. Conversion of prothrombin to thrombin.

   b. Generation of thromboplastin.

   c. Initiation of the intrinsic system.

   d. Conversion of fibrinogen to fibrin.

13–2. Mrs. Rodriguez has a malabsorption syndrome that makes fat absorption difficult. How would this pathological condition affect the prothrombin time (PT)?

    a. The percentage and time in seconds will both be increased.

    b. The percentage and time will both be decreased.

    c. The percentage will be increased and the time decreased.

    d. The percentage will be decreased and the time increased.

13–3. The charge nurse is quickly scanning the laboratory reports that were just sent to the unit. A prothrombin time (PT) of 25% and 24 seconds (with a control of 12 seconds) would not be indicative of pathology if the report was for which of the following patients?

    a. Mr. Ramos, who is on coumarin therapy.

    b. Mr. Ringer, who has cirrhosis of the liver.

    c. Mrs. Saxon, who is on long-term antibiotic therapy.

    d. Mrs. Java, who has obstructive jaundice of unknown etiology.

13–4. A prophylactic injection of vitamin K_1, is given to newborns for which of the following reasons?

    a. The prothrombin time (PT) of newborns is increased in seconds.

    b. The fibrinogen level of newborns is decreased.

    c. The platelet count may be lowered in some cases.

    d. All of the above.

13–5. Vitamin K injections are less likely to return the prothrombin time (PT) to normal for which patient?

    a. Mr. Ramos, who is on coumarin therapy.

    b. Mr. Ringer, who has cirrhosis of the liver.

    c. Mrs. Saxon, who is on long-term antibiotic therapy.

    d. Mrs. Java, who has obstructive jaundice of unknown etiology.

13–6. Mr. Ringer, a patient with cirrhosis, has had two episodes of slight gastrointestinal bleeding, but he seems stabilized now. He still has an abnormal prothrombin time (PT) and a low platelet count. He is on a regular diet. What should the nurse teach Mr. Ringer?

    a. Increase his dietary intake of vitamin K, by giving him a list of foods.

    b. Check his pulse several times a day. (Have him do a repeat performance.)

    c. Be sure and drink a glass of milk when he takes aspirin.

    d. Report any signs of bleeding, no matter how slight.

13–7. Mr. Ramos is being discharged on long-term coumarin therapy. The nurse should assess to make sure the patient understands which of the following?

a. The necessity of carrying identification that he is on long-term coumarin therapy.

b. The critical importance of having periodic prothrombin times (PT) drawn.

c. The interaction of many nonprescription drugs with coumarin.

d. All of the above are essential to emphasize before the patient is discharged.

13–8. Mr. Cristophos is due to receive another dose of heparin via heparin lock at 12 PM. An activated PTT was done one hour before the 8 AM dose. Which of these reports should be reported to the physician before the next dose of heparin is given? The reference value for control was 30 seconds.

a. PTT of 35 seconds.   c. PTT of 65 seconds.

b. PTT of 55 seconds.   d. None of the above.

13–9. The nurse is preparing a dose of heparin (5,000 units) to be given subcutaneously. This mini-dose has been ordered to decrease the possibility of a pulmonary embolus after surgery. The dose is given every 12 hours. Which laboratory test should the nurse check before giving the heparin?

a. Prothrombin time (PT).

b. Partial thromboplastin time (PTT).

c. Lee-White coagulation time.

d. None of the above.

13–10. Prothrombin time (PT) and partial thromboplastin time (PTT) are similar in that both tests:

a. test for the intrinsic clotting system.

b. are reported in seconds that are compared to controls.

c. can be used to monitor heparin therapy.

d. can be affected by vitamin K.

13–11. The primary goal of the nurse in caring for a patient with a decreased PT and/or PTT is minimizing which of the following possibilities?

a. Bleeding.   c. Venous thrombosis.

b. Arterial thrombosis.   d. Overhydration.

13–12. Classical hemophilia (hemophilia A) is confirmed by the laboratory test for which?

a. PTT.   c. Factor IX assay.

b. Factor VIII assay.   d. Clot retraction.

13–13. Both the patient with thrombocytopenia and the patient with thrombocytosis should be assessed for which of the following?

a. Effects of bone marrow depression. **c.** Possible bleeding episodes.

b. Possible thrombus formation. **d.** Possible infection.

13–14. Sally, age 21, has a low platelet count. Medical interventions that are done specifically to counteract thrombocytopenia include all except which?

a. Administration of corticosteroids. **c.** Splenectomy.

b. Administration of aspirin. **d.** Platelet transfusions.

13–15. Which of the following nursing actions is probably the most appropriate for Mrs. Jonson, who is complaining of a headache and asking if she can take some aspirin for her headache? Her platelet count is 50,000/mm^3.

a. Assess for any changes in her level of consciousness.

b. Offer her fluids frequently to decrease the viscosity of the blood.

c. See if she can have some aspirin for the headache.

d. All of the above.

13–16. Which of the following changes in laboratory tests are most indicative of the complex bleeding disorder that is called disseminated intravascular clotting (DIC) or consumption coagulopathy?

a. Increased prothrombin time (PT), increased partial thromboplastin time (PTT), and increased platelet count.

b. Decreased prothrombin time (PT), decreased partial thromboplastin time (PTT), and decreased fibrinogen levels.

c. Increased prothrombin time (PT), decreased platelet count, and increased fibrinogen levels.

d. Increased prothrombin time (PT), decreased platelet count, and decreased fibrinogen levels.

13–17. Important facts about the guaiac test (Hemoccult) for stool are all the following *except* which?

a. Meat may cause false positive results in the feces.

b. The test is very useful as a screening test for cancer of the colon.

c. The stool specimen must be tested within two to four hours after collection.

d. A blue color indicates a positive reaction for the presence of blood.

REFERENCES

Boutaugh, Michelle and Peterson, Phyllis. "Summer Camp for Hemophiliacs," *American Journal of Nursing* 77 (August 1977): 1288–1289.

Bynum, Lincoln *et al*. "Diagnostic Value of Tests of Fibrin Metabolism in Patients Predisposed to Pulmonary Embolism," *Archives of Internal Medicine* 139 (January 1979): 283–285.

Byrne, Judith. ''Tests of Plasma Clotting Factor,'' *Nursing '77* 7 (June 1977): 24–25.

DeMeester, Tom *et al.* ''Pulmonary Embolism Therapy,'' *Patient Care* 12 (March 15, 1978): 14–71.

Dressler, Diane. ''Understanding and Treating Hemophilia,'' *Nursing '80* 10 (August 1980): 72–73.

Glouberman, Stephen and Szokol, Attila. ''Melena and Occult Blood in the Stool,'' *Arizona Medicine* 35 (June 1978): 399–400.

Hernandez, Bernadita. ''Platelets: A Short Course,'' *RN* 43 (June 1980): 35–41.

Howie, P. W. ''Blood Clotting and Fibrinolysis in Pregnancy,'' *Post Graduate Medical Journal* 55 (May 1979): 362–366.

Jensen, Margaret *et al. Maternity Care: The Nurse and the Family,* 2nd ed. St. Louis: C. V. Mosby Co., 1981.

Koepke, John. ''Chapter 14: Abnormal Bleeding'' in *Guide to Clinical Laboratory Diagnosis,* 2nd ed. New York: Appleton-Century-Crofts, 1979.

Loebl, Suzanne *et al. The Nurses' Drug Handbook.* New York: John Wiley & Sons, Inc., 1977.

Luckmann, Joan and Sorenson, Karen. *Medical-Surgical Nursing: A Psychophysiologic Approach,* 2nd ed. Philadelphia: W. B. Saunders Company, 1980.

Mar, Dexter. Drug Data, ''Cimitidine Update,'' American Journal of Nursing 81 (May, 1981): 1026–1027.

Miller, S. F. and Knight, R. ''Early Detection of Colon-Rectal Cancer,'' *Ca* 40 (1977): 945–949.

O'Brien, Bonnie and Woods, Susan. ''The Paradox of DIC,'' *American Journal of Nursing* 78 (November 1978): 1878–1880.

Price, Sylvia and Wilson, Lorraine. Chapter 18: ''Coagulation'' in *Pathophysiology: Clinical Concepts of Disease Processes.* New York: McGraw-Hill Book Co., 1978.

Ravel, Richard. *Clinical Laboratory Medicine* 3d ed. Chicago: Year Book Medical Publishers, Inc., 1978.

Redman, C. W. ''Coagulation Problems in Pregnancy,'' *Post Graduate Medical Journal* 55 (May 1979): 367–371.

Shapiro, Ruth. ''Anticoagulant Therapy,'' *American Journal of Nursing* 74 (March 1974): 439–444.

Sherry, Sol. *Low Dose Heparin Therapy: A Retrospective Review.* Princeton, N.J.: Excerpta Medica Offices, 1976.

SmithKline Diagnostics. *Product Instructions: Hemoccult Slides* and *Tape.* Sunnyvale, Cal: SmithKline Diagnostics, 1975.

Sohn, Catherine. ''Rescind the Risks in Administering Anticoagulants,'' *Nursing '81* (October 1981): 34–41.

Wroblewski, Sandra and Wroblewski, Shelia. ''Caring for the Patient with Chemotherapy-Induced Thrombocytopenia,'' *American Journal of Nursing* 81 (April 1981): 746–749.

CHAPTER FOURTEEN

Serological Tests

Objectives

1. Explain the basic procedures used for serological tests for blood bank procedures, microbiology, and immunology.
2. Describe the role of the nurse in the prevention and assessment of transfusion reactions from ABO incompatibility.
3. Explain the rationale for the administration of Rh immunoglobulins (RhoGam) after certain deliveries.
4. Identify the most important nursing implications when a patient has a positive report for HB_sAG (hepatitis B surface antigen) or for hepatitis A.
5. Describe what a patient should be taught about the various serological tests for syphilis (STS).
6. Describe the clinical usefulness of serological tests for common bacterial, viral, fungal, and rickettsial diseases.
7. Describe the information that should be given to a woman of childbearing age who has a negative titer of rubella antibodies.
8. Explain why positive serology tests or skin tests may not be indicative of an active infection.
9. Describe how C_3 and C_4, two components of the complement system, are altered by antigen–antibody reactions.
10. Describe how humoral antibodies, such as RF, ANA, and others, are useful in assessing possible autoimmune pathology.

The category of serology tests is very broad, including blood bank procedures (immunohematology), identification of antibodies against infectious diseases (microbiology), and studies of immune diseases (immunology). The basic principle underlying serology tests is that a reaction between an antibody and antigen results in a recordable event. In some tests, the patient's blood sample is mixed with an antigen to see if there are antibodies in the serum. In other tests, antibodies may be added to the blood sample to see if the antigen exists.

Serological tests alone, however, are usually not specific enough to establish a diagnosis. For example, patients may have antibodies against an infectious agent, such as a fungus, but they may not have the disease when the test is administered. As another example, two patients may both have a high level of the rheumatic factor (RF), which is a type of immunoglobulin. Yet one patient has all the symptoms of rheumatoid arthritis, while the other has no symptoms. Likewise, some patients with syphilis may be what is termed "seronegative," while some who do not have the disease are "seropositive." This lack of total specificity is a common problem of all serological tests. Drugs, infections, and such diseases as carcinomas often cause unpredictable changes in immunological response.

The first part of this chapter covers the techniques used in blood banking procedures. The blood types of ABO demonstrate in a dramatic way the antigen–antibody basis for tests. Blood cross matching also uses several antibody titer tests.

The second part of the chapter discusses the common serology tests used in microbiology. (Specific microbiological tests, such as cultures and microscopic examinations, are covered in Chapter 16.) Serology tests are only indirect tests for the presence of an organism, such as a virus, which may have many different antigens. Laboratory tests can detect specific antibodies to a bacterial, viral, fungal, protozoan, or rickettsial antigen or antigens.

The last part of the chapter contains a discussion on the common serology tests used to assess immunological diseases, such as systemic lupus erythematous (SLE). Serological testing in autoimmune diseases is rapidly growing more common, as research discovers more about the antigen–antibody reactions that occur in these baffling diseases. This chapter may be viewed as a continuum in that tests of antigen–antibody reactions in ABO typing are very predictable, while tests such as the new ones for ANA (antinuclear antibodies) are much less predictable in clinical use.

COMMON TECHNIQUES IN SEROLOGICAL TESTING

The basic principle underlying serological testing is the fact that an antigen–antibody reaction causes an observable event. From a nursing point of view, the exact testing technique is not of prime interest. Nonetheless, to understand the description of the test, nurses do need to be familiar with the general meaning of the techniques. Five different techniques are commonly used in serological tests:

1. agglutinations and titer levels,
2. complement fixation (CF),
3. immunofluorescence antibody tests (IFA),
4. radioimmunoassay (RIA), and
5. enzyme-linked immunoabsorbent assay (ELISA).

Agglutination and Titer Levels. Agglutination or clumping, which often occurs when antibodies attach to an antigen, is the most basic type of serology testing. Febrile agglutins, cold agglutins, and the Coombs test are three examples of an observable clumping of cells in the blood sample when there is a certain ratio of antibodies to antigens.

The serum is diluted with normal saline in graduated amounts. For many serological tests, rather than reporting just agglutination (positive) or no agglutination (negative), the laboratory represents the results as a certain *titer,* which is the last dilution at which a reaction occurred. For example, the laboratory would use the standard dilutions in Table 14-1 to test for antibodies against an antigen streptolysin-O that is produced by group A-beta hemolytic streptococci. In the example in the table, the last dilution to cause a reaction was 1:170, which would be the titer reported. In essence, this finding means that the patient's serum contained enough antibodies to still cause a reaction with the antigenic material when the serum was diluted 1:170.

One titer does not give as much information as do two titers separated by a time interval, because a *rise* in titer is more significant than any one high number. So, to catch a rise or fall, the timing of titers is very important. A fourfold increase in titer between an acute and a convalescent sample is usually necessary to confirm the presence of an infection (Weinstein 1979:1099). The time interval between acute and convalescent phase depends on the organism causing the disease.

Complement Fixation (CF). Complement factors are a group of proteins in the bloodstream that enter into certain antigen–antibody reactions. One or more of the constituents of complement (see the test for C_3 and C_4) can be consumed during an antibody–antigen reaction. Since the complement used in the reaction is fixed, it cannot be used again. The tests using complement fixation are hard to standardize, so the newer techniques of IFA, RIA, and ELISA are being used if the laboratory is equipped to do these newer tests. The now out-dated Wasserman test for syphilis is an example of a test using CF.

Immunofluorescence Antibody Tests (IFA). The IFA test can be direct or indirect. In the direct method, an antibody labelled with a fluorescent dye (fluorescein) is mixed with a

TABLE 14-1.   TITER DILUTION CHART FOR ASO
(Anti-Streptolysin O Antibodies)

1:60	Positive
1:85	Positive
1:120	Positive
1:170	Positive
1:240	Negative
1:340	
1:480	
1:680	
1:960	
1:1360	
1:2720	

Note that an antibody titer is reported as the last dilution that causes an antigen–antibody reaction or agglutinzation. Thus, in this example, the laboratory report would read "ASO titer 1:170." See text for further explanation.

sample of blood from the patient. If an antigen is present, the antigen–antibody complex can be seen under a microscope with an ultraviolet light source. With the indirect method, the known antigen is mixed with the serum and any antigen–antibody complex is then mixed with fluorescein-labeled anti-immunoglobulin antibodies.

An example of a fluorescent type of test is the FTA-ABS for syphilis. The "FTA" stands for fluorescent treponemal antibody, and the "ABS" stands for a special absorption technique that helps to get rid of some of the nonspecific antibodies that may also get stained with the fluorescent dye. Another example of an immunofluorescence antibody test (IFA) discussed in this chapter is the IFA for toxoplasmosis. The IFA test can be falsely positive if the serum contains antinuclear antibodies. (See the ANA test at end of the chapter.)

Radioimmunoassay (RIA). The use of radioactive-tagged antigens is discussed in Chapter 15 in relation to hormone assay.

Enzyme-Linked Immunoabsorbent Assay (ELISA). The use of enzymes to tag antigens is also briefly discussed in Chapter 15.

Immunoglobulin Electrophoresis. See Chapter 10 for a discussion on how gamma globulins can be separated into patterns on a graph. The specific identification of immunoglobulins is a direct method of identifying immunological problems that can help to supplement the information gained from serological testing.

IMMUNOHEMATOLOGY TESTS

The tests done on blood used for transfusions are often given the name "immunohematology," rather than the broader term of "serology." See Table 14–2 for a list of the routine tests done on donor blood and for typing and cross matching.

Screening Blood for Transfusions
Five routine laboratory tests are done on a donor unit of blood:

   1. typing by the ABO system,
   2. typing as Rh positive or negative,
   3. serological test for syphilis (STS), and
   4. screening for hepatitis B surface antigen (HB$_s$Ag),
   5. antibody screening.

Each of these tests is discussed in detail in this chapter. Since transmission by syphilis is possible only in fresh blood that is less than three days old, the need for routine STS is being reevaluated (Kazak 1979).

Blood banks take several precautions to ensure not only that donor blood is safe to give to a patient, but also that it is safe for the person to donate blood. For example, the donor must weigh at least 110 lbs (50 k) and have a hemoglobin level of 13.5 g for men and 12.5 g for women. (See Chapter 2 on the measurement of hemoglobin levels.) The

TABLE 14-2.   ROUTINE TESTS ON DONOR BLOOD
AND FOR TYPE AND CROSS MATCHING*

Donor Blood:
1. ABO typing
2. Rh factor and other variations
3. STS
4. HB_s Ag
5. Antibody screening

Type and Cross Matching:
1. ABO typing (compatability)
2. Rh typing (compatability)
3. Direct Coombs
4. Antibody screening
5. Antibody titer
6. Identification of unusual antibodies and antigens

* See text for explanation of each test.

donor must have a temperature no higher than 98.6°F (37°C), a heart rate of 50 to 100 with no irregularities, and a blood pressure between 200/100 to 100/50. The blood bank physician may modify these guidelines depending on the individual situation. Overall, the donor must be in generally good health with no upper respiratory infections or allergies. Blood donations are not taken from people who have ever had hepatitis, malaria, jaundice, or a venereal disease. Pregnancy or a blood transfusion excludes donors for 6 months. Travel to other countries also excludes donors for 6 months. (Note that the incubation period for hepatitis B is 6 months.) Dental surgery or teeth extraction in the 72 hours prior to the donation excludes a donor. [See Chapter 16 on how even minor dental work can cause transient bacteria in the bloodstream (bacteremia).]

Typing and Cross Matching of Blood (T&C). To do a type and cross match, (T&C), the laboratory needs at least 45 minutes to make sure that the donor unit of blood is compatible with the blood of the recipient (Strand 1980). The patient's blood type and Rh factor are determined so that a matching unit of blood can be taken from the blood bank. Yet It Is never safe to assume that any unit of A positive blood can be given to any patient with A positive blood. So the cross match mixes a small sample of the two bloods to see if any clumping occurs. When the two serums and cells are combined and incubated, compatibility is demonstrated by the absence of clumping. The full range of tests for a type and cross matching include:

1. ABO grouping,
2. Rh typing,
3. direct antiglobulin test (Coombs),
4. antibody screen,
5. determination of antibody titer, and
6. identification of unusual antibodies and antigens.

In an emergency, the laboratory may do a less-than-full cross match by eliminating items 5 and 6. The physician, however, must notify the blood bank that the shortened version of the cross match is permissible for an emergency case.

Typing and Screening (T&S). If there is only a faint possibility of the blood being needed, the physician may order a typing and screening (T&S) rather than a cross match. In a screening, the patient's blood is tested, so that, if blood is needed, the actual cross matching can be done in less than 30 minutes. The advantage of the screening is that it does not tie up a unit of blood when the potential need is slight. For example, if two units of blood are typed and cross matched for a surgical patient, those two units of blood cannot be used for another patient until the surgery is done and the blood is released for re-cross matching with another patient. In one study, 4,762 units of blood were cross matched for elective surgical procedures, and only 200 were actually needed (Lang 1979).

Typing for Packed Cells. If the patient needs red blood cells but not serum, the physician orders a unit of packed cells. A unit of packed red blood cells contains only about a third of the amount of plasma as a unit of blood. Typing and cross matching are just as necessary for packed cells as for whole blood. Packed cells are now more commonly used for blood transfusions than whole blood. The major advantage of packed cells is the prevention of volume overload (Buickus 1979). In this discussion a "blood transfusion" refers to either whole blood or packed cells.

Preparation of Patient

There is no special preparation of the patient either for type and cross matching or for type and screening. For either procedure, the laboratory needs 10 ml of whole blood. Dextran, a plasma expander, should not be started before a type and cross match because it will interfere with the cross matching.

ABO GROUPING

All humans can be grouped into four major blood types—A, B, AB, and O—which are genetically determined. Even though Type A has subgroups, one can generally speak of only four types (Ravel 1978:84), the frequency of which is shown in Table 14–3, along with a description of the antigens and antibodies in each type. Besides the ABO grouping, which is the most important variable, the matching of donor and recipient must take into account many other factors.

Understanding the concept of the universal donor and recipient may help the nurse visualize, in a simple way, the significance of antibody–antigen response in immunological testing. Type O blood is theoretically the "universal donor" because there are none of the major antigens on the red blood cells of people with type O blood. Type O blood does have antibodies against A and B, but, in one unit of donor blood, the donor antibodies become so diluted in the plasma of the recipient that the antibodies are of minor importance. The person with AB has both A and B antigens on the red blood cells, so the plasma contains no antibodies against A or B antigens. Thus Type AB people are sometimes called "universal recipients." It is interesting to note that a person born with one type of

TABLE 14-3. ABO BLOOD TYPING

Estimated Percentage of Population	Type	Description
46%	O	No A or B antigens on RBCs. Antibodies against A and B antigens.*
41%	A	Antigen A on RBCs. Antibodies against B antigens.
9%	B	Antigen B on RBCs. Antibodies against A antigen.
4%	AB	Antigens A and B on RBCs. No antibodies against A or B antigens.

*From birth, the person has the antibodies, even with no exposure to the antigens. In contrast, the Rh negative person does not have antibodies against the RH factor until exposed to the factor.

ABO antigens has the antibodies against the other antigens, even though the person has never had contact with the other types of blood. In contrast, an Rh negative person does not have antibodies against the Rh factor until there is sensitization. (The Rh factor which, like ABO types, is genetically determined, is discussed later in this chapter.)

Nursing Implications. Patients must *never* be given a type of blood that contains foreign A and/or B antigens. For example, a patient with Type A blood who is given a unit of Type B blood would undergo a severe hemolytic reaction. The antibodies against the B antigen, which are present in the A patient, attack the red blood cells of the Type B donor blood. The hemolysis of the red blood cells causes the release, directly into the bloodstream, of free hemoglobin, which can be very damaging to the renal tubules. The end result of a transfusion of incompatible blood may be renal failure and death.

In most institutions, at least two people must check the patient's nameband against the unit of blood to be administered. Obviously, typing and cross matching are of no value if the blood is inadvertently given to the wrong patient. Not only the patient's name, but the medical record number too, must match the identification number of the unit of blood. After the unit of blood is hung, the nurse's responsibility is to see that the blood is given correctly. Buickus (1979) gives an excellent description of the nurse's role in administering not only whole blood, but also various other blood components. (See also Chapter 13 for a discussion on platelet transfusion and Chapter 2 for leukocyte replacement.)

Assessing for Complications. The nurse must also be aware of the signs and symptoms of an adverse reaction to a blood transfusion. The most severe hemolytic reaction is due to donor-recipient ABO incompatibilities. Rh and other factors may also cause some hemolysis, but usually not as pronounced. (See the next section on laboratory tests done after a hemolytic transfusion reaction.) Checking of vital signs before and during the blood transfusion is the basic nursing action. Also, running the blood slowly for the first 20 minutes minimizes the severity of a reaction, should it occur. Cullins (1979) describes the nurse's role in the detection and treatment of hemolytic transfusion reactions, as well as of other transfusion reactions, such as allergic reactions, febrile reactions, circulatory overload, and air embolism.

Laboratory Tests for Hemolytic Transfusion Reactions. If a patient begins to exhibit symptoms such as fever, chills, and low back pain, it is essential that the nurse not let the transfusion continue. Normal saline can be infused to keep the intravenous patent when the unit of blood is discontinued.

The unfinished unit of blood must be sent back to the laboratory, along with another specimen of the patient's blood, for the laboratory to try to determine what caused the reaction. The patient's blood and the donor's blood are re-cross matched to see if they are truely incompatible.

Since one of the dreaded complications of an incompatible blood transfusions is renal failure, the laboratory also needs a urine specimen to check for the presence of hemoglobin in the urine. The patient should be on strict intake and output, and all urine should be saved for laboratory examination for at least 24 hours.

The laboratory also checks for free hemoglobin in the plasma, as well as for other substances, such as indirect bilirubin and haptoglobin, that would indicate hemolysis. (See Chapter 11 for an explanation of why the indirect bilirubin is elevated with hemolysis.) Haptoglobin is a serum glycoprotein whose role is to bind free hemoglobin released from destroyed red blood cells. Evidently, haptoglobin is diminished in severe hemolysis because it cannot be replaced quickly enough.

Assessing for and Preventing Bacterial Contamination. In addition to the tests for hemolysis, the laboratory may also do a blood culture from the donor bag. (See Chapter 16 on culture reports from blood specimens.) Blood at room temperature becomes a very attractive culture medium for bacteria. Nursing actions to prevent sepsis from blood transfusions include the aseptic technique for starting the transfusion, hanging the blood within 15 minutes after it is taken from the blood bank, and ensuring that the entire unit is transfused within two to four hours.

Rh FACTOR

The Rh factor is named after the rhesus monkey used in the original research on this factor. Actually, several different Rh factors have been identified, but usually only the main factor is significant. The Rh factor, like the ABO types, is genetically determined.

There are two different nomenclatures for the Rh factors. In the Weiner system the main Rh factor is Rh_0. In the Fisher-Rose system, the main Rh factor is called D. In the literature, "Rh_0" or "D" is often just called the "Rh factor." In this discussion, the term "Rh factor" specifies the main factor involved when one speaks of Rh positive or Rh negative blood. (See Table 14-4 for a description of Rh positive and Rh negative.)

Normally, the person with Rh negative blood does not have any antibodies against the Rh factor. The Rh negative male can become sensitized (that is, develop antibodies against the Rh factor) by transfusion with Rh positive blood. The Rh negative female can develop antibodies against the Rh factor not only through blood transfusions with Rh positive factors, but also through a pregnancy where the fetus is Rh positive. Once the Rh negative person has developed antibodies against the Rh factor, another transfusion with Rh positive blood, or another pregnancy with a Rh positive fetus, can have serious consequences. The specific nursing implications for blood transfusions and for the Rh factor in pregnancy are discussed next.

TABLE 14–4. Rh FACTOR

Estimated Percentage of Population	Type	Description
85–90%	Rh+	Rh antigen on RBCs. No antibodies against Rh factor.
10–15%	Rh–	No Rh antigen on RBCs. Develops antibodies against Rh factor if sensitized by transfusion of Rh positive blood. Also, the pregnant woman can be sensitized by an Rh positive infant (see text).

Rh Factor in Blood Transfusions

Nursing Implications. To keep the Rh negative person from developing antibodies against the Rh factor, the Rh negative person is given only Rh negative blood. Hence Rh typing is one of the components of cross matching. The administration of Rh positive blood to a Rh negative person who had developed antibodies against the Rh factor (that is, who is sensitized) causes a hemolytic reaction because the person's antibodies attack the red blood cells that contain the Rh factor. The severity of this hemolytic reaction is usually not as great as it is in ABO incompatibility, but it is nevertheless to be avoided. (See the nursing implications above when a patient has any kind of transfusion reaction.)

Rh Factor in Pregnancy

Nursing Implications. An Rh negative mother and an Rh positive father can produce either a Rh negative or Rh positive baby, depending on the gene passed from the father. Laboratory tests can be done to determine if the Rh positive father has either two positive genes for Rh or one positive and one negative. (Note that an Rh positive mother can carry an Rh negative fetus without any problem Rh-related.)

A potential problem occurs when an Rh negative mother is carrying an Rh positive child. Hemolytic disease of the newborn, formerly called erythroblastosis fetalis, occurs when an Rh negative mother produces antibodies against the Rh positive red blood cells of her fetus. With the first pregnancy, the fetus is usually not affected because the mother has not had time to build antibodies against the Rh factor. However, at the time of the infant's separation from the placenta (a full-term birth or an abortion), some of the red blood cells from the fetus enter the mother's general circulation and trigger the production of antibodies against the Rh factor. Subsequent pregnancies with another Rh positive fetus may present problems because the woman's serum is now sensitized against Rh positive antigens.

Use of RhoGam. About 10% of all Rh negative mothers become sensitized (that is, they develop antibodies against the Rh factor) by their first pregnancy with a Rh positive fetus. If the woman is not immunized by the administration of Rh immunoglobulins (RhoGam is the brand name), each subsequent pregnancy with an Rh positive fetus incurs a further 10% risk of starting antibody production (Ortho Diagnostics, 1969). The use of Rh immunoglobulins is based on the principle of passive immunity. Because the mother has been given a dose of antibodies against the Rh factor, her body is not stimulated to begin an active production of antibodies against the Rh factor. RhoGam provides the needed temporary serum level of antibodies to block the effect of the antigen from the fetus, so the mother is not stimulated to begin producing her own antibodies. With each subsequent pregnancy with an Rh positive fetus, the Rh negative mother must receive RhoGam after delivery or an abortion. To be effective, RhoGam must be given within 72 hours after a birth or an abortion. RhoGam is not useful if the mother has already developed Rh antibodies, which can be measured in the serum. (The Rh antibody test is discussed later in this chapter.)

Nurses who work with women in the childbearing years should have a good understanding of the Rh factor so that they can help these women understand the possible implications in relation to pregnancy. The laws of some states make it mandatory that any woman who is bloodtyped must be told the results of the Rh factor. For the Rh negative pregnant women, Ortho Diagnostics (1969) has a pamphlet that explains, in lay terms, the necessity of RhoGam following each Rh positive pregnancy, including abortions.

Rh ANTIBODY TITER TEST

The Rh antibody titer test is used to monitor the course of the Rh negative woman who is carrying an Rh positive fetus. If the mother is in a second pregnancy and did not receive RhoGam after a first pregnancy or abortion, the rise of the titer helps to determine the need for medical interventions, such as exchange transfusions or an early delivery.

Preparation of Patient
And Collection of Sample
The laboratory needs 10 ml of blood. Note that this test may also be done on a sample of cord blood.

Reference Values

The normal Rh antibody titer is negative. A titer above 1:64 may indicate the need for immediate medical intervention to prevent serious damage to the fetus or newborn.

DIRECT ANTIGLOBULIN (COOMBS) TEST

In certain types of sensitization, such as to the Rh factor, the erythrocytes become coated with antibodies or immunoglobulins. The Coombs test is used as a screening test to detect whether immunoglobulins have become attached to the red blood cells.

The test is referred to as a "direct" antiglobulin test (as opposed to the indirect or antibody screening test discussed next), because the red blood cells are tested without any intervening manipulations. A sample of the patient's blood is mixed with Coombs serum, which is a rabbit serum that has antibodies against human globulins. If the patient's red blood cells are coated with immunoglobulins, agglutination occurs. The Coombs test is done:

1. To screen blood for cross matching: If a patient's erythrocytes have been exposed to incompatible blood, the erythrocytes are coated with an antibody or globulin complex.
2. To check for hemolytic transfusion reactions.
3. To assess hemolytic disease in the newborn: In hemolytic disease of the newborn, the antibodies from a sensitized Rh negative mother cross the placenta and coat the fetal red cells.

Other factors may also cause the patient's red blood cells to be coated with immunoglobulins. For example, many drugs, as well as autoimmune diseases that cause hemolytic anemia, may cause a positive Coombs reaction. If necessary, further testing can be done to identify the specific immunoglobulins present. (See Chapter 10 on immunoglobulin testing.)

Preparation of Patient
And Collection of Sample
In the newborn, the blood sample is taken directly from the umbilical cord. In children and adults, a venous sample is used. Note that this test is routine for one aspect of typing and cross matching, which requires 10 ml.

Reference Values

The Coombs test should be negative. A positive test indicates that some type of globulin is coating the red blood cells.

ANTIBODY SCREENING TEST

This test used to be called the "indirect" Coombs because the serum is subjected to several different conditions to detect various antibodies. It is a screening test because it does not directly identify specific antibodies. However, by observing which types of mixtures cause agglutinations, the laboratory can identify specific antibodies indirectly. If there is a positive result from the antibody screening, the laboratory may do more tests to identify the specific antibodies.

Preparation of Patient
And Collection of Sample
This test is usually done as part of a cross match. The laboratory uses 10 ml of venous blood.

Reference Values

The antibody screening test should be negative.

MICROBIOLOGY SEROLOGICAL TESTS

The tests in this section are used for various types of diseases with infectious agents. See Table 14–5 for an overview.

Serological Tests for Hepatitis

The several different forms of viral hepatitis are designated as hepatitis A (formerly called infectious hepatitis), hepatitis B (formerly called serum hepatitis), and Non-A/Non-B hepatitis. There are at least two different types of Non-A/Non-B hepatitis. Zuckerman (1979) describes a wide array of the tests presently being used to detect hepatitis A and hepatitis B. At the present time, there are no tests to detect Non-A/Non-B hepatitis.

HEPATITIS B SURFACE ANTIGEN (HB$_s$AG)
AND ANTIBODIES AGAINST HB$_s$AG

The virus that causes hepatitis B was discovered in 1965 in an Australian man. It was originally named the ''Australian'' antigen, and some of the literature may still use this name rather than the newer name of hepatitis B surface antigen (HB$_s$Ag). Since a typical virus has many different antigens, a surface antigen is but one component of the hepatitis B virus. Numerous types of tests are now available to identify the hepatitis B surface antigen. One of the most popular methods is the enzyme-linked immunosorbent assay. (See Chapter 16 for a brief explanation of enzyme and radioimmunoassay.)

The detection of hepatitis B surface antigen in a person's serum means either the patient is that ill with the disease or a carrier. In either case, the blood is a possible source of infection for other people. Evidently most people do not carry the virus after the disease is over. London (1977) states that in about 90% of hepatitis B patients the antigen disappears from the serum in about 6 weeks. Hepatitis B is spread primarily by blood or blood products. Since the incubation period is 50 to 180 days, a patient who gets hepatitis B from a blood transfusion may not show symptoms for up to 6 months. Thus no one who has had a blood transfusion can donate blood for 6 months. Tests of HB$_s$Ag have become very useful in screening blood donors, many of whom would not be aware that they are carriers. (Note that, since blood also transmits Non-A/Non-B hepatitis, hepatitis is still a possibility after any blood transfusion.)

In addition to testing for the presence of the HB$_s$Ag, the laboratory can also test for antibodies against the hepatitis B antigen. A person who has antibodies against HB$_s$Ag is presumed to be immune to hepatitis B, but not necessarily to other types of hepatitis.

Preparation of Patient
And Collection of Sample

The laboratory uses venous blood to test for hepatitis B. The exact amount needed depends on the specific test used. Anyone drawing blood for hepatitis B testing should be aware of the danger of hepatitis. When drawing blood, wear gloves. See the note under nursing implications.

TABLE 14–5. COMMON SEROLOGICAL TESTS USED IN MICROBIOLOGY

Test	Organism	Remarks*
VDRL RPR FTA-ABS MHA	*Treponema pallidum,* which causes syphilis.	Confirming tests are done if screening tests are positive.
HB$_S$Ag	Hepatitis B virus (formerly called serum hepatitis).	Can also measure antibodies against HB$_S$Ag.
Hepatitis A antigens	Hepatitis A virus (formerly called infectious hepatitis).	Tests for A are not common yet Also, no tests for Non-A/Non-B.
Cold agglutinins	Eaton agent or pleuropneumonia-like organism [PPLO] may cause atypical pneumonia.	Positive in some cases, not all.
Febrile agglutinins	Paratyphoid fever Typhoid fever (salmonella organisms) Tularemia (rabbit fever) Brucellosis (undulant fever)	Often these infectious diseases cause fever of undetermined origin (FUO).
HAT Monospot Monoscreen Monotest	Epstein-Barr virus of infectious mononucleosis	Also see WBC with differential in Chapter 2.
1. ASO 2. Anti-DNase B 3. Streptozyme	Group A-beta hemolytic streptococci	Measures antibodies *after* an acute infection with streptococci. Not useful during initial infectious stage.
Rubella	Rubella virus (3-day measles).	Even low-antibody titer probably indicates immunity.
TPM	Toxoplasma gondi, a protozoan that causes toxoplasmosis.	Most tests are indirect measurements of the protozoan.
Hemagglutination for amoebiasis	Entameba histolytica (causes amebic dysentery and hepatic abcess).	Stool cultures also done (see Chapter 16).
Fungus antibody tests	Histoplasmosis Coccidioidomycosis Blastomycosis	Cultures also done (see Chapter 16).
Proteus Ox19 Ox2 OxK	Rickettsial disease such as *Ricketessia, akeri* which causes Rocky Mountain spotted fever, and *Rickettiae prowazukki,* which causes epidemic typhus	Rickettslae can be cultured, but the reaction to Proteus is an easier method to get presumptive evidence.

*See text for full explanation.

Reference Values

A positive HB$_s$Ag indicates either active hepatitis or a carrier state. In either case, the patient's blood may be a source of infection.

A positive antibody titer to HB$_s$Ag presumably indicates immunity to hepatitis B.

Both a negative antigen and an antibody test for HB$_s$Ag indicate the person is susceptible to hepatitis B.

Positive HB$_s$Ag

Possible Nursing Implications. Because hepatitis B is spread by the parenteral route (blood and blood products), nurses must use blood precautions when hepatitis B is suspected or confirmed by testing. They should wear gloves to draw blood, to start an intravenous, or to handle any blood-contamined articles. Nurses in other areas, such as blood laboratories, operating rooms, and delivery rooms, must also be aware of the risk in handling blood. All cuts, skin breaks, or injuries with a needle should be avoided or reported if they do occur.

Bauer (1980) outlines a specific program for regular serological testing in renal dialysis units because the incidence of hepatitis B is high for both staff and patients. Both patients and staff may be routinely monitored by the HB$_s$Ag test and the HB$_s$Ag antibody test. Patients and staff who are identified as carriers of HB$_s$Ag are then separated from patients who do not have antibodies against HB$_s$Ag.

Gamma globulin is used to lessen the severity of hepatitis A, but it is not generally used to lessen the impact of hepatitis B. Hepatitis B immune globulin, which differs from the standard gamma globulin, is available (Cutter 1979). A vaccine to protect against hepatitis B has been developed to provide active immunity against hepatitis B (Roche 1981).

See the discussion under hepatitis A and on bilirubin levels (Chapter 11) and transaminase levels (Chapter 12) for more information on the nursing care of patients with hepatitis.

HEPATITIS A ANTIGEN

Hepatitis A is primarily spread by the oral-fecal route. It is often spread by food handlers or by sexual contact. The incubation period is about 15 to 45 days, which is much shorter than the 50 to 180 days of hepatitis B. The tests to identify hepatitis A include electron microscopy, agglutination tests, the RAI (radioimmunoassay), and EIA (enzyme immunoassay). In the early stages of the disease, virus particles can be identified in the feces. Zuckerman (1979:876) states that various tests for hepatitis A have shown that hepatitis A is endemic all over the world, that it is not transmitted by blood transfusions, and that there is no evidence of progression to chronic liver disease. Much research is now being done to find out how Non-A/Non-B hepatitis differs from the clinical entity called hepatitis A.

Preparation of Patient
And Collection of Sample

The amount of venous blood needed depends on the type of hepatitis A antigen test done by a given laboratory. Since some types of hepatitis are spread through the blood products, the laboratory should be warned that the patient is suspected of having hepatitis.

Reference Values

All groups	A positive test for hepatitis A means an active disease state since it is believed that there is no carrier state for A. Note that recent research is giving support to the idea that Non-A/Non-B hepatitis may exist in a carrier state (Zuckerman 1979). Since the tests for hepatitis A are not yet standard in most laboratories, the usual practice is to conclude that a patient with clinical signs of hepatitis has A, or Non-A/Non-B, if the test for HB_sAg is negative.

Positive Hepatitis A Test

Possible Nursing Implications. The major nursing implication is to initiate enteric precautions so that feces-to-oral transmission of the virus does not occur. Isolation is usually not necessary if the person is a responsible adult who can do thorough handwashing after touching the perineal area. The person should not be allowed to handle or prepare any food for others. The disease can also be transmitted by sexual contact. If there is a possibility that the infected person may have infected others by food handling or by intimate contact, the contacts may be offered gamma globulin. Gamma globulin or (Gamastan) is also recommended for persons who plan to travel in areas where hepatitis A is common (Cutter 1979). Gamma globulin, which can be given up to two weeks after exposure, does not prevent the disease, but it may lessen the severity. The immune serum globulin against hepatitis A comes from human sources (Gamastan). The product information sheet gives the recommended dosages based on weight. Note that anaphylactic reactions, although very rare, can occur.

Since there is no drug to cure hepatitis, the mainstays of treatment are rest and a nutritious diet to promote liver regeneration. Bilirubin levels (Chapter 11) and transaminase levels (Chapter 12) are used to monitor the progress of the patient.

SEROLOGIC TESTS FOR SYPHILIS (STS)

Except for the common cold and flu, venereal diseases are the most common infectious diseases in the United States. Although gonorrhea is more common than syphilis, syphilis is the more dangerous if left undetected and thus untreated. There is no serological test for gonorrhea (see Chapter 17 for the smear and culture tests for gonorrhea).

Although the sphirochete, *Treponema pallidum,* that causes syphilis may occasionally be identified from a syphilitic sore or chancre, syphilis is more commonly diagnosed by a serology test. Testing for syphilis may be divided into tests done for screening and those done for a confirmation of a positive screening test. The VDRL or RPR are screening tests, while the FTA-ABS and the MHA are confirmatory tests for syphilis. The Wasserman test, which used a complement fixation technique, was the first serological test for syphilis, but it is no longer used.

VDRL (Veneral Disease Research Laboratory) and RPR (Rapid Plasma Reagen)

The VDRL is named for the research laboratory that perfected this flocculation test for syphilis. The test measures a globulin complex called reagen that appears early in the course of syphilis. If the globulin complex reagen is present, an aggregation occurs that can be reported as either negative, weakly reactive, or reactive. The RPR rapid plasma reagen uses the VDRL antigen, but it adds some carbon particles so that the flocculation can be seen on a plastic card.

The VDRL and variations of it are indirect tests for syphilis because they are tests for a reaction to a globulin, not to the sphirochete itself. Thus a person who is treated for syphilis may still have antibodies in the serum for an indefinite time. Also, a person who has just contracted syphilis may not have had time to build up antibodies against *Treponema pallidum*. The tests usually become positive in three to four weeks after exposure. Because the screening tests react to abnormal globulins, other types of pathology, such as some connective tissue disorders, may cause false positives.

FTA-ABS and MHA

The fluorescent treponemal antibody absorption test (FTA-ABS) is used to confirm an infection with the sphirochete that causes syphilis. It tests for the specific antibodies against *Treponema pallidum*. The laboratory prepares a slide and stains it to make the antibodies show up as a yellow-green color under an ultraviolet microscope. Technical difficulties are involved in doing the test, and false positives can occur.

Another confirming test being studied is the microhemagglutination (MHA) test. Ravel (1979:388) states that the MHA may be substituted for the FTA-ABS in certain situations to confirm the diagnosis of syphilis. The MHA is easier to perform and costs less than the FTA-ABS.

Preparation of Patient And Collection of Specimen

The laboratory uses 4 ml of venous blood for serological tests for syphilis (STS). No special preparation of the patient is necessary.

Reference Values

These tests should be negative.

Note that various conditions may cause false positives in the screening test as explained in the text. Also note that the tests will be the most strongly positive four to six weeks after exposure.

Positive Serological Test for Syphilis

Nursing Implications. Anyone who is sexually active should be aware of the early symptoms of syphilis. If not detected in the early stages, syphilis may eventually spread, causing severe neurological problems, blindness, and even death. Luckmann (1980) describes the characteristic signs and symptoms of primary, secondary, and tertiary syphilis. The treatment of syphilis is extremely easy: penicillin by injection. Other antibiotics are used if the person is allergic to penicillin.

As a communicable disease, syphilis must be reported to the public health department. Venereal disease clinics and public health departments have staffs who follow up the sexual contacts of the person who has a positive STS. Nurses may take an active role in educating the public about the importance of screening people who may have been exposed to the disease. Nurses working with patients who have a positive STS can help impress upon them the importance of early detection and early treatment. Obviously, nurses need to be nonjudgmental in their approach.

Since syphilis can be passed to a fetus, it is extremely important that a pregnant woman be treated for syphilis. The American College of Obstetricians and Gynecologists publishes a patient information booklet (ACOG 1978) that explains the important facts about venereal disease and pregnancy. The nurse working in a prenatal clinic can help to explain to patients why a STS is done in early pregnancy.

COLD AGGLUTININS OR COLD HEMAGGLUTININS

In some disease states, antibodies cause clumping of the patient's blood when the blood is refrigerated at a certain temperature. When a patient has a respiratory infection with *Mycoplasma pneumoniae,* there is often an increase in cold agglutinins. Hence this test of cold agglutinins is primarily used to assess for the possibility of primary atypical pneumonia. Mycoplasma pneumonia is caused by a pleuropneumonia-like organism (PPLO) that has characteristics of both a virus and a bacteria (Ravel 1978:187). *Mycoplasma pneumoniae* is also called the Eaton agent. The PPLO can be cultured, but it takes about a week, so a rising titer of cold agglutinins helps with the diagnosis sooner. Other conditions, such as severe anemia, congenital syphilis, hepatitis, and cirrhosis, may also cause cold agglutinins. Antibiotic therapy may interfere with the formation of the cold agglutinins.

Preparation of Patient
And Collection of Sample
The test requires 10 ml of whole blood. The blood is drawn into a warm tube or syringe and immediately put into a 37°C (98.6°F) water bath for transportation to the laboratory. The specimen should be hand-carried to the laboratory.

Reference Values

All groups	Titers over 1:32 are considered abnormal. A rising titer is more significant than just one high titer.
Aged	Titer is higher in older people.

Positive Cold Agglutinins

Possible Nursing Implications. Since the patient who has cold agglutinins ordered usually has a respiratory infection, general nursing care takes the form of the standard care for the patient with pneumonia. Antibiotics, such as erythromycin or one of the tetracyclines, may be ordered for atypical pneumonia by the Eaton agent. Respiratory isolation is needed.

FEBRILE AGGLUTININS FOR TYPHOID FEVER, PARATYPHOID, BRUCELLOSIS, AND TULAREMIA

Febrile agglutinins are antibodies that are produced in response to certain bacterial infections that cause fever in the patient. Although cold agglutinins are tested by cooling the blood sample, febrile agglutinins are not tested by heating the sample. A specific bacterial cell antigen is mixed with the sample of blood from the patient to see if agglutination occurs. For example, the Widal test uses the Salmonella antigen to test for typhoid and paratyphoid fever. Two other common tests using specific bacterial antigens are for tularemia (rabbit fever) and brucellosis (undulant fever). With simple slide agglutination techniques for these bacterial infections, the laboratory can easily do the test of "febrile agglutinins." In fevers of undetermined origin (FUO), the febrile agglutinins may be very useful because this battery of tests includes the common infections usually considered in FUOs that may be bacterial (Ravel 1979:161).

Preparation of Patient
And Collection of Sample
The laboratory needs 6 ml of whole blood. At least two samples are needed, one during the acute stage and one during the convalescent stage.

Reference Values

A fourfold rise in titer is considered strong evidence of infection with the specific bacteria being tested.

Possible Nursing Implications. Nursing care depends on the type of infection. (See Chapter 16 for some general nursing implications for any patient with a bacterial infection.) Refer to nursing texts for the care of the patient with typhoid fever or other febrile diseases caused by various bacteria.

INFECTIOUS MONONUCLEOSIS

Heterophil Antibody Titer (HAT)
The heterophil antibody titer (HAT) is a screening test for infectious mononucleosis, a viral disease. The word "heterophil" refers to having an affinity for more than one group or species. Normally humans do not have antibodies against the red blood cells of sheep, but patients with infectious mononucleosis do develop antibodies that agglutinate the red blood cells of sheep.

The test, however, is not specifically diagnostic since other factors may also cause an increase in heterophile antibodies. For example, allergic reactions, such as serum sickness, cause an increased HAT. Also, some patients with infectious mononucleosis may not have a significant heterophil titer. The older version of the HAT, sometimes called the Paul-Bunnell test, is no longer done, since the diagnostic kits can obtain results in one or two minutes.

Diagnostic Kits for Infectious Mononucleosis

Spot tests for infectious mononucleosis include Monospot (Ortho Diagnostics), Monotest (Wampole), and Monoscreen (Smith Kline & French). The "spot" test uses a saline suspension of antigen derived from horses' red blood cells. The mixture of the test material with a drop of the patient's serum causes a coarse granulation if the patient has infectious mononucleosis. The spot tests are rapid, specific, and sensitive as screening tests, and they are valuable in supporting a clinical diagnosis of infectious mononucleosis. Yet they do not positively identify the Epstein-Barr virus of infectious mononucleosis. Other criteria for diagnosing infectious mononucleosis include lymphocytosis and the presence of atypical lymphocytes in the serum. (See Chapter 2 for a discussion of lymphocytes as part of a differential WBC).

Preparation of Patient
And Collection of Sample

The screening tests require *1 to 2 ml* of blood. A WBC with differential is also ordered.

Positive HAT or Spot Test

Possible Nursing Implications. Nursing care for patients with infectious mononucleosis includes providing rest and other general measures to help them overcome a viral infection. Although infectious mononucleosis is sometimes called the "kissing disease," the exact mode of transmission is unknown. Isolation is not necessary, but the patient needs to avoid strenuous exercise since rupture of the spleen can occur as a complication (Luckmann 1980). Transaminase levels (Chapter 12) and bilirubin levels (Chapter 11) are used to assess the degree of liver dysfunction.

STREPTOCOCCI INFECTIONS

Definition and Purpose

Three tests are used to identify a recent infection with group A-beta hemolytic streptococci:

  1. anti-streptolysin-O (ASO),
  2. anti-streptodornase-B (anti-DNase B), and
  3. streptozyme.

Group A-beta hemolytic streptococci produce several substances (antigens) that induce the formation of measurable antibodies in the serum. Because the aftermath of group A streptococci infections may be such diseases as rheumatic fever or glomerulonephritis, one or more of these three streptococcal antigen tests is used to help in confirming that the patient did have a streptococci infection in the recent past. Rheumatic fever is becoming rarer due to early recognition and treatment of streptocci infections such as strep throat. (See Chapter 16 on the importance of throat cultures to identify strep throat.) In patients with rheumatic fever, 95% show an elevated titer to one or more of the streptococcal antigen tests (Fitzmaurice 1980:14). A rising titer suggests a very recent infection, while a stable titer indicates previous exposure to the streptococci antigens.

Anti-Streptolysin-O (ASO). The antibodies to streptolysin-O appear about seven days after an acute streptococcal infection. The antibodies peak two to four weeks later, remaining high for weeks to months. The test may not always be elevated with streptococci infections, and other disease conditions, such as liver disease, may make the test falsely positive.

Anti-Streptolysin-B (Anti-DNase-B). Anti-DNase B measures the antibodies formed against another of the streptococcal enzymes called streptodornase-B. It may be used in conjunction with the other two tests for streptococci antigens.

Streptozyme Test. This test is more general than the ASO or Anti-DNase-B. It measures antibodies against five different streptococcal enzymes: (1) streptolysis-O, (2) deoxyribonuclease-B, (3) hyalurodinase, (4) streptikinase, and (5) nicotinamide afemine dinucleotidase. This test may be more sensitive than the other tests, but false positives can also occur.

Preparation of Patient
And Collection of Sample

These tests require venous blood. Make a note on the lab slip if the patient was on antibiotics, since titers may not increase if the patient has been on antibiotics.

Reference Values

	ASO Titers
Preschool	1:85
Age 5–18	1:170
Adults	1:85
	Anti-DNase-B Titers
Preschool	1:60
Age 5–18	1:170
Adults	1:85

Streptozyme Titers. Check with individual laboratory.

Positive for Streptococci Infection

Clinical Significance. Titers above the dilutions set for each age group are possible evidence of recent infection with the group A-beta hemolytic streptococcus.

Possible Nursing Implications. Nursing care is based on the underlying pathophysiology that may have occurred due to a recent streptococcal infection. See nursing texts for the care of the patient with rheumatic fever or glomerulonephritis. Note that throat cultures (Chapter 16) are useful in detecting streptoccal infections at the time of the infection. These serological tests are done *after* the acute infection has subsided, since the antibodies are elevated after the bacteria are no longer present.

RUBELLA

The Rubacell test detects antibodies against rubella. Rubella (also called "three-day measles") is usually of no significance unless it occurs in a pregnant woman. Rubella may cause a miscarriage, or it may bring about congenital heart disease, cataracts, deafness, and brain damage in the fetus. Thus, it is important to assess whether women who are to become pregnant have an immunity against rubella.

The laboratory uses either hemagglutination inhibition (HI) or complement fixation serology tests to assess for the presence of antibodies against the rubella virus. Antibodies appear within a week or less after the rash. Once the person has had the disease, an elevated titer of antibodies persists for many years or perhaps for life (Ravel 1980:178). Even a small amount of antibodies indicates some immunity from the disease. Women who are not immune to rubella (that is, who have no antibody titer) should be vaccinated before becoming pregnant. The rubella test for antibodies is one of the blood tests necessary to obtain a marriage license.

Preparation of Patient
And Collection of Sample
The test requires venous blood.

Reference Values

Evidently, even a 1:8 titer indicates immunity, although newer studies suggest that a 1:8 or 1:10 indicates only marginal immunity and that a 1:64 is more desirable for continued protection (Claypool 1981:54).

Negative Titer

Possible Nursing Implications. The lack of a titer to rubella is significant in women who may become pregnant. Since 1969, when the first rubella vaccine was licensed in the United States, there has been a mass immunization program for school-aged children. However, there are still women in their childbearing years who are susceptible to rubella. At the present time, a single dose of rubella vaccine is recommended not only for children more than 12 months old, but also for any woman who has no antibody titer for rubella and who may become pregnant (Abramowicz 1979:54).

Whether some action should be taken may be a very disturbing question for the woman who contacts rubella during her pregnancy. If a pregnant woman is suspected of having contacted rubella, a fourfold rise in titer would be evidence of recent infection. The patient needs to confer with the physician about the possible damage to the fetus.

Health care workers must take all measures necessary to prevent susceptible pregnant women from contacting rubella. All health workers who might transmit rubella to pregnant women should also be immunized against the disease. Claypool (1981) describes a program that was used in a health agency to establish rubella protection. The policy at the agency included immunization for all health workers who did not have evidence of a positive rubella titer within the past five years. The immunization requirement was also for nursing students who had clinical experience with the agency.

Nurses should be aware that adult women who are given the vaccine should avoid pregnancy for three months. Giving the patient information about reliable birth control may be necessary. Also, since the vaccine can cause some joint symptoms, particularly in adults, the possible side effects of the vaccine need to be explained. (Check the product information for a specific vaccine.)

TOXOPLASMOSIS

Toxoplasmosis is caused by an infection with the protozoan *Toxoplasma gondi,* which is found in raw or poorly cooked meat and in the feces of cats. The infection causes fatigue, fever, and lymph gland swelling. The oldest test for toxoplasmosis is the Sabin-Feldman, which uses a dye to stain the organism. Other tests for toxoplasmosis use serological tests of antibodies. The immunofluorescent antibody test (IFA) is considered almost diagnostic if one other test, such as the indirect hemagglutination (IHA) or complement fixation (CF), is positive (Lake 1979). Toxoplasmosis can be treated by certain drugs so that usually the infection is not too serious in an adult. However, toxoplasmosis can be passed to the fetus and cause various types of neurologic damage and eye problems.

Preparation of Patient
And Collection of Sample
Check with the laboratory for the specific type of serological test being used. Most of the tests for toxoplasmosis require about 4 ml of whole blood. Pertinent history includes whether the patient has been exposed to cats or may be pregnant.

Reference Values

Immunofluorescent antibody test (IFA) titer of 1:10 is considered almost diagnostic if one other test is up, such as the indirect hemagglutination (INA) or the complement fixation (CF).

Note that the IFA is falsely positive if the serum contains antinuclear antibodies (ANA), which is discussed later in this chapter.

Infants may have an increased titer due to the transfer of antibodies from the mother. Infants need to be retested later.

Positive Titer

Possible Nursing Implications. People should be aware that poorly cooked or raw meat can introduce organisms into the human body. Also the importance of avoiding hand contamination from the feces of cats should be made common knowledge. Since cats are the host, the pregnant women needs to be careful about handling the feces of a cat and certainly to avoid strange cats. A veterinarian can be contacted about the health status of a house cat.

The presence of lymphadenopathy (enlarged lymph glands) and vague symptoms in an otherwise healthy person may suggest a viral infection. The patient with suspected toxoplasmosis may also have tests done for infectious mononucleosis. Unlike infectious mononucleosis, there is no elevated heterophil antibody test. (See earlier in this chapter for the discussion of the HAT.) Until the diagnosis is made by the physician, the patient may be alarmed that the lymph gland swelling is due to a malignancy and is likely to be very relieved to find out that the problem is an infection with a protozoan. The drugs used for treatment include pyrimethamine, sulfonamide, and sometimes clindomycin (Lake 1979).

AMEBIASIS

Entamoeba histolytica is an ameba that causes amebic dysentary and hepatic abcesses. The ameba can be identified by microscopic examination. (See Chapter 16 for the technique used to obtain a stool culture for ameba.) The stool examination is the most definitive test for ameba, but it is technically difficult to obtain live ameba for direct examination. An indirect hemagglutination technique can identify antibodies to *Entamoeba histolytica,* which are present in 95% of patients with a hepatic abcess due to the ameba and in 85% of patients with an intestinal infection of *Entamoeba histolytica* (Weinstein 1979:1114).

Preparation of Patient
And Collection of Sample
The test requires venous blood. Check with the laboratory for the exact amount.

Reference Values

Increasing titers may indicate infections with the ameba. Antibody levels persist for some time after an active infestation.

Increasing Titer

Possible Nursing Implications. See Chapter 16 for the patient teaching needed when a patient must be on enteric precautions.

FUNGAL ANTIBODIES

By use of the complement fixation (CF) technique, the laboratory can identify antibodies that occur in response to fungus diseases, such as histoplasmosis, coccidioidomycosis, and blastomycosis. Histoplasmosis is particularly found in the Ohio Valley area, and coccidioidomycosis (valley fever or desert fever) is prominent in the San Joaquin Valley of California. Because many people who live in an area where a fungus is endemic may have positive serologic tests from past exposures, one titer is not enough to be diagnostic. A fourfold rise in titer would be evidence of a present infection. Although certain types of fungus are endemic in certain areas, in this age of jet travel, patients with the disease may be far from the origin. A travel history is mandatory when a fungus is suspected (Einstein 1980).

Skin testing and cultures may also be used to identify the particular fungus causing the systemic infection. (See Chapter 16 for some tips on cultures for fungus.) A positive skin test does not indicate that an infection is currently present, since the antibodies may be from past exposure. More significant is a conversion of a negative skin test to a positive one. Since skin tests can also cause a serological test to become positive, they should be started after the blood is drawn for serological tests for fungus antibodies.

Preparation of Patient
And Collection of Sample

The test requires 5 ml of venous blood, which should be drawn before any skin testing is done.

Rising Titers

Nursing Implications. The nurse should confer with the physician to see if the patient presents any danger to other patients or to the staff. Refer to a nursing text for detailed information on the care of patients with fungus disease. Nurses may administer ordered skin tests for fungus. The technique for intradermal injection, the dilutent strength of the antigen, and the times to read the results are clearly explained with the product information that comes with the test material.

RICKETTSIAL DISEASE:
PROTEUS OX 19, PROTEUS OX 2, AND PROTEUS OX K

The nonpathogenic organism, Proteus Ox 19, is agglutinated by the serum of people with certain rickettsial diseases, such as Rocky Mountain spotted fever and typhus. This reaction is called the Weil-Felix reaction. Other types of Proteus, such as Ox 2 or Ox K, may be used to determine other specific types of infection with rickettsiae. Culturing the rickettsiae is possible, but it must be done in a special viral laboratory. Any laboratory, on the other hand, can do serological testing. So the Proteus test is commonly used when a rickettsial disease is suspected.

Preparation of Patient
And Collection of Sample

The test requires 6 ml of venous blood. Since the Weil-Felix reaction involves a reaction to the Proteus antigen, the test is not indicative of rickettsial disease if the patient has an infection with certain pathogenic strains of Proteus. Note the possibility of any Proteus infections. (See Chapter 16 for a discussion on Proteus infections of the urinary tract, respiratory tract, and wounds.)

All rickettsiae are spread by vectors. For example, epidemic typhus is spread by body lice, and Rocky Mountain spotted fever is spread by a tick. The laboratory needs to know of possible exposure to these vectors.

Reference Values

A titer of 1:40 or 1:80 is considered possible evidence of rickettsial disease.

A titer of 1:160 or above is presumptive evidence of infection with one of the rickettsiae.

Other diseases, such as typhoid, may occasionally cause agglutinations of Proteux OX 19 too (Koepke 1979:277).

Rickettsial Positive Tests

Possible Nursing Implications. Nursing care is based on caring for the patient with an infection. Since transmission requires a vector, the patient is not infectious to others. Refer to current literature for details on diseases caused by rickettsiae.

IMMUNOLOGICAL TESTS

The few tests discussed in this section are used primarily to assess for diseases such as systemic lupus erythematous (SLE), rheumatoid arthritis (RA), or other autoimmune reactions. See Table 14–6 for a list of the common serological tests used in immunology.

C-REACTIVE PROTEIN

The C-reactive protein, not normally present in the blood, appears with inflammatory processes or with tissue destruction. It is not elevated in viral infections. Sometimes this test is used to monitor rheumatic fever or rheumatoid arthritis. Like the ESR (erythrocyte sedimentation rate), the C-reactive protein is a very nonspecific test that indicates only an inflammation. The C-reactive protein may rise sooner than the ESR, and different clinicians may choose to use either the ESR or the C-reactive protein. (See Chapter 2 for the discussion on ESR as the more common test used to monitor rheumatoid arthritis.)

Preparation of Patient
And Collection of Sample

The test requires 3 ml of venous blood.

TABLE 14–6.   COMMON SEROLOGICAL TESTS USED IN IMMUNOLOGY

Test	Description*
C-reactive protein	Measures an abnormal protein found in the serum in certain inflammations. Compare to ESR in Chapter 2.
Complement activity	Measures activity of the complement system.
C_3 and C_4	Specific measurements of the amount of two of the complement factors.
LE prep	Examination for a particular type of cell in SLE.
ANA	Measures antinuclear antibodies, which are sometimes increased in SLE.
Anti-DNA, Anti-DNP	Other humoral antibodies, which are sometimes elevated in SLE.
RF	Measurement of antibodies, which may be elevated in rheumatoid arthritis.
Thyroid colloid and microsomal antigen tests	Measurement of antibodies, which may be elevated in certain types of thyroditis.

*See text for further explanation.

Reference Values: C-Reactive Protein

Should be negative except in pregnancy.
Oral contraceptive pills may cause an increase.

Possible Nursing Implications. See the discussion in Chapter 2 on the use of the ESR (erythrocyte sedimentation rate).

Complement Activity and C_3 and C_4 Measurements

The complement system is comprised of several proteins that are active in producing the inflammatory response sometimes following an antigen–antibody reaction. The final reaction of the complement system produces a complex protein capable of lyzing cell membranes (Koffler 1979:4).

The total amount of complement activity may be measured by a hemolytic assay and expressed in units as compared to a normal standard. The test of total complement activity is difficult to do and to standardize since it must use fresh human or guinea pig complement. A much simpler test involves measuring two of the components of the complement system. These two components, C_3 and C_4, as well as the other components of the complement system, are used up in the very complicated series of reactions that follow some antibody–antigen reactions. In certain of the rheumatoid diseases, tests of complement activity help clinicians to judge the amount of immune complexes occurring. Immune complexes appear to be the primary mediators of tissue injury in systemic lupus ertythematous (SLE), rheumatoid arthritis, and polyarteritis nodosa (Koffler 1979:11).

Preparation of Patient
And Collection of Sample

Both these tests require 10 ml of venous blood. The specimen for total hemolytic activity must be sent on ice.

Reference Values

Complement, total hemolytic activity	150–250 U/ml
C_3	55–120 mg/dl
C_4	20–50 mg/dl

Clinical Significance. An increase in the total complement activity occurs in some acute inflammatory diseases. Decreased serum levels of C_3 and C_4 indicate the presence of immune complexes that have used up the complement factors (assuming no inherited complement deficiencies).

Possible Nursing Implications. Although an increase in the amount of complement activity and a decrease in serum C_3 and C_4 indicate that immune complexes are being formed, the actual diagnosis may be very difficult to establish. These tests are likely to be only part of the assessment needed to help the physician establish a diagnosis of a rheumatoid disease. (See the following discussion on LE prep, ANA, and RF.)

A normal level of serum complement levels does not rule out the possibility of an immune reaction, since some antigen–antibody responses do not cause an activation and depletion of the complement factors. Much research is presently being done on the very complicated picture of immune response. Nurses must read current articles to obtain up-to-date information on the current status of immunological tests.

LE PREP

The LE prep is a microscopic examination for a particular type of neutrophil that has been changed due to the LE factor in the rheumatoid disease called systemic lupus erythematous (SLE). The LE factor evidently consists of antibodies that react with the cells. A direct test for antibodies to native DNA is a more sensitive test for SLE (Koffler 1979:14). Not all patients with SLE have a positive LE prep, and patients with other diseases, such as rheumatoid arthritis, may also have a positive test.

Preparation of Patient
And Collection of Sample

The test requires 5 ml of whole blood, which should be drawn in the early morning.

Reference Values

The test should be negative.

Possible Nursing Implications. This is only one of several tests and assessments to diagnose systemic lupus erythematous (SLE). Refer to a pathophysiology text for a detailed accoun of SLE.

ANTINUCLEAR ANTIBODIES (ANA)

Antinuclear antibodies are gamma globulins found in patients with certain types of autoimmune diseases. The test is typically used to rule out systemic lupus erythematous since most patients with SLE have a positive ANA. However, the test is not specific for SLE since the test may also be positive in rheumatoid arthritis, scleroderma, carcinoma, tuberculosis, and hepatitis. Various drugs may also cause an increased ANA.

Preparation of Patient
And Collection of Sample
The test requires 10 ml of clotted blood, which should be sent to the laboratory immediately.

Reference Values

Test is considered positive if detected with serum diluted 1:10.

Aged   ANA levels seem to increase with age even in people without immune diseases.

ANTI-DNA, ANTI-NATIVE DNA, AND ANTI-DNP

In addition to the antinuclear antibodies (ANA) test, several other tests of humoral antibodies, such as anti-DNA, anti-native DNA, and anti-DNP, are used to diagnose various immune diseases. Consult the current literature to find out more about the recent advances in the use of these tests. What is research today will perhaps be a common laboratory test in a few years.

Immunoelectrophoresis. The advent of immunoelectrophoresis has made it possible to identify many patterns of antibody activity in various pathological states (Cawley 1978). (See Chapter 10 for a discussion on immunoglobins.)

Rheumatoid Factor
(Latex Fixation or Agglutination Tests)
The rheumatoid factor is a test of abnormal proteins found in the serum of many patients with rheumatoid arthritis. Evidently the rheumatoid factor really consists of different types of IgM antibodies. (See Chapter 10 for the measurement of IgM.) Although the RF is present with other diseases, the highest titers are found in patients with rheumatoid arthritis. Koffler (1979) states that the RF is present in approximately 75% of patients with rheumatoid arthritis, but it does not always correlate with the severity of the disease activity.

These tests, which may involve agglutination either of sensitized sheep red blood cells or of latex particles covered with an antigen, are not specific for rheumatoid arthritis. Some "normal" people, particularly the elderly, may have the factor. Patients with tuberculosis, bacterial endocarditis, syphilis, and collagen diseases may have the RF. The RF also commonly occurs in both B and non-B hepatitis (London 1977).

Preparation of Patient
And Collection of Sample

Check with the laboratory for the type of test being done. Rheumaton (Wampole) is a diagnostic kit for testing for the RF.

Reference Values

Titers of 1:80 may be diagnostic of rheumatoid arthritis if other clinical data shows evidence of the disease.

Possible Nursing Implications. The patient with rheumatoid arthritis needs a lot of nursing care both during the acute stages and during remissions. Brown-Skeers (1979) gives some excellent tips on how nurse practitioners can manage patients with rheumatoid arthritis. The basis triad of treatment includes (1) physical therapy and exercises, (2) emotional and psychological support, and (3) monitoring of anti-inflammatory drug therapy. The erythrocyte sedimentation rate (ESR) (Chapter 2) is used to follow the disease process. The C-reactive protein may also be used to monitor the amount of inflammatory response over time.

THYROID COLLOID AND MICROSOMAL ANTIGEN TESTS

In certain types of thyroid disorders, the body produces antibodies against certain thyroid constituents. The end result is inflammation and destruction of the thyroid gland. Although the level of antibodies does not exactly correlate with the severity of the symptoms, identifying the probable cause of thyroid dysfunction is a help. (See Chapter 15 for a complete discussion on hypo- and hyperthyroidism, along with the tests used.) Relatives of patients with thyroid autoimmunity problems may also have high titers of the thyroid antibodies. Since other diseases, such as the collagen diseases, may cause increased titers too, the patient may also have other types of antibody tests.

Preparation of Patient
And Collection of Sample

The test requires 2 ml of serum. Because oral contraceptives may cause titers to become detectable, note whether the patient is on birth control pills.

Reference Values

Women	Titers should be absent or below 1:20. Have higher titers than men.
Aged	Titers increase with age, particularly in women.

Possible Nursing Implications. Nursing care depends on the underlying pathophysiology. See Chapter 15 for some general notes on care of the patient with a thyroid disorder that causes hyper- or hypothyroidism.

Questions

14–1. Serological tests for blood banking, microbiology, and immunology are based on which of the following principles?

   a. Antigens are always introduced into the body by an outside force, such as bacteria or foreign proteins.

   b. A seronegative test demonstrates probable immunity from a disease.

   c. A seropositive test is evidence of an existing antigen in the serum.

   d. A reaction between an antibody and antigen results in a recordable event.

14–2. A serological test reports a positive titer of 1:240. The number 1:240 is a measurement of the:

   a. number of the antibodies in the serum sample.

   b. last dilution at which a reaction took place between the diluted serum and the test antigen.

   c. ratio of antigens to antibodies in the serum.

   d. amount of antigen that was needed to cause a positive result in the blood sample.

14–3. Which of the following tests is not routinely done on a unit of donor blood?

   a. HB_sAg (hepatitis B surface antigen).

   b. Coombs (antibody screening).

   c. ANA (antinuclear antibodies).

   d. STS (serologic test for syphilis).

14–4. Mr. Royal has type AB blood. Theoretically, based on just the ABO typing, Mr. Royal could receive any type of blood because he has which of the following?

   a. No A or B antigens.

   b. No antibodies against A and B antigens.

   c. Only antibodies against O.

   d. Only AB antibodies.

14–5. Mrs. Tudor had a hemolytic transfusion reaction, possibly due to incompatible blood. She had fever, chills, and low back pain. The unit of blood was stopped and returned to the laboratory. The nurse should also save all urine voided for which reason?

      a. The urine needs to be checked for free hemoglobin.

      b. Dehydration must be prevented.

      c. A bilirubin test should be done stat.

      d. Circulatory overload may require use of a diuretic.

14-6. Mrs. Sanchez, who is Rh negative, just delivered a healthy 8-lb baby boy who is Rh positive. She was given an injection of RhoGam. She asks the nurse shy she had the shot. Which of the following explanations by the nurse is accurate? ''This shot . . .

      a. prevents you from having any problems with any other pregnancies because it eliminates the Rh factor.''

      b. gives you temporary antibodies against the Rh factor so that your body won't make any on your own, which could still be present if you have another Rh positive pregnancy.''

      c. helps to eliminate any antibodies that you might have gotten from this pregnancy so that the next pregnancy will be normal.''

      d. helps your body to manufacture antibodies, so that if you have another pregnancy with a Rh baby there won't be any problems.''

14-7. A positive Coombs test indicates coating of the erythrocytes by some type of globulin. Which of the following clinical situations is *not* assessed for by a positive Coombs test?

      a. Hemolytic disease of the newborn.

      b. Autoimmune hemolytic anemias.

      c. Hemolytic transfusion reactions.

      d. Administration of gamma globulin.

14-8. Mr. Wayler is a patient receiving renal dialysis three times a week. His laboratory test shows a positive report for HB_sAg (hepatitis B surface antigen). Mr. Wayler does not have any symptoms of hepatitis. Based on this data, which precaution should be instituted?

      a. None, since he has no evidence of clinical disease.

      b. Good handwashing technique after contact with Mr. Wayler.

      c. Use of gloves when any blood-contaminated articles must be handled.

      d. Administration of gamma globulin to staff who must work directly with Mr. Wayler.

14-9. Serologic tests for syphilis (STS) include screening tests and confirmatory tests. The test commonly used to confirm a positive screening test is which of the following?

      a. VDRL.   **c.** Wasserman.

      b. RPR.   **d.** FTA-ABS.

14–10. The school nurse has been asked to provide some information about syphilis to a group of teenage girls. Which of the following statements is *not* correct?

　　a. A blood test for syphilis should be done on anyone who had sexual contact with a person who has syphilis.

　　b. Syphilis is treated with a penicillin injection, or with other antibiotics if the person is allergic to penicillin.

　　c. Syphilis is a communicable disease that must be reported to the health department.

　　d. A positive laboratory test for syphilis is always indicative of active infection.

14–11. Mrs. Ritter has an acute respiratory infection. She is to have blood drawn for cold agglutinins, because she may have primary atypical pneumonia due to an infection with a PPLO (pleuropneumonia-like organism). Preparation for the cold agglutinins test includes which of the following?

　　a. NPO for eight hours.

　　b. Placement of blood sample into a 37°C bath for transport to the laboratory.

　　c. No special preparation.

　　d. Checking the patient's temperature and drawing the blood when there is a fever spike.

14–12. Febrile agglutinins are produced in response to certain types of bacterial infections, such as typhoid fever, brucellosis, or tularemia. What degree of change in titer is considered evidence of an acute infection?

　　a. A fourfold rise in titer.

　　b. A threefold rise in titer.

　　c. A twofold rise in titer.

　　d. Any increase in titer above a baseline.

14–13. Shirley Bowden is a college freshman who has been weak and very tired for a week. She has swollen lymph glands and a slight fever (100.6°F). The nurse practitioner in the student health service thinks Shirley may have infectious mononucleosis. Which of these laboratory tests is not used to help establish a diagnosis of infectious mononucleosis?

　　a. Heterophil antibody test (HAT).

　　b. Spot tests for mono.

　　c. WBC with a differential.

　　d. C-reactive protein.

14-14. ASO, anti-DNase B, and streptozyme (the serological tests for antibodies against group A-beta hemolytic streptococci) may be part of the data base for all the following pediatric patients except which?

a. Carolyn, age 10, who has just been diagnosed as having "strep" throat.

b. Billy, age 8, who has symptoms of possible rheumatic fever.

c. Tommy, age 14, who has acute glomerulonephritis.

d. Barbara, age 9, who has a history of repeated sore throats and joint pains.

14-15. Martha Leahy, age 25, is getting married next week. Her premarital blood test showed a negative titer of rubella antibodies. What should Martha do before she becomes pregnant?

a. Nothing, because a negative titer shows immunity to rubella.

b. Try to catch rubella by exposure to young children with measles.

c. Consult her physician about receiving the rubella vaccine if she becomes pregnant.

d. Ask her physician to give her the rubella vaccine now and practice some form of birth control for at least three months.

14-16. Ginny Jasper is to have a serology test for toxoplasmosis. Which of the following is a significant factor in her health history in relationship to the test for TPM?

a. Has had a tick bite.

b. Just moved from the San Joaquin Valley.

c. Has a cat.

d. Likes raw fruits and vegetables.

14-17. In the Ohio Valley area, where the fungus histoplasmosis is endemic, people who have positive skin and serology tests for histoplasmosis are:

a. highly susceptible to the fungus.

b. always carriers of the fungal disease.

c. always infected with the fungus.

d. showing evidence of some exposure to the fungus.

14-18. The laboratory test, Proteus Ox 19, is an indirect test for which?

a. Proteus infections.

b. Rickettsial diseases.

c. Protozoan infestations.

d. *Entamoeba histolytica.*

14-19. Which of the following tests is an alternative to the C-reactive protein test?

a. ESR (erythrocyte sedimentation rate).

b. ANA (antinuclear antibodies).

c. LE prep (lupus erythematous prep).

d. RF (rheumatoid factor).

14-20. Assuming that the patient does not have an inherited deficiency, a decrease in C_3 and C_4 serum levels indicates which of the following?

    a. An inability of the body to produce antibodies.

    b. The amount of antigen–antibody reactions that is occurring.

    c. The severity of the hemolysis of red blood cells.

    d. Decreased stimulation from antigens.

14-21. Which of the following is not used for assessment of the patient with possible systemic lupus erythematous (SLE)?

    a. LE prep.

    b. ANA (antinuclear antibodies).

    c. Anti-native DNA.

    d. Complement activity.

14-22. Patients with rheumatoid arthritis often have an increase of the rheumatoid factor (RF test), which is probably a type of IgM antibody. Patients with certain types of thyroiditis have antibodies against certain thyroid antigens (thyroid colloid and microsomal antigen test). Common to both of these tests of humoral antibodies is the fact that both of the tests are:

    a. diagnostic proof of a specific disease.

    b. directly correlated with the severity of the symptoms.

    c. thought to be evidence of some autoimmune process that is destructive in nature.

    d. no longer used for clinical assessment because they are totally nonspecific.

REFERENCES

Abramowicz, Mark. "The New Rubella Vaccine," *The Medical Letter on Drugs and Therapeutics* 21 (June 29, 1979): 53-54.

ACOG, Commission on Patient Education. *Important Facts About Veneral Diseases.* Chicago: American College of Obstetricians and Gynecologists, 1978.

Bauer, Deborah. "Preventing the Spread of Hepatitis B in Dialysis Units," *American Journal of Nursing* 80 (February 1980): 260-261.

Brown-Skeers, Vicki. "How the Nurse Practitioner Manages the Rheumatoid Arthritis Patient," *Nursing* 79 (June 1979): 26-35.

Buickus, Barbara. "Administering Blood Components," *American Journal of Nursing* 79 (May 1979): 937-941.

Cawley, Leo *et al. Electrophoresis and Immunochemical Reactions in Gel.* Chicago: American Society of Clinical Pathologists, 1978.

Claypool, Janet. "Rubella Protection for Maternal Child Health Care Providers" *Maternal Child Nursing* 6 (January/February): 1981.

Cullins, Laura. "Preventing and Treating Transfusion Reactions," *American Journal of Nursing* 79 (May 1979): 935-937.

Cutter Laboratory, "Product Information on Gamastan." Berkeley, Ca.: Cutter Biologicals, 1979.

Einstein, Hans. "Coccidioidomycosis," *Basics of RD* 9 (November 1980): 1-6.

Fitzmaurice, Joan. *Rheumatic Heart Disease and Mitral Valve Disease.* New York: Appleton-Century-Crofts, 1980.

Kazak, Aldona. "Processing Blood for Transfusion," *American Journal of Nursing* 79 (May 1979): 931-934.

Koepke, John. *A Guide to Clinical Laboratory Diagnosis,* 2nd ed. New York: Appleton-Century-Crofts, 1979.

Koffler, David. "The Immunology of Rheumatoid Disease," *Ciba's Clinical Symposia* 31 (4) (November 1979).

Lang, Gordon and Drozda, Edward. "Survey of Blood Ordering Practices for 12 Elective Surgical Procedures." *Wisconsin Medical Journal* 78: 27-31 January, 1979.

Lake, Kevin. "Lympho-glandular Toxoplasmosis: A Diagnosis Often Missed," *Post-Graduate Medicine* 65 (January 1979): 110-117.

London, W. T. "Hepatitis B Virus and Antigen-Antibody Complex Diseases," *New England Journal of Medicine* 296 (1977): 1528.

Luckmann, Joan and Sorensen, Karen. *Medical-Surgical Nursing,* 2nd ed. Philadelphia: W. B. Saunders Company, 1980.

Ortho Diagnostics. *The Rh Negative Mother Asks About RhoGam.* Raritan, N.J.: Ortho Diagnostics, 1969.

Ravel, Richard. *Clinical Laboratory Medicine,* 3rd ed. Chicago: Year Book Medical Publishers, Inc., 1979.

Roche, Christine. "At Last! Reliable Protection from Hepatitis B," *RN* 44 (September 1981): 79.

Strand, Marcella and Elmer, Lucille. *Clinical Laboratory Tests: A Manual for Nurses.* St. Louis, Mo.: C. V. Mosby Co., 1980.

Weinstein, Allan and Farkas, Stephen. "Serological Tests in Infectious Diseases: Clinical Utility and Interpretation," *Medical Clinics of North America* 62 (September 1979): 1099-1117.

Zuckerman, Arie. "Specific Serological Diagnosis of Viral Hepatitis," *British Medical Journal* 2 (6182) (July 14, 1979): 84-86.

CHAPTER FIFTEEN

Endocrine Tests

Objectives

1. Explain the concepts of negative feedback, circadian rhythms, and ectopic hormone production.
2. Give examples of how laboratory tests are used to assess the relationship of the anterior pituitary gland to other endocrine glands.
3. Determine the appropriate nursing assessments and interventions for a patient with increased or decreased serum cortisol levels.
4. Devise a teaching plan for parents who have a child with adrenogenital syndrome.
5. Identify the characteristic clinical manifestations of increased and decreased levels of serum aldosterone, including changes in renin activity.
6. Explain the purpose of 24-hour urine specimens for vanillylmandelic acid (VMA) and metanephrines.
7. Describe the clinical effect of an increased level of parathormone (PTH) and the major nursing intervention needed.
8. Explain the usefulness of TSH, T_4, T_3, and T_3 resin uptake in evaluating patients with hyper- or hypothyroidism.
9. Determine the appropriate nursing assessments and interventions for patients with increased or decreased serum thyroid hormones.
10. Explain why infants who may have hypothyroidism (cretinism) need immediate medical evaluation and treatment.
11. Identify the key nursing implication when a patient has altered levels of the sex hormones.

The brief discussions on the negative feedback system, circadian rhythms, ectopic hormone production, and other physiological information in this chapter should help the reader to better understand the tests that are done to measure hormone levels. In addition, the techniques for doing radioimmunoassay (RIA) and enzyme immunoassay (EIA) are briefly described since immunoassay methods have made it possible to measure all hormones by direct, rather than by indirect, methods.

Except for ectopic hormone production (discussed later) each hormone is produced by a specific endocrine gland, and each has a very specific function or functions. These functions are briefly discussed in relationship to the tests for each hormone. Refer to a physiology book for a detailed review of the functions of each hormone, if needed.

Table 15-1 gives an overview of the endocrine glands, the hormones produced by each gland, and how the hormones are tested by specific laboratory tests of blood and urine samples. The releasing factors (discussed in the following section) are not included in this table since, they are not normally measured.

TABLE 15-1. COMMONLY MEASURED HORMONES

Source of Hormone	Name of Hormone	Tests Used to Assess Hormone Levels
Anterior pituitary	1. Growth hormone (GH) or somatotropin (STH)	Serum GH levels
	2. Adrenocorticotropin (ACTH)	Serum ACTH levels; see section on adrenal gland for ACTH suppression and stimulation tests.
	3. Thyrotrophin (TSH)	Serum TSH levels; see section on tests of thyroid gland.
	4. Follicle-stimulating hormone (FSH) (one of the gonadotropins)	Serum and urine FSH levels; see section on sex hormones.
	5. Leutinizing hormone (LH); sometimes called interstitial-cell-stimulating hormone (ICSH) in male (the other gonadotropin).	Serum and urine levels; see section on sex hormones.
	6. Prolactin (PRL)	Serum prolactin not commonly done; see discussion on anterior pituitary.
	7. Melanocyte-stimulating hormone (MSH)	Serum MSH not usually measured directly; see discussion about increase of MSH with cortical lack.
Posterior pituitary	1. Antidiuretic hormone (ADH) or argine vasopressin (AVP)	Not commonly measured; see Chapter 4 on serum and urine osmolality.
	2. Pitressin or oxytocin	Not measured as diagnostic test; note that oxytocin is used in obstetrics as drug to induce labor.

(continued)

TABLE 15-1. *Continued*

Source of Hormone	Name of Hormone	Tests Used to Assess Hormone Levels
Adrenal cortex	1. Glucocorticoids (cortisol as major one)	Plasma and urine cortisol; 17-hydroxysteroids (17OHCS) or Porter-Silber test; see ACTH tests also.
	2. Mineralocorticoids (aldosterone as major one)	Serum and urine aldosterone levels; tests for renin activity; saralassin test; see Chapter 5 for serum levels of sodium and potassium.
	3. Sex hormones (androgens, progesterone, and estrogen)	Pregnanetriol in urine; 17 ketosteroids (17 KS) in urine.
Adrenal medulla	1. Norepinephrine	Catecholamines in urine; metaphrines in urine; vanillymandelic acid (VMA) in urine; norepinephrine and epinephrine are not commonly measured in serum; pharmacologic tests not commonly done anymore (i.e., Regitine).
	2. Epinephrine	
Parathyroid	1. Parathormone (PTH)	Serum PTH; serum and urine calcium and phosphate levels; see Chapter 7.
Thyroid	1. Calcitonin	Calcitonin not commonly measured; see Chapter 7 on serum calcium.
	2. L-thyroxine (T_4) and triiodothyronine (T_3)	T_4; T_3 resin uptake; T_3; free thyroxin index (FTI); TSH levels.
Pancreas	1. Insulin	See Chapter 8 for tests on glucose metabolisms.
	2. Glucogen	
Testes	1. Androgens	Serum testosterone; see 17 KS urine test for androgens.
	2. Estrogen and progesterone in minute amounts	Serum estrodial; see also tests for FSH and LH.
Ovaries	1. Estrogens	Serum estrodial; serum and urine estriol in pregnancy (see Chapter 18).
	2. Progesterone	Pregnanediol in urine.
	3. Androgens in minute amounts	17 KS for androgens; see also tests for FSH and LH.

BACKGROUND INFORMATION

Releasing Factors That Stimulate Anterior Pituitary

The central nervous system is very closely connected to the endocrine system because some releasing factors from the hypothalmus are carried to the pituitary gland through the venous system that connects the hypothalmus and the pituitary gland. Since hypophysis is another name for the pituitary gland, this venous system is thus called the *hypophyseal portal system*. These releasing factors from the hypothalmus stimulate the pituitary to release certain hormones. For example, thyrotrophin releasing factor (TRF) is sent from the hypothalmus to the pituitary gland. The pituitary gland is thus stimulated to release thyrotrophin-stimulating hormone (TSF), which in turns acts upon the thyroid gland to produce thyroxin.

At the present time, the existence of some of these factors has been documented, and it is hypothesized that there is probably some type of hypothalmus control for all the pituitary hormones (Juebiz 1979:8). Two of the releasing factors have been used diagnostically: the releasing factor for the gonadotropin hormones (FSH and LH) and the releasing factor for thyrotropin (TSH).

Currently, several releasing factors from the hypothalmus are being extensively studied in relation to the effect of various drugs. Locke (1978) names over thirty drugs that may affect the secretion of anterior pituitary hormones. The susceptibility of the hypothalmus–anterior pituitary system to drugs is taking on major clinical importance as more is being learned about the interaction of drugs and hormone levels.

Negative Feedback System for Endocrine Functioning

The anterior pituitary gland secretes hormones that act on specific target organs to cause the release of other hormones. For example, the pituitary releases ACTH, which then stimulates the adrenal gland to produce cortisol. When the cortisol reaches a certain level in the bloodstream, there is a suppression of continued secretion of ACTH from the pituitary. In other words, a high level of cortisol turns off the secretion of ACTH. Conversely, a low level of serum cortisol is a stimulus for the increased production of ACTH. This interplay, in which the increased level of one hormone causes a decrease in the level of the other hormone, is called *negative feedback*. The hormones from the adrenal cortex, thyroid gland, ovaries, and testes all have negative feedback systems with hormones from the anterior pituitary gland. Understanding negative feedback is important since tests for the suppression or stimulation of hormones are based on this physiological principle that levels of one hormone should change the level of another hormone.

Other Methods to Control Hormone Production

Not all hormones are controlled by a negative feedback system through the pituitary gland. For example, parathyroid hormone (PTH) is regulated by the serum calcium and phosphorus levels (see Chapter 7). A high level of serum calcium causes a suppression of the parathyroid hormone from the parathyroid gland. A decrease in the serum calcium level causes an increased production of the parathyroid hormone (PTH).

The intricate balance between too much and too little of a hormone is one of the wonders of the human body. In a healthy state, all hormones are kept within a precise range that can fluctuate as the body needs change. All hormones are interrelated to some degree, so changes in one hormone may affect the level of others, although not in as direct a fashion as in negative feedback.

Circadian Rhythms and Other Rhythms

A change in the levels of a hormone every 24 hours is called a *circadian* (around the day) *rhythm*. For example, cortisol is higher in the morning than in the evening. While cortisol seems to be relatively independent of the sleep pattern, growth hormone is strongly bound to the sleep pattern (Krieger 1979:36). Much research is being done to investigate which factors, other than activity patterns and sleep, regulate the normal variations every 24 hours. In addition to cortisol and growth hormone, aldosterone, prolactin, thyrotropin, testosterone, LH, and FSH all vary considerably during each 24-hour period. Krieger (1979) gives a detailed account of studies being done on the rhythms of hormones. Because the hormones do fluctuate, more than one blood sample or one urine specimen may be needed to get an accurate reflection of an individual's hormone level.

The female hormones, estrogen and progesterone, are, of course, on another rhythm that must also be taken into account in comparing reference values. Rhythms that are longer than circadian (24-hours) rhythms are termed *intradian rhythms*. In adult women, the menstrual cycle is an intradian rhythm, because the variations in FSH and LH are on a monthly, not on a daily, cycle. Besides the sex hormones, other hormones may fluctuate with menstrual cycles (Krieger 1979:267). In adult women, therefore, various hormones must be considered in relation to the menstrual cycle.

Ectopic Hormone Production

Most elevations of serum hormone levels are due to an overproduction by the specific endocrine gland. They can also occur if there is production of the hormone from a nonendocrine source. Hormones from nonendocrine sources are called *ectopic hormones* because they come from the wrong place or originate outside the normal pathway. For example, certain benign and malignant tumors are able to manufacture hormones that are very similar to the hormone produced by the endocrine gland. Certain types of neoplasms of the lung can secrete a form of ACTH. ACTH, MSH, gonadotropins, ADH, and PTH are the five most common ectopic hormones. Ryan (1979:41) lists seventeen different polypeptide hormones that can be produced by nonendocrine neoplasms.

In certain malignant states, hormones tests may be done to see if some of the symptoms are due to ectopic hormone production. For example, a tumor that produces parathyroid hormone (PTH) may cause symptoms of hypercalcemia. (See Chapter 7 for a discussion about hypercalcemia.) The physician may have to order a variety of tests to determine whether the symptoms of a hormone imbalance are due to the malignancy or to primary dysfunction of the endocrine gland.

Screening Tests and Definitive Tests for
Primary and Secondary Imbalances

In general, screening tests for hormone imbalances are done by measuring the concentration of the hormone in the serum. If the serum level is above or below the reference values, more definitive tests are done to find out whether the problem is in the gland itself. If the disorder is due to a problem in the gland itself, the disorder is called *primary*. If the endocrine imbalance is due to other causes, such as pituitary dysfunction, the endocrine disorder is termed *secondary*. For example, if hypothyroidism is due to the malfunction of the thyroid gland, the disorder is called primary hypothyroidism. If the hypothyroidism is due to pituitary insufficiency, the disorder is called secondary hypothyroidism. Laboratory tests that use drugs to stimulate or to suppress hormone production are useful in determining whether the disorder is primary or secondary (see Table 15–2).

The Technique of Radioimmunoassay (RIA)

By being able to identify very small amounts of chemicals, such as hormones or drugs, in the bloodstream, the laboratory technique of radioimmunoassay (RIA) has revolutionized the laboratory approach to testing for hormones. Rosalyn Yalow received a share of the 1977 Nobel Prize in Medicine and Physics for the development of the technique (Holum 1979:530). The method is considered very valuable because, before RIA, many substances, such as hormones, could not be detected by chemical means because the amounts in the serum are so small. Four elements are required for RIA:

1. an antibody to the hormone to be measured (the antigen),
2. a labelled or radio-tagged hormone,
3. a highly purified hormone standard, and
4. a method to separate the bound from the free hormone (Juebiz 1979:345).

Antigen. The hormone to be measured in the patient's blood is termed the antigen. Any substance can become an antigen if it is in pure enough form to elicit *specific antibodies* from the immune system. Thus drugs are also measured by the technique of RIA (see Chapter 17 on toxicology). The antibodies against the specific hormone (or other substances, such as drugs) are obtained by giving the antigen (hormone or drug) to animals, such as rabbits or guinea pigs.

Radio-Tagged Hormone. In addition to the antibodies to a specific hormone, the laboratory uses a small amount of radioactive material to tag a measured amount of the antigen.

TABLE 15–2.   SCREENING AND DEFINITIVE TESTS OF HORMONE FUNCTION

Screening Tests	Definitive Tests
Usually just measure the amounts of hormone in the serum.	Tests to suppress hormone function. Example, Dexamethasone to suppress cortisol production.
If hormone is elevated . . .	
If hormone is decreased . . .	
If hormone is normal, no further testing, unless clinical symptoms indicate (see text).	Tests to stimulate endocrine gland. Example, ACTH stimulation test of adrenal cortex.

Samples of the antibody and tagged antigen are mixed with a sample of the patient's blood. If the patient's sample has little of the hormone (antigen), most of the antigen–antibody complex is composed of the radioactive antigen. On the other hand, if the patient's blood sample contains a lot of hormone (antigen), this untagged hormone is what reacts with the antibody. So the antibody–antigen complex does not contain much of the radioactive-tagged antigen.

Hormone Standard. The laboratory has then to determine exactly what amount of the antibody–antigen reaction is due to antigens from the patient and what amount is due to the tagged antigen. To make that determination the laboratory technician measures the radioactivity of the antibody–antigen complex and compares this with known standards.

Extremely small amounts of hormones or other substances can be detected by RIA. These very small amounts are expressed as nanograms (10^9 g) or picograms (10^{12} g). A picogram is 1/10,000,000,000,000 of a gram! It seems incredible that such a tiny amount can be accurately measured, but with RIA even very minute amounts of an antigen are locked into the antigen–antibody complex.

Enzyme Immunoassay (EIA)

Laboratories may also use enzymes as labels in antibody–antigen reactions. The enzyme is tagged either to the antigen or to the antibody before they are mixed with the blood sample from the patient. The use of an enzyme as a tagging agent eliminates the need for a radioactive tag, and the tests are as sensitive to small amounts of the antigen (hormone or drug) as the radioactive assay. The enzyme method, as described by Galen (1978), has made it possible to make a test for thyroid hormone part of an automated system.

ANTERIOR PITUITARY GLAND

The seven different hormones secreted by the anterior pituitary gland are listed in Table 12–2. Two of these hormones, prolactin and MSH, are not discussed in this chapter since they are not routinely tested. Since prolactin is an essential hormone for breast feeding, studies of factors affecting breast feeding may require measurements of prolactin. Melanocyte-stimulating hormone (MSH) causes pigmentation of the skin. The clinical significance of increases in MSH, which occur in Addison's disease, is found in the section on the lack of cortisol (Addison's disease).

Four of the hormones from the anterior pituitary gland are stimulating hormones for other specific endocrine glands: ACTH for the adrenal gland, TSH for the thyroid gland, and FSH and LH for the ovaries and testes. Each of these four pituitary hormones has major clinical significance in testing done on the target glands. (See the discussion for each specific gland.) The last of the seven anterior pituitary hormones, growth hormone, is discussed before the others since it is not connected to a specific target gland.

GROWTH HORMONE (GH) OR SOMATROPIN

Growth hormone (GH), produced by the anterior pituitary, stimulates the growth of bone and other tissue. GH affects metabolism by increasing protein synthesis, decreasing carbohydrate utilization, and increasing fat mobilization. GH is higher in children, but it is present in smaller amounts all through life. GH levels are done to evaluate a lack of growth in the child. For the adult, measurement of GH is done as one assessment of pituitary function.

Several factors influence the production of GH. Diets low in protein cause an increased production of the hormone. Hypoglycemia also causes an increased surge of GH in the serum, and hyperglycemia causes a decreased production of it. Because GH production is suppressed by hyperglycemia and stimulated by hypoglycemia, tests for GH may involve the administration of a glucose load or an insulin injection. Since exercise and sleep also cause variations in plasma GH levels, the activity of the patient and the timing of the specimen are important to note. (For reasons that are still unknown, GH increases during sleep.)

Preparation of Patient
And Collection of Sample

The laboratory needs 1 ml of serum. The activity of the patient, including sleep patterns, needs to be normal. A baseline level is done with the patient fasting and at rest, although the patient should have been on a regular diet before the fasting period.

GH levels may also be drawn after the patient has been given L-dopa or an insulin injection. Several serum blood samples are drawn after the administration of insulin or L-dopa to see how much the GH increases. The problem with giving a test dose of insulin is that the patient may have symptoms of hypoglycemia (see Chapter 8 for symptoms of hypoglycemia).

In patients with GH excess, a glucose load may be given to demonstrate that the GH cannot be suppressed. The procedure may consist of a glucose tolerance test with simultaneous glucose and GH measurement. (See Chapter 8 for the procedure for glucose tolerance tests.)

Reference Values

Newborns	30–180 ng/ml
Children	Over 10 ng/ml
Adults (fasting and at rest)	Below 5 ng/ml See Appendix A for values after exercise and glucose loads.
Note	In adults, the usual values may be so low that the hormone cannot be detected by radioimmunoassay. Stimulation by L-dopa or insulin should increase GH to measurable levels.

With sample drawn at 8 AM after normal sleep.

Increased Level of Growth Hormone (GH)

Clinical Significance. Severe malnutritional states cause a prolonged elevation of GH. Various types of tumors, either benign or malignant, can cause excess secretion of GH. In children, an abnormal increase of GH causes *gigantism*. Increased GH after puberty brings about a distortion of bony structures since the bones are stimulated to grow. Growth hormone excess in the adult is called *acromegaly*.

Possible Nursing Implications. The patient with a pituitary tumor may have radiation or surgery to remove the tumor. Refer to nursing texts, such as Krueger (1976), for details on care of patients with pituitary disorders. An important point to remember in relation to increased GH levels is that hyperglycemia may be a clinical problem. An increased level of GH decreases the body's ability to handle glucose. (See Chapter 8 for more discussion on hyperglycemia.)

Decreased GH Serum Level

Clinical Significance. Lack of GH is due to hypofunction of the pituitary gland, which can result from a tumor, from trauma, or from an unknown cause. In the child, a lack of GH causes *dwarfism*. In the adult, although the lack of GH does not cause clinical symptoms, it may be associated with deficiencies of other pituitary hormones, so symptoms are related to the other deficiencies. Usually the lack of pituitary function in an adult is in the order of lack of growth hormone, hypogonadism, hypothyroidism, and adrenal insufficiency (Price 1978:688). Thus the first symptom of pituitary insufficiency may be related to the lack of production of the normal sex hormones. Hence a measurement of GH may be used to help in assessing the presence of hypopituitarism in the adult.

Sheehan's syndrome is a type of hypopituitarism that sometimes occurs after a complicated delivery with bleeding and shock. During the postpartum period, a thrombus may occur in the hypophyseal vessels, which causes a destruction of the pituitary gland.

Possible Nursing Implications. In the child, a lack of GH is treated medically by injections of GH so that the child develops normally. In infants, a lack of GH may create an immediate problem by causing hypoglycemia (Kaplan 1979:7). Older patients with a lack of GH may show symptoms of hypoglycemia only if they are fasting. Adults are not given injections of GH, but they may need replacement of other pituitary hormones, all of which can be replaced by parenteral injection. Also, the hormones from specific glands, such as thyroid, may be given. The nursing implications for specific hormone therapy are briefly covered in the discussion for each hormone.

ADRENAL CORTEX

The adrenal cortex secretes three types of hormones (see Table 15–3):

1. *The glucocorticoids:* The glucocorticoid that is usually measured in the plasma is cortisol, and free cortisol can also be measured in the urine. Also, various metabolites of the glucocorticoids can be measured in the urine as 17-hydroxysteroids (17-OHCS).
2. *The mineral corticoids:* The mineralocorticoid that is measured in the serum is aldosterone.
3. *The sex hormones:* The sex hormones that are produced by the adrenal cortex

TABLE 15-3. MAJOR EFFECTS OF THREE TYPES OF
HORMONES FROM ADRENAL CORTEX

Hormone	Major Effects
1. Glucocorticoids (cortisol)	Major effects on metabolism of carbohydrates, fats, and proteins. Suppresses immune response.
2. Mineralcorticoids (aldosterone)	Major effect on fluid and electrolyte balance. Increased retention of sodium and water. Decreased retention of potassium.
3. Sex hormones (androgens, progesterone, and estrogen)	Affect secondary sex characteristics but not as significantly as hormones from ovaries and testes.

include the androgens, progesterone, and estrogen. Both males and females have the male hormone (androgens, such as testosterone) and the female hormones (progesterone and estrogen). A measurement of androgens becomes important when there is hyperplasia of the adrenal gland, which increases the production of the sex hormones. A urine test, 17-ketosteroids (17-KS) is one way to determine an increase of sex hormones from the adrenal gland.

ACTH ADRENAL AXIS

Production of cortisol by the adrenal cortex is controlled by the ACTH-adrenal axis. Since ACTH and cortisol are related by the concept of a negative feedback system, when the plasma cortisol level is low, the pituitary is stimulated to produce ACTH. ACTH then causes an increased production of cortisol by the adrenal cortex. The increasing plasma cortisol level becomes the stimulus for the pituitary to discontinue the high levels of ACTH production. Homeostasis is maintained by the increases and decreases of ACTH, which keep a certain balance of cortisol in the serum. ACTH also causes an increased production of the sex hormones by the adrenal cortex, but this effect is usually not significant except in certain adrenogenital syndromes. (Androgen excess is discussed in the section on the clinical significance of decreased cortisol levels.) ACTH has little or no effect on the serum levels of the third type of adrenal cortex hormones, the mineralocorticosteroids, or aldosterone. Aldosterone is controlled by the renin-angiotension system, which is explained under the section on aldosterone.

ADRENOCORTITROPHIC HORMONE (ACTH)

The level of ACTH can be measured directly by radioimmunoassay (RIA). A measurement of ACTH helps to determine whether the lack of serum cortisol is due to hypofunction either of the adrenal cortex or of the pituitary. A baseline measurement may be done to help in assessing whether changes in serum cortisol are related to pituitary dysfunction.

The administration of certain drugs, such as insulin, dexamethasone (Decadron), and metryapone, are used either to stimulate or to suppress the production of ACTH. Each of these tests is discussed briefly, along with a summary of the clinical significance of the findings.

Collection of Sample
And Preparation of Patient

The baseline specimen is usually collected in the morning, for which the laboratory needs 5 ml of plasma. The specimen should be put on ice and sent to the laboratory immediately.

Reference Value

15–70 pg/ml

ACTH Stimulation Test
With Metyrapone

Metyrapone is a drug that interferes with the normal production of cortisol by blocking some enzymatic actions so that compound S is not converted to cortisol. Due to the negative feedback, a fall in plasma cortisol level should cause an increase in the level of circulating ACTH. If patients have pituitary insufficiency, however, the ACTH level is *not* increased, even with the blockage of cortisol production by metyrapone. Because several ACTH levels may be drawn after the administration of metyrapone, nurses must check with the individual laboratory for the exact timing of the specimens. Phenytoin (Dilantin) interferes with the test because the drug has a variety of endocrine effects. Estrogen compounds also interfere with the test.

ACTH Stimulation with Insulin

Because a drop in blood sugar normally causes an increased production of ACTH, insulin can be used to stimulate the production of ACTH. Insulin, however, is not used as frequently as metyrapone. One of the problems with using insulin as a test drug is that the patient must be watched carefully so that the hypoglycemia is not too severe. (See Chapter 8 for the symptoms and treatment of hypoglycemia.)

ACTH Suppression Test
With Dexamethasone (Decadron)

Normally, high plasma corticosteroid levels suppress the formation of ACTH (the negative feedback concept again). Dexamethasone (Decadron), which is a potent corticosteroid that suppresses the formation of ACTH, is given as a test to determine whether the patient continues to produce large amounts of cortisol after ACTH is suppressed. Patients with a hyperactive adrenal cortex (Cushing's syndrome) do continue to have high serum cortisol levels because the suppression of pituitary ACTH does not affect the hyperactive adrenal gland.

For screening purposes, 1 mg of dexamethasone is given orally at 11 PM (a patient who weighs more than 200 lbs takes a larger dose) to suppress ACTH formation. A serum cortisol is drawn the next morning at 8 AM. The plasma levels of cortisol should drop below 5 μg/100 ml. Urine levels of cortisol and other metabolites may be measured too.

(These tests are discussed later.) To confirm that ACTH suppression is not causing the expected drop in serum cortisol levels, the dexamethasone dosage may be increased and given for several days. Sometimes a barbiturate is given with the test dose so that stress is reduced (Ravel 1978:357).

Use of ACTH to Stimulate
Cortisol Production

Patients with suspected diseases of the adrenal cortex can be given a test dose of ACTH to determine whether ACTH causes an increased production of cortisol in the serum. A synthetic type of ACTH, called cosyntropin, may be given intravenously, intramuscularly, or, sometimes, infused over a period of hours. While the dosages used and the timing of the serum samples vary, nurses must follow the exact procedure for a particular institution. The administration of ACTH should stimulate the adrenal cortex to produce a plasma cortisol level of at least 30 to 45 μg/100ml. A lack of response to ACTH indicates primary hypofunction of the adrenal cortex.

CORTISOL PLASMA LEVELS

Cortisol is the glucocorticoid that is found in the largest concentration in the serum. Thus it is the one usually measured to gain information about the functioning of the adrenal cortex. Plasma cortisol has a diurnal variation, its levels being higher in the morning than in the evening. Baseline readings are done in the morning with the patient at rest. The timing of cortisol levels with suppression and stimulation tests are determined by the procedure of the particular laboratory.

Preparation of Patient
And Collection of Sample

The laboratory needs 1 cc of plasma. The specimen is usually drawn in the morning after the patient has been fasting. Evening samples may also require about three hours of fasting. Water is allowed. Because activity increases the level, the patient needs to be supine for two hours before the test. The administration of estrogens in contraceptive pills causes an increase in cortisol levels. Spironlactone (Aldactone) may also cause false positives.

Reference Values

There are no age or sex differences. Obese people do have higher levels. Activity also increases levels.

8 AM (patient at rest)   8 PM Below 10 μg/100 ml
5-25 μg/100 ml

Dexamethasone suppression should decrease cortisol levels to below 5 μg/100 ml.

ACTH stimulation should increase 8 AM cortisol levels 30–45 μg/100 ml.

Increased Serum Cortisol Level

Clinical Significance. Tests for ACTH suppression are necessary to distinguish whether the increased cortisol level is due either to ACTH overproduction by the pituitary or to increased production by the adrenal gland itself. An increase in cortisol can be either ACTH-dependent or ACTH-independent. A pituitary tumor can cause an increase of ACTH, which in turn causes an increased cortisol level. This type of cortisol increase is ACTH-dependent, and it is sometimes called Cushing's disease. Increases of serum cortisol from other causes are called Cushing's syndrome. (Cushing was an American endocrinologist who first described the characteristic signs and symptoms of cortisol excess.)

Plasma cortisol levels are increased independently of the pituitary gland when there is hyperplasia of the adrenal cortex. Hypersecreting tumors of the adrenal cortex may be malignant or benign.

Certain nonendocrine malignancies can also secrete ACTH, which can result in increased serum cortisol levels. (Note the earlier discussion on ectopic hormones.) Cushing's syndrome, or high plasma cortisol levels, can also be caused by the administration of corticosteroids over a long period of time. Long-term administration of cortisone causes a suppression of ACTH and an eventual atropy of the adrenal glands.

Possible Nursing Implications. The specific medical treatment for elevated cortisol levels depends on the etiology. The patient may have a battery of tests to determine whether there is a tumor of the pituitary or of the adrenal gland. If Cushing's syndrome is due to exogenous cortisol administration, the dosage of cortisone may be decreased. However, until the specific treatment is effective, the patient may have several problems related to the effects of cortisol excess. Sometimes difficult medical decisions must be made regarding the continuation of cortisone therapy. The problems created by the disease condition must be weighed against the untoward effects of the therapy.

Although detailed discussion of all the signs and symptoms of Cushing's syndrome is beyond the scope of this text, some of the most important implications for treating patients with elevated cortisol levels follow:

Decreased Resistance to Infection. Nurses must recognize that patients with cortisol elevations do not have a normal response to infections. Cortisol impairs antibody production and cellular immunity, qualities that are beneficial in the treatment of abnormal inflammatory responses, but detrimental in the face of an infection. Such patients may have little elevation of temperature or other response to a bacterial invasion. So they must be taught to avoid possible sources of infection.

Tendency for Hyperglycemia. Cortisol stimulates the formation of glucose from other substances, such as protein (gluconeogenesis), and it also interferes with the action of insulin. Patients may thus have problems with hyperglycemia. (See Chapter 8 for nursing implications with hyperglycemia.)

Negative Nitrogen Balance. High levels of cortisol cause a reduction in protein stores and, in children, suppression of growth. Wound healing is delayed. If cortisol levels are elevated for more than six months, the matrix of the bone may be upset, and calcium is lost, leading to osteoporosis (Blount 1974) With their healing diminished, patients need to be protected from falls or wounds.

Potential for Gastric Ulcers. Increased cortisol levels cause an increased secretion of hydrochloric acid and pepsinogen. There is also an inhibition of collagen formation and of other protective proteins in the gastric mucosa. The exact cause of gastric ulcers is not known, but ulcers are a risk of high cortisol levels. To protect the stomach mucosa, patients may be given antacids. Any signs of gastrointestinal bleeding should be reported at once. (See Chapter 13 for guaiac for occult gastrointestinal bleeding.)

Fluid and Electrolyte Imbalance. Depending on the level of cortisol increase, patients may have sodium retention and potassium excretion. (See the discussion on the effects of aldosterone.) They may also have elevated blood pressure, weight gain, and edema. (See Chapter 5 for the nursing implications for the patient with hypernatremia and/or hypokalemia.)

Changes in Body Image. Elevated cortisol levels cause a round, full face ("moon face") and a redistribution of fat deposits. Patients may have a buffalo hump on the back. Their trunks are obese, while their wasted muscles make the extremities thin. Females may become masculinized with unwanted hair and acne. All in all, the person is not what is usually considered physically attractive. Treatment helps to correct most of these body changes, but patients need help to cope with their altered body images.

Changes in Mood. Increased cortisol levels tend to cause hyperactivity. Patients may need to be cautioned about too much activity. There is an increased stimulation of the central nervous system, which can lead to convulsions. The person may have dramatic mood changes. Euphoria is often present, and psychotic behavior may occur. The family may need help in learning to deal with such wide mood changes.

Decreased Serum Cortisol Level

Clinical Significance. A subnormal level of cortisol in the plasma is known as Addison's disease. (One way to remember that Addison's disease involves a lack of cortisone is to remember that in *Add*ison's disease, one must *add* some cortisone.) The lack of cortisol in the serum may be due to primary hypofunction of the adrenal cortex, or it may be secondary to hypofunctioning of the pituitary. Infections such as tuberculosis may invade the adrenal cortex. Often the reason for the failure of the adrenal cortex cannot be discovered. These patients are likely to have symptoms not only of cortisol lack, but also of aldosterone deficiency.

Long-term administration of high doses of corticosteroids causes suppression of ACTH production and a resulting inactivity of these patients' own adrenal glands. There is some atrophy of the adrenal cortex so that the glands do not respond normally to the need for more cortisone in stesss. The inability of the adrenal cortex to increase production of cortisol during stress may cause a collection of symptoms known as an *Addisonian crisis*. If cortisol drugs are not withdrawn gradually (tapered off), the patient may have a lowered cortisol level before the adrenal glands can begin to function normally again.

See the separate section on congenital adrenocortical hyperplasia for an explanation of cortisol lack in newborns and young children.

Possible Nursing Implications. Patients with borderline adrenal cortex functioning may not have problems until they are faced with a stressful situation, such as surgery or some other physical or psychological trauma. Once the symptoms of a lack of cortisol and aldosterone are recognized and confirmed, replacement therapy is started. Until the hormones are replaced, or when the need is greater than the supply, these patients may have problems related to the lack of cortisol and aldosterone (Elliott 1974). Some of the nursing implications are described in relation to the potential problems.

Hypovolemia Due to Lack of Retention of Sodium and Water. A lack of cortisol and of the mineralcorticoid aldosterone causes low serum sodium levels, which may lead to hypovolemia. Thus patients with a lack of cortisol tend to get dizzy, and they may faint if they are gotten out of bed rapidly (postural hypotension). In more advanced cases, the lack of sodium retention can lead to hypovolemia that is severe enough to cause shock. (See Chapter 5 for the nursing implications for patients with hyponatremia.)

Hyperkalemia Due to Retention of Potassium. Cortisol and, even more so, aldosterone, cause sodium retention and potassium excretion. So in Addison's disease, when cortisol is low, not only is the serum sodium low, but the serum potassium rises. The serum potassium may or may not be high enough to cause symptoms. Certainly the patient should not be given additional potassium. (See Chapter 5 for the nursing implications for hyperkalemia.)

Hypoglycemia with Fasting States. Patients with a lack of cortisol are less able to maintain a normal blood sugar when there is no continual replacement of glucose. Thus patients with suspected cortisol deficiency may have symptoms of hypoglycemia if they fast. (See Chapter 8 for the signs, symptoms, and treatment of hypoglycemic episodes.)

Inability to Handle Stress (Addisonian Crisis). Patients with slightly low cortisol levels may be asymptomatic until faced with stress: They cannot cope with a crisis. The patient needs to be protected not only from physical stress, such as infections, but also from psychological stress, such as high levels of anxiety. In either case, since the adrenal cortex cannot produce enough cortisol and aldosterone, the person has an Addisonian crisis. The symptoms of an Addisonian crisis are the extreme of the problems already described. The patients become shocky from the lack of sodium and water in the plasma, while their serum potassium level increases. They have pain, nausea, and vomiting. Circulatory collapse and death can occur. Treatment of an Addisonian crisis includes the administration of cortisol intravenously, along with the replacement of sodium, chloride, and water.

Changes in Body Image. On the whole, a lack of cortisol does not cause as many physical changes as does an excess of cortisol. One characteristic of a lack of cortisol is pigmentation of the skin, because the lack triggers the release of the melanocyte-stimulating hormone (MSH). The exact reasons for the increase in MSH are not well understood. It is hypothesized that the lowered cortisol triggers the pituitary to produce not only more ACTH, but also MSH. Patients can be told that the darkening of the skin will fade when the cortisol level is brought back to normal.

If the cortisol lack is associated with a lack of androgens, there may not be many changes since most sex hormones are produced by the gonads. However, if only cortisol is lacking, the adrenal cortex may be stimulated to increase the production of androgens. This increase causes a collection of symptoms known as adrenogenital syndrome, which causes the masculization of females. (See the section on androgen levels.) In infants and children, congenital hyperplasia of the adrenal due to cortisol lack causes many body changes, as described in the section on adrenogenital syndrome.

Health Teaching on Life-Long Replacement Therapy. Patients with a lack of cortisol are placed on cortisone supplements. The majority of the dose is usually given in the morning since this is in keeping with the normal rhythm of the hormone (Grotch 1981). They may be taught to take the cortisone replacement with food or antacid. (See the discussion under excess cortisol for the symptoms possible with too high levels of cortisol.)

A mineralocorticoid may also be needed; fluorohydrocortidone (Florinef) is one that is given orally, while desoxycorticosterone (DOCA) is another that is given parenterally. The mineralocorticoid replacement is needed only when patients are deficient in aldosterone as well as in cortisol.

These patients need to carry identification that notes the need for extra cortisone in times of stress. They may also keep parenteral cortisone (Solu-Cortef) for emergency replacement. They may be taught to double their doses for minor stress and triple them for major stress, such as surgery (Burnett 1980:1308). The adult patient needs to know exactly how to recognize the need for more cortisone. Also parents need to know when to give extra medication to children. (See the discussion on congenital adrenal hyperplasia.)

ADRENOGENITAL SYNDROME DUE TO CONGENITAL ADRENOCORTICAL HYPERPLASIA

A congenital lack of certain enzymes can cause a decreased production of cortisol and sometimes of mineralocorticoids. At least six different inherited genetic defects cause a decreased synthesis of cortisol, and some of these defects also cause a lack of mineralocorticoids. Burnett (1980) describes in detail all six genetic defects.

The lack of cortisol causes an increased production of ACTH and hyperplasia of the adrenal gland. Even when the adrenal gland enlarges, it does not produce more cortisone, due to the genetic defect in manufacturing cortisol. However, the adrenal cortex is stimulated to produce more androgens and the precursors of hydrocortisone. In the infant or in the young child, while the increase in estrogens is not apparent, the increase in androgens causes masculization of the female and signs of early puberty in the male. In addition to the genetic defect that causes a lack of manufacturing of cortisol, there may be an associated inability to produce aldosterone. The children who also lack aldosterone are called *salt losers* because they are unable to retain sodium and water.

Nursing Implications.

Examining Newborns. Nursery nurses need to examine each newborn's genitalia for any abnormalities. Sometimes the female is incorrectly assumed to be a male. The infant may fail to thrive and have milk intolerances. The salt loser may have a very poor appetite, frequent vomiting, and other symptoms of severe fluid and electrolyte imbalance.

Assisting with the Assessments and Treatment of Older Children. Some children may seem normal at birth but show symptoms of a very early puberty. In these cases, diagnosing the lack of cortisol is important so that the increased androgen level does not create secondary sex characteristics. The female child may need surgery later, to repair an enlarged clitoris or fused vagina. The parents need reassurance that normal sexual functioning can be expected later. The child is tested for serum cortisol levels, which will be low. Urine tests are also done to evaluate the presence of metabolites of the glucocorticoids and the androgens in the urine. (These urine tests are covered next.) Treatment with cortisol and, if necessary, with a mineralcorticoid, reduces the level of ACTH and thus the hyperplasia of the adrenal cortex causing the excess of androgens.

Patient Teaching. Children with a cortisol lack and their parents need careful instruction on how to manage the replacement of cortisol. It is recommended that families always keep a plastic syringe, two needles, and an ampule of hydrocortisone (Solu-Cortef) in their automobiles and homes for emergency injections. Parents are told that a dose of Solu-Cortef, given unnecessarily, does not harm the child, but a delay in giving a dose could be fatal (McFarlane 1976:1292). Older children can be taught to recognize symptoms that indicate a need for more hydrocortisone. Burnett (1980) describes a case study of a child with cortisol lack and how he managed to live with the disease.

URINARY MEASUREMENT OF
THE ADRENAL CORTEX STEROIDS

Free urinary cortisol, as well as various metabolites of the adrenal cortex hormones, can be measured by 24-hour urine specimens. In general, the urine excretion of steroids is increased when the serum levels of the steroids are increased and decreased when the steroids are low in the serum. Sometimes creatinine measurements are done on the urine sample too, to ensure that the volume of urine is normal.

Very important is that all urine for 24 hours be saved (see details for urine collections in Chapter 3.) The nurse should check with the laboratory to see if any preservative is needed. The urine specimens are kept cold to decrease bacterial growth. These urine specimens may be ordered as part of the test of ACTH suppression or ACTH stimulation.

URINARY CORTISOL LEVELS

This test, which measures cortisol itself rather than the metabolites, may be preferable in certain types of screening for Cushing's syndrome. It is a rather expensive test, and various drugs may interfere with the results.

Reference Values

20–70 μg/24 hours

17-HYDROXYSTEROIDS (17-OHCS)
(PORTER-SILBER TEST)

This urine test, sometimes called the Porter-Silber test, measures several of the metabolites of both the glucocorticoids and aldosterone. These metabolites are increased in Cushing's syndrome. The administration of ACTH should cause a rise in the 17-OHCS too. These metabolites are decreased in Addison's disease and in the adrenogenital syndrome of lack of cortisol. Abnormal values can be caused by hepatic or renal dysfunctions. Chlorpromazine and related drugs interfere with assay. The specimen should be kept cold.

Reference Values

All groups	3–8 mg/24-hour urine specimen
Females	Slightly lower than males due to less muscle mass and body weight.

17-KETOSTEROIDS (17-KS)

The 17-ketosteroids are metabolites of the steroids from both the adrenal cortex and the testes. Thus the values for men are considerably higher after puberty. The values are increased in tumors when production of hormones from the adrenal cortex or the testes is increased. These metabolites are also increased in the adrenogenital syndrome. Hypofunctioning of the adrenal gland and certain adrenal adenomas cause a decrease. Meprobamate and many other drugs may make the test invalid. So check for possible drug interferences if the patient is receiving any drugs. The urine should be kept cold.

Reference Values

	Male	Female
	(mg/24-hour urine specimen)	
Age 10	1–4	1–4
20	6–21	4–16
30	8–26	4–14
50	5–18	3–9
70	2–10	1–7

17-KETOGENIC STEROIDS (17-KGS)

The 17-KGS test measures several of the glucocorticoid derivatives, as well as pregnanetriol, which is a precursor in adrenal corticoid synthesis. The 17-KGS are elevated when there is increased production by the adrenal gland, whereas they are low if there is hypofunction of the adrenal cortex. Since 17-KGS include the 17-OHCS, they are reflective of a more total steroid measurement.

Reference Values

All groups	5–20 mg/24 hours

URINARY PREGNANETRIOL

Since pregnanetriol is a precursor in adrenal corticoid synthesis, this test is useful in confirming the presence of the adrenogenital syndrome due to a lack of an enzyme to make cortisol. (Pregnane*di*ol is a test of progesterone. See the section on gonadtropins.)

Reference Values

Adults	4 mg/24-hour urine specimen
Children:	
2 weeks to 2 years	0–0.2 mg/24-hour specimen
Ages 2–16	0.3–1.1 mg/24-hour specimen

ALDOSTERONE

Aldosterone, a hormone produced by the adrenal cortex, is a mineralocorticoid. Increases in aldosterone cause an increase in the extracellular fluid volume because aldosterone increases the reabsorption of sodium and chloride by the proximal renal tubules, while increasing the excretion of potassium and hydrogen ions.

Aldosterone is not regulated by ACTH, as are the glucocorticoids. A decrease in extracellular fluid causes an increased production of aldosterone through stimulation of the renin-angiotensin system. A decreased flow of blood through the kidney is a stimulus for the production of renin, a hormone secreted by the kidney. Renin, when secreted into the bloodstream, acts on angiotensinogen to form angiotensin. (Angiotensinogen is formed in the liver and circulates in the plasma.) Angiotensin then stimulates the adrenal cortex to increase production of aldosterone. Thus a drop in extracellular volume is corrected by the final action of retaining more sodium and water in the plasma. Conversely, an increased extracellular volume is a signal for less production of renin. Without renin, angiotensinogen is not converted to the active form of angiotensin, so the adrenal cortex decreases production of aldosterone. Less aldosterone means less sodium (and water) retention, and so the extracellular fluid volume is decreased to normal again. See Table 15-4 for a simple diagram of the regulation of aldosterone and the related laboratory tests.

Preparation of Patient
and Collection of Samples

The patient needs to be on a regular diet with the usual intake of sodium and potassium. The patient may be put on a specific sodium diet of 10 mEq, 110 mEq, or 210 mEq. With

TABLE 15–4.   THE RENIN ANGIOTENSIN CONTROL OF ALDOSTERONE*

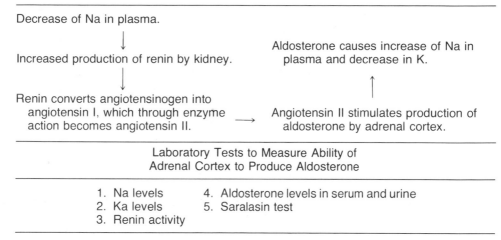

Decrease of Na in plasma.

Increased production of renin by kidney.

Renin converts angiotensinogen into
angiotensin I, which through enzyme
action becomes angiotensin II.

Aldosterone causes increase of Na in
plasma and decrease in K.

Angiotensin II stimulates production of
aldosterone by adrenal cortex.

Laboratory Tests to Measure Ability of
Adrenal Cortex to Produce Aldosterone

1. Na levels
2. Ka levels
3. Renin activity

4. Aldosterone levels in serum and urine
5. Saralasin test

*See Cryer (1979) for more detail.

more sodium in the diet, the reference values are lower. The dietician must plan the diet if a specific sodium intake is to be followed before the urine and plasma samples are collected.

The laboratory needs 3 ml of plasma or serum for the specimen. The plasma specimen is taken after the patient has been resting in the supine position for at least two hours. The peak concentration of aldosterone is in the early morning sample. A 24-hour urine specimen may also be collected, and it needs to be kept cold. (See Chapter 3 on 24-hour urine collection.)

Reference Values

All groups	Fasting, at rest, 110 mEq sodium diet. Values differ with various intakes of sodium.
Plasma level	107 ± 45 pg/ml
Urinary excretion for 24 hours	5–19 μg

Note: In addition to direct measurement of aldosterone levels, serum and urine levels of sodium and potassium are measured too. (See Chapter 5 on electrolyte measurements in serum and urine.)

Increased Aldosterone Levels in Serum and Urine (Hyperaldosteronism)

Clinical Significance.   Increased levels of the hormone aldosterone can be either primary or secondary. In primary hyperaldosteronism, a tumor of the adrenal cortex causes an increased secretion of aldosterone. The renin level in the serum is low because the increased production of the hormone is not due to the renin-angiotensin mechanism. (The test for renin is discussed next.) Note that oral contraceptives may also cause an increase aldosterone level. (See Appendix D.)

Secondary hyperaldosteronism is a much more common clinical problem (Ryan 1980). In this type of hyperaldosteronism, the oversecretion of aldosterone is due to the continual activity of the renin-angiotensin system. This constant stimulation of the system occurs when the perfusion to the kidneys is not adequate. For example, patients with congestive heart failure (CHF) often have poor renal perfusion. A lack of pressure in the juxtaglomerular apparatus causes the kidney to secrete more renin because the kidneys interpret the lack of perfusion as a lack of extracellular fluid. Renin activates angiotensin, which stimulates aldosterone production. Unfortunately, in congestive failure, the extracellular fluid is already in abundance. So the increased aldosterone level, as a response to poor renal perfusion, does not correct the underlying problem. With secondary hyperaldosteronism, the renin level is therefore high.

Not all cases of increased aldosterone are so simple. Sometimes drugs, such as oral contraceptives, cause an increase in aldosterone levels, although the exact mechanism is not well understood. Patients with severe liver dysfunction, such as in cirrhosis, tend to have elevated aldosterone levels too, which are partly related to poor renal perfusion. Also, if a failing liver can no longer detoxify aldosterone, levels of serum aldosterone remain higher for longer periods.

Nursing Implications.

Assisting with Diagnostic Work-Ups for Primary Aldosteronism. The patient may have several tests done, such as the renin level (discussed next), to determine whether the increased aldosterone is due to a primary cause. Electrolytes (Chapter 5) are closely monitored, and nursing is geared to correcting any imbalance. The adrenal gland may be tested by scans to detect tumors. Surgery is done for primary aldosteronism.

Ways to Prevent Edema with Secondary Aldosteronism. The testing for aldosterone is more of academic interest than of clinical usefulness in patients with such diseases as congestive heart failures. Nursing is based on the standard care for patients with poor cardiac function. Because aldosterone causes increased sodium and water retention, these patients need to have their blood pressure monitored.

If the increased aldosterone level is due to secondary causes, edema is usually a clinical problem. (See Chapter 5 for a discussion of the nursing implications when a patient has edema and needs to be on a restricted sodium diet.) Diuretics may be particularly useful for secondary hyperaldosteronism. The type of diuretic often used is spironolactone because this drug is an aldosterone-blocking agent. Spironolactone (Aldactone) is a steroid compound that presumably acts by competing with aldosterone for cellular receptor sites in the tubules. Thus it promotes sodium and water excretion without a loss of potassium.

Decreased Aldosterone Levels

Clinical Significance. The decrease in aldosterone is often part of a generalized hypofunctioning of the adrenal gland. The causes of Addison's disease were discussed in the section on cortisol deficiencies. In congenital adrenal hyperplasia, the infant lacks an enzyme needed to manufacture cortisol from cholesterol, and this deficiency may or may not be associated with a deficiency of aldosterone. In the most common type of genetic defect that causes a lack of cortisol, about one-third of the patients are also deficient in mineralocorticoid or aldosterone (Burnett 1980). The lack of aldosterone gives the symptoms of "salt wasting" seen in some genetic defects and in Addison's disease.

Possible Nursing Implications. Patients with decreased aldosterone levels are unable to maintain normal serum sodium levels. (See the discussion on Addisonian crisis under the section on low cortisol levels.) They must therefore have salt, water, and mineralocorticoid replacement. If they lack aldosterone, they must take fluorocortisone (Florinef) orally or desoxycorticosterone (DOCA) parenterally to ensure mineralocorticoid activity. These medications are continued for life. Because a lack of mineralocorticoid activity may also be part of the adrenogenital syndrome, children who experience salt wasting as part of their congenital problem must have replacement too. Children born with severe lacks of mineralocorticoids may die, however, before the defect is recognized (Kaplan 1980).

RENIN

Renin is an enzyme produced by the juxtaglomerular apparatus in response to a decreased blood flow through the kidneys. A change from the recumbent position to upright also causes an increased production. A high-sodium diet causes a decrease in renin. Thus diet and the position of the patient must be taken into account when using reference values for renin activity.

Preparation of Patient
And Collection of Sample

Because the values of renin are normally higher in the morning, the test is done early. The patient is usually in the supine position when the blood is drawn. The laboratory needs 4 ml of plasma, which is put into a tube with EDTA as an anticoagulant (lavender Vacutainer). The specimen should be iced. Diuretics cause changes in the values; so make note of the use of any medications on the lab slip. Also note the sodium content of the diet.

Reference Values

Supine	1.1+ or −0.8 ng/ml/h
Upright	1.9+ or −1.7 ng/ml/h

* Low-sodium diets cause an increased production of renin activity.

Changes in Renin Activity

Clinical Significance. Renal disease and low renal perfusion cause an increase in renin activity.

Use of Saralasin to Assess Renin Activity. Saralasin, a competitive antagonist of angiotensin II, is sometimes used as a clinical bioassay of the renin system. Weber (1979) describes the use of saralasin testing for renin-dependent hypertension. A drop in blood pressure is expected if the hypertension is renin-dependent.

ADRENAL MEDULLA:
CATECHOLAMINES AND THE
METABOLITES OF THE CATECHOLAMINES

The adrenal medulla secretes epinephrine and norepinephrine, both of which are essential in assisting the body for the "fight-or-flight" response to stress. These two hormones, called the catecholamines, are usually measured in 24-hour urine samples rather than in plasma samples.

Catecholamines are broken down into intermediate metabolites, which are called normetanephine and metanephrines. Laboratories may also measure these intermediate metabolites in the urine. The main product of catecholamine breakdown is an acid called vanillylmandelic acid (VMA). Since the VMA test is easier to do than the other urine tests for catecholamines, the laboratory may use the VMA as the screening procedure. The other tests of metabolites, such as the metanephrines, may be elevated even if the VMA is not. Thus more than one of the urine tests may be done to confirm a diagnosis of increased catecholamine secretion (Juebiz 1979).

Preparation of Patient
And Collection of 24-hour Urine Specimen

All the tests for the metabolites of the catecholamines require that the urine remain very acid with a pH of 3 or below. Usually 12 ml of hydrochloric acid (HCl) is added to the 24-hour specimen bottle. The usual procedure for collecting urine for 24 hours is followed (see Chapter 3).

The patient needs to be relatively free of stress. Vigorous exercise causes an elevation of catecholamines.

Nurses must validate the need for restriction of certain foods by checking with the specific laboratory doing the test. The patient should be on a regular diet since fasting increases catecholamines. Depending on the procedure used by the laboratory, certain foods must be restricted in the diet. For example, coffee, tea, chocolate, bananas, avocados, and anything with vanilla interferes with the VMA results. Newer laboratory methods are not affected by food intake.

A multitude of drugs also lead to confusing results. Drugs that act via the sympathetic nervous system, such as some antihypertensives and antidepressants, make the test invalid. Ideally, the patient needs to be off all drugs for three to seven days before the test. Nurses must check with the individual physician to see which drugs can be given.

Reference Values

Catecholamines in Urine	
Epinephrine	Under 20 μg/24-hour urine specimen
Norepinephrine	Under 100 μg/24-hour urine specimen
Metanephrines	0.3–0.9 mg/24-hour urine specimen
Vanillylmandelic Acid (VMA)	
Up to 9 mg/24-hour urine specimen	

Increased Catecholamines in Urine

Clinical Significance. Mild elevations of the catecholamines and of their metabolites can be due to stress such as surgery, burns, or childbirth. (Obviously, any endocrine response cannot be effectively evaluated during stress.) A marked increase in the catecholamines has two major causes: The first, a tumor of the adrenal medulla called a pheochromocytoma, causes a marked elevation of the catecholamines. The other comes from certain types of malignancies, called neuroblastomas, which arise from primitive sympathetic tissue (Kaplan 1979). Other tests, such as scans, help to pinpoint the presence of a tumor.

Pharmacologic Tests for Diagnosing Pheochromocytoma

One of the effects of catecholamines, as adrenergic substances, is to elevate the blood pressure. So a test for the presence of elevated catecholamines involves the administration of an adrenergic-blocking agent such as phenlolamine (Regitine). Such an agent should cause a significant drop in elevated blood pressure that is due to high levels of norepinephrine and epinephrine (adrenalin) in the bloodstream. Other drugs can be used to cause an additional release of the catecholamines. These pharmacological tests are difficult to standardize, and the results are not always reliable as a diagnostic aid. In addition, patients run some risk when their blood pressure suddenly decreases or increases. Since catecholamines and their metabolites can now be accurately measured in the urine, these older, less reliable drug tests are rarely indicated (Cryer 1979:131). Older nursing textbooks may still refer to Regitine tests.

Elevated Catecholamines

Possible Nursing Implications.

Assessing for the Effects of Increased Catecholamines. Patients with elevated catecholamines have symptoms reflective of the stimulating effects of epinephrine and norepinephrine. Often their symptoms can be attributed to other causes. Some of the outstanding symptoms are increased blood pressure and pulse. Since patients may feel very jittery and notice heart palpitations, their symptoms may be wrongly ascribed to an anxiety attack. The surge of catecholamines may be intermittent, so that, during an attack, the blood pressure may become very high and the patient can have pounding headaches, nausea, and vomiting. The high levels of epinephrine can cause hyperglycemia and glycosuria, and the patient may be suspected of having diabetes. (See Chapter 8 on symptoms of hyperglycemia.)

Nurses should carefully monitor the blood pressure and pulse of any patient with suspected catecholamine increase due to pheochromocytoma or a childhood neuroblastoma. They need to watch for any symptoms that help to confirm the presence of high levels of catecholamines. A blood or urine sample, taken during or soon after an attack, may demonstrate the presence of high levels of catecholamines.

Assisting with Surgical Interventions. Once a tumor has been diagnosed, the patient has surgery, and care is based on the standard postoperative needs of the patient (Tucker 1980).

Catecholamine Deficiency

Clinical Significance. Even when the adrenal medulla is hypofunctional or destroyed by disease or surgery, the patient does not have any symptoms of catecholamine deficiency because catecholamines are also produced by the autonomic nerve endings (Juebiz 1979:370).

PARATHORMONE (PTH)

Parathyroid hormone, or parathormone (PTH), is produced by the parathyroid glands—the only hormone secreted by these glands. The parathyroid glands, usually four in number, are located in the vicinity of the thyroid gland. Unlike many of the other hormones, the level of PTH is not under the influence of the pituitary gland.

The function of PTH is to control serum calcium and phosphorus levels (see Table 15–5). Hence the level of PTH depends on the serum calcium and phosphorus levels. A lowered serum calcium level is a stimulus for the release of more PTH to keep the serum calcium level normal. PTH works various ways to keep a constant serum calcium level and a correspondingly normal phosphorus level:

1. It works in concert with vitamin D to stimulate calcium and phosphorus absorption via the intestinal mucosa.
2. It causes mobilization of calcium from the bone.
3. It also causes increased excretion of phosphorus in the urine.

An abnormal elevation or decrease in PTH always causes changes in the serum calcium and phosphorus levels. (See Chapter 7 for a detailed discussion of the effects of PTH on serum calcium and phosphorus levels. Note that phosphorus is measured as phosphate in the serum.)

Preparation of Patient
And Collection of Sample
The patient does not have to be fasting. Collect an AM sample. The laboratory needs 5 ml of plasma, which should be kept on ice in all cases or, if it must be sent a distance, frozen. (Samples are often shipped because the test is difficult to do in most laboratories.)

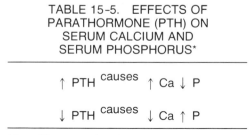

TABLE 15–5. EFFECTS OF
PARATHORMONE (PTH) ON
SERUM CALCIUM AND
SERUM PHOSPHORUS*

$$\uparrow \text{PTH} \xrightarrow{\text{causes}} \uparrow \text{Ca} \downarrow \text{P}$$

$$\downarrow \text{PTH} \xrightarrow{\text{causes}} \downarrow \text{Ca} \uparrow \text{P}$$

*See Chapter 7 for discussion of calcium and phosphorus levels in serum.

Reference Values

All groups	Less than 10 μEq/ml

Increased PTH Serum Level

Clinical Significance. Increased PTH levels may indicate primary hyperparathyroidism. Tumors of the parathyroid, which are usually benign, cause increased secretion of PTH. These patients have symptoms of high serum calcium levels and low phosphate levels (as discussed in Chapter 7). A persistently low serum calcium level or a high phosphate level causes a secondary rise in PTH. Also, malignant tumors from nonendocrine sources can secrete PTH. (See the discussion on ectopic hormones.)

Possible Nursing Implications.

Assessing for the Effects of Hypercalcemia. Since an elevated PTH causes an increased serum calcium level and a decreased serum phosphate level, the nursing implications are based on these imbalances. (See Chapter 7 for the nursing implications when a patient has hypercalcemia.)

Assisting with Surgical Inventions. If the patient has a parathyroid adenoma, surgery is done. Tucker (1980) gives standard guidelines for the postoperative parathyroidectomy patient.

Decreased PTH Serum Level

Clinical Significance. Decreased levels of PTH can be due to trauma to the parathyroid glands during a thyroidectomy. Infections or other traumas may affect the parathyroid gland. Tumors of the gland usually also cause an increase in hormone production, but some tumors may cause a decreased function of the gland. Since the levels of PTH are normally low in the serum, a low level may not be helpful in diagnosis.

Possible Nursing Implications.

Assessing for Hypocalcemia. The symptoms and clinical manifestations of a lack of PTH are reflected in low serum calcium levels and in high phosphate levels. Severe hypocalcemia causes tetany. (See Chapter 7 for a detailed description of tetany.)

Assisting with Replacement of Calcium and Vitamin D. A lack of PTH is treated by the administration of vitamin D and calcium salts. (See Chapter 7 on the treatment of low serum calcium levels and possible patient teaching.)

THE THYROID GLAND

The thyroid gland secretes three hormones: T_3, T_4, and calcitonin. Calcitonin lowers the plasma calcium level by inhibiting mobilization of calcium from the bone. (See Chapter 7 on the role of calcitonin in the regulation of calcium levels.) The other two of these hormones, T_3 and T_4, are forms of thyroxine, and they are usually called the *thyroid hormones*. (The T_3 contains *three* iodine molecules, and T_4 contains *four* iodine molecules in an atom.) An adequate intake of iodine is necessary for the continual formation of T_3 and T_4. As with the other hormones, protein intake must be normal too. In many countries, table salt has been iodized so that people have an adequate intake of iodine.

Most of the thyroid's output is in the form of T_4; only a small amount is in the form of T_3, but T_3 is much more potent than T_4. Both T_4 and T_3 can be measured directly. Also, the amount of T_4 can be calculated by other tests such as the T_3 resin uptake. Each of these tests is discussed individually later in this section. The thyroid hormones, T_4 (L-thyroxine) and T_3 (triiodothyronine), have several functions:

1. They potentiate the effects of epinephrine and decrease the serum cholesterol level.
2. They are necessary for normal development of the central nervous system.
3. They stimulate growth and normal metabolism in all cells.

Tests to Diagnose
Hypothyroidism and Hyperthyroidism

No one diagnostic test can be used alone to diagnose hypo- or hyperthyroidism. (Table 15–6 summarizes changes in various tests of thyroid function.) Also, thyroid tests are not useful for several months after I_{131} therapy (Soler 1979). T_4 is considered to be the basic screening test in most cases of suspected thyroid disease. In addition to the T_4, T_3, T_3 resin uptake, and TSH, the patient may also have thyroid scans and radioactive iodine uptakes done. Cancer of the thyroid is suggested by cold nodules on a thyroid scan and not by thyroid tests (Guimond 1979).

Older tests, such as the protein bound iodine (PBI) and the basal metabolic rate (BMR), have become obsolete since T_3 and T_4 can be measured directly. Hence they are not discussed in this book. Nonetheless, since PBI and BMR were once used to diagnose hyper- and hypothyroidism, older nursing texts may still mention them.

Because the thyroid hormones increase the metabolism of cholesterol, patients with

TABLE 15–6. TESTS OF THYROID FUNCTION

Test	Hypothyroidism	Hyperthyroidism
TSH (thyroid-stimulating hormone)	↓ or ↑ (see text)	↑ or ↓ (see text)
T_4 (L-thyroxine)	↓	↑
T_3 (triiodothyronine)	Not usually done	↑
T_3 resin uptake	↓	↑
FTI (free thyroxin index)	↓	↑
RAI (radioactive iodine uptake)	↓	↑
Thyroid scans	Used to identify nodules not hypo or hyper states per se.	

hyperthyroidism tend to have low serum cholesterol levels, and patients with hypothyroidism tend to have high serum cholesterol levels. (See Chapter 9 on cholesterol tests.) Yet the cholesterol level is not particularly helpful in confirming the presence of a thyroid disorder.

Certain types of thyroid inflammations are associated with increased amounts of antibodies. (See Chapter 14 for a discussion on auto-antibodies against thyroid tissue, the antimicrosomal antibodies.)

THYROID-STIMULATING HORMONE (TSH)

The production of the thyroid hormones, T_4 and T_3 (but not calcitonin), is controlled by the thyroid-stimulating hormone (TSH) from the anterior pituitary gland. In turn, TSH is released from the pituitary in response to the thyrotrophic-releasing hormone (TRH) in the hypothalmus. Thus, like most of the other anterior pituitary hormones, TSH is sensitive to nervous response from the hypothalmus. Measurement of TSH is useful in determining whether hypothyroidism is due to primary hypofunction of the thyroid gland or to secondary hypofunction of the anterior pituitary gland. In sophisticated endocrine work-ups, the thyrotopin-releasing factor (TRH) from the hypothalmus can be measured too (Juebiz 1979).

Preparation of Patient
And Collection of Sample
The laboratory requires 2 ml of serum. The patient does not need to be fasting.

Reference Values	
All groups	0.5 to 3.5 μU/ml

Increased or Decreased TSH

Clinical Significance. The purpose of measuring TSH is to evaluate the possibility of pituitary failure as the cause of hypothyroidism. A low TSH is an indication for further investigation of pituitary disorders. Primary hypothyroidism, due to insufficiency of the thyroid gland itself, is a much more common cause of hypothyroidism. In primary hypothyroidism, the TSH level becomes greatly elevated in an attempt to stimulate the failing thyroid gland. In hyperthyroidism, the TSH level is suppressed due to the negative feedback system. Yet this test is not useful as a diagnosis of hyperthyroidism because in some people with normal thyroid functioning (euthyroid) the TSH is barely if at all detectable. Cryer (1979) discusses in detail the use of a TSH stimulation test and the use of thyrotropin-releasing hormone (TRH). The TSH measurement is done on newborns who have low T_4 levels as confirmation of primary hypothyroidism (Fisher 1979).

L-THYROXINE (T_4) SERUM CONCENTRATION

T_4, the thyroxine with four iodine molecules, is the most abundant of the thyroid hormones. The test of T_4 measures both free thyroxine and the portion carried by the thyroid-binding plasma proteins. (See the test for thyroid-binding globulins.) The T_4 is the test used most often for screening and follow-up of patients who have been diagnosed as having either hypo- or hyperthyroidism.

T_4 can be measured by radio- or enzyme immunoassay. Radioimmunoassay is the more costly of the two methods and it does include a radioactive drug in a several-step procedure. The advantage of the enzyme method is it can be done by an automated system. The development of an enzyme-based test for thyroxine marked the first time that screening for thyroid disorders could be part of an automatic screening profile done by computer (Galen 1978). T_4, which can be done with a filter paper, is useful for newborn screening (see Chapter 18).

Preparation of Patient
And Collection of Sample

The laboratory requires 1 ml of plasma. The sample is not affected by food or iodine ingestion, but, if the patient is taking a thyroid preparation, this should be noted on the requisition slip. Note that many drugs may interfere with the test results.

Reference Values

All groups	4–12 μg/dl by RIA
	Values vary due to different laboratory methods.
Pregnancy	Causes an increase.
	A decrease in plasma proteins lowers values.

Decreases and Increases in T_4

Clinical Significance. The hormone is increased in hyperthyroidism and decreased in hypothyroidism. The nursing implications for these two conditions are summarized later in this chapter. In patients with hydatidiform mole, the T_4 may be very elevated. Evidently, there is an increase of some TSH activity from the molar tissue (Hyten 1975:74). Oral contraceptives and pregnancy also cause an increase of thyroxine (see Appendix D).

TRIIODOTHYRONINE (T_3) SERUM CONCENTRATION (T_3-RIA)

The test for triiodothyronine (T_3) is sometimes called T_3-RIA to denote that the hormone is measured by radioimmunoassay. The use of the letters ''RIA'' also helps to distinguish this test from the T_3 resin uptake (discussed next). T_3 is more biologically active than T_4, but both hormones have similar actions in the body. So the T_3 is not usually used in confirming the diagnosis of suspected hypothyroidism because other tests can demonstrate hypofunction of the thyroid gland. The T_4 is usually adequate as a screen for hyperthyroidism. Sometimes, however, a patient may have clinical signs of thyrotoxicosis with a normal T_4. Measurement of the T_3 is then needed, since T_3 may be elevated in thyrotoxicosis while other thyroid tests are still in the normal range (Soler 1979).

Preparation of Patient
And Collection of Sample

The preparation and collection instructions are the same as those for the T_4 test. *

Reference Values

All groups	70–190 ng/dl by RIA
Pregnancy and oral contraceptives	Tend to increase the values. A decrease in plasma proteins causes lowered values.

T_3 RESIN UPTAKE
(PERCENTAGE OF T_3 UPTAKE)

T_3 resin uptake measures the amount of T_4 indirectly by measuring the amount of T_3 that can be attached to the proteins that bind the thyroid hormones. Normally, almost all the thyroxin (T_4) is attached to thyroid-binding globulins (TBG). With a lack of T_4, the thyroid-binding globulins are able to absorb more T_3 that is added to a blood sample. With an increase in T_4, the thyroid-binding globulins are oversaturated with the T_4 and unable to carry much additional T_3. The resin uptake test does not measure the amount of T_3 taken up by the thyroid-binding globulins. Instead, it measures the amount of T_3 left over and thus free to bind to the resin added to the blood sample.

In the T_3 resin uptake, a measured amount of radioactive tagged T_3 and resin is added to a sample of the patient's blood. The resin is put into the test tube to absorb any of the radioactive-tagged T_3 that cannot be taken up by the thyroid-binding globulins in the blood sample. In other words, the resin is the ''sponge'' that takes up all the tagged T_3 that cannot bind with the globulins. Since hypothyroid states create a lot of ''vacant'' thyroid-binding globulins, the tagged T_3 is attached to the thyroid-binding globulins and less is taken up by the resin. In hyperthyroid states, the thyroid-binding globulins are saturated with T_4; so they have little binding capacity for the additional T_3. Thus the added tagged T_3 must go to the secondary binding site, which is the resin. The laboratory measures the amount of T_3 that is taken up by the resin and reports the results in percentages.

Reference Values

25–35% of the tagged T_3 is taken up by the resin. The rest of the T_3 is assumed to be bound to the thyroid-binding globulins.

Values in hyperthyroidism	There is little room for the tagged T_3, so more T_3 goes to the resin. The resin uptake is above 35%.
Values in hypothyroidism	More of the T_3 can be attached to thyroid-binding globulins, so less tagged T_3 is absorbed by the resin. The uptake by the resin is below 25%.

Note: This test is based on the amount of thyroid-binding globulins. So increases in globulins cause more uptake of T_3 on globulins and less by the resin. The resin uptake seems abnormally low when thyroid-binding globulins are elevated in pregnancy and by drugs such as estrogens.

A decrease in plasma proteins means less binding capacity and thus an increased uptake by the resin. Thus in patients with severe liver disease or nephrosis, the lack of plasma proteins causes an unusually high T_3 uptake by the resin (Hallal 1977).

The important thing to remember is that any changes in plasma proteins invalidate the results of the T_3 resin uptake. To overcome the problems of unknown changes in the amount of plasma proteins, the T_3 resin uptake can be compared to other thyroid tests. One way to make the tests of T_3 resin uptake and T_4 more accurate is to use these two tests to calculate the free thyroxin index (FTI).

FREE THYROXIN INDEX (FTI)

The FTI is not a test; it is a calculated value based on the results of the T_4 and T_3 resin uptake tests. The calculated value is obtained by multiplying the T_4 by the T_3 resin uptake. This value shows the ratio of total thyroxine (T_4) to the total available binding sites (T_3 resin uptake). For example, a normal T_4 would be 6 μg and a T_3 resin uptake should be about 25%. So the FTI is:

$$6 \ \mu g \ (T_4) \times 25\% \ (T_3 \text{ resin uptake}) = 1.5 \ (\text{FTI})$$

Reference Values

1 to 4 mg (based on the reference values for T_4 and T_3 resin uptakes in the example in the text.)

As explained in the reference values for T_3 uptake, the FTI makes corrections when the plasma proteins are not normal or when there is a change in the binding sites rather than in the amount of thyroxine. High amounts of free thyroxine, as shown by the FIT, are highly suggestive of hyperthyroidism. Low values for the FTI are suggestive of hypothyroidism. The clinician must also look at both the T_4 and the T_3 resin uptake as individual tests too.

THYROID-BINDING GLOBULINS CAPACITY (TBG)

Some laboratories may do direct measurement of the globulins involved in thyroid binding to check on the validity of other tests done for thyroid function.

Preparation of Patient
And Collection of Sample
The laboratory needs 2 ml of serum.

Reference Values

15–25 pg of T_4/100 ml

Elevated Thyroid Tests

Clinical Significance. A diagnosis of hyperthyroidism is made when the patient has an elevation of several of the tests discussed in this chapter. (One test alone may not be diagnostic.) Table 15-6 shows which of the common tests of thyroid function are usually elevated in hyperthyroidism, which is also called thyrotoxicosis. An excess of thyroid hormone can result from inflammation, tumors, or autoimmune disorders of the thyroid gland. Often the cause of the hyperthyroidism is unknown (that is, it is idiopathic). A hyperthyroid state associated with goiter and a bulging of the eyes (exophthalmos) is called Grave's disease, which is considered the most fully developed hyperthryoid state and the cause of which is not known. It sometimes follows an infection, physical stress, or emotional crisis. Clearly, TSH is not responsible for the hyperthyroid state (Juebiz 1979:50). Hyperthyroidism is rare in infants, but it does occur in children and particularly in adolescents. Hyperthyroidism is much more common in girls than in boys (Heagerty 1980:358).

Possible Nursing Implications.

Assisting with Medical Interventions. Once the patient is definitely diagnosed as having hyperthyroidism, treatment may include the use of antithyroid drugs, such as methimanzole (Tapazole), therapy with radioactive iodine, or surgical intervention. Hallal (1977) is an excellent review of the pathophysiology of hyperthyroidism, the treatments used, and the nursing care needed. The goal of treatment is to bring the patient back to a "euthyroid," or normal thyroid, balance. The patient needs help from the nurse and from others in learning to cope with the manifestations of thyrotoxicosis.

Assessing for Symptoms of Hyperthyroidism or Thyrotoxicosis. In general, most of the symptoms of hyperthyroidism are due to the accelerated metabolism that results from an excess of circulating thyroid hormones. These patients have tachycardia and often arrhythmias, such as atrial fibrillation. Even their resting pulses may be over 90. Extreme thyrotoxicosis can even cause heart failure. Although these patients have voracious appetites, they lose weight, become weak, and are easily fatigued, despite an increased intake of calories. Their symptoms of central nervous system irritability include nervousness, an inability to sleep, and tremors of muscles. Diarrhea may also be a problem. Heat intolerance and excessive perspiration are common.

Providing Adequate Food and Fluid Intake. These patients' increased metabolism make them hungry most of the time. They need a well-balanced diet with extra calories, as well as between-meal snacks. Extra fluids are needed due to the diaphoresis. Stimulants, such as coffee, should be avoided. The patient should be weighed periodically to see that weight loss is not continuing. If diarrhea is a problem, the diet should avoid foods that tend to aggrevate the hyperactive bowel.

Maintaining a Cool, Quiet Environment. These patients have a heat intolerance, so the room should be kept a little cool. Besides being cool, the environment should not be filled with a lot of noise or confusion. Patients need a quiet and relaxing atmosphere, and perhaps sedatives, to sleep.

Monitoring for Tachycardia, Arrhythmias, or Cardiovascular Failure. The high pulse rate decreases as the thyroid gland is brought under control (Krueger 1976), but the pulse rate should be checked to see how well these patients can tolerate activity. They need adequate rest between activities so that the cardiovascular system is not overtaxed. They may be taught to take their own pulses to monitor the effectiveness of the antithyroid medication.

Helping the Patient Cope with Exophthalmos. Exophthalmos is an abnormal protrusion of the eye that sometimes occurs with hyperthyroidism. Pathologically, lymphocytes and mucopolysaccharides collect behind the eyeball. This collection may be unilateral or bilateral. The treatment of hyperthyroidism does not seem to have an appreciable influence on the progression or regression of the exophthalmos (Ryan 1980:61). The key thing is to prevent trauma to the eyes and to help patients adjust to the altered body image.

Helping Significant Others Understand the Symptoms of Thyrotoxicosis. Family, coworkers, and friends may find it hard to understand the actions of a patient who has hyperthyroidism symptoms. Nurses may be very helpful in explaining in simple terms why these patients fuss about heat, noise, or whatever. Jenkins (1980) gives a personal account of the frustrations of learning to live with thyrotoxicosis and how this has affected her jobs in nursing. Control of a hormone imbalance is not always achieved in a short time. It may take months to years to gain really adequate balance.

Decreased Level of Serum Thyroid Levels

Clinical Significance. The findings of the several tests used to confirm the suspected diagnosis of hypothyroidism are summarized in Table 15–6. In the adult, the presence of hypothyroidism is called myxedema. The failure of the thyroid gland to produce thyroid hormones is usually a primary dysfunction of the gland itself. However, hypothyroidism can also result from a lack of TSH (as discussed in the section on TSH). Diets deficient in iodine also cause a lack of thyroid hormone and an enlargement of the thyroid gland (goiter). Inflammations and autoimmune responses may cause insufficiency of the gland, but often the hypofunctioning cannot be linked to a causative factor.

In congenital hypothyroidism, the lack of the thyroid hormone can cause cretinism. Lack of thyroid in newborns causes growth failure and mental retardation. The symptoms of hypothyroidism may not be present at birth because the fetus has some thyroid hormones from the mother. Recent studies (Fisher 1979) have concluded that T_4 should be a screening device for all newborns, so that congenital hypothyroidism can be detected. (See Chapter 18 on newborn screening.) Hypothyroidism may also develop later in childhood.

Possible Nursing Implications.
Assessing for Hypothyroidism in Infants. Nurses must be aware of the symptoms of hypothyroidism in newborns and in adults, because they may be involved in case finding. Case finding in infants is very important since mental retardation occurs if the infant is not treated within two to three months after birth (Heagerty 1979:359) and sometimes the effects of lack of thyroid may not be prominent at birth because the fetus has some thyroid hormones from the mother. Some of the outstanding characteristics of a lack of thyroid in a newborn are protruding tongue, a broad flattened nose, a protruding abdomen with an umbilical hernia, and a generalized muscle hypotonia. The baby has a hoarse cry and may be a very poor feeder. The heart rate is slow.

Once the infant is diagnosed as having hypothyroidism, treatment is begun with thyroid replacement. The medication helps the infant to grow and to develop normally.

The parents need careful teaching in the importance of life-long administration of the hormone.

Assessing for Symptoms in Older Children and Adults. Symptoms of hypothyroidism, or myxedema, in the person beyond infancy are due to the slowing down of metabolism that occurs with insufficient thyroid hormone. These patients may have only slight symptoms so that the disease can be overlooked (Guthrie 1979). They typically have fatigue, lethargy, and an intolerance to cold (Krueger 1976). Their hair is coarse and their skin is very dry. They gain weight even on a limited diet. Constipation may be a problem. Their blood pressure and pulse are low. They may have memory impairment or a definite slowness in mental ability.

Providing a Warm, Relaxed, and Slow-Paced Environment. Patients with hypothyroidism have a cold intolerance, so the environment needs to be warm. The nurse can provide extra clothing, such as heavy socks. The environment needs to be warm in the psychological sense too. These patients may be slower in doing activities, so the nurse needs to let them proceed at their own pace. They may need help to adjust to fast-moving situations. Because inactivity may create more lethargy and dullness, some sensory stimulation is needed. In the home setting, the family may need help in making the environment warm, relaxed, and relatively quiet for the patient.

Helping the Patient with Dietary Problems. These patients may need to be on a diet that is low in calories due to their weight gain. The nurse should see that their diets contain all the essential nutrients and vitamins. Patients can be assured that, when their thyroid level is returned to normal, their excess poundage should be easier to lose. (In fact, thyroid pills have been used as a type of diet pill. Obviously, thyroid intake by a patient who is euthyroid is not a physiologically sound way to lose weight.) Plenty of fluids and roughage in the diet helps to decrease the problem of constipation.

Recognizing the Patient's Intolerance for Sedatives and Narcotics. Since these patients have a slower-than-normal metabolism, sedatives and narcotics may have a much more profound effect. So these types of drugs should be used with caution, if at all (Hallal 1977).

Helping with Skin Care and Hair Care. Patients may be distressed by the rough skin and coarse hair they develop. They may need to use hair conditioners and plenty of skin lotion to keep their skin and hair attractive-looking. These skin and hair problems fade as the hormonal balance is restored.

Teaching the Patient about the Effects of Thyroid Replacement. Refer to a pharmacology text for a detailed discussion about thyroid replacement. The patient needs to know the signs of overdosage of the drugs. (See the discussion on the symptoms of hyperthyroidism.) A resting pulse above 90 is an indicator of possibly too much thyroid replacement. Patients can be taught to check their own pulses.

GONADOTROPINS AND THE SEX-RELATED HORMONES

The sex-related hormones include the gonadotropins from the anterior pituitary gland (FSH and LH), along with estrogen, progesterone, and the androgens from the ovaries, testes, and adrenal cortex. Both the ovaries and testes produce progesterone, estrogen and the androgens but in markedly different proportions in males and females. The sex hormones from the adrenal cortex are in minute amounts in both sexes.

Infertility, the lack of development of secondary sex characteristics, and changes in sexual characteristics or sexual functioning are common reasons for measuring the sex hormones. The gonadatropins are measured directly in the serum and in 24-hour urine specimens. Testosterone, the main androgen, can be measured in the serum. Also, the metabolites of the androgens from the testes and from the adrenal cortex can be measured in the urine. (See the 17-ketosteroids test in this chapter.) Progesterone and estrogen are not usually measured in the serum, but rather as various metabolites in the urine.

Only the more common urine and serum laboratory tests for the sex hormones are discussed in this chapter. The clinical significance of the change in each of the different hormones is beyond the scope of this book. Refer to the references at the end of this chapter for detailed information about various disorders that can cause changes in the sex-related hormones.

FOLLICLE-STIMULATING HORMONE (FSH)

FSH from the anterior pituitary gland controls the growth and maturation of the ovarian follicles in the female for ovulation. FSH also controls the secretion of estrogen in the female. In the male, FSH stimulates the testes to produce sperm.

Preparation of Patient
And Collection of Samples
There is no special preparation of the patient. The laboratory needs 2 ml of serum or plasma for the blood test. A 24-hour urine specimen may be done. (See Chapter 3 for hints on urine collections.) The urine specimen should be kept cold to prevent bacterial growth.

Reference Values

Plasma FSH	
Adult male	4–15 mIU/ml
Adult female	4–25 mIU/ml depending on time in menstrual cycle
Prepubertal male	2–10 mIU/ml
Prepubertal female	3–7 mIU/ml
Postmenopausal	30–200 mIU/ml
Urine FSH—24-Hour Specimens	
Adult male	5–25 IU
Adult female	5–60 IU depending on time in menstrual cycle
Pregnancy	2,000–50,000 IU

(*continued*)

Reference Values (*continued*)

Prepubertal child	None detectable in urine
Postmenopausal	50–100 IU

LUETENIZING HORMONES (LH)

LH is the second gonadotrophic hormone secreted by the anterior pituitary gland. In the female, LH, along with FSH, is necessary for ovulation to take place. After ovulation, LH stimulates the ruptured follicle to secrete increasing amounts of progesterone. In males, LH stimulates the production of androgens, which are important in determining the secondary sex characteristics. LH in the male is sometimes referred to as the interstitial cell-stimulating hormone (ICSH).

Preparation of the Patient
And Collection of the Sample

The preparation of the patient for serum or urine specimens for LH is the same as the preparation for FSH.

Reference Values

Serum Levels of LH	
Adult males	6–18 mU/ml
Females	5–22 mU/ml pre- and postovulation 30–250 mU/ml, mid-cycle peaks
Children	2–12 mU/ml
Postmenopausal	30–200 mU/ml

Urine Levels of LH (24-Hour Urine Specimen)

Varies with technique used. Serum levels are usually considered more accurate.

Changes in FSH and LH Serum and Urine Levels

Clinical Significance. Syndromes of excessive gonadatropins are extremely infrequent, if they exist at all (Cryer 1979). FSH and LH levels are measured to see whether patients with hypogonadism have a primary gonad problem or a secondary problem of pituitary insufficiency. Pituitary insufficiency may be first manifested by a lack of function of the testes or ovaries. The LH and FSH are low if the gonads' failure is due to pituitary insufficiency (secondary hypogonadism). The levels of FSH and LH in serum and urine are high if the gonads' failure is primary failure of the ovaries or testes. Drugs, such as clomiphene (Clomid) or gonadotropin-releasing factor (GRH), may be given to see if the level of gonadotropins increases. Increased levels of FSH are also used to verify that a woman is undergoing menopause.

ESTRADIOL AND OTHER FORMS OF ESTROGEN

Different forms of the estrogens, including estradiol, estrone, and estriol, can be measured. Estriol is the estrogen present in largest amounts of pregnancy. (See Chapter 18 for the use of estriol as a test of fetal well-being during pregnancy.) Since estrogens are produced not only by the ovaries but also by the adrenal cortex and the testes, estradiol levels may be useful to assess pathology in all three glands.

The level of estradiol is increased in males who have testicular or adrenal tumors. In women, the increased estradiol arises from estrogen-secreting ovarian tumors. Decreases of estradiol in the female, or a lack of increase during a menstrual cycle, can be due either to ovarian failure or to pituitary insufficiency. Hepatic and renal failure can cause abnormal levels of estrogens in the serum. Females may show no symptoms when estrogens are increased. Males may exhibit feminizing signs, such as an enlarged breast, when any of the estrogens is increased.

PREGNANEDIOL (PROGESTERONE METABOLITE)

Pregnanediol is the principle form of progesterone in the urine. (Note that pregnane*triol* is another urine test done to evaluate adrenocortical function. See the discussion earlier in this chapter.) In the female, the level of pregnanediol rises rapidly in the urine after ovulation and steadily during pregnancy. The 24-hour urine specimen may be done to evaluate the need for progesterone replacement.

Reference Values

Children	0.4–1.0 mg/24-hour specimen
Men	0.5–1.5 mg/24-hour specimen
Women:	
Pregnancy, 28–32 weeks	27–47 mg/24-hour specimen
Nonpregnant	0.5–7.0 mg/24-hour specimen
Lueteal phase	2.0–7.0 mg/24-hour specimen
Postmenopausal	0.3–1.5 mg/24-hour specimen

TESTOSTERONE AND OTHER ANDROGENS

The male sex hormones, the androgens, are produced by the adrenal cortex, the testes, and the ovaries. The most powerful of the androgens, testosterone, comes mainly from the testes. Adult males with increased testosterone levels do not have any symptoms. In male children before puberty, there is precocious development of secondary sex characteristics (Guthrie 1979). In females of all ages, there is masculization. The adrenogenital syndrome, which occurs due to a lack of cortisol and an abundance of androgens, was discussed earlier in this chapter. In the adult male, a lack of testosterone, which can be due to primary failure of the testes or secondary to pituitary insufficiency, causes feminization.

Reference Values

Adult male	300–1000 ng/100 ml
Adult female	25–90 ng/100 ml
Adolescent males	Over 100 ng/100 ml

Some laboratories have 250 ng as the lower limit in adult males.

Imbalances in Sex Hormones

Possible Nursing Implications.

Helping Patients Cope with Changes in Body Image. Hormones are very potent in shaping and maintaining secondary sex characteristics. For example, a female who has an increase of testosterone develops more facial hair, more muscle mass, and a deeper voice. The key nursing implication for patients undergoing sex hormone changes due to pathology is to help them cope with the disturbance in their body images. Alterations in sexual characteristics are corrected if the hormone balance can be established. The mood changes and depression may be due both to hormonal influences and to the effect of the physical changes. Nurses can help these patients play down the unwanted characteristics. Even little details, such as helping the woman find a place to have unwanted hair removed, can mean a lot.

Specific Interventions for Malignancies. Several of the tumors that cause masculinizing features in the female or feminizing features in male are due to a malignancy. Nurses must be aware of the specific nursing care guidelines related to the pathophysiology of the tumor. Also, some types of cancer are treated by hormone therapy, which causes an imbalance of sex hormones and permanent changes in the body image.

Referring for Counseling. A change in sexual functioning may occur due to sex hormone changes. The person may need professional counseling to deal with problems related to sexual functioning. Hogan (1980) contains a chapter devoted to the nursing implications for the patient with different types of impaired hormonal function. The major emphasis for any sex hormonal change is to help the patient deal with a decreased sexual self-concept. If hormone tests are being done as part of an infertility work-up, the nurse needs to be sensitive to the anxiety of the couple who have not been able to conceive a child.

Helping Parents Cope with Precocious Puberty in Children. The problem of mistaken sexual identity in newborns was discussed earlier in the section on adrenogenital syndrome. (See the section on cortisol.) A masculinization of the female child or precocious puberty in either sex is disturbing for the child and probably much more so for the parents. Endocrine problems in children are usually treated by specialists who can also help the parents deal with the frightening changes in their child. A visiting nurse may be very useful in assessing the adjustment of the child and family to these changes. School nurses can be instrumental too, in recognizing children who may need counseling to deal with the physical and psychological problems of early maturity. Sexual precocity is three times more prevalent in girls than in boys (Hogan 1980:344); some girls are capable of reproduction at age 8 or 9. Refer to pediatric texts for a more detailed discussion on the psychological effects of sexual changes and precocious puberty in children.

Questions

15–1. Which of the following illustrates the concept of a negative feedback system for control of serum cortisol?

    a. An increase of serum cortisol when ACTH secretion is increased.

    b. A decreased level of serum cortisol when ACTH secretion is decreased.

    c. A decreased secretion of ACTH when serum cortisol is increased.

    d. An increased secretion of ACTH when serum cortisol is increased.

15–2. If a hormone has a circadian rhythm, its reference values for the laboratory test of the hormone:

    a. will vary predictably in each 24-hour period.

    b. will be lower when the patient sleeps.

    c. will change from day to day.

    d. are established to account for ectopic hormone production.

15–3. *Anterior* pituitary hypofunction is usually manifested first as a deficiency of the gonadotropins (LH, FSH) and of:

    a. growth hormone (GH).

    b. thyroid-stimulating hormone (TSH).

    c. adrenocorticotropic hormone (ACTH).

    d. antidiuretic hormone (ADH).

15–4. The purpose of doing an ACTH suppression test with dexamethasone (Decadron) is to assess which of the following?

    a. Whether aldosterone levels remain elevated after suppression of ACTH.

    b. Whether the adrenogenital syndrome is due to anterior pituitary hyperfunction of ACTH.

    c. If ACTH is still produced by the anterior pituitary.

    d. Whether the adrenal cortex continues to secrete cortisol after ACTH is suppressed.

15–5. Mrs. Wu has an elevated serum cortisol level. This patient has a tentative diagnosis of Cushing's syndrome due to an adrenal cortex tumor. Which nursing action would be appropriate?

a. Observing and reporting any gastric distress, since gastric ulcers may develop.

b. Assessing for potential renal failure due to high serum potassium levels (hyperkalemia).

c. Recognizing that an extremely elevated temperature may occur with even minor infections.

d. Encouraging physical activity to counteract the lethargy and boredom.

15–6. Mr. Lee has a lower-than-normal serum cortisol level. Which nursing action would *not* be appropriate for this patient with a tentative diagnosis of Addison's disease?

a. Assuring the patient that his increased skin pigmentation will fade when the cortisol hormone replacement is adequate.

b. Checking the urine for sugar and acetone, since hyperglycemia is a potential problem.

c. Helping Mr. Lee to prevent postural hypotension by teaching him to get out of bed slowly.

d. Encouraging rest and relaxation to decrease physical and physiological stress.

15–7. Bobby, age 5, has been referred to an endocrinologist because he has an enlarged penis and other secondary sex characteristics. His serum sodium was low, and his serum potassium was elevated. A 24-hour urine for 17-ketosteroids (17-KS) was elevated. The increased elevation of serum androgens in adrenogenital syndrome is due to a basic lack of which of the following?

a. ACTH production. c. Gonadatropic hormones.

b. Cortisol production. d. Testosterone.

15–8. Mrs. Rodriquez has congestive heart failure with secondary aldosteronism. An elevation of the mineralocorticoid aldosterone may cause all of Mrs. Rodriquez's symptoms except which?

a. BP of 170/100.

b. Serum potassium of 3.0 mEq/l.

c. Pitting edema of the ankles.

d. Polyuria (urine output of 2,000 cc in 24 hours).

15–9. Barbara, age 16, has an elevated blood pressure due to a tumor of the adrenal cortex. Her serum aldosterone level is increased. Because Barbara has primary hyperaldostonerism, one would expect her renin level to be which of the following?

a. Markedly increased. c. Normal.

b. Slightly increased. d. Slightly decreased.

15–10. Urine testing for metanephrine and for vanillylmandelic acid (VMA) are two of the screening tests for tumors of the

    a. Adrenal cortex.   **c.** Pituitary gland.

    b. Adrenal medulla.   **d.** Parathyroid gland.

15–11. An increased level of parathormone (PTH) causes an increased serum level of which?

    a. Sodium.   **b.** Potassium.   **c.** Phosphorus.   **d.** Calcium.

15–12. The test most often used to follow patients with hyper- or hypothyroidism is which of the following?

    a. TSH (thyroid stimulating hormone test).

    b. T_4 (L-thyroxine).

    c. T_3 (triiodothyronine).

    d. T_3 resin uptake.

15–13. Mrs. Graves has been admitted to the hospital because of suspected hyperthyroidism. Her T_4 level was normal but her T_3 was elevated. Which of the following nursing actions would *not* be appropriate in caring for Mrs. Graves?

    a. Seeing that she has between-meal snacks.

    b. Keeping her room slightly warmer than usual.

    c. Allowing her time to rest between activities.

    d. Checking an apical pulse when vital signs are done.

15–14. Mr. Lane has come to the clinic to begin tests for hypothyroidism because symptoms were noted by a public health nurse who was visiting the Lane family. Which of the following symptoms is not characteristic of a patient with suspected hypothyroidism?

    a. Memory impairment.   **c.** Intolerance to cold.

    b. Constipation.   **d.** Weight loss.

15–15. Baby Finley, age 2 months, has been diagnosed as having congenital hypothyroidism. The baby has been started on a thyroid preparation. If hypothyroidism is not picked up in early infancy (two to three months), the infant will develop which of the following?

    a. Mental retardation.   **c.** Generalized muscle hypertrophy.

    b. Cardiovascular problems.   **d.** Vision abnormalities.

15–16. Increased gonadatropin (LH and FSH) levels would be expected in all of the following patients except which?

    a. Mrs. Rachter, who is undergoing menopause.

    b. Mrs. Lax, who is taking clomiphene (Clomid).

    c. Mr. Faber, who has a suspected pituitary insufficiency.

    d. Mr. Wolf, who has primary hypofunction of the testes.

15-17. The key nursing implication for patients with alterations in their sex hormones is to be aware that they often need help in coping with which of the following?

    a. Decreased appetite and weight loss.

    b. Changes in secondary sex characteristics.

    c. Changes in energy level.

    d. Physical stress, such as an infection.

REFERENCES

Blount, Mary and Kinney, Anna. "Chronic Steroid Therapy," *American Journal of Nursing* 74 (September 1974): 1626-1631.

Burnett, Joanne. "Congenital Adrenocortical Hyplerplasia: The Syndrome and Nursing Interventions," *American Journal of Nursing* 80 (July 1980): 1306-1311.

Cryer, Philip. *Diagnostic Endocrinology*. New York: Oxford University Press, 1979.

Elliott, Diane. "Adrenocortical Insufficiency: A Self Instruction Unit," *American Journal of Nursing* 74 (June 1974): 1115-1130.

Fisher, Delbert, *et al.* "Screening for Congenital Hypothyroidism: Results of Screening One Million North American Infants," *Journal of Pediatrics* 94 (May 1979): 700-705.

Galen, Robert. "Thyroxine as a Routine Screening Test," *Diagnostic Medicine* 1 (April 1978): 89-90.

Gotch, Paula. "Teaching Patients About Adrenal Corticosteroids," *American Journal of Nursing* 81: 78-81, Januray 1981.

Guimond, Joyce and Wilson, Susan. "Postirridation Thyroid Disorders," *American Journal of Nursing* 79 (July 1979): 1256-1258.

Guthrie, Diana. "The Endocrine System," Chapter 17 in Armstrong, Margaret, ed. *Handbook of Clinical Nursing*. New York: McGraw-Hill Book Co., 1979.

Hallal, Janice. "Thyroid Disorders," *American Journal of Nursing* 77 (March 1977): 418-431.

Heagarty, Margaret *et al. Child Health: Basics for Primary Care*. New York: Appleton-Century-Crofts, 1980.

Hogan, Rosemarie. *Human Sexuality: A Nursing Perspective*. New York: Appleton-Century-Crofts, 1980.

Holum, John. *Elements of General and Biological Chemistry*, 5th ed. New York: John Wiley & Sons, Inc., 1979.

Hytten, Frank and Lind, Tom. *Diagnostic Indices in Pregnancy*. Summit, N.J.: Ciba-Geigy Corp., 1975.

Jenkins, Elda. "Living with Thyrotoxicosis," *American Journal of Nursing* 80 (May 1980): 956-958.

Juebiz, William. *Endocrinology: A Logical Approach for Clinicians*. New York: McGraw-Hill Book Co., 1979.

Kaplan, Solomon *et al.* "Symposium on Pediatric Endocrinology," *Pediatric Clinics of North America* 26 (February 1979): 1-247.

Koepke, John. *Guide to Clinical Laboratory Diagnosis,* 2nd ed. New York: Appleton-Century-Crofts, 1979.

Krieger, Dorothy, ed. *Comprehensive Endocrinology: Endocrine Rhythms*. New York: Raven Press, 1979.

Krueger, Judith and Ray, Janis. *Endocrine Problems in Nursing: A Physiologic Approach*. St Louis, Mo.: C. V. Mosby Co., 1976.

Locke, William. "Control of Anterior Pituitary Function," *Archives of Internal Medicine* 138 (October 1978): 1541–1545.

McFarlane, Judith. "Congenital Adrenal Hyperplasia," *American Journal of Nursing* 76 (August 1976): 1290–1292.

Price, Sylvia and Wilson, Lorraine. *Pathphysiology: Clinical Concepts of Disease Processes.* New York: McGraw-Hill Book Co., 1978.

Ravel, Richard. *Clinical Laboratory Medicine,* 3rd ed. Chicago: Year Book Medical Publishers, Inc., 1979.

Ryan, Will. *Endocrine Disorders: A Pathophysiologic Approach.* Chicago: Year Book Medical Publishers, Inc., 1980.

Soler, Norman *et al.,* "Isolated High Serum Triiodothyronine Levels," *Archives of Internal Medicine* 139 (January 1979): 38–39.

Tucker, Susan *et al. Patient Care Standards.* St. Louis, Mo.: C. V. Mosby Co., 1980.

Weber, Michael. "Saralasin Testing for Renin-Dependent Hypertension," *Archives of Internal Medicine* 139 (January 1979): 93–95.

CHAPTER SIXTEEN

Culture and Sensitivity Tests

Objectives

1. Describe the classification system used by the laboratory to identify bacteria.
2. Interpret the clinical significance of C&S and MIC reports.
3. Identify the general nursing implications when a patient has cultures ordered for a possible bacterial infection.
4. Describe in detail the various ways urine is collected for urine cultures.
5. Explain the procedures used to obtain blood cultures, as well as the timing of preliminary and final reports.
6. Describe what the nurse should teach the patient to obtain a useful sputum specimen.
7. Explain why it may be important to do throat cultures for children with sore throats.
8. Describe the correct procedure to obtain a wound culture and what should be taught to the patient.
9. Describe how gonorrhea is detected by laboratory methods.
10. Describe the proper procedure for collecting a stool specimen for bacterial culture of *Salmonella* or *Shigella*.

The first part of this chapter provides some background information about the classification of bacteria, as well as how the laboratory does cultures and sensitivities on clinical specimens. Specific nursing implications for culture collections are outlined. In addition, the nurse's role in caring for patients with infections is reviewed. The last part of the chapter outlines in detail the purpose, procedure, and preparation of the patient for each type of common culture.

CLASSIFICATION OF BACTERIA BY MICROSCOPIC EXAM

Bacteria can be classified into groups according to:

1. whether the bacteria takes a gram stain,
2. the shape of the bacteria—round (cocci), rod-shaped (bacilli), or spiral-shaped (spirilla), and
3. whether the bacteria thrives with oxygen (aerobic) or without (anaerobic).

The distribution of the cocci in pairs (diploccoci), in a string (streptococci), or in a cluster (staphylococci) also helps the microbiologist to classify bacteria. A preliminary stain may not identify the exact bacteria, but it can help to make a presumptive diagnosis as well as rule out what the bacteria are not. For example, if the Gram stain shows gram-negative diplococci, gonorrhea is most likely the causitive organism. If the Gram stain reveals gram-negative rods, the infection may be caused by organisms such as *Escherichia coli* or *Pseudomonas*. (See Table 16-1 for the classification of some of the *common* bacteria that are identified in laboratory specimens.)

TABLE 16-1. EXAMPLES OF COMMON BACTERIA FOUND IN CULTURES*

	Commonly Found in Cultures of . . .
I. *Aerobic Organisms*	
A. Gram-positive cocci	
1. *Staphylococcus aureus* (coagulase, positive)	Blood, wound, sputum
2. *Streptococcus* (A-beta hemolytic)	Throat, wound, sputum
3. *Streptococcus pneumoniae* (Pneumococcus)	Sputum, CSF in adult
B. Gram-negative cocci	
1. *Neisseria meningitidis* (meningococcus)	CSF, throat
2. *Neisseria gonorrhea* (gonococcus)	Urethra, endocervix, throat
C. Gram-negative rods or bacilli	
1. *Escherichia coli* (many strains)	Urine, blood, wound
2. Proteus species	Urine, sputum, wound
3. *Enterobacteria-Klebsiella*	Urine, sputum, wound
4. *Pseudomonas*	Sputum, urine, wound
5. *Salmonella*	Stool
6. *Shigella*	Stool
II. *Anaerobic Organisms*	
A. Gram-positive cocci	
1. Anaerobic streptococci	Wound, stool, vagina
B. Gram-positive bacillus	
1. Clostridium group	Wounds, stool
C. Gram-negative bacillus	
1. Bacteroides	Wound, stool
III. Acid-fast bacillus	
A. Mycobacterium tuberculosis	Sputum, gastric contents, CSF

*Information compiled from various references. See text. A Clinician's Dictionary Guide to Bacteria and Fungi (Mickat 1976) can be obtained free from Eli Lilly Company.

The trained laboratory technician also notes other details, such as the number of different bacteria present, to estimate the probability of an infection. The technician is able to note that the specimen is grossly contaminated with "normal" flora too.

Gram stains are particularly useful, for the presumptive identification of gonorrhea in endocervical smears in women and urethral smears in men and for meningitis in cerebrospinal fluid. Yet Gram stains for stool and urine may or may not be helpful, and in several areas, such as sputum smears, the usefulness of a Gram stain is controversial (Ravel 1978).

CULTURE GROWTHS

A stain is only a presumptive identification of the bacteria. A culture allows the bacteria to grow and to multiply so that the exact organism can be identified by various methods of analysis. The laboratory usually takes two or more days to make a final identification of the organisms present in a specimen. For some specimens it may be six to ten days. The growth on the culture takes about 24 hours. The laboratory must then use various tests to determine the exact species of bacteria present. Various methods, such as the addition of sugars, are used to identify different strains of a species. These tests to positively identify a specific type of bacteria may take another 24 hours or more.

The amount of growth on the culture varies with the organism. For example, some bacteria, such as *Escherichia coli,* reproduce every 20 minutes. At the other extreme, the organism that cause tuberculosis, *Mycobacterium tuberculosis,* reproduces only about once a day. Thus a final report of a culture for tuberculosis may take 3 to 8 weeks. [See the section on sputum collection for acid-fast bacillus (AFB).]

For most of the commonly cultured organisms (Table 16-1), a report is ready in the usual 2 to 3 days. Before the culture results are known, the physician chooses an antibiotic or antibiotics that are most likely to help. For example, antibiotics, such as penicillin, are used for most gram-positive cocci and aminoglycosides for gram-negative bacilli (Lee 1973).

Anaerobic Cultures

Without a specific order to the contrary, bacterial cultures are usually done under aerobic conditions because the majority of disease-causing organisms require oxygen. However, if the patient may possibly have an infection with an anaerobic organism, the specimen must be cultured without oxygen. For example, a deep wound may be infected with both anaerobic and aerobic organisms, and thus two culture specimens should be obtained. For an anaerobic specimen, the nurse should call the laboratory to obtain the needed container, which may be a tube filled with carbon dioxide rather than oxygen. The tube can be opened long enough to put in the swab that has the material to be cultured. Since carbon dioxide is heavier than air, it remains in the tube as long as the tube is held upright (Marchiondo 1979:38). The specimen should be sent immediately to the laboratory. With blood cultures, the routine is to put the blood specimens into two different containers so that an anaerobic culture can be done as well as an aerobic culture. Two laboratory requisitions should be sent with the two specimens so the laboratory is aware of the need to do both types of culture.

Besides wound and blood cultures, cerebral spinal fluid and feces may also commonly be cultured for anaerobic organisms. The female genital tract can also harbor anaerobic organisms, but this is not a common culture.

Cultures for Fungus

Cultures for fungus require specific culture media. With swabs moistened with saline (dry swabs are used for Gram stains of bacteria), small scrapings may be taken from a lesion. The nurse should consult with the laboratory on exactly how to collect the specimen.

The cultures for fungus take a long time to grow, and they must be handled carefully because the spores from the fungus can get into the air. For most of the systemic fungus diseases, such as histoplasmosis, various serology tests are done. (See Chapter 14 on serology tests.) Skin tests are also used to identify patients who have antibodies against certain fungus infections. (Skin tests for fungus diseases are covered in pharmacology books.)

Cultures for Viruses

The laboratory identification of viral diseases is usually done by serology tests since a culture of a virus requires a living cell culture, which demands the services of a specialized laboratory. Recently some viruses have been identified with the electron microscope, but the positive identification of certain viruses is still done only in large medical centers. So, if a specimen is to be transported elsewhere, the nurse must check with the specific laboratory about how to collect it. Some specimens can be frozen for later analysis. (See Chapter 14 for serology tests for viral diseases, such as infectious mononucleosis or rubella.)

Culture and Sensitivity Tests (C&S)

Sometimes, in addition to knowing the exact organism causing the infection, it is necessary to demonstrate if the organism is sensitive to a certain antibiotic. In regard to C&S, *sensitivity* refers to the ability of the antibiotic to inhibit the growth of the bacteria. Sensitivity has an entirely different connotation when describing the reaction of a patient to an antibiotic. A patient who is allergic to a drug is said to be "sensitive" or "hypersensitive" to the drug. Obviously, sensitivity of the *patient* to the drug is very undesirable, while sensitivity of the *organism* to the antibiotic is essential. If the antibiotic does not inhibit the growth of the bacteria, the organism is said to be "resistant" to the antibiotic.

The most common way that the laboratory checks the sensitivity of organisms to specific antibiotics is to put various disks of paper impregnated with antibiotics in a culture. If the growth of an organism is retarded, the report is an "S" for sensitive or susceptible. If the antibiotic disk does not retard the growth of the specific bacteria in the culture, the report is "R" for resistant. An "I" on a report means that the results are in an intermediate zone or inconclusive of growth retardation. Some laboratories place an intermediate growth into the resistant category. Usually the laboratory uses only one member of an antibiotic family since sensitive differences are usually minor. See Table 16-2 for an example of the antibiotics that may be used for antibiotic sensitivity testing.

The purpose of doing a C&S is to ensure that the patient is receiving the correct antibiotic for the particular organism causing the infection. For example, suppose a patient was receiving ampicillin. If a report came back that showed the organisms to be resistant to ampicillin but sensitive to other antibiotics, the physician must change the antibiotic

TABLE 16-2. EXAMPLE OF CULTURE AND SENSITIVITIES REPORT

Preliminary Culture Report

_____ No Growth _____ Too Early to Interpret

Neg.	Pos.	Final Report
√		Culpak Strep
√		G C Culture
√		Salmonella, Shigella, Arizona
	1 & 2	Growth
		Normal Flora

1. _Escherichia coli_
2. _Pseudomonas aeruginosa_

Sensitivity

1	2	
S	S	Amikacin
R	R	Ampicillin
S	S	Bacitracin
R	R	Cephalothin
S	S	Chloramphenical
S	S	Colistin
R	R	Erythromycin
S	S	Gentamycin
R	S	Kanamycin
R	R	Methicillin
		Nalidixic Acid
		Neomycin
R	R	Nitrofurantoin
R	R	Penicillin G
		Streptomycin
		Sulfathiazole
		Tetracycline
S	S	Tobramycin

order. (See Table 16-2 for an example of a C&S report that would necessitate notification of the physician before the next dose of ampicillin was given.) Culture and sensitivities are particularly useful when the patient is not responding to therapeutic dosages of antibiotics. A routine sensitivity for every culture may not be needed and could be an unnecessary health cost to the patient. The physician must determine if a culture _and_ sensitivity are cost-effective in a particular situation.

MIC

Minimal inhibitory concentration (MIC) is a report of the amount of concentration of an antibiotic that inhibits the growth or that kills the organism. Venous blood containing the microorganism is put into liquid culture mediums, each containing an antibiotic concentration. Hewitt (1978) cautions that the MIC which is effective in vitro (the test tube) may not always correlate well with the effectiveness in vivo. See Table 16-3 for the range of testing for some antibiotics. The concentration of antibiotic that inhibits the growth of the microorganism in vitro is then noted. The MIC may help the physician adjust the dosage of antibiotics. Antibiotic levels may be measured directly in the serum (see Chapter 17). For an organism to be considered sensitive to an antibiotic, attainable blood or urine levels should be at least 2 to 4× the MIC.

TABLE 16-3. RANGES TESTED FOR MINIMAL INHIBITORY CONCENTRATION (MIC) BY LABORATORY*

Antibiotics (range tested)	Representative Adult Dose Grams	Approximate Blood Levels mcg/ml	Approximate Urine Levels mcg/ml
Clindamycin (.25–16)	PO.15–.3q6h IV.3–.6q6–8h	2–4 4–8	30–90 45–240
Erythromycin (.25–16)	PO.25–.5q6h IV.3q4–6h	1–4 10–20	(5%)
Methicillin (.25–16)	(OxPO.25–.5q4–6h) IV1–2q4h	(1.5–4) 10–40	(30–40%)
Penicillin (.06–4)	(VK.25–.5q6h) 1–2 milq4h	1.5–4 20–40	300–450 3000–5000
Ampicillin (.12–8, g. pos.) (.25–16, g. neg.)	PO.25–1.5q6h IV1–2q4h	1.5–4 15–30	50–100 200–400
Cephalothin (1–64)	PO.25–5q6h IV1–2q4h	2–15 25–85	300–1000 800–2000
Gentamicin (.25–16)	IM,IVq8–12h (3–5mg/kg/d)	5–10	65–300
Tetracycline (.25–16)	PO.25–.5q6h IV0.5q6–12h	1.5–4 10–20	200–800 600–1000
Carbenicillin (8–512)	PO1q6h IV4q4h	5–10 125–175	350–1400 2000–10,000
Chloramphenicol (.5–32)	PO.25–.5q6h IV.5–1q6h	1.5–4 10–20	200–700 500–1400
Kanamycin (1–64)	IM,IV5q12h (15mg/kg/d)	15–20	100–200

(*continued*)

TABLE 16-3 *Continued*

Antibiotics (range tested)	Representative Adult Dose Grams	Approximate Blood Levels mcg/ml	Approximate Urine Levels mcg/ml
Tobramycin (.25-16)	IM,IVq8-12h (3-5 mg/kg/d)	5-10	65-300
Amikacin (1-64)	IM,IVq8-12h (15mg/kg/d)	16-21	700-830
Trimeth/Sulfa .5/9.5-32/608	PO160/800ql q12h		200/(90-100)
Colistin 4	—	—	—
Nitrofurantoin 64	PO.1q6h		100-200
Sulfisoxazole	—	—	—
Streptomycin	—	—	—
Nalidixic Acid 1	—	—	—

Reprinted laboratory report courtesy of Kaiser Hospital, San Francisco, Ca. See text for explanation of use of MIC.

COLLECTING SPECIMENS FOR CULTURE

General Nursing Implications
Specific information about each type of common culture is covered in the second half of this chapter. This section presents general guidelines for the collection of all specimens for bacterial culture:

1. *Collect specimens before giving antibiotics.* If possible, cultures should be collected before the antibiotic is begun. If the patient is already on antibiotics, the laboratory should be notified since techniques to counteract the effect of the antibiotic, such as adding penicillinase, may be done.
2. *Use the correct specimen container.* All specimens, except stool, must be collected in a sterile container, and anaerobic specimens must be collected in oxygen-free containers. Some cultures, such as throat cultures, may be transferred to the culture media immediately. The nurse should call the laboratory if there is any doubt about the type of culture medium to be used. For example, the laboratory has specific cultures for blood, and it may be desirable to have the blood transferred to the culture medium as soon as it is drawn. In other settings, the laboratory may prefer to receive the blood in tubes and make the transfer to

the culture medium in the laboratory. If the specimen is not placed in the correct medium, it may be useless.

3. *Know how much of the specimen is needed.* For example, the laboratory can do a culture on just a few ml of sputum, so it would be useless to keep the container longer to try to get a larger amount. See Table 16–4 for a list of the amounts needed for each type of specimen. Information on the amount needed for each type of specimen is also covered under the discussion on the specific test.

4. *Do not expose others to the infectious material.* Meticulous hand washing before and after obtaining a culture is essential. The nurse must make sure that the outside of the specimen container does not get contaminated with the contents inside it. Since the contents are potentially infectious, the personnel handling the container must be protected. If the outside of the container does become contaminated, the nurse can use gloves to transfer the contents to another container. As an alternative, the nurse might also put the container into a bag and note that the outside of the container has been contaminated. Thus laboratory personnel will not touch the outside of the container with their bare hands.

5. *Make sure that the specimen is properly labeled.* The laboratory requisition must be filled out correctly. A specimen that is not properly identified is useless. If the specimen is for an outpatient, making sure that the home phone of the person is available is very important. Information required on the laboratory slip includes the patient's name and other identification, such as medical number, hospital room number, or clinic site. The type and *source* of the specimen, as well as the date and time collected, are essential. Sometimes laboratories receive a yellow liquid marked for C&S. The laboratory cannot assume that this is urine. Even if it is marked urine, the technicians have no idea whether it is from a Foley, a clean catch, or whatever. Other items, such as the need for an anaerobic report or whether the patient is on antibiotics, should be noted too.

6. *Send the culture to the laboratory as soon as possible.* All cultures should be sent to the laboratory immediately, but some specimens, such as urine, can be refrigerated if there is a delay in transporting the specimen. Some commercial kits contain an ampule of transport medium that keeps samples moist for as long as 72 hours. For some specimens, such as a culture of cerebrospinal fluid, the laboratory needs to be called before the culture is sent, so that the personnel are available to begin immediate examination of the fluid when it arrives at the laboratory. In the hospital setting, cultures are not usually collected on the evening or night shift unless the laboratory provides 24-hour service. If specimens are collected in a home setting, the nurse must check with the laboratory to see how the specimen can be transported without causing the death of the organism to be cultured.

WHEN A CULTURE AND SENSITIVITY IS ORDERED

General Nursing Implications

Besides the nurse's most obvious role of making sure that the specimen is collected properly, the nurse should consider several other possible actions once the culture has been sent to the laboratory.

TABLE 16-4.   AMOUNTS NEEDED FOR CULTURES AND TIPS FOR COLLECTION*

Type of Culture	Amount Needed	Special Notes (See Text)
Urine	2-3 ml in sterile container. (If also for urinalysis, send 15-30 ml.)	Must be clean catch or catheterized specimen so not contaminated by perineal flora.
Blood	10 ml by venipuncture. Keep in syringe or put into culture at bedside—5 ml aerobic, 5 ml anaerobic.	Be sure not contaminated with skin flora.
Sputum	2-3 ml in sterile container.	Sputum, *not* saliva.
Throat	One swab put in prepared culture (Culpak).	Touch back of throat only.
Nasopharyngeal	One swab in test tube.	Do gently.
Wound	One swab in test tube. May do syringe for anaerobic.	Clean skin around wound first.
Eye	One swab.	Careful not to touch cornea.
Vaginal	One swab. If anaerobic, need special container.	Need to do cervical for gonorrhea
Urethral	One swab.	See text for other ways to detect gonorrhea in males.
Stool	One-inch lump (walnut size) or 20 ml if diarrhea.	Only culture specimen not collected in sterile container.
CSF (pleural fluid; peritoneal fluid)	1 ml—aerobic and anaerobic.	Need to notify lab that CSF is coming. CSF, pleural, or peritoneal fluid is collected in other tubes for other types of analysis.

Information compiled from various references.

1. *Conferring with the physician about the possible need for isolation until the results of the C&S are known.* Depending on the type of potential infection, putting the patient into isolation until the definitive diagnosis is made may or may not be warranted. Hospitals have specific procedures for wound isolation, respiratory isolation, or enteric precautions depending on the type of suspected infection. The hospital should also have a written policy on criteria that designate when a patient should be isolated. If the policies are written, the nurse is given backing to isolate patients independently, without waiting for a physician's order (Aspinall 1978:1704). Although unnecessary isolation procedures are costly, as well as potentially upsetting to the patient, the decision not to isolate the patient until a culture is reported positive may expose other patients, family members, and staff to the risk of a serious infection.

Whatever the level of isolation needed, the patient should be taught how to decrease the chances of spreading a potential infection to others. Simple things, such as a paper bag for contaminated tissues, may be overlooked. Or nurses and physicians may handle dressings or wounds without using gloves. Handwashing should be routine after physical care of any patient, but staff seem to forget this "obvious" way to prevent the spread of bacteria from one patient to another. Patients may not be washing their hands after defecating either. Unless the nurse carefully surveys the environmental setting, all these breaks in technique can occur. In the home setting, the other family members need to be taught how to protect themselves from the spread of a possible infection.

2. *Preventing nosocomial infections.* A nosocomial infection is one that is acquired as a result of hospitalization or of treatment received in the hospital. During the last decades, the pool of nosocomial pathogens have changed. Reinarz (1978) notes that, despite some effective control measures, penicillinase-producing staphylococci (that is, staph resistant to penicillin) continue to be the most frequent cause of hospital-related infections. In fact, maybe "staph" infections should be spelled "staff" infections, since too often the staff of a hospital are responsible for the hospital-acquired infection. The second type of hospital-generated infection is due to gram-negative bacilla, which in the past few years have also become resistant to antiobiotics. More recently, the fungi, especially the *Candida* species, have also become important as a cause of hospital infections. Unnecessary use of antibiotics can contribute to the development of resistant strains of bacteria. Usually harmless organisms, such as fungus and some protozoans, have also begun to fill the ecological void created by the effects of antimicrobial therapy (Reinarz 1978:3).

Although nurses are not prescribing antibiotics, they should be aware of the problems so they can teach patients about the proper use of antibiotics. Patients may save antibiotics to take for another infection, or they may demand a penicillin shot for a cold. (Antibiotics are not used for viral infections.) Health teaching about the proper use of antibiotics can help to prevent abuse and misuse of antibiotics. Even more basic to nursing is the fact that nurses can help to prevent nosocomial infections by the use of proper techniques for the care of Foley catheters, the suctioning of tracheotomies, or the care of intravenous equipment. All the nursing measures that decrease the chance of the patient's developing an infection mean less need for the physician to resort to antibiotics. Aspinall (1978) gives several specific ways on how nurses can score against nosocomial infections. Basic to any successful prevention of bacterial spread is proper handwashing technique. Again and again, it must be stressed, all staff must wash their hands before and after caring for all patients.

Poor techniques by health professionals are not always to blame when patients get an infection in the hospital or nursing home. Always present in our environment are opportunistic pathogens, which do not usually cause an infection unless the resistance of the host is low. (See the discussion in Chapter 2 about the controversy of using isolation procedures to protect the patient who is severely immunosuppressed.) Reducing all possible pathogens in an environment may be very difficult. For example, food is not sterile. Salad is a notorious source of organisms, and even pepper has been shown to have potential pathogens (Kuhn 1978). So to prevent infection, rather than concentrating only on antibiotics and isolation procedures, the nurse may see that the patient has as high a resistance to organisms as possible by a good diet, plenty of rest, and other measures that promote optimum levels of well-being.

3. *Assisting the patient to combat infection.* Too often health professionals consider that the administration of antibiotics is the *only* way to treat infections, but a holistic approach to the treatment of an infection includes more. Increased fluids, a diet adequate in protein, and plenty of rest are other ways to help the body combat a bacterial invasion. The patient may need antipyretic drugs to reduce the fever, if the fever is over 102° F. Aspirin or acetaminophen (Tylenol, Datril, and the like) are two drugs prescribed to reduce high fevers. However, a moderate increase in temperature is considered useful in helping the body mobilize the defense against bacterial invasion. The natural defenses of the body to infection need to be encouraged, along with the proper use of antibiotics. Stress reduction should also be employed, so the body is free to mobilize against the infection.

4. *Assessing for characteristic signs and symptoms of infection.* Often the nurse may be the first one to detect that the patient may be getting an infection, and thus a culture should be done. For example, a nurse in a nursing home may note that the urine in a drainage bag is cloudy and has a foul odor. A pediatric nurse may note that the lungs of a child are congested and that the child has a fever. A nurse making a home visit may note that a wound appears inflamed and sore to the touch.

Although fever is usually present in infections, in some patients, particularly the elderly, fever may be absent and the WBC and differential normal. (See Chapter 2 for a discussion on the "shift to the left" as a characteristic sign of a developing bacterial infection.) The elderly who complain of "not feeling good" or who are weak or lethargic may need a complete physical to rule out the possibility of an unnoticed infection (Deal 1979:77). In the very young, laboratory reports such as the white blood count (WBC) may not be elevated, but an increase in the sedimentation rate and the bands (see Chapter 2) may be important in screening for newborn sepsis (Grylack 1979). If the patient has a potential infection, a culture is the diagnostic proof of an infection. The collection of a culture depends on the likely site of the infection, such as blood cultures for possible septicemia or a throat culture for a complaint of a sore throat.

URINE CULTURES

General Indications

On a routine urinalysis, the findings that suggest a urinary tract infection are the presence of a large number of WBCs and bacteria in the urine. Many organisms that cause urinary infections also cause an alkaline pH because the bacteria break down urea into ammonia. If the urine is not grossly contaminated with perineal secretions, a microscopic exam, which is much cheaper than a urine culture, may be enough to establish the presence of a urinary tract infection. If the urinary tract infection (UTI) does not respond quickly to medication, the culture may be needed to determine appropriate therapy (Deal 1979). The most common organism causing such infections is *Escherichia coli*. Other gram-negative rods, such as the Proteus or Pseudomonas group, are occasionally present in UTI.

Females are particularly susceptible to urinary tract infections due to the short distance of the urethra and the possible contamination from perineal organisms. ("Honeymoon" cystitis often occurs when sexual activity introduces organisms into the urinary tract). Young female children are also much more likely to have UTI than are male children. Catheterization procedures for either sex are very likely to result in a UTI unless sterile technique is used.

Frequency of urination, burning during urination, and a low-grade fever may be indicators of a urinary tract infection. If the infection is rampant, the urine may be cloudy in color and have a foul odor. See the discussion under nursing implications for the differences between lower urinary tract infection (cystitis) and upper urinary tract infections (pyelonephritis). More commonly, a UTI is of the lower urinary tract.

Preparation of Patient
And Collection of Urine Sample

Ideally, urine for cultures should be the early morning specimen since the urine is more concentrated. However, urine can be collected at any time for a culture. In addition to the general requirements for specimens noted earlier, the laboratory slip should note whether the patient is on a forced fluid regime. Most laboratories consider a clean catch midstream urine as the best method to collect urine for a culture. The laboratory needs only 1 ml to do the culture, so the urine can be transmitted by syringe if it is removed from a Foley. (See discussion on Foley specimens.) If a routine urinalysis is to be done before a C&S, the laboratory needs at least 15 ml.

There are various diagnostic kits for doing urine cultures, such as Microstix (Ames), Clinicult (Smith, Kline & French), and Uricult (Medical Technology). Patients may be taught to use these at home. (See Chapter 1 for a discussion on diagnostic kits and Chapter 3 for a screening test for nitrites as an indication of a urine infection.)

Clean Catch or Midstream Specimens. The problem in collecting urine for culture and sensitivity is that the urine may be contaminated with the bacteria normally present in the perineal area. Thus the perineal area needs to be cleansed thoroughly before the urine is collected. In one study, patient instruction with diagrams on how to use iodophor-soaked tissues as a cleanser did reduce the number of nonpathogens that often contaminate a urine specimen (McGuckin 1981). The vulvular area in the female or the tip of the penis in the male must be cleansed well with soap and water and/or a disinfectant, such as an iodine solution.

In addition, the urine is collected midstream so it contains fewer of the bacteria that reside on the perineal surfaces near the urinary meatus. To collect a midstream specimen, the patient must be able to stop the urine flow after it is begun and then urinate into a sterile cup or directly onto a dipstick for culture. The female needs to hold the labia separated so that the urinary meatus is clear. If the patient is unable to do the cleansing, the nurse can cleanse around the meatus. (A nonsterile glove can be used to protect the nurse who washes the perineal area.) In an uncircumsized male, the foreskin must stay retracted during the procedure.

Collecting Urine by Straight Catheterization. In the past, urine specimens for culture were often done by a straight catheterization to make sure that the specimen did not get contaminated from perineal secretions. For example, if a woman has a heavy menstrual flow, the urine may be contaminated with blood. However, the danger of subsequent infection as a result of catheterization is a reason to try to get urine by clean catch whenever possible. During the menstrual flow, or with vaginal secretions, the patient can clean the perineal area, insert a tampon, and then clean around the meatus again before urinating. If, for some reason, catheterizing a patient, for a urine specimen is necessary, strict aseptic technique must be followed.

Collecting Urine from a Foley Catheter. If the patient has an indwelling (Foley) catheter, urine can be collected from it. The Foley catheter must be clamped so that urine can accumulate in the bladder. Urine taken from a drainage bag is never suitable for a culture because the urine is not fresh. The newer Foley catheter drainage tubings have a special sample port for inserting a needle and syringe to remove a few cc of urine for tests. The tubing below the area may be bent back on itself so that urine collects near the port. Some tubings have a special clamp with the tubing.

In Foleys without the special vent, a 25-gauge needle can be inserted into the catheter and a small amount of urine drawn into a syringe. The catheter site or sample port should be cleansed with alcohol before the needle is inserted. It is important to make sure that the catheter is the type that reseals after a puncture. Until a few years ago, the usual practice was just to disconnect the Foley from the drainage tubing and allow some urine to drip into a sterile container. Opening the system should no longer be done due to the increased chance of contamination.

Culturing the Tip of the Foley When Removed. Sometimes the tip of the Foley catheter is cultured after the Foley is removed. If the tip of the catheter is to be cultured, it must not touch the bed or perineal area as the catheter is being withdrawn. Once the catheter is removed, it is held suspended in the air or placed on a sterile towel placed between the patient's legs. The tip of the catheter is cut off with sterile scissors and placed into the specimen container. Some clinicians feel that culturing of the Foley indicates whether a urinary tract infection is developing. However, since the catheter tip may pick up bacteria as it is withdrawn through the meatus, the findings may not be conclusive. It may be preferable just to collect a urine sample at the time the Foley is removed.

Collecting Urine in Young Children. For very young children, the perineal area is cleansed and a sterile collection bag is secured around the meatus. Obviously, this procedure is easier for male than for female infants. In older children, the perineal area can be cleansed and a urine specimen collected as for an adult. La Fave (1979) has suggested that screening procedures for urinary tract infections in young children can be done just by

Reference Values

Urine is sterile in the bladder, but it becomes contaminated with organisms normally present in the perineal area. The amount of organisms are counted and usually interpreted as follows:

Less than 10,000 organisms/ml	Unlikely UTI, probable contamination.
10,000 to 100,000 organisms/ml	Probable UTI, particularly if urine specimen is from a catheter.
More than 100,000 organisms/ml	Definite UTI.

These numbers are excluding the presence of normal genital flora such as lactobacilli.
In low-grade pyelonephritis, the urine culture may be negative even though bacteria are present in the pelvis of the kidney.
See Chapter 3 for the nitrite dipstick test as a screening test for urinary infection. A urine culture may be done in conjunction with the dipstick test.

having mothers collect a voided specimen in a clean Dixie cup. If doing so is essential, children can also be catheterized to obtain a urine specimen.

Positive Urine Culture

Nursing Implications. The key measure to assist the patient in overcoming a urinary tract infection is to keep the urine as dilute as possible so that bacteria cannot multiply rapidly. Keeping the urine acidic may also be helpful for certain bacterial infections. (See Chapter 3 on the use of cranberry juice to make the urine more acidic.) The patient needs to know exactly how much fluid should be consumed each day. The physician may prescribe sulfa drugs or antibiotics, such as ampicillin, depending on the causitive organism for the UTI, and the patient should know the possible side effects of the drugs. In addition, the nurse should make sure that the patient knows ways to prevent infections in the future by continuing adequate fluid intake. Also, some women are not aware that wiping the perineal area should be frontwards to back so that bowel bacteria are not transmitted to the meatus.

As a general rule, a patient who has a urinary tract infection has just an infection of the bladder, not of the upper portion of the urinary tract, although an infection can ascend if not properly treated. Symptoms of a lower urinary tract infection (cystitis) include frequency of urination and burning, and the urine may smell foul and look cloudy. These symptoms should subside as therapy is begun. Symptoms of flank pain, high fever, and overall malaise may indicate that the urinary tract infection has ascended and is now pyelonephritis.

BLOOD CULTURES

General Indications

Blood cultures are ordered when the patient is suspected of having septicema. In many localized infections, a few bacteria may enter the bloodstream (bacteremia), but they are usually not sufficient to cause symptoms of sepsis (septicemia). The patient with septicemia is usually severely ill with fever, chills, and other signs of a serious infection. The spikes of fever may be related to the release into the bloodstream of more bacteria. So sometimes blood cultures are ordered to be done when the patient has another spike in temperature.

Bacteria can enter the bloodstream from infections in soft tissues, from contaminated intravenous lines, such as those used for hyperalimentation, or even from minor surgical procedures, such as a tooth extraction or instrumentation by endoscopes, particularly cystoscopes. Bacteremia in elderly patients can result from pneumococcal pneumonia (Deal 1979). In adults the most common organisms causing septicemia are gram-negative rods, such as *Escherichia coli* or Aerobacter species, which can enter the bloodstream due to urinary tract infection or instrumentation of the urinary tract. *Staphlococcus aureus* may also cause septicemia. In newborns, *Escherichia coli* and B-hemolytic streptococcus are the two most frequent causes of septicemia. In the newborn, sepsis is often a result of prolonged and early rupture of the membranes (more than 24 hours before delivery), maternal infection (proven or suspected), and neonatal aspiration (Grylack 1979:222).

Preparation of Patient And Collection of Sample

Usually blood samples for blood cultures are drawn at least two different times and in both arms to increase the chance of detecting any organisms. For example, the order may read,

"Blood cultures now and in three hours. If the patient has another temperature spike, draw blood cultures immediately." The physician, nurse, or laboratory technician may draw the blood for the cultures.

Usually 10 ml are obtained from one venipuncture. Half of the specimen (5 ml) is put into a culture for anaerobic bacteria and 5 ml into a culture for aerobic bacteria. Some laboratories have the person who draws the blood add the blood directly to the culture mediums. Other laboratories prefer that the blood sample be sent directly to the laboratory and that the transfer to culture be made by the bacteriology technician.

The major problem with blood cultures is that the specimen is often contaminated with bacteria from the environment (McGuckin 1976). Hence the drawing of venous blood for blood culture is done under aseptic conditions. The skin is specially prepped before the venipuncture is done. The prep, much like a surgical prep, consists of thorough cleansing with iodine and alcohol solutions. The skin over the vein must not be touched after the prep is completed. If the skin over the vein must be probed, the person drawing the blood uses a sterile glove. The transfer of the blood sample to the culture medium must also be done as a sterile procedure. For infants, a heel stick may be done to obtain blood for a culture.

Culturing of Catheter Tip. Sometimes septicemia can result from an indwelling intravenous catheter, particularly a central venous catheter used to deliver hyperalimentation fluids. The high glucose content of hyperalimentation fluids supports bacterial growth. Sometimes when the intravenous catheter is removed, the tip is cut off with sterile scissors and sent to the laboratory for culturing. The tip should not be allowed to touch the patient's skin or the bedclothes. A sterile towel can be used to catch the catheter when it is removed.

Reference Values

Any bacteria in the blood is clinically significant. Yet, since there is always the possibility of contamination from the skin, the bacteriologist may make an interpretation of possible contaminants if certain skin bacteria are present in small amounts. Another blood culture may be ordered to determine if bacteria are actually in the blood. A final diagnosis from a blood culture may take seven to ten days. However, if the laboratory identifies the presence of certain pathogens, even in small amounts, it issues a preliminary positive report so that the physician can order appropriate antibiotics. *Escherichia coli* is a common pathogen in both adults and children. Other pathogens may be *Staphylococcus aureus* and various streptococci. (See discussion under general indications.)

If an intravenous catheter tip is cultured, a count of 15 or fewer colonies is usually not significant. A count of more than 15 colonies on the culture suggests the catheter as the source of the septicemia (Reinarz 1978:16).

Positive Blood Culture

Possible Nursing Implications. Patients with septicemia often have low resistance to infection because they are already critically ill from other causes. So most of the appropriate nursing care is that given to acutely ill patients. Refer to nursing texts for care of septicemia patients. Septic shock may occur and be fatal. Usually patients with septicemia are not a source of infection for others, but this possibility should be carefully assessed. In the infant, hypoglycemia (Chapter 8) and hyperbilirubinemia (Chapter 11) are often concurrent problems with septicemia.

SPUTUM CULTURES

General Indications

Sputum cultures are often ordered when the patient has lung congestion (rales), elevated temperature, and other signs of a probable respiratory infection. Respiratory infections cause an increased secretion of respiratory secretions or sputum. Sputum originates in the bronchi, not in the upper respiratory tract. Different bacteria cause the sputum to be greenish, yellowish, or rust-colored. The sputum may have a foul smell.

Almost all of the bacteria that cause respiratory infections are normally present in the respiratory tract in small amounts. In healthy people, these organisms, such as *Klebsiella* or *Staphylococcus,* do not cause disease because they are present in small amounts. Yet when an organism has a chance to grow quickly due to stagnant respiratory secretions, the patient can get pneumonia. Three of the organisms that often cause pneumonia are *Pneumonococcus, Staphylococcus aureus,* and *Hemophilus influenza.* Sputum cultures can identify which organism is in abundance and thus the cause of the respiratory problem. If tuberculosis is suspected, a special type of culture for AFB (acid-fast bacillus) is done.

Preparation of Patient
And Collection of Sample

The laboratory needs only a few milliliters of sputum for a culture. Sputum, however, is not the same thing as saliva. The sputum specimen must be from the bronchial tree, not just saliva from the mouth.Having patients rinse out their mouths before the sputum is obtained is a good idea, so that the sputum is not contaminated with saliva and mouth bacteria. An early morning specimen is ideal because the sputum is more concentrated then. Early morning sputum also tends to be more plentiful if the patient has been sleeping through the night and the secretions have tended to pool. Sometimes the sputum culture is ordered ''×3,'' which means that three different collections should be made, not three at one time!

Sputum from the bronchial tree can be obtained in several ways. If at all possible, the patient should be allowed to cough up the sputum. If the patient is unable to cough, suctioning can be done with a special catheter that allows some of the secretions to be caught in a special reservoir. Sputum cultures are also obtained by the use of a bronchoscope.

If the purpose is to determine the presence of the acid-fast bacillus (AFB) that causes tuberculosis, the culture may be done at least three different days. If no sputum can be obtained, the physician may order a gastric analysis since *Mycobacterium tuberculosis* is acid-resistant and thus not destroyed by the gastric acidity. Urine may be cultured for AFB too if tuberculosis of the kidney is suspected.

Reference Values

Various organisms, if present in large amounts, can cause acute respiratory infections. The laboratory reports the predominant organism or organisms present in the sputum. Common organisms include *Pneumonococci, Staphlococcus aureus,* and *Hemophilus influenza.*

Various gram-negative bacilli may also cause respiratory infections. The culture for these common bacteria is completed in 24 to 48 hours.

A culture for tuberculosis (AFB culture) grows very slowly. It may take three to eight weeks to get a final report. Yet sometimes the laboratory is able to report a positive smear for AFB, so treatment can be initiated before the final growth is documented.

Positive Sputum Culture

Possible Nursing Implications. As with other types of positive cultures antibiotics are given. Patients need encouragement to do deep breathing and coughing exercises. They may also need intensive respiratory therapy by suctioning or some type of postural drainage. The nurse needs to make sure that hydration is adequate because without adequate fluids the sputum becomes very tenacious. The nurse also needs to teach patients how to safely dispose of the sputum that is excreted. If patients are coughing up large amounts of sputum, cleaning an emesis basin is easier if the basin is first lined with tissues. Otherwise sputum tends to become encrusted in the basin. Teaching patients to cover their mouths when coughing seems common sense, but the nurse may have to remind patients. As a general rule, patients with most types of pneumonia are not put on isolation. However, depending on the type of organism in the sputum, respiratory isolation might be justified. Coagulase-positive staphylcoccal and group A streptococcal pneumonias are two organisms that require isolation.

For patients with tuberculosis (positive AFB culture), the nursing care is based on the standard care for tuberculosis patients. Refer to a nursing text on the current treatment of tuberculosis in this country. The patient needs to be on respiratory isolation as soon as a positive AFB is known.

THROAT CULTURES

Throat cultures are the only reliable means for differentiating strep throats from viral sore throats. Most sore throats are caused by viruses; only about 15% of them in children are caused by group A beta hemolytic streptococci (Wang 1977:1797). Yet identifying whether the patient has group A beta hemolytic streptococci is important because rheumatic fever and glomerulonephritis may follow such infections. (Streptococci are classified according to the antigens. Some are not considered particularly pathogenic as is group A beta hemolytic strep.) (See Chapter 14 on the streptococcal antigen–antibody tests of ASO, anti-DNase-B, and streptoenzyme.) Occasionally a throat culture for gonorrhea may be done if the patient has been engaging in oral sex with a partner with gonorrhea.

Certain clinical signs and symptoms should alert nurses to the possibility that a sore throat is indeed a bacterial infection rather than a viral one. Usually, with bacterial infections:

1. Temperatures are higher than with viral infections.
2. The symptoms usually occur more abruptly and the patient seems more ill.
3. Also, the patches on the throat are more distinctive.
4. The white blood count (WBC) is characteristically elevated—not so with viral infections. (See Chapter 2 on the significance of the WBC in bacterial infections.)

Wang (1977) provides an excellent comparison of the physical findings for viral and bacterial sore throats.

Preparation of Patient
And Collection of Sample

Throat cultures are done with a swab that is immediately placed into a test tube or kit with a special medium for the growth of streptococci (Culpak). The tongue is depressed with a tongue blade and a flashlight used to visualize the inflamed area of the throat. The sterile swab is rubbed over each tonsilar area and the posterior pharynx without touching the lips or tongue. Any white patch should be cultured. If throat cultures are done on an outpatient basis, it is important to get a phone number so the patient can be reached if the culture is positive for "strep" throat or for group A beta hemolytic streptococci.

Reference Values

The diagnosis of strep throat is based on finding group A beta hemolytic streptococcus in a culture. Other possible pathogens can be *Hemophilus influenza, Corynbacterium diphtheriae,* Gonococcus, or Meningcoccus.

Positive Throat Culture for
Streptococci Group A

Possible Nursing Implications. If streptococci are the cause of the sore throat, the patient is put on penicillin, or erthyromycin in the case of a penicillin allergy. If all signs and symptoms point to a diagnosis of strep throat, the physician may order antibiotics before the 18 to 24 hours that it takes to get a culture result.

People sometimes discontinue antibiotics after they begin to feel better. Yet antibiotic therapy for strep throat must be continued for at least ten days as a minimum (Wang 1977:1798), regardless of how well the patient feels. So the nurse may assess to make sure that the parents, or the patients themselves, understand the reason why the antibiotic is to be continued for ten or so days. Either the physician or the nurse may have to explain to the parents that undertreating "strep" throat increases the possibility of the later development of rheumatic fever.

Patients with strep throat are not isolated since they are considered noninfectious a few hours after antibiotic therapy is begun. Wang (1977) reports that about half of the siblings and nearly one-fourth of the parents of a child with strep throat have the organism too. Since streptococci are transmitted in the droplets from the respiratory tract, the infected person should not cough or breathe on others. The nurse may become involved with follow-up contacts for other family members. In a school setting, the school nurse or public health nurse can be very effective in both detecting and preventing the spread of strep throat in a population. Preventing strep infections helps to prevent rheumatic fever, of which approximately 100,000 new cases occur in this country each year (Fitzmaurice 1980:1). Rheumatic heart disease is the only major form of cardiovascular disease that is potentially preventable at the present time. (See Chapter 14 on the streptococci antigen tests used to assess for previous acute infections with streptococci.)

NASOPHARYNGEAL CULTURES

General Indications
Nasal cultures may be done to identify suspected carriers of organisms, such as *Staphylococcuc aureus,* which are also called coag-positive. The differentiation between carrier state and infection is often difficult since some pathogens do transiently appear in the normal human pharynx (Shelter 1980). Health workers in such areas as newborn nurseries or operating rooms may have nasal cultures to screen out potential sources of disease to patients. The exact meaning of a carrier state, however, is often hard to assess.

Preparation of Patient
And Collection of Sample
A flexible swab is inserted gently into the nose and rotated against the anterior nares. The flexible swab makes it possible to culture the posterior pharynx also. The swab is placed into a tube of transport medium and sent to the laboratory. Identification of particular strains of staphylococcus may require special laboratory resources not found in all institutions.

Reference Values

Pathogens such as streptococcus, pneumonococcus, or *Neisseria meningitis* may or may not be clinically significant. Coag-positive staphylococcus may be present in 50% of people who have nasopharyngeal cultures done (Ravel 1978:145).

Positive Nasal Cultures
Possible Nursing Implications. If a health worker has a positive culture, the physician must evaluate the importance of the person as a carrier. The health worker who is a potential source of pathogens may be assigned to areas where the risk of infecting others is minimized. The actual danger to others is somewhat controversial since many pathogens are always present to some degree and become disease-producing only when the opportunity arises. These opportunistic pathogens are probably dangerous for the already ill and immuno-deficient person (Kuhn, 1978). Many hospitals have an infection control nurse as part of an infection control team. As employees, nurses should seek out information about how their institutions handle the problem of carriers. How to treat a positive nasal culture is a medical decision.

WOUND CULTURES

General Indications
Normally wounds should not be infected with any organisms. Yet once the integrity of the skin is broken, there is a direct pathway for skin flora to reach tissue. An infected wound is usually obvious even to the untrained eye. The characteristic signs are redness, heat, and swelling. There may also be drainage that contains pus (purulent) and that may have a foul smell. If the wound cannot drain, the infection can cause pain and swelling, such as in

an abscess. The wounds of surgical patients should be inspected daily for any sign of infection. Patients with burns, abrasions, or bedsores (decubiti) are also very susceptible to infections of the open skin areas.

Preparation of Patient
And Collection of Wound Culture

In collecting a specimen for culture from a wound, nurses must not contaminate the specimen with the normal skin flora. The skin around the wound should be cleansed to eliminate any flora present. The swab should be put deep into the wound without touching the skin around the wound, and it should be directed to the area where the purulent drainage is the most profuse. It is permissible, and indeed necessary, to make sure that the swab is in direct contact with the infected area. If the infected area is contained in a pocket or abcess, the physician has to do an incision and drainage (I&D) to obtain material for culturing. (The I&D is also therapeutic in that it allows the infected material to be removed.)

As with the collection of other specimens, nurses must be sure to prevent the spread of the infection. After using the swab to collect the specimen, they should immediately place it into a culture tube. One swab, well soaked with wound drainage, is usually sufficient. If there is the possibility of a fungus infection, a swab should be wet with sterile, normal saline before the culture is done. Swabs made for wound culture have an area above the stopper that can be touched by the nurse. If the swab is not attached to a stopper, the nurse can break off the part of the swab that was touched.

For an anaerobic culture, some wound drainage can be collected in a syringe. All of the air should be expelled from the syringe and the sample sent to the laboratory in the syringe (Marchiondo 1979).

Reference Values

Common organisms found in wounds are *Staphylococcus aureus,* group A streptococci, gram-negative bacilli, and fungi. If the wound is deep and hence not in direct contact with the air, anaerobic bacteria such as *Clostridium* or anaerobic streptococci may also thrive. The culture and sensitivity is very useful in assisting the physician to select an effective antibiotic.

Possible Nursing Implications. If the wound is completely covered and is not draining to the outside, simple wound isolation is needed. In essence, wound isolation means using a gown and gloves when the wound must be dressed. Sometimes staff tend to become careless in using sterile technique when the patient has a wound infection. A break in sterile technique is shrugged off as being not too important because "the patient already has an infected wound." Obviously this kind of thinking is not justifiable because, no matter how infected a wound may be, adding other organisms to it is still possible. Dressing changes of an infected wound require the same careful sterile technique as do wounds that are not already infected.

If the wound is draining enough so that the dressings become soaked, the patient may become a source of infection to others. So more extreme isolation procedures may need to be carried out. Refer to the specific policies of a given institution. Many hospitals now have an infection control nurse who can help nursing personnel decide what level of isolation is required for the hospitalized patient with a wound infection. In the home setting, the nurse needs to teach the patient how to avoid transmitting the infection to others. Because proper wound healing requires good nutrition, the dietary needs of the patient should be assessed. (See the ideas discussed earlier in this chapter about ways to increase a person's resistance to infection.)

EYE CULTURES

Though the eye contains few bacteria, the bathing of the eye with tears usually keeps the actual count of bacteria very low. An infected eye is easy to see even by the lay person. The physician may wish to determine whether an eye discharge is due to a viral or bacterial invasion.

Preparation of Patient
And Collection of Sample
A sterile swab is used to collect some of the purulent matter from the eye. The patient should be told to look up while the nurse gently pulls down on the cheek. The swab can be placed on the conjunctiva. Not touching the cornea with the swab is important. After the specimen is collected, it is put into a sterile culture tube.

Reference Values

Staphylococcus aureus and *Pseudomonas aerogenosa* are two bacteria that may cause eye infections. In the newborn, *Gonococcus neisseria* can be transmitted when the baby goes through the birth canal. To prevent this transmission of gonorrhea, some state laws require delivery room personnel to instill silver nitrate or an antibiotic ointment in every newborn's eyes.

Possible Nursing Implications. Patients should be taught not to wipe the infected eye. They must also avoid transmitting the infection to the other eye. Dark glasses may offer some comfort to patients, if they need to be outdoors. They may also need instructions on the proper way to instill eye drops.

VAGINAL AND URETHRAL SMEARS

The vagina normally contains such bacteria as *Lactobacillus, Staphylococci, Escherichia coli,* and some yeast. Most commonly, vaginal infections are due to *Trichomonas vaginalis* or to the fungus *Candida albicans.* If gonorrhea is suspected in a female, an endocervical smear is done. In the male, smears or cultures of the drainage from the urethra may be done for gonorrhea. Also in the male, centrifuged urine may be cultured for gonorrhea.

Gonorrhea is the most common sexually transmitted disease in the United States. About half of the cases of pelvic inflammatory disease (PID) in women are due to gonorrhea. Smears and/or cultures may be done to identify the gram-negative diplococci, *Neisseria gonorrhaeae.* Hansfield (1978:932) states that, if a highly experienced technician is examining the smear, smears alone are often adequate to detect gonorrhea. Any patient who is shown to have the gram-negative diplococci, but who does not respond to antibiotic therapy, is cultured to determine if the infection is due to a penicillin-resistant strain of gonorrhea.

Oropharyngeal and rectal smears may need to be done if the patient has had oral or rectal sex with an infected person.

Preparation of Patient
And Collection of Sample

Vaginal and Endocervical Smears in Females. To obtain a vaginal smear or culture, the swab needs to be inserted well into the vagina. The patient or the nurse needs to hold the labia apart so that the swab does not touch the outer lips. If the nurse must separate the lips of the vagina, a nonsterile glove should be used. An endocervical specimen, necessary for suspected gonorrhea, requires the use of a speculum as for other pelvic examinations. Only water is used to lubricate the speculum. Excess cervical mucus is wiped off with a dry cotton ball and then a cotton tipped swab is inserted in the endocervical canal for 30 seconds to absorb any organisms. Two specimens are put on one special culture medium. (If an anal specimen is collected it is put on a separate culture.) A smear for *Trichomonas* is obtained on a wet saline swab for immediate transport to the laboratory.

Urethral Smears in Males. Collection of urethral smears in the male is often done at the time the physician is examining the patient for complaints of discharge from the penis. The exudate is collected on a swab which is rolled, not rubbed, on a slide. A special loop swab can be gently inserted into the urinary meatus to obtain exudate. If the patient has no discharge from the penis, a urine specimen may be centrifuged to obtain a smear or culture for possible gonorrhea.

Reference Values

The presence of gram-negative cocci on a smear is considered diagnostic of gonorrhea. A culture may or may not be needed to confirm the identification of the *Gonococcus.* Vaginal smears can identify other organisms, such as fungus (*Candida*) or protozoan (*Trichomonas*), that may be causing vaginitis.

Positive Vaginal or
Urethral Smear or Culture

Possible Nursing Implications. Gonorrhea is a communicable disease that needs to be reported to the health department, which employs people to serve as case finders. Alhtough the sexual contacts of these patients need to be examined to do case finding, patients may or may not wish to name their sexual partners. The nurse can be sensitive to their needs and yet also impress upon them the importance of the disease as a public health problem. These patients need clear instructions from the physician or from other health professionals about the restrictions that should be put on sexual contact until the disease is cured. Penicillin is the usual treatment. Repeat smears and/or cultures (in women) are done 3–5 days after therapy as a test of cure.

Other diseases, such as *Trichimonas,* do not require reporting but its spread from person to person is also of concern. The female may keep getting reinfected from a male partner unless he too is cultured and treated (the ping-pong effect). Thus treatment of any infection of the genitourinary tract involves not only the person, but also the person or persons who have been and who will be sexual partners of the patient. The nurse can help set a climate that is conducive to assisting these patients to help themselves and others. A punitive, noncaring, or hostile environment alienates persons who come to seek help.

Female patients may need specific instructions on how to insert vaginal suppositories or to administer douches, if medicine is ordered in these forms. Again, the nurse must foster a climate that helps patients feel comfortable about discussing intimate details.

STOOL CULTURES

Many normal bacteria live in the feces. In fact, a large percentage of the weight of feces is from bacteria. Most of the organisms in the bowel are many types of gram-negative bacilli. For example, *Escherichia coli* is a common normal inhabitant in adults. (In children under one year of age, *Escherichia coli* can be pathogenic.) Bacterial cultures for stool are routinely checked for *Staphylococcus aureus, Salmonella, Shigella* and other enteropathogens. If anaerobic organisms are suspected, such as botulism, an anaerobic culture is done too.

In addition to cultures for bacteria, stool specimens may also be collected to identify parasites that can be protozoa or worms (helminths). If the laboratory is checking for protozoa such as *Entamoeba histolytica,* the nurse must collect several specimens over a period of days. Since the protozoan parasites have cyclical lifestyles, multiple collections increase the chance of spotting a parasite (Shelter 1980). (See Chapter 14 for a serology test done for amebas.)

Two other methods to collect stool specimens for examination involve cellophane tape and a rectal swab. The cellophane tape may be pressed over the perineal area to pick up pinworms, which are very small intestinal worms. Rectal swabs are sometimes done for *Shigella* and for gonorrhea, if this disease is suspected. Yet few organisms live in the rectal wall; the mass of bacteria or parasites is in the feces.

Preparation of Patient
And Collection of Sample

For bacterial or protozoan cultures, a walnut-sized piece of feces is all that is needed. Diarrhea stool can also be cultured; only about 15 to 20 ml are needed. The rest of the stool is discarded. The specimen should be sent to the laboratory immediately. Check with the laboratory for the time span permissible.

The patient must defecate into a clean bedpan. Urine in the bedpan may kill some of the growth. A tongue blade can be used to transfer the small amount of stool to the stool container. Commercial kits contain small spoons inside a specimen container. When handling the bedpan, the nurse should wear disposable nonsterile gloves. Since parasites or bacteria may often be harbored in mucus or in streaks of blood, some of this material should be included in the sample. The stool specimen is put into a waxed container with a tight-fitting lid. It is important not to contaminate the outside of the specimen container. Patients may collect a stool specimen at home. If so, they need to be taught how to properly collect the specimen and how to properly wash their hands so that the outside of the container is not contaminated. Enteric diseases are spread by oral-fecal transmission. For children, a container can be put under the toilet seat so the child can sit on the toilet.

If a rectal swab or cellophane tape is used to collect material from the rectal area, the nurse should wear a glove when touching the perineal area. A sterile cotton-tipped swab is inserted 1 inch into the anal canal. The swab should be moved side to side and left for 30 seconds for the absorption of organisms. Note on the laboratory slip whether the patient is on antibiotics since these drugs change the flora in the intestines. Also, the use of antacids may change the pH of the stool and affect bacterial growth.

If the fat content of the stool is to be measured due to malabsorption problems, the *entire* stool for one to three days is sent to the laboratory. The patient would be on a 100-g fat diet. (See Appendix A, Table 6 for values.)

Reference Values

The laboratory may issue a preliminary report of probable findings of *Salmonella* or *Shigella,* so that enteric precautions can be started. Parasites or worms may be immediately identified by examination. The two major protozoa infections in the United States are amebiasis and giandiasis (John 1981).

Positive Stool Culture

Possible Nursing Implications. Regardless of the type of pathogen in the stool, the nurse must make sure that the patient does not spread the pathogens to others. Isolation is usually not required if patients can wash their hands properly and if the feces can quickly be flushed into the sewage system. The nurse should be aware that the collection of stool and the focus on the anal area is often a source of embarrassment for the individual. (Saving a stool has been frowned upon since the age of 2 and the anal stage.) The patient should not be made to feel "unclean" due to the extra precautions needed to protect others. Others in the family need to be checked for pathogens too. Children are very prone to spread disease due to poor hygiene.

Once appropriate therapy has been started, patients need follow-up stool samples to evaluate the effectiveness of the therapy. Some of the drugs used for intestinal pathogens cause gastrointestinal symptoms; so it is important that patients know what may be expected from the drug and what may be an indication that therapy is not being effective. Later stool samples may show a second type of pathogen also present.

CULTURES OF CEREBROSPINAL FLUID

Specimens of cerebrospinal fluid (CSF) are obtained by lumbar puncture. CSF is sterile, and it is collected under sterile conditions. Various organisms may be responsible for meningitis, including *Hemophilus meningitis, Neisseria meningitidis,* and *Pneumococcus.* The first is common in infants and the last in adults (McGuckin 1976:17).

The laboratory does an immediate smear to see if any organisms exist. The laboratory should be notified that CSF is going to the laboratory so that immediate analysis can begin. The specific identifications of the organism may take 48 to 72 hours. Refer to a nursing text for the care of patients with suspected or diagnosed meningitis.

CULTURES OF PLEURAL FLUID, PERITONEAL FLUID, AND JOINT FLUID

Pleural fluid, obtained from a thoracentesis, can be cultured for possible bacterial growth as can peritoneal fluid from a paracentesis. Joint fluid from a joint aspiration may also be cultured. The role of the nurse in carefully marking the specimens and sending them to the laboratory was discussed in the beginning of this chapter. Careful labeling is necessary for *all* specimens, and, if a urine specimen is not labeled correctly, it is usually possible to obtain another specimen. But it may be much less feasible to obtain a second specimen of any fluid that requires an invasive technique.

Questions

16-1. The laboratory reports a large number of gram-negative rods *are* present on the preliminary stain of a urine specimen. Which one of the following organisms could not be present if all the organisms are gram-negative rods?

    a. *Escherichia coli.*   **c.** *Neisseria gonorrhea.*

    b. *Proteus* species.   **d.** *Pseudomonas* species.

16-2. An anaerobic collection of a specimen is necessary if the suspected organism is/are which of the following?

    a. Acid-fast bacillus (AFB).   **c.** Bacteroides.

    b. *Staphylococcus aureus.*   **d.** Hemophilus influenza.

16-3. Mrs. Siegel's urine was sent to the laboratory for a C&S (culture and sensitivity). The report notes an "S" next to all the listed antibiotics except penicillin, which is marked with an "R." An "R" next to the penicillin indicates what?

    a. Penicillin is the right drug for the urine infection.

    b. Mrs. Siegel is resistant to penicillin.

    c. Penicillin must be increased to obtain a successful urine level.

    d. The organisms in the culture were resistant to penicillin.

16-4. Which of the following is *not* a standard procedure when collecting a specimen for culture?

    a. Administering the first dose of the antibiotic prior to collecting the specimen.

    b. Collecting all specimens, except stool, by sterile technique.

    c. Sending the specimen to the laboratory as soon as possible.

    d. Marking the source of the specimen on the laboratory requisition.

16-5. Common bacteria that cause noscomial infections are staphylococci and gram-negative rods. Which nursing action would be the most effective way to *prevent* these noscomial infections?

    a. Administering all prescribed antibiotics on time.

    b. Emphasizing handwashing before and after caring for every patient.

    c. Isolating all patients with fevers of undetermined origin (FUO).

    d. Culturing all open wounds.

16–6. Mrs. Mozian, age 78, has had cultures done of blood, urine, and sputum due to a persistent fever and general malaise. In planning care for Mrs. Mozian, the nurse in the nursing home should do all the following *except* which?

    a. Assess the fluid intake and determine how much PO fluids should be taken daily.

    b. Consult with the physician to see if there is any need for isolation procedures.

    c. Promote periods of rest so that Mrs. Mozian does not become fatigued.

    d. Use aspirin PRN to keep the temperature at a normal level.

16–7. Which of the following is a correct statement about the collection of urine for urine cultures?

    a. The meatus of the male requires more cleansing than does the meatus of the female.

    b. A disinfectant should never be used to cleanse the genital area before a clean catch is done.

    c. A clean catch urine requires that the urine be caught in midstream.

    d. Only a catheterized urine specimen is suitable for urine culture.

16–8. According to the laboratory report, Mary Jones has a probable urinary tract infection. This classification of ''probable'' is based on which finding?

    a. Only a few organisms/ml.

    b. Less than 10,000 organisms/ml.

    c. 10,000 to 100,000 organisms/ml.

    d. More than 100,000 organisms/ml.

16–9. Mr. Edwards has been having fever and chills from an unknown cause. He is to have blood cultures drawn ×2. The nurse should be aware of which of the following?

    a. The skin over the venipuncture site must be prepped with an iodine preparation to reduce contamination by skin flora.

    b. Both blood cultures can be drawn at the same time if the specimens are put into two different test tubes.

    c. Blood cultures should not be drawn after a spike of fever or a chill.

    d. A positive confirmation of a diagnosis can be made in 24 hours.

16–10. Mrs. Solado has had a central venous catheter in place for several days for hyperalimentation. The physician is removing the catheter because of possible sepsis.

The catheter is to be cultured. How should the nurse prepare the specimen for the laboratory?

   a. Wrap the entire catheter in a sterile towel and send to the lab.

   b. Cut off the tip of the catheter with sterile scissors, put the tip into a sterile container, and send it to the lab.

   c. Cut off the tip of the catheter with bandage scissors, put the tip in a clean test tube, and send it to the lab.

   d. Put a sterile swab inside the tip of the catheter and then send the swab to the lab.

16-11. Mr. McKay is to have a sputum specimen obtained due to lung congestion and fever. Which of the following instructions by the nurse is correct to tell Mr. McKay?

   a. "Save as much sputum as you can in the next two hours since the laboratory needs at least an ounce (30 ml) of sputum."

   b. "Discard the first specimen in the morning because the secretions will not be fresh."

   c. "Saliva will be all right for a specimen if it hurts to do a deep cough."

   d. "Rinse out your mouth before obtaining the specimen so bacteria from the mouth will be less numerous."

16-12. Mrs. Gardeni is to have sputum specimens ×3 for AFB. If the preliminary report comes back positive, she may be on respiratory isolation to prevent the spread of what?

   a. Tuberculosis.   **c.** Influenza.

   b. Pneumonia.   **d.** All of the above.

16-13. Timmy, age 10, has come to see the school nurse for a "sore throat." The nurse decides to do a throat culture. The concern for correctly identifying the cause of the sore throat is important because rheumatic fever or glomerulonephritis sometimes occurs after infection with which organism?

   a. A virus.

   b. Group A-beta hemolytic streptococcus.

   c. Staphylococcus aureus.

   d. Any of the streptococci.

16-14. In a hospital setting, nasopharyngeal cultures are used mainly to do which of the following?

   a. Diagnose respiratory infections in children.

   b. Confirm the organisms causing meningitis in newborns.

   c. Diagnose pneumonia in adults.

   d. Identify carriers of pathogens such as *Staphylococcus aureus*.

16-15. Mr. Jason has a Penrose drain from an abdominal stab wound. The nurse is to obtain a culture of the wound. Which action by the nurse is *not* appropriate?

    a. Using sterile gloves to obtain the specimen.

    b. Cleansing the skin around the drain before obtaining the specimen.

    c. Inserting the swab deep into the wound to get the specimen.

    d. Obtaining a second culture from the wound after the wound has been irrigated.

16-16. Mr. Rabinowitz has an infected eye. Which of the following actions by the visiting nurse is *not* appropriate?

    a. Using a sterile swab to collect some exudate and putting the swab into culture media supplied by the laboratory.

    b. Lightly touching the cornea with the swab to get the specimen.

    c. Instructing the patient not to rub his eye with his fingers.

    d. Showing the patient how to rinse off the exudate without contaminating the other eye.

16-17. Johnny Phillips, age 17, is concerned that he may have gonorrhea. He asks the nurse in the clinic how gonorrhea can be detected. The nurse should explain to Johnny that the test for gonorrhea involves which of the following?

    a. Drawing blood by venipuncture for a serology test.

    b. Obtaining some secretions from the end of the penis for a microscopic exam.

    c. Both urine and blood tests.

    d. Only a fingerstick for a blood sample.

16-18. Mr. Cohen is to have a stool specimen collected due to a possible *Salmonella* infection. He just had a bowel movement in the bedside commode. Which action by the nurse is appropriate?

    a. Send a small portion of the stool in a waxed container to the laboratory.

    b. Discard the stool since it was diarrhea rather than formed stool.

    c. Use sterile gloves to transfer all of the stool to a sterile container and send it to the laboratory.

    d. Send the entire stool in a waxed container to the laboratory.

REFERENCES

Aspinall, Mary J. "Scoring Against Nosocomial Infections," *American Journal of Nursing* 78 (October 1978): 1704-1707.

Deal, William. "Unusual Manifestations of Infectious Diseases in the Aging," *Geriatrics* 34 (May 1979): 77-84.

Fitzmaurice, Joan. *Rheumatic Heart Disease and Mitral Valve Disease*. New York: Appleton-Century Crofts, 1980.

Grylack, Lawrence and Scanlon, John. "Practical Evaluation of Historical Data and Laboratory Screening Procedures For Recognition of Newborn Sepsis," *Clinical Pediatrics* 18 (April 1979): 227-231.

Hansfield, Hunter. "Gonorrhea and Nongonoccal Urethritis, Recent Advances," *Medical Clinics of North America* 62 (September 1978): 925-943.

Hewitt, William and McHenry, Martin. "Blood Level Determinations of Antimicrobial Drugs" *Medical Clinics of North America* 62: 1119-1137, September, 1978.

Kuhn, Phyllis. "Opportunistic Pathogens, Microbes with a Potential for Violence," *Diagnostic Medicine* 1 (November 1978): 80-92.

LaFave, John *et al.* "Office Screening for Asymptomatic Urinary Tract Infections," *Clinical Pediatrics* 18 (January 1979): 53-59.

John, Rita Marie. "Giardiasis and Amebiasis", *RN* 44 (April 1981): 53-57.

Lee, Richard. "Antimicrobial Therapy," *American Journal of Nursing* 73 (December 1973): 2044-2048.

McGuckin, Maryanne. "Microbiologic Studies, Part 2: Improving Your Role in Blood Culture Procedures," *Nursing '76* 6 (January 1976): 16-17.

McGuckin, Maryanne. "Tips for Assisting with Cultures of CSF and Other Body Fluids," *Nursing '76* 6 (April 1976): 17-20.

McGuckin, Maryanne. "Getting Better Urine Specimens with the Clean Catch Midstream Technique" *Nursing 81* 11: 72-73, January, 1981.

Marchiondo, Kathleen. "Collecting Culture Specimens," *Nursing '79* 9 (April 1979): 34-43.

Mikat, Dorothy and Mikat, Kurt. *A Clinician's Guide to Bacteria and Fungi,* 3rd ed. Indianapolis: Eli Lilly Company, 1976.

Ravel, Richard. *Clinical Laboratory Medicine.* Chicago: Yearbook Medical Publishers, Inc., 3rd ed., 1978.

Reinarz, James. "Nosocomial Infections," *Ciba Clinical Symptoms* 30 (1978): 6.

Shelter, Mary and Bartos, Harriet. "Stool Specimens: Key to Detecting Intestinal Invaders," *RN* 43 (October 1980): 50-53.

Shelter, Mary and Bartos, Harriet. "Respiratory Tract Cultures," *RN* 43 (November 1980): 52-53.

Wang, Rosalind. "Streptococcal Sore Throat," *American Journal of Nursing '77* (November 1977): 1797-1798.

CHAPTER SEVENTEEN

Clinical Toxicology Tests

Objectives

1. Explain the rationale for drug monitoring by plasma drug levels, including the use of peak and trough levels.
2. Describe how plasma drug levels are used to monitor aminoglycoside levels.
3. Name four anticonvulsants that are sometimes monitored by serum levels, and indicate the clinical symptoms of each that may indicate toxicity.
4. Identify the antipsychotic drug that must be monitored by serum drug levels to avoid toxicity.
5. Identify the two major clinical problems that may develop if a patient has a serum theophylline level above the therapeutic range.
6. Identify which cardiac drugs are most commonly monitored by serum drug levels, along with the key nursing implications for each drug.
7. Describe three different clinical situations in which aspirin (ASA) serum levels are useful.
8. Identify the important facts that emergency room nurses should know about blood alcohol levels and other depressant drugs.
9. Identify the usual medication history of a patient who develops bromide toxicity.
10. Identify the major source for lead poisoning in young children.

Clinical toxicology involves the study of drugs that are therapeutic as well as those that are toxic. In clinical practice, the line between therapeutic effects and toxic effects may be narrow. The cardinal principle of experimental toxicology, derived from a sixteenth-century physician and alchemist, is that only the *dose* differentiates between a poison and a remedy (Scala 1978:774). For example, digoxin in the correct dosage for an individual is therapeutic, but, if the dose is increased even slightly, the drug may be extremely toxic. Measurements of arsenic, carbon monoxide, or mercury (all poisons) are traditional examples of toxicology (Miller 1978). Therapeutic drug monitoring is a type of clinical toxicology. Toxicology departments in general hospitals have expanded in the last few years because more and more drugs can be easily measured in the serum. The radioimmunoassay method (RIA) and the enzyme methods (discussed in Chapter 15) have made it possible for the laboratory to detect even very small amounts of a drug or toxic substance in the bloodstream.

Although any drug can be measured in the serum, this chapter focuses on the drugs that are commonly measured and that have clinical significance for the nurse. Some general reasons for monitoring drugs, some of the pitfalls of using drug levels as assessment tools, and the general nursing implications when drug levels are used are discussed at the beginning of the chapter. Tests for specific drugs, along with any needed precautions about collection of the sample and about the specific nursing implications, are listed separately in the second part of the chapter.

PLASMA DRUG LEVELS

Reasons for Monitoring

Richens and Warrington (1979:493) list seven reasons why plasma drug levels need to be measured. In addition, two other reasons for monitoring are discussed.

1. *When the rate of a drug's metabolism has a wide interindividual variation.* Many drugs are given at about the same dosage for all people because the rate of metabolism does not vary much from person to person. For other drugs, such as theophylline, the rate of metabolism may vary greatly, depending on many metabolic variations in the individual. With regard to theophylline, the Federal Drug Administration has put out specific guidelines for dosage based on weight, age, smoker/nonsmoker, and presence of certain diseases (FDA Bulletin, February 1980). The dosage of theophylline must be tailored to fit the particular individual. For example, if a smoker becomes a nonsmoker, the theophylline dose may need to be decreased. The serum theophylline concentration can be measured to make sure that the dosage is maintaining the correct serum level.

2. *When saturation kinetics occur.* For some drugs, such as phenytoin (Dilantin), an increase in dosage beyond a certain point does not increase the effectiveness of the drug because the body is saturated. The actual pharmacokinetics of a drug may be very complex, and they are used to determine the serum level considered therapeutically effective. On the other hand, for some drugs, the serum level is not at all reliable because the main action of the drug may be in tissues.

3. *When the therapeutic ratio of the drug is close to the toxic level.* If a drug leaves a lot of leeway between its therapeutic effect and its toxic effect, carefully monitoring it by *serum* levels is usually not considered necessary. Digoxin, however, is a good example of a drug that has a narrow margin of safety and that must be monitored.

4. *When signs of toxicity are difficult to recognize clinically.* Serum levels for certain drugs help to detect or to prevent toxicity that might otherwise not be noticed because of other clinical problems. In way of illustration, an antiarrhythmic drug, such as quinidine, may depress the myocardium and cause symptoms that could be wrongly attributed to a worsening of the underlying cardiac disease, rather than to the toxicity from the drug.

5. *When gastrointestinal, hepatic, or renal disease is present.* If gastrointestinal

problems are present, any oral medication may have an erratic drug absorption. (Usually the drug would be ordered parenterally to avoid this problem.) If hepatic disease is present, drugs that are metabolized by the liver—and almost all are—are not cleared from the serum normally. (See Chapter 11 for the role of the liver in conjugating drugs and other substances, such as bilirubin or BSP dye.) Finally, since most drugs are excreted in the urine, renal disease means a problem with excretion. For example, the aminoglycoside antibiotics, if given at all, must be carefully monitored by serum levels when renal disease is present.

6. *When drug interactions result from the use of several drugs.* Patients with epilepsy may be on several types of anticonvulsants, most of which can cause central nervous system symptoms, such as lethargy and depression. It may not be at all clear which drug or combination of drugs is causing the toxic effects. A serum level of the drugs helps to pinpoint the culprit.

7. *When noncompliance is suspected.* "Noncompliance" means that a patient is not taking a drug as ordered. The reasons for not taking a drug can be varied, including such a simple thing as a misunderstanding of the need. Patients who are put on certain drugs may be overly afraid of side effects, so they cut down on the amount of drug that was prescribed or they "forget" to take the pill at certain times. The physician and nurse may be surprised that the patient has not had a therapeutic effect from the drug. A serum level of the drug helps to determine whether the present regime is adequate to maintain a certain blood level. Sometimes, when patients are admitted to the hospital, they become toxic to a drug, such as digoxin, because in the hospital they are given it religiously every day as ordered. At home, the administration may not have been on schedule. A community health nurse can be of valuable assistance in visiting patients at home to determine whether noncompliance is a reason for erratic serum drug levels.

8. *When an overdose of an unknown substance or substances has occurred.* Therapeutic drugs, such as aspirin or barbiturates, are often taken in toxic amounts either accidentally (poisoning) or deliberately as a suicidal gesture. With drug experimentation, the patient may have inhaled, ingested, or injected a variety of different drugs. The laboratory can do screens of serum, urine, and gastric contents to identify the chemicals present. In chronic poisoning with heavy metals, such as lead, the laboratory can identify the toxic substance in both the serum and urine.

9. *To detect abuse of drugs for legal prosecution.* The legal implications of the blood alcohol test are discussed under the section on alcohol tests. Other legal problems are discussed in the section on opiate abuse.

Reasons for Not Monitoring

Although there are many reasons to monitor drugs, there are also reasons not to monitor them. One good reason is cost. If the drug is not particularly toxic, and if the patient responds well to the usual prescribed dosage, a serum drug level is unnecessary (Conrad 1978). The nurse can help to explain to patients in simple terms why drug monitoring either is or is not necessary. For some drugs, the effect of the drug on other laboratory tests is more important than the actual serum level of the drug. For example, if the patient is on anticoagulants, either the PTT (for heparin) or the PT (for coumarin) is used to monitor the dosage of the respective anticoagulants. (See Chapter 13 on tests for coagulation.) If the patient is on insulin therapy, the laboratory tests the blood for glucose and the urine for sugar and acetone, but not the insulin level per se. (See Chapter 8 on glucose, and Chapter 3 on urine tests.)

Caution in Interpretation

Because serum drug levels reflect only the amount of the drug in the plasma at a given time, the level may not reflect the actual physiological activity of the drug. Laboratory tests of serum drugs measure both the bound and unbound parts of the drug. A patient with less albumin in the serum may thus have a larger amount of "free" drug in the serum. With some tests, the clinician has to take into account the conjugated and unconjugated portions of the drug or the amount of plasma proteins available for binding. (See Chapter 10 on the measurement of albumin.)

Variation in results due to a lack of standardization in different laboratories is also a problem. McCormick (1978) found a wide range of test results when three different laboratories ran tests on standardized samples of digoxin, phenobarbital, and phenytoin. Although laboratory error is not a nursing problem, the potential for laboratory error must be kept in mind when serum drug levels do not correlate well with the clinical picture.

General Nursing Implications

Correct Sample Timing: Peaks, Troughs, and Steady States. Serum samples of drug levels may be ordered as peak levels, as trough levels, or after obtaining a steady state. For serum drug levels, *peak* times refer to measurements of the highest level of drug reached in the serum; *trough* times represent the lowest levels. Some laboratories may refer to the trough levels as "residuals."

The *steady state* of a drug refers to the time when the plasma level has been stabilized by a maintenance dose. For some drugs, a steady state is not obtained for several weeks. The patient may have periodic samples drawn to check on the exact "steady rate" that is being maintained with a specific dosage level. Information about the steady state of an individual drug is included in the discussion on specific drugs.

The trough or residual level is usually drawn just before the next dose of the drug is given. The timing for the peak level drawing is based on the knowledge about when the particular drug is usually at a peak in the serum. Hence, for a particular drug, the physician and/or the laboratory determine the time to draw the peak. Information about peak and trough levels are included with the specific drug test when appropriate.

Controversy exists about whether peak or trough levels are better indicators of toxicity for specific drugs. In general, the peak is a determination of the rate of absorption of the drug, while the trough is a measurement of the drug's rate of elimination. (A timetable for drawing peak and trough levels for gentamicin is shown in Table 17–1.)

Peak and trough levels of serum drug levels are meaningless unless it is known when the drug was given, the amount given, and the route. Knowing what other drugs are being taken by the patient is also important, since they may interfere with some tests. If the patient is being assessed for a steady state of the drug, make note not only of this information, but also of the daily dosage that has been maintained over a certain period. (Also, question the patient and make sure that the ordered dosage was in fact the dosage being taken at home.) In summary, the laboratory needs the following information:

   1. the exact timing of the last dose of the drug,
   2. the exact amount of the drug given,
   3. the route of the drug (peak times change dramatically between oral and par-
      enteral administration),
   4. how long the patient has been on a certain dosage (if the patient is being assessed
      for a steady state level), and
   5. other medications that may interfere with the specific test (check with the indi-
      vidual laboratory to determine this).

If the drug is not given on time, the entire schedule for drawing peak and trough
levels must be changed. For example, if a patient is receiving an intravenous antibiotic
and the intravenous becomes infiltrated, the peak level for the drug does not reflect the
usual peak. The laboratory must be notified and the test rescheduled. If an outpatient is to
have a serum drug level drawn, assessing whether the prescribed drug was taken at the
prescribed time or times is important. If not, doing a test that has no real meaning is
useless and expensive. Patient teaching is very important when serum drug levels are to be
monitored on an outpatient basis.

Assessing the Therapeutic and Toxic Effects of Drugs. The patient who is being
monitored by serum drug levels still needs to be observed by the nurse for symptoms of
therapeutic or toxic effects of the drug. Serum drug monitoring can never replace the
clinical assessment of the patient. For example, a patient may have adequate levels of
gentamicin in the serum, but still have a raging fever and other signs that the infection is
not responding to the antibiotic. As another example, the digoxin level may be within the
''normal'' range, and yet the patient has a pulse below 60 and other symptoms of digoxin
toxicity. (See Chapter 16 for tests on minimal inhibitory concentration (MIC) and culture
and sensitivities (C&S) as ways to assess whether specific bacteria are sensitive to specific
antibiotics.)
   The nurse must be aware of both the desired or therapeutic effects of the drug, as well
as of the side effects or toxic effects of the drug. In this chapter, some of the more
outstanding nursing assessments are mentioned in connection with the specific test for the
drug. Refer to pharmacology books such as Loebel (1977) or Govoni and Hayes (1978)
for detailed nursing implications when a particular drug is being given.

TABLE 17-1.   PEAK AND TROUGH LEVELS

Timing of Medication	Peak to Be Drawn 15 Minutes After IV Completed	Trough to Be Drawn Less Than One Hour Before Next Dose
Gentamicin 80 mg in 100 ml of D_5W q8 h. intravenously over 1 hour:		
8 AM–9 AM	Draw sample at 9:15 AM	Draw sample at 7:45 AM
	or	or
4 PM–5 PM	5:15 PM	3:45 PM
	or	or
12 midnight–1 AM	1:15 AM	11:45 PM

Reason for Tests and Deviations from Reference Values. The information gained by serum drug levels is used primarily by the physician who readjusts the dosages if needed. Nurses need to be aware of the reference values used in a particular setting, so that deviations from normal can be reported before another drug dosage is given. For example, if a trough level shows a range as high, or nearly as high, as the expected peak, continuing with the drug may be dangerous. Contacting the physician before the next dose of the drug is administered would be wise. Unless the information from the laboratory report is utilized, the serum drug levels are just a costly academic exercise that are of no benefit to the patient.

ANTIBIOTIC LEVELS: EMPHASIS ON AMINOGLYCOSIDES

Serum antibiotic levels are not routinely done if the antibiotic is not usually toxic, if the infection is responding appropriately, and if the patient does not have liver or renal dysfunction. For example, since penicillin and the cephalosporins have a much wider range between therapeutic doses and toxic doses than do the antibiotics that are classified as aminoglycosides, patients who are on penicillin or the cephalosporins are not routinely followed by serum antibiotic levels.

All aminoglycosides have a central amino sugar—hence the name aminoglycoside (sugar). These antibiotics are used for serious infections with gram-negative bacteria, such as *Esterichia coli* and *Pseudomonas*. (See Chapter 16 on cultures and sensitivities.) The amnioglycosides that are commonly monitored by serum levels are gentamicin (Garamycin), tobramycin (Tobicin) and amikacin (Amikin). Langslet (1981) gives an excellent summary about aminoglycosides and appropriate nursing actions.

The nurse needs to be aware that the aminoglycosides have the potential for nerve damage (neurotoxicity). The eighth cranial nerve is often affected by this group of antibiotics. Impairment may involve both the auditory branch (ototoxicity) and the vestibular branch. Involvement of the vestibular branch causes a lack of equilibrium. The patient may complain of a lack of balance and dizziness. If patients are on aminoglycosides for more than ten days without having their serum levels monitored, they may be given hearing tests to check for ototoxicity (Yoshikawa 1980:12).

Aminoglycosides may also cause kidney damage (nephrotoxicity). Neurotoxicity is more likely if renal function is not normal. BUN and/or creatinine tests are often used to monitor renal function while the patient is on aminoglycosides. (See Chapter 4 on BUN and creatinine.) If the laboratory is equipped to do serum antibiotic levels, the physician may prefer to follow the course of aminoglycoside therapy by monitoring the actual level in the bloodstream. If a patient has liver, or particularly renal, dysfunction, the serum levels may be the only way to safely give aminoglycoside antibiotics (Hewitt 1978:113).

Controversy surrounds the question of how well serum antibiotic levels correlate with clinical effects. It is not correct to assume that a certain blood level is a true reflection of the biological activity of the drug in the patient. A therapeutic level for one patient may not be a therapeutic level for another, due to individual variations in the metabolism of the drug. (See Chapter 16 for a discussion about the minimal inhibitory concentration as another way to gauge the effectiveness of an antibiotic.) At best, a serum sample shows only the concentration of the drug at that moment. If the serum antibiotic levels are accurately timed, appropriately performed, and carefully interpreted, the laboratory report can be useful for the physician who is regulating the dosage schedule. Hewitt (1978) discusses the correlation of serum antibiotic levels with clinical considerations, and he cautions that serum antibiotic levels must always be correlated with the clinical picture of the patient.

Preparation of Patient
And Collection of Sample
The laboratory needs 1 ml of serum. Usually blood samples for peak levels of antibiotics are drawn 45 to 60 minutes after an intramuscular (IM) injection or 15 minutes after completion of an intravenous (IV) antibiotic. The trough or residual level is done about 15 minutes before the next dose of antibiotic is due. The nurse should check with the physician about exact trough and peak times. Table 17–1 gives an example of the timing of levels for gentamicin. In general, peak levels are used to determine whether the dosage is adequate, while trough levels aid in ascertaining whether there is too much drug accumulation (Yoshikawa 1980:128).

Reference Values

Gentamicin (Garamicin) and tobramycin (Nebein)	Therapeutic, 4–8 μg/ml Peak, below 12 μg/ml Trough, below 2 μg/ml
Amikacin (Amikin) and kanamycin (Kantrex)	Therapeutic, 8–16 μg/ml Peak, below 35 μg/ml Trough, below 10 μg/ml

ANTIBACTERIALS: SULFA DRUGS

Sulfa drugs are antibacterials, not antibiotics (which are obatined from living organisms). Sulfa drugs are usually not measured in the serum since the concentration in the urine is usually a more useful assessment of therapeutic effectiveness (Hewitt 1978:1131). Occasionally sulfa drugs may be measured in the serum if renal function is not optimal.

Preparation of Patient
And Collection of Sample
The laboratory needs 2 ml of serum or urine.

Reference Values

Therapeutic level:	
In serum	5–15 mg/dl
In urine	15–20 mg/ml

ANTICONVULSANTS:
PHENYTOIN OR DIPHYNYLDANTOIN

Phenytoin, formerly called diphynyhydantoin (Dilantin), is the most common drug used to treat various types of epilepsy. It may be used alone or in combination with the other anticonvulsants in this section. Phenytoin is also used as an antiarrhythmic for certain types of cardiac irregularities. (See the section on antiarrhythmic drugs.)

Patients may have serum phenytoin levels done to determine the proper dose level for long-term therapy. Since it takes at least a week or two to achieve stable serum phenytoin levels, during this time the patient may have blood samples drawn several times. As with most other serum drug levels, the level per se is not always a prediction of toxicity from the drug.

Serum levels are related to certain side effects. In general, nystagmus (involuntary rapid movements of the eyeballs) appears when serum phenytoin levels are above 20 μg/ml. Gait ataxia occurs at about 30, and constant lethargy if the level is above 40 (Govoni 1978:573).

Preparation of Patient
And Collection of Sample
The laboratory needs 3 ml of serum. Note the time of the last dose, the route, and the amount of phenytoin. Intramuscular injection of phenytoin, rather than oral administration, reduces blood levels about 50%. Levels are usually drawn about 3 hours after the last dose.

Reference Values

10–20 μg/ml	As an anticonvulsant
10–18 μg/ml	As an antiarrhythmic

ANTICONVULSANTS:
PRIMIDONE (MYSOLINE, PRIMOLINE)

Primidone is not a barbiturate, but it is closely related with similar actions. Primidone is used for the control of certain types of epilepsy. Doses higher than the therapeutic range can, however, cause significant ataxia and lethargy.

Preparation of Patient
And Collection of Sample
The laboratory needs 3 ml of serum. Note the time and dosage of the drug.

Reference Values

Therapeutic level	4–12 μg/ml

ANTICONVULSANTS:
VALPROIC ACID (DEPAKENE)

Valproic acid (Depakene) is a relatively new anticonvulsant that is given orally. Since valproic acid has a short biological half-life, the time of the last dose and the time of the sampling must be considered carefully when judging the clinical effect from a certain concentration. A short half-life means that it is cleared from the serum in a short time. A steady state of valporic is reached in about 40 hours.

Preparation of Patient
And Collection of Sample
The Laboratory needs 1 ml of serum. The dose, the time of last dose, and the time of the sampling should be entered on the requisition.

Reference Value

Therapeutic range	50–100 μg/ml

ANTICONVULSANTS:
PHENOBARBITAL (LUMINAL)

Phenobarbital is a long-acting barbituate (see later discussion of barbituate panel) that is sometimes used in conjunction with other anticonvulsants. Phenobarbital is also given as treatment for neonatal bilirubinemia (see Chapter 11).

Preparation of Patient
And Collection of Sample
The laboratory needs 5 ml of serum. The dose, the time of the last dose, and the time of the sampling should be noted. Since phenobarbital is long-acting and cumulative, the daily dose of the patient should also be noted. Patients can develop a tolerance to high levels of phenobarbital if the increase is gradual.

Reference Values

Therapeutic range	for anticonvulsant control 15–40 μg/ml
Newborns	Levels over 40 μg cause apnea.

ANTIPSYCHOTIC AGENT:
LITHIUM CARBONATE

Lithium (Lithane, Eskalith, Lithonate) is a psychotherapeutic agent used to treat manic patients with certain types of bipolar depression (manic depressives). When the dosage is being adjusted, blood samples are done one to two times a week. The serum lithium level may be drawn eight to twelve hours after the dosage is given. After a therapeutic dosage level has been established, the patient may have serum lithium levels done on a monthly basis. Newman (1979:701) has suggested that red cell lithium levels may be more reliable of incipient toxicity than serum levels. Electroencephalographs (EEG) may also be done to evaluate the neurotoxicity from lithium.

Lithium toxicity is a very serious problem. In some patients, particularly the elderly, neurotoxicity can develop even with normal serum lithium levels. Hence patients must be assessed for such symptoms as diarrhea, vomiting, muscle weakness, and incoordination. Another nursing implication is to make sure that these patients have normal amounts of salt, since lithium toxicity may be greater if serum sodium levels are low (Loebel 1977:386). (See Chapter 5 on diets with high sodium content.)

Preparation of Patient
And Collection of Sample

The laboratory needs 1 ml of serum. Lithium samples are drawn 8 to 12 hours after the dosage. Note the amount, the route, and the time of the last dosage on the laboratory request.

Reference Values

Notify the physician if level is above 1.6 mEq/l.

Toxic level   Considered to be above 2 mEq/l, but it may be less in some individuals.

BRONCHODILATORS:
THEOPHYLLINE PRODUCTS

Theophylline and its derivatives, such as aminophylline, dyphylline, and oxtriphylline, are all used as bronchodilators. For example, theophylline or a theophylline derivative is usually the primary drug for the treatment of asthma. There are many brand names for theophylline and the derivatives: Aminodur, Theodur, Choledyl, Bronkodyl, Elixophyllin and various others. Consult a pharmacology text for peak times and durations of the various products. The timing of the serum samples varies with the exact form of theophylline or theophylline derivative used. For example, since aminophylline is 85% theophylline (Govoni 1978:22), aminophylline causes different theophylline levels than do other theophylline products.

If theophylline products are being given in high doses for an acute asthmatic attack, serum level monitoring is crucial. Because high serum levels of theophylline can result in life-threatening cardiac arrhythmias and seizures (FDA Drug Bulletin, February 1980), the Federal Drug Administration recommends that the safest approach to individualize dosages of theophylline or theophylline products is to monitor serum levels. For patients who are on chronic theophylline therapy, measurement of trough levels as well as peak levels should be made. Patients who have abnormal liver function, who have congestive failure, or who are very young or very old may need very close monitoring of serum theophylline levels.

Nurses should be aware of early clinical symptoms of theophylline overdose. Because theophylline is a xanthine, as is caffeine, some of the early symptoms of theophylline toxicity resemble a "coffee jag." Patients may have tachycardia with skipped beats. They may also be very nervous and jittery, with tremors of the hands. The dosage of theophylline must be readjusted to prevent further development of lethal cardiac arrhythmias and/or seizures.

Preparation of Patient
And Collection of Sample

The laboratory needs 3 ml of serum. The dose, the route, and the time of the last dose should be entered on the requisition. Note the specific times to draw peak and trough levels, which vary depending on the theophylline product being monitored. Since both theophylline and caffeine are xanthines, the patient should not have coffee, colas, tea, chocolate, or any other sources of caffeine for several hours before the serum specimen is drawn.

Reference Values

Therapeutic range	10–20 µg/ml
Risk of toxicity	Over 20 µg/ml

CARDIAC DRUGS: DIGOXIN

Digoxin (Lanoxin) is a cardiotonic used to prevent or to treat congestive heart failure (CHF). Digoxin is also used to treat various types of atrial arrhythmias, such as atrial fibrillation (AF). Digoxin and the other forms of digitalis are all cumulative in action, and thus serious toxicity can occur over time.

To prevent digitalis toxicity, the key nursing implication is to monitor the patient's pulse before digoxin is given. Digoxin, or other digitalis products, should be withheld and the doctor notified if the adult's pulse is below 60. Usually a pulse below 70 is the guideline for children, but this criterion varies depending on age. Patients should be taught to take their own pulses because, once digoxin is begun, it is usually continued on a long-term basis. Other symptoms of digitalis toxicity—such as nausea and vomiting, diarrhea, headaches, and visual disturbance—are also sometimes relied upon to signal digitalis toxicity. An electrocardiogram (EKG) also helps the clinician determine whether there is a toxic effect from digoxin. However, the symptoms of mild toxicity from digoxin may not be readily noted by clinical assessment or EKG data. A measurement of serum levels of digoxin therefore aids in determining whether symptoms are due to a higher-than-necessary digoxin level.

Other laboratory tests that are important in assessing for potential digitalis toxicity are the serum potassium and the serum calcium levels. The nurse needs to be aware that a low serum potassium or a high serum calcium level tends to increase the risk of digitalis toxicity, even though the serum digoxin levels are not high. (See Chapter 5 on potassium and Chapter 7 on calcium levels.) Since digoxin is excreted by the kidneys, patients with poor renal function are also more prone to develop digitalis toxicity. (See Chapter 4 for tests of renal function, BUN and creatinine.)

Preparation of Patient
And Collection of Sample

The laboratory needs 1 ml of serum. The dosage of digoxin, the route, and the time of the last dose should be included on the requisition. (Digoxin is given only orally or intravenously because the intramuscular route has an erratic absorption rate.) The serum level is usually drawn at a minimum of 16 hours after either an oral or intravenous dose because it takes at least this long for the drug to equilibrate in the tissues. Often the level is not drawn until just prior to the next dose.

Reference Values*

Therapeutic range:

With dosage of 0.25 mg/day	0.8–1.6 ng/ml
With dosage of 0.5 mg/day	1.1–1.9 ng/ml

Some sources give a wider range of 1-3 ng/ml, with much emphasis on clinical data to substantiate toxicity.

ANTIARRHYTHMIC DRUGS: QUINIDINE

Quinidine (Quinoglute, Cin-Quin, Quindex, Cardioquin, and others) is an alkaloid obtained from the bark of the cinchona tree. Hence toxicity from quinidine products is sometimes referred to as cinchonism. Since quinidine depresses the excitability of the heart, it is used as an antiarrhythmic drug. It can be given intravenously for acute states or orally as a long-term maintenance drug.

Nurses should be aware that quinidine, particularly in the intravenous form, can cause severe bradycardia and hypotension. Hypersensitivity reactions, gastrointestinal upsets, and central nervous system effects, such as tremors or even coma, can occur with quinidine toxicity. When a dosage schedule is being started, these patients need to have their pulses and blood pressures closely monitored.

Serum quinidine levels help the clinician to adjust the dosage to the correct amount for the individual patient. In fact, quinidine is the antiarrhythmic drug that is most often monitored by serum levels. Since the toxicity from chronic use may not be readily apparent or may be attributed to other causes, peak and trough levels can be used to ascertain whether patients are in a therapeutic range.

Preparation of Patient
And Collection of Sample

The dosage, the time of the last dose, and the route should all be noted on the lab requisition. The peak level for quinidine occurs about 2 hours after the dose. The laboratory needs 1 ml of serum.

Reference Values

Therapeutic range	1.5–3 μg/ml
Toxic range	5–6 μg/ml

ANTIARRHYTHMIC DRUGS: PROCAINAMIDE

Procainamide (Pronestyl) is usually given orally for long-term prevention of arrhythmias. As with quinidine products, serum peak and trough levels help to prevent toxicity such as myocardial depression.

Preparation of Patient
And Collection of Sample
The dosage, the route, and the time of the last dose should be noted on the laboratory request. The level is usually drawn about 3 hours after the last dose.

Reference Values

Therapeutic level	4–8 μg/ml

ANTIARRHYTHMIC DRUGS: PHENYTOIN

Although phenytoin (Dilantin) is more commonly used as an anticonvulsant, it is also sometimes used to control cardiac arrhythmias, such as those caused by digitalis toxicity. It is not, however, as commonly used as procainamide or quinimide for long-term prevention of arrhythmias. (See the reference values under anticonvulsant drugs.)

ANTIARRHYTHMIC DRUGS: PROPRANOLOL

Propranolol (Inderal) is used for the treatment of certain arrhythmias because it is a beta adrenergic blocker. Since propranolol decreases the rate and the force of heart contraction, hypotension and bradycardia are serious side effects. Propranolol is used in combination with other drugs for the treatment of hypertension.

Serum levels of propranolol may occasionally be drawn, but doing so is not a common practice since a wide range is included in the therapeutic index (Conrad 1978).

Preparation of Patient
And Collection of Sample
The dosage, the route, and the time of the last dose should be noted on the laboratory slip. Check with the laboratory on the timing of the sample, which is usually drawn 4 hours after the last dose.

Reference Value

Therapeutic range	ng/ml
	100–300

ANTIARRHYTHMIC DRUGS: LIDOCAINE

Lidocaine (Xylocaine) is given intravenously for the immediate control of premature ventricular contractions (PVCs). Because lidocaine is usually given only on an intermittent basis when the need arises, lidocaine levels are seldom measured. If patients have a continuous lidocaine drop, there may be a need to monitor serum levels.

Preparation of Patient And Collection of Sample

Note the concentration of the drug and the rate of intravenous administration on the laboratory request.

Reference Value

Therapeutic range	1.5–6 μg/ml

SALICYLATES: ACETYLSALICYLIC ACID (ASA)

Acetylsalicyclic acid, or aspirin, is used as an analgesic, as an antiinflammatory agent, and as an anticoagulant. Many over-the-counter (OTC) pain relievers contain ASA, such as Anacin, Bufferin, Excedrin, and many others. Aspirin poisoning is the most common type of poisoning in children. Adults may also take ASA or ASA-containing drugs in a suicidal gesture. In an overdose case, the laboratory can do a screen of a serum sample to see whether ASA is the culprit. (If an overdose has occurred, gastric contents and urine specimens should also be sent to the laboratory, if available.)

Mild intoxication, or salicyclism, causes a ringing in the ears (tinnitus) and gastric upsets. Since ASA acts as a respiratory stimulant, the hyperventilation that may result from aspirin overdose can cause respiratory alkalosis. (See Chapter 6 on acid–base balance.) Large doses of ASA may also cause gastrointestinal bleeding, which is due to the irritant effect on the gastric mucosa and to the interference with coagulation factors.

With its anticoagulant properties, ASA is sometimes used as a regular medication for patients who have a high potential for thromboembolic episodes. Serum ASA levels may be done to prevent ASA toxicity.

ASA is also commonly used in high doses for patients who may benefit from the antiinflammatory properties of ASA. For example, patients with rheumatoid arthritis may be on large doses of ASA over a long period of time. It may take 12 to 20 grV aspirin tablets to keep the serum level around 20 mg/dl. Serum ASA levels may be done periodically to aid in maintaining the patient in a therapeutic, but not a toxic range. Sometimes patients are afraid to take enough ASA to really ever achieve therapeutic benefit. Serum levels may be used to evaluate whether they are complying with the plan.

Preparation of Patient
And Collection of Sample

The laboratory needs 5 ml of serum, collected in a heparin (green Vacutainer) or EDTA tube (lavender Vacutainer). In the case of an overdose patient, urine, any vomitus, or gastric lavage should be saved for laboratory analysis too. For a routine assessment of salicyclate level, the total daily dosage of ASA should be noted, as well as the time and amount of the last dose. Note exactly how many *tablets* the patient says he or she takes a day. Do not rely on what the physician has ordered and assume that the patient has followed this dose at home.

Reference Values

Therapeutic range
(three hours after dose):

Children to age 10	25–30 mg/100 ml
Adults	20–25 mg/100 ml

Toxic range:

Children and adults	Over 30 mg/100 ml
After age 60	Over 20 mg/100 ml

Lethal range may be around 60 mg/100 ml.

Urine Testing for Salicylate Intoxication

Phenistix (Ames Product Information, 1978) are reagent strips used primarily to test for phenylketones in the urine. (See Chapter 18 for a discussion on PKU.) However, metabolites of aspirin, other salicylates, and phenothiazines also cause color changes in Phenistix. The color chart used to detect salicylates or phenothiazines shows tan for small amounts and brown for large amounts. (The color change for PKU uses a different color chart.) Phenistix can be used as a screening device of urine to check for overdose with aspirin or phenothiazines. (Phenothiazine testing is covered later in this chapter.)

BLOOD ALCOHOL TESTS

Ethanol, or grain alcohol, is the type of alcohol in alcoholic beverages. Ethanol, undoubtedly the most commonly abused drug, may often be one of the drugs involved in an overdose (Mukherjee 1979:171). As part of a toxicology screen, the laboratory may do an alcohol panel that, in addition to ethanol, includes methanol (wood alcohol), isopropyl (rubbing alcohol), and acetone (an alcohol-related compound). Alcohol and related toxic compounds may be ingested by drinking undrinkable solutions such as cleaning fluids, shaving lotions, or disinfectants. Methanol is particularly dangerous since it can result in convulsions, blindness, and possibly death.

In addition to determining the cause of a coma, blood alcohol tests are also used to determine whether the person driving the car was intoxicated at the time of an accident. The drawing of the blood specimen must be done in a medically suitable environment following the legal requirements of the state. (Breath analyzers are done at the scene of the accident, so nurses are not involved in obtaining samples.) Nurses who are trained in venipuncture may draw the blood for alcohol blood samples when the patient is brought to the emergency room for medical treatment. George (1976) has stated that many hospitals do not permit nurses or technicians to obtain specimens at the request of the police. The reluctance to involve hospital staff in drawing blood for legal evidence is based on the facts that the persons drawing the blood may not know the exact legal ramifications of the procedure and that they will probably be subpoenaed to testify in a court case. Although it is permissible for qualified nurses to draw blood for the alcohol test, it is important that they understand the legal ramifications of the procedure and the policy for nurses in a particular institution.

Legal Definitions of Intoxication

Each state determines the exact blood alcohol level that is considered legally permissible for driving. Levels over 0.10% are usually considered proof of intoxication. Some people may not be sober with very low blood alcohol levels, but the exact line for sobriety is disputable. Holum (1978:243) notes that as little as 0.05% means the person is no longer sober and that the risk of an auto accident for a driver with 0.2% alcohol in the blood is a hundred times higher than the sober driver.

With regard to the legal meaning of a blood alcohol level, the recommendation of the National Safety Council on alcohol and drugs is:

1. Less than 0.05%: No influence by alcohol within the meaning of the law.
2. *Between 0.05% and 0.10%:* Alcohol influence is usually present, but courts of law are advised to consider the person's behavior and circumstances that led to the arrest.
3. *Above 0.10%:* Definite evidence of being "under the influence" (Ravel 1978:433).

Relationship of Alcohol to
Other Laboratory Tests

In addition to the usual symptoms of alcohol intoxication, the patient with alcohol abuse may have severe hypoglycemia, since alcohol tends to inhibit the formation of glucose. (See Chapter 8 for symptoms and treatment of hypoglycemia.) Alcohol-induced hypoglycemia carries a high mortality if not identified and corrected. The mortality is particularly high for children (Dipp 1978:651). High blood alcohol levels are also a major cause of secondary hyperlipidemia. (See Chapter 9 on serum triglyceride levels.)

Preparation of Patient
And Collection of Blood Sample

The patient needs to give consent for a blood specimen. Be aware of the legal ramifications, state requirements, and the individual hospital's policy. No alcohol, such as alcohol wipes, should be used to obtain the blood specimen. An aqueous germicidial solution, such as benzalkonium, can be used. Tinctures should not be used, since they have an alcohol base. The laboratory needs 2 ml of blood in an oxalated tube (black Vacutainer). The specimen should be refrigerated if it cannot be sent to the laboratory immediately.

Reference Values

Ethanol or Ethyl (Grain) Alcohol	
0.0%–0.5%	Sobriety is presumed
0.05%–0.1%	"Gray zone"
0.10%–0.15%	Legal limit, depending on state law
0.30%–0.40%	Marked intoxication
0.40%–0.50%	Severe toxic effects with alcoholic stupor
0.50%–over	Coma and death possible
Methanol or Methyl (Wood) Alcohol	
25 mg/dl	Toxic level
80–115 mg/dl	Lethal

BARBITURATE PANEL FOR OVERDOSES

The barbiturates are used as anticonvulsants, as sedatives, and as hypnotics. The most severe effect of overdosage with barbiturates is respiratory failure followed by circulatory collapse. Because the various barbituates are often used in overdoses, the laboratory runs a barbiturate panel when patients are comatose from an unknown cause. The five barbiturates usually measured are:

1. the short-acting ones—pentobarbital (Nembutal) and secobarbital (Seconal);
2. the intermediate-acting ones—amobarbital (Amytal) and butabarbital (Butisol, Butacaps); and
3. the long-acting one, phenobarbital (Luminal, Eskabarb).

A smaller amount of the short-acting barbiturates, as opposed to a larger amount for the long-acting barbiturate, causes coma. A toxicology screen for barbiturate overdose also includes an analysis of urine samples and gastric contents. So any vomitus or gastric lavage products should be saved for laboratory analysis.

Preparation of Patient
And Collection of Blood Sample
The laboratory needs 5 ml of serum. Note any drugs that the patient may have taken. Theophylline, for example, can cause a false elevation of the barbiturate level.

Reference Value

Short-acting barbiturates	Coma level at about 1–3 mg/dl
Long-acting barbiturates	Coma level at about 9–10 mg/dl

See the section on anticonvulsants for the measurement of therapeutic levels of phenobarbital.

Sedatives and Hypnotics Other Than Barbiturates

In addition to barbiturates, several other sedative/hypnotic drugs have the potential for overdosage by drug abuse practices. Laboratories screen for these sedative/hypnotics when the cause of the overdose is not known. The four common hypnotic drugs that can cause coma are glutethimide (Doriden), methyprylon (Noludar), ethchorvynol (Placidyl), and methaqualone (Quaalude, Sopor). All four of these drugs are prescribed in small doses to aid sleep (hypnotic), and so they should not be present in large amounts in the serum.

MINOR TRANQUILIZERS AND PROPOXYPHENE

Three minor tranquilizers or antianxiety agents may be associated with drug abuse. These three minor tranquilizers are diazepam (Valium), meprobamate (Equanil, Miltown, and others), and chlordiazepoxide (Librium). For several years, diazepam (Valium) has been the most frequently prescribed prescription drug. Reports from the Drug Abuse Warning Network (FDA Drug Bulletin, February 1980) show that, in 1978, diazepam ranked second only to alcohol as the drug most often combined with other drugs in drug abuse episodes treated in emergency rooms.

Propoxyphene (Darvon) is a prescription analgesic that is often associated with drug deaths. Many of these deaths are in association with alcohol and tranquilizers. Patients at particular risk of propoxyphene-associated deaths include adolescents and young adults who engage in multidrug abuse. Also, patients with chronic pain and depression are likely to use propoxyphene in deliberate overuse or abuse (FDA Drug Bulletin, July 1980).

OPIATE ABUSE

Opiates, such as morphine or methadone, can be measured in the urine as well as in the serum. Opiates are measured in the serum to see if they are present in a high enough level to be the cause of coma. Narcotic antagonists can then be used to reverse a narcotic coma. For detecting chronic abuse, urine tests may be used. Detecting opiate abuse by laboratory methods is difficult since patients may refrain from drugs if they are to have testing done. Recently, the analysis of human hair by radioimmunoassay has been developed as a way to detect opiate use (See Chapter 15 for the RIA method). Baumgartner (1979) discusses the impact of the test (Abuscan I-123 by Roche Diagnostics) that can detect morphine content for the life of the hair. Obviously, many legal and ethical considerations come into play when patients who are not comatose are tested for suspected drug abuse. Refer to texts on drug abuse for specific nursing implications in dealing with the complex problem of suspected or known drug abuse.

BROMIDE LEVELS IN OTC DRUGS

Bromide is an ingredient in several over-the-counter (OTC) drugs that are used as sleeping aids and "nerve tonics." Too often, the patients and the health professionals, consider all over-the-counter drugs as harmless. Bromide, a central nervous system depressant, in large doses can cause toxicity, which is called bromism. Patients with inadequate renal function are particularly susceptible to bromide overdosage.

The symptoms of bromism are nonspecific, but they usually include signs and symptoms of central nervous system toxicity, such as muscle incoordination and impaired intellectual functioning. The patient may have vomiting and a rash. A public health nurse or clinic nurse may detect patients with symptoms of bromism. A health history should contain a list of all over-the-counter drugs that these patients take.

Preparation of Patient
And Collection of Sample

The laboratory needs 3 ml of serum. All medications that contain bromide should be noted.

Reference Values

Toxic level in serum	Above 17 mEq/l

MAJOR TRANQUILIZERS: PHENOTHIAZINES

Phenothiazines are used in high dosages as antipsychotic agents. The phenothiazine most often used for schizophrenic patients is chlorpromazine (Thorazine). Other phenothiazines commonly used as major tranquilizers include fluphenazine (Prolixin), trifluoperazine (Stelazine), thioridiazine (Mellaril), and promazine (Sparine). Serum levels of phenothiazines are not used to regulate dosage because the serum levels do not correlate well either with toxic or with therapeutic effects of the drugs. Phenothiazines are occasionally monitored in the urine, and, in the case of a suspected overdose, the laboratory can screen the urine for the presence of phenothiazines. (See the discussion on Phenistix, which is a quick method to screen for phenothiazines.)

HEAVY METAL POISONING: LEAD

Heavy metal poisoning can result from the ingestion or inhalation of zinc, mercury, arsenic, or lead that is used in paint, in insecticides, or in other substances. To discover the presence of a heavy metal, laboratories do screening tests of urine.

Of particular interest to nurses, particularly public health and pediatric nurses, is lead poisoning. Exposure to lead is an occupational hazard for some adults. The person usually has a variety of chronic symptoms, such as abdominal pain, weakness, and eventually neurological dysfunction, with the potential for permanent brain damage. Since lead interferes with the normal synthesis of red blood cells, patients have anemia and characteristic changes in the peripheral blood smear (Ravel 1978:430).

In the past few years, nurses have been involved in doing lead screening for children who may have chronic lead poisoning. The child most likely to get lead poisoning is a preschool child who lives in a poorly maintained house. Before World War II, lead paints were customarily used; so older houses that have not been repainted may still contain lead paint. Lead screening programs have been done by the government in areas where the prevalence of lead poisoning is great. Croft and Frenkel (1975) report about the lead screening and treatment program for children in a southern city, describing in detail the role of the nurses in a community survey.

The treatment of lead poisoning is a process called *chelation*. For deleading by chelation, the patient is given the calcium salt of a chemical called EDTA. Lead replaces the calcium, and the lead-EDTA is excreted in the urine. (Note that other heavy metal poisoning may also be treated with various types of chelating products.)

Preparation of Patient
And Collection of Sample

The laboratory needs 2 ml of blood. It is very important that all the blood drawing equipment be free from lead or lead particles. Special tubes from Vacutainer have brown tops to notify they are lead free. A complete history is needed concerning the patient's exposure to toxic chemicals, etc. Most public health surveys will have a definite assessment guide which is to be followed when interviewing patients. The possible exposure of other people in the patient's environment must be considered, too. Industrial pollution can be a major public health problem.

Reference Values

For serum lead levels	0–39 μg/100 ml is within normal range. Some references consider up to 50 μg to be normal.
	40–60 μg/100 ml. Careful watching with repeated levels done frequently.
Children	If over 60 μg/100 ml, chelation therapy is needed (see text).
Adults	Toxic symptoms may occur when the level is above 80 μg/ml.

ALA-D Tests for Lead Poisoning and FEP

Laboratories may do screens for lead poisoning by enzyme testing of ALA-D (aminolevulinic acid delta), an enzyme that is increased after lead exposure. The free erythrocyte porphyrins (FEP) is another screening test that requires only a drop of blood on a filter paper. Enzyme levels and porphyrins may also be measured in the urine. The actual confirmation of lead toxicity may be difficult when the exposure to lead is either too small or not current enough to change serum lead levels. (See Chapter 3 for a discussion on the 24-hour urine specimen for delta-aminolevulinic acid (ΔALA) and porphyrins.

Questions

17-1. Which of these situations is not an indication for monitoring plasma drug levels? The use of a drug:

    a. with a wide range between therapeutic and toxic effect.

    b. whose toxic symptoms may be difficult to recognize from clinical assessment.

    c. in combination with other drugs that may all cause side effects.

    d. that has interindividual variation in the metabolism of the drug.

17-2. Serum levels of drugs may be needed when the risk of toxicity from a drug is increased. Factors that increase the toxicity of most drugs include all *except* which?

    a. Increase in dosage.

    b. Use of intravenous rather than intramuscular or oral route.

    c. Hepatic dysfunction.

    d. Increased urine output due to increased intake of fluids.

17-3. Which of the following is not necessary to note on the laboratory requisition when the patient is to have serum drug levels drawn?

    a. The exact timing of the last dose of drug.

    b. The exact amount of the drug.

    c. The route of administration.

    d. The reason patient is on the drug.

17-4. Serum trough levels of drugs are used primarily to do which of the following?

    a. Estimate the therapeutic effect of the drug.

    b. Determine the residual drug in the serum before the next dose is given.

    c. Conclusively determine the toxicity of a drug.

    d. Establish that the drug has reached a steady state.

17-5. Mr. Telerechio is having blood drawn for peak and trough serum antibiotic levels. The nurse should be aware that the type of antibiotics that are commonly monitored by serum levels are the:

    a. penicillins.   **c.** aminoglycosides.

    b. cephalosporins.   **d.** any of the above.

17-6. Mrs. Gray is receiving gentamicin (Garamycin) 80 mg q 8 hours intravenously at 8 AM, 4 PM, and 12 midnight. The 80 mg of gentamicin is added to a 100 ml of fluid and given "piggyback" over a one-hour period. Serum peak levels would best be assessed by a blood sample drawn at which time?

    a. 8:30 AM.   **b.** 9:15 AM.   **c.** 3:45 PM.   **d.** 4:15 PM

17-7. Which one of the following anticonvulsants is likely to have an erratic or widely fluctuating serum level due to the short half-life of the drug?

    a. Phenytoin (Dilantin).

    b. Phenobarbital (Luminal, Eskabarbs).

    c. Valproic acid (Depakane).

    d. Primidone (Mysoline, Primoline).

17-8. Bobby, age 13, is an epileptic whose seizures are controlled by phenytoin (Dilantin). A serum phenytoin level drawn today was 23 μg/ml. Because he is slightly above the therapeutic range of 10-20 μg/ml, he may begin to show a symptom of early phenytoin toxicity, which is:

    a. severe lethargy.

    b. cardiac arrhythmias.

    c. gait ataxia.

    d. nystagmus (involuntary rapid movements of the eyeballs).

17-9. Molley Faber is a psychiatric patient being observed in a mental health clinic. Which of the following antipsychotic drugs requires monitoring by serum levels?

    a. Chloropromazine (Thorazine).   **c.** Fluphenazine (Prolixin).

    b. Lithium carbonate (Lithane).   **d.** Thioridiazine (Mellaril).

17-10. Johnny, age 8, is receiving aminophylline 20 mg an hour via the intravenous route for treatment of an acute asthmatic attack. Because aminophylline is a theophylline derivative, serum theophylline levels have been measured. His latest level of 30 μg/ml is considerably higher than the desired therapeutic range of 10-20 μg/ml. The nurse needs to make assessments of the patient and be prepared for potential·

    a. cardiac arrhythmias and seizures.   **c.** renal and hepatic failure.

    b. bronchospasms and dyspnea.   **d.** hypertension crisis and stroke.

17-11. Johnny has recovered from his acute asthmatic attack. He is being discharged with instructions to take a theophylline suspension (Elixophyllin 50 mg) q 6 hours. Johnny and his parents need to be taught that early symptoms of overdose from this drug may be similar to which of the following?

    a. Deep sleep.   **c.** Another asthmatic attack.

    b. Overuse of coffee.   **d.** Cold or flu.

17-12. Mr. Gardener is a 78-year-old man who is on digoxin 0.25 mg/day due to congestive heart failure (CHF). He is being visited by a community health nurse. Which of the following information in Mr. Gardener's health history should alert the nurse to the fact that this patient should be closely watched for digoxin toxicity?

   a. Large intake of sodium in the diet, refusal of visit from dietician.

   b. Slightly low-serum calcium level due to possible endocrine problem, work-up in progress.

   c. Poor renal function as evidenced by increased serum creatinine.

   d. History of noncompliance with physician's orders.

17-13. Serum monitoring is most commonly done for which of the following antiarrhythmic drugs?

   a. Quinidine (Quiniglute and others).   **c.** Lidocaine (Xylocaine).

   b. Propanalol (Inderal).   **d.** Phenytoin (Dilantin).

17-14. Mrs. Ramos has a serum quinidine level of 4 μg/ml which is higher than the therapeutic range of 1.5 to 3 μg/ml. Because there may be possible toxic effects from the quinidine, the nurse should assess and record which of the following?

   a. Level of consciousness every two hours.

   b. Blood pressure and pulse every two hours.

   c. Lack of appetite or other gastrointestinal symptoms.

   d. Hourly urine output.

17-15. Serum aspirin (ASA) levels may be part of the necessary clinical assessment for all of the following patients *except* which?

   a. Mr. Fink, who uses ASA PRN for a headache.

   b. Sally, age 2½, who was found in the bathroom playing with an empty bottle of Bufferin.

   c. Mrs. Catalina, who takes ASA gr X q i d for treatment of rheumatoid arthritis.

   d. Mr. Weber, who is on ASA gr X b i d for an anticoagulant effect and who is complaining of ringing in his ears (tinnitus).

17-16. In relation to blood alcohol levels, the emergency room nurse should know that all of the following are true *except* which?

   a. Alcohol should not be used to wipe the skin before the blood specimen is drawn.

   b. A blood alcohol over 0.10% is usually considered legal evidence of intoxication, but this criterion may vary from state to state.

   c. The patient's permission does not need to be obtained for a blood specimen.

   d. The person who draws the blood may be subpoenaed to testify in a court case.

17-17. Identify the type of drug, second to alcohol, that is most often combined with other drugs in drug abuse episodes treated in emergency rooms.

    a. Morphine or other opiates.

    b. Diazepam (Valium), an antianxiety drug.

    c. Short-acting barbiturates, secobarbital (Seconal), or pentobarbitol (Nembutal).

    d. Amphetamines (Dexedrine and others).

17-18. If a patient has taken an overdose of barbiturates or other hypnotics, the nurse should be prepared to assist with measures to treat:

    a. convulsions.   **c.** respiratory depression.

    b. cardiac arrhythmias.   **d.** hypertension.

17-19. Mrs. Gearhart is a 78-year-old woman who uses various over-the-counter (OTC) sleeping medications and nerve tonics. Mrs. Gearhart's niece reports to the visiting nurse that her aunt has become very forgetful and irritable since she increased her nerve tonic. The niece thinks her aunt is taking "too much nonprescribed medicine." After looking at the ingredients in the OTC medicine, the nurse may need to refer Mrs. Gearhart for a medical evaluation of possible:

    a. salicylism (aspirin toxicity).   **c.** plumbism (lead poisoning).

    b. cinchonism (quinidine toxicity).   **d.** bromism (bromide toxicity).

17-20. A public health nurse should know that the major source for lead poisoning in young children is which of the following?

    a. Contaminated food.   **c.** Polluted water.

    b. Lead-based paint.   **d.** Fumes from industrial plants.

REFERENCES

Ames Product Information, *Phenistix Reagent Strips*. Elkhart, Ind.: Ames Company, Miles Laboratories, 1978.

Baumgartner, Annette et al. "Radioimmunoassay of Hair for Determining Opiate Abuse Histories," *Journal of Nuclear Medicine* 20 (July 1979): 748–752.

Conrad, Kenneth. "Measurement of Drug Levels in Clinical Practice," *Arizona Medicine* 35 (November 1978): 747–748.

Croft, Harriet and Frenkel, Sallie. "Children and Lead Poisoning," *American Journal of Nursing* 75 (January 1975): 102–104.

Dipp, Stephen. "Metabolic Effects of Alcohol," *Arizona Medicine* 35 (October 1978): 651–652.

Federal Drug Administration, "Prescribing of Minor Tranquilizers," *FDA Drug Bulletin* 10 (February 1980): 2–3.

Federal Drug Administration, "Dosage Guidelines for Theophylline Products," *FDA Drug Bulletin* 10 (February 1980): 4–6.

Federal Drug Administration, "Propoxyphene Prescriptions," *FDA Drug Bulletin* 10 (July 1980): 11.

George, James E. "Blood Alcohol Tests," *Journal of Emergency Nursing* 2: 2 (March–April 1976): 7.

Govoni, Laura and Hayes, Janice. *Drugs and Nursing Implications,* New York: Appleton-Century-Crofts, 1978.

Hewitt, Williams and McHenry, Martin, "Blood Level Determinations of Antimicrobial Drugs," *Medical Clinics of North America* 62 (September 1978): 1119–1137.

Holum, John. *Elements of General and Biological Chemistry,* 5th ed. New York: John Wiley & Sons, Inc., 1979.

Loebel, Suzanne *et al. The Nurse's Drug Handbook.* New York: John Wiley & Sons, Inc., 1977.

McCormick, William *et al.* "Errors in Measuring Drug Concentrations," *New England Journal of Medicine* 299: 20 (November 16, 1978): 1118–1121.

Miller, Benjamin and Keane, Claire. "Reference Values for Therapeutic Drug Monitoring," p. 1143, *Encyclopedia and Dictionary of Medicine, Nursing and Allied Health,* Philadelphia: W. B. Saunders Company, 1978.

Mukherjee, Kana, *Review of Clinical Laboratory Methods.* St. Louis, Mo.: C. V. Mosby Co., 1979.

Langslet, Julie and Habel, Maureen. "The Aminoglycoside Antibiotics," *American Journal of Nursing* 81 (June 1981): 1144–1146.

Newman, Paul. "Lithium Neurotoxicity," *Postgraduate Medical Journal* 55 (October 1979): 701–703.

Ravel, Richard. *Clinical Laboratory Medicine,* 3rd ed. Chicago: Year Book Medical Publishers, Inc., 1978.

Richens, Alan and Warrington, Steven. "When Should Plasma Drug Levels Be Monitored," *Drugs* 17 (January 1979): 488–500.

Scala, Robert. "The Duty to Report Hazards: A Toxicologist's View," *Bulletin of New York Academy of Medicine* 54 (September 1978): 774–781.

Yoshikawa, Thomas. "Proper Use of Aminoglycosides," *American Family Physician* 21 (May 1980): 125–130.

CHAPTER EIGHTEEN

Tests Done in Pregnancy And the Newborn Period

Objectives

1. Identify how a normal pregnancy changes the values of common laboratory tests, as compared to the woman's prepregnancy values.
2. Explain the basic immunological principle of tests for pregnancy.
3. Explain which of the autosomal recessive genetic diseases are commonly tested by screening programs for certain ethnic groups.
4. Explain why PKU, galactesemia, and hypothyroidism are done as routine screening tests for newborns even though the infants appear healthy.
5. Describe the appropriate nursing functions for a community health nurse who is following a family that has a child with a genetic defect.

All prior chapters integrate information about the effects of pregnancy or of newborn status with information on tests that are not essentially related to pregnancy or infants (see Table 18–1). Appendix D summarizes the expected changes in laboratory values in a normal pregnancy and some of the changes that occur with oral contraceptives. Although integration of content from all clinical settings is stressed in this book, some tests pertain *only* to the pregnant or to the newborn state. This chapter therefore focuses on common laboratory tests that are unique in maternal child health settings.

Pregnancy tests, including the now historical biological methods, are discussed. Since home pregnancy tests have become popular in the last few years, nurses need to have some basic knowledge about how these tests are used. Understanding about human chorionic gonadotrophin (HCG) is also useful in caring for patients with certain types of tumors.

Blood tests for carriers of sickle cell anemia, thalassemia, Tay-Sachs disease, and PKU are included because all four of these autosomal recessive genetic diseases can be detected by screening tests.

A test of fetal maturity, estriol levels, is detailed.

TABLE 18-1. ROUTINE TESTS DONE DURING PREGNANCY

Name of Test	Assessment	Location in Book
Hb-Hct	Anemia	Chap. 2 on CBC
Microscopic Urinalysis	Possible urinary tract infection (UTI)	Chap. 3 on routine urinalysis
Urine for protein	Possible toxemia	Chap. 3 on proteinuria
Urine for glucose	Possible diabetes	Chap. 8 for diabetes and pregnancy
Rh typing and unexpected antibody screen	Possible hemolytic disease of newborn (HDN)	Chap. 14 for Rh factor in pregnancy
STS	Possible congenital syphilis	Chap. 16 on syphilis and pregnancy
Rubella titer (done *before* pregnancy)	Immunity to 3-day measles	Chap. 14 on why rubella titers are done *before* pregnancy

The last few tests in this chapter are for newborn screening, and they include detection of PKU, galactosemia, and hypothyroidism. Early detection of these three diseases prevents the mental retardation that can occur. The sweat test for CF is also briefly discussed.

Interwoven with all these advanced methods of testing is the nurse's involvement with the patient as a person. The premise of this chapter is that pregnancy and childbirth should be joyous and healthy events for a couple. If tests must be used for a pregnancy, then health professionals need to make sure that such tests are as unthreatening as possible. So the focus can be on what is normal about the pregnancy, not what may be abnormal.

PREGNANCY TESTS

Although pregnancy has early presumptive signs and symptoms, such as amenorrhea, nausea and vomiting, and skin changes, the positive signs are rarely present until the fifth or sixth month of pregnancy. Any one of the following signs is both legal and medical proof of pregnancy:

"(1) fetal heartbeat, (2) palpation of fetal outline, (3) recognition of fetal movements by someone other than the mother, and (4) ultrasonographic demonstration of the fetus [Jensen 1981:270]."

In today's modern world, few, if any, women are willing to wait a few months to know for sure if they are pregnant. The desire to know as soon as possible is strong, both for the woman who desires a child and for the woman who may choose to terminate the pregnancy if it is present. This desire has prompted the commercial success of home pregnancy kits, which were put on the market in 1976.

All the pregnancy tests are based on detecting the presence of human chorionic gonadotropin (HCG) in the urine or serum of the pregnant woman. HCG, produced by the trophoblast cell component of the fetal placental tissue, can be measured as subunits of alpha and beta. The beta subunit is probably similar to the luteinizing hormona (LH) (Jensen 1981). HCG is present in the serum within 10 days after implantation, peaks in 12 to 14 weeks, and remains elevated all during pregnancy. Since HCG is also produced by certain types of tumors of the testes or placenta, this test is used to assess these conditions too. (See the quantitative test for HCG.) Although HCG can be measured directly in the serum to detect pregnancy (see the qualitative test for HCG), most pregnancy tests rely on indirect measurements of the amount of HCG in the urine.

BIOLOGICAL TESTS FOR PREGNANCY

The older pregnancy tests used animals to test for pregnancy: Some of the woman's urine was injected into mice, rabbits, or frogs, and various changes in the animals were evidence that HCG was present. For example, HCG in the injected urine causes ovarian changes in rabbits (Friedman test) and in mice (Achheim-Zondek AZ test). In frogs (Galli-Mainini test), sperm are found in the frog's urine if the injected urine contains HCG. With the advent of immunological techniques, these older, biological tests for pregnancy are mostly of historical interest.

IMMUNOLOGICAL TESTS FOR PREGNANCY

Direct Agglutination Versus Agglutination-Inhibition Techniques

In the *direct agglutination techniques,* indicator cells from animals or latex particles are coated with HCG antibodies. If HCG is in the urine specimen, it causes an agglutination when the sample of the urine is mixed with the anti-HCG serum. The agglutination can be seen on a slide or in a test tube. The test is not as sensitive as the indirect or agglutination-inhibition technique.

With the two-step *agglutination-inhibition technique,* the urine specimen is first mixed with a commercial preparation of HCG antibodies. If the urine contains HCG, the preparation uses up the antibodies and neutralizes the serum. The serum that has been mixed with the urine is then mixed with the indicator cells, which are coated with HCG. If HCG was in the urine, then it should have neutralized the serum, so that there should be no reaction with the HCG cells. If there is no such reaction, the agglutination is inhibited and thus a *positive* for pregnancy. For this two-step technique, a reaction or clumping is a *negative* test for pregnancy.

Home Pregnancy Tests

Kits that can be used at home to detect pregnancy were introduced in 1976. Various manufacturers make the tests, such as EPT Early Pregnancy Test (Warner/Chicott), Gravindex (Ortho Diagnostics), and Daisy 2 (Bio-Dynamics Home Healthcare, Inc.). Some of these tests can detect pregnancy as early as 6 days after the expected period. Although each manufacturer claims a high degree of accuracy, each also acknowledges that false readings can occur.

Each kit has very specific directions. With these home pregnancy tests it is important to follow the directions exactly and determine whether the technique being used means that agglutination is a positive or negative result. Most require two drops of urine. One kit (Daisy 2) boasts that the result is ready in 1 hour rather than the 2 hours for the other tests. (Women want to know early, but their need is perhaps not *that* extreme!) All the tests recommend a second test if the first test is negative and if menses does not begin within a week. A second test may be needed because the urine did not have enough HCG yet, or because the woman may have miscalculated her period. If the test is positive, the woman can call her physician or clinic to have definite confirmation of the pregnancy.

All the kits stress the fact that the kit does not replace the advice or care of a physician. If repeated tests are negative, the woman has saved the expense and time of consulting the health care system. Advertisements for the kits also make the point that a pregnancy test at home provides a way for a couple to discover the good news together. A test done at home means no waiting for appointments and no suspense in waiting for an answer. A home pregnancy test may be a way for a woman to establish right from the beginning that the baby belongs to her—not to a health professional. On the other hand, health professionals express concern that a woman may not do the test correctly and thus function under the false assumption that she is not pregnant, continuing to take medicines that could be dangerous to the fetus.

HCG PREGNANCY TEST (HCG QUALITATIVE)

The laboratory can use radioimmunoassay to detect small amounts of HCG in the serum. (The technique of radioimmunoassay or RIA is described in Chapter 15.) There is some cross sensitivity with the luteinizing hormone (LH), and certain drugs may also interfere with the test. Even with these limitations, however, RIA pregnancy tests are the most reliable of laboratory assessments.

Preparation of Patient
And Collection of Sample
The test requires 0.5 ml of serum.

Reference Values

The laboratory reports either positive or negative for pregnancy.

TESTING OF BETA SUBUNIT
(HCG QUANTITATIVE TEST)

Since HCG can be increased due to certain tumors, it could come from a hydatidiform mole (a benign adenoma) of the placenta, from a choriocarcinoma (malignancy) of placenta-like tissue, or from certain types of testicular carcinoma. If any of these conditions is suspected, the HCG levels help to confirm a diagnosis. Serial HCG levels are also used to monitor the response to surgical therapy or chemotherapy. For these pathological conditions, it is not enough to just know whether HCG is present. The physician needs to know whether the levels are increasing or decreasing.

Preparation of Patient
And Collection of Sample
The test requires 0.5 ml of serum.

Reference Values

Less than 5 mIU/ml	Not significant
5–40 mIU/ml	Possible cross reaction with LH
Above 40 mIU/ml	Significant

Postmenopausal women or women who have had their ovaries removed may show positive HCG due to the cross reaction with LH. (See Chapter 15 for a discussion about LH, the luteinizing hormone and how this hormone increases at menopause.)

ALPHA-FETOPROTEIN (AFP)
IN THE SERUM

By about 16 to 18 weeks of pregnancy, alpha-fetoprotein (AFP) can be measured in the mother's blood. Presently, a maternal blood test for AFP is the *only* screening test that can be done of the pregnant woman's blood as a check for genetic defects in the child. (See Table 18–2).

Unfortunately, high levels of AFP in pregnant women do not always indicate a problem with neural tube defects because the fetal age may be incorrectly estimated, the woman may be bearing twins, or the rise could be due to other reasons that are not yet well understood (Kimball 1977). If the AFP blood screening test is elevated, a repeat is done. If the test is positive on a second blood sample, the woman has an ultrasonogram. If there is still doubt about the possibility of a defect, an amniocentesis is done.

Even with its drawbacks, AFP blood screening is offered to pregnant women in certain screening programs in the United States. AFP screening is already being done routinely in other countries, such as England and Australia. Since AFP blood testing is the first large-scale screening test offered to any woman, there are concerns about how the test is conducted and about whether the couple will have the benefit of informed advice. At the present time, the proposed FDA regulations are that the sale of AFP materials to laboratories should be available only when physicians are participating in comprehensive screening programs (Chedd 1981). Opponents of mass screening say that testing of all pregnant women causes a great deal of unnecessary anxiety, particularly if one does not believe in terminating any pregnancy. It will be interesting to see what develops with AFP as the first maternal blood test to screen for genetic disease.

TESTS TO SCREEN CARRIERS OF GENETIC DEFECTS

Laboratory tests can be done to detect whether parents are carriers of certain autosomal recessive genetic defects. If both parents are carriers, the fetus has a one-in-four chance of

TABLE 18-2.　COMMON GENETIC DISEASES THAT MAY BE DETECTED BY SCREENING

Defect	Types of Screening				Comments
	Detected in Carrier State by Blood Samples of Both Parents	Screening of Maternal Blood after Woman Is Pregnant	Amniocentesis	Fetal Blood Sampling (Research Studies)	
1. Sickle cell anemia	X			X	Most common in black families. May be difficult to accurately diagnose in fetus or newborn, but new tests on cord blood are being tried.
2. Tay-Sachs disease	X		X		Most common in Jewish families of Eastern European origin. Wide scale testing is done for Jewish populations.
3. Neural tube defects (alpha-fetoprotein tests)		X	X		At the present time, only genetic defect that can be screened for in maternal blood.* Can occur in any pregnancy.
4. Cystic fibrosis					*No prenatal tests.* See sweat test. More common in Caucasians.
5. Galactosemia			X		Tests of newborns required by law in some states.
6. Hemophilia				X	Sex-linked gene. Amniocentesis cannot determine if disease present, but can do so indirectly by determining sex of fetus.
7. Down's syndrome			X		Incidence increases with maternal age. Most common reason for amniocentesis is to check for Down's syndrome.
8. Thalassemia (beta)	X			X	Most common in families of Mediterranean descent. Screening of carriers not commonly done on large-scale basis.
9. PKU	X				Screening of carriers not common. More common in Caucasians. Almost all states require newborn screening.

*Updates on genetic diseases are available from the National Clearinghouse for Human Genetic Disease. (See the HHS reference, Publication 79-5132.)

438

having the genetic defect. (See Table 18–3 for the probability when each parent has an autosomal recessive gene for a specific disease.) For the fetus to have the defect, both parents must contribute the recessive gene. This one-in-four chance refers to autosomal recessive traits, not to sex-linked recessive traits or to dominant traits. At the present time, two common tests are done to identify carrier states for sickle cell anemia and Tay-Sachs disease, both of which are predominant in specific ethnic groups. Intermarriage eventually changes the gene pool for various ethnic groups. Two other tests for carrier states are sometimes done, namely thalassemia and PKU, but not on wide-scale screening. See Table 18–2 for common genetic diseases detected by screening.

SICKLE CELL ANEMIA

Sickle cell anemia results from an autosomal recessive gene that produces an abnormal type of hemoglobin called *hemoglobin S*. (See Chapter 2 for tests on hemoglobin.) Hemoglobin S does not function as normal hemoglobin. The red blood cells have a sickle

TABLE 18–3.   PROBABILITY OF AUTOSOMAL RECESSIVE GENETIC DISEASES WHEN BOTH PARENTS ARE CARRIERS

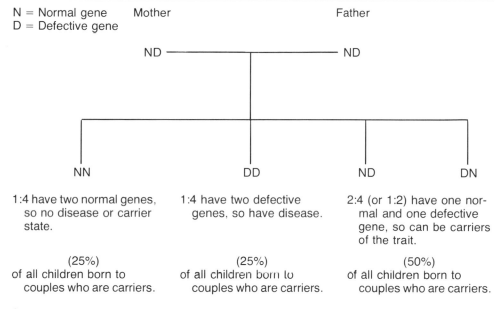

Autosomal recessive diseases discussed in the chapter include:

1. PKU	3. Sickle cell anemia
2. Cystic fibrosis	4. Tay-Sachs
	5. Thalassemia (Cooley's anemia)

Note that sex-linked recessive traits occur in different patterns. See the text for a discussion of hemophilia, which is transmitted by X chromosome.

form, particularly when they are exposed to low oxygen concentrations or if the person is dehydrated. The abnormal cells are hemolyzed at an increased rate. Also, the capillaries can become occluded by these sickled cells.

A person can either be a carrier or have the disease. If the person has only one recessive gene for sickle cell, the person is a carrier who has the sickle cell trait. The person with sickle cell trait usually has no symptoms, although exposure to very low oxygen concentrations may cause minor symptoms. However, the effect of the trait, if any, is being studied at the present time since in the past some people with the trait were denied jobs, such as piloting planes. If only one person is a carrier, there is no difficulty. If both parents are carriers, they face the one-in-four risk, for each pregnancy, that their child will have the disease. As shown in Table 18–3, the risk is also one-in-four that the child will not receive the trait from either parent, and the chance is one-in-two that the child will be a carrier. The carrier state is estimated to be present in 7 to 8% of American blacks and the disease to be present in about one in 600 blacks (Heagarty 1980:312).

Prospective black parents can be given the screening test for sickle cell anemia. The quick screening tests for sickle cell trait (Sickledex, Ortho Diagnostics) do not distinguish whether a person has the trait or the disease. So the actual diagnosis of sickle cell anemia is made with hemoglobin electrophoresis. In recent years, prominent black people have done a lot to see that the test is made available to all who desire it. For example, a traveling van in San Francisco, sponsored by Sickle Cell Anemia Research and Education, Inc. (SCARE), goes to neighborhoods to educate the community and to identify carriers of the disease. *Mandatory* screening of children is potentially harmful if a careful follow-up is not done to explain about the meaning of the trait. The addresses of regional centers for sickle cell anemia testing are available from the Department of Health and Human Services (DHHS 80–5135).

In the newborn period, the amount of fetal hemoglobin present makes it technically difficult to determine whether the disease is present (Widmann 1979). New techniques being developed are making it possible to identify sickle cell anemia from samples of cord blood in the newborn. Also research is also being done to test blood obtained by fetoscopy. Much of this research is at Yale and the University of California at San Francisco and is being made known to the public (*Time* March 24, 1980).

THALASSEMIA (COOLEY'S ANEMIA)

Thalassemia, like sickle cell anemia, is transmitted by autosomal recessive genes. Yet screening for this disease is not done on a wide-scale basis. Both the carrier state (thalassemia minor) and the presence of two recessive genes (thalassemia major) can be detected by hemoglobin electrophoresis. Thalassemia major is a chronic disease that causes severe anemia and mongoloid faces. Thalessemia minor is characterized by mild to moderate hemolytic anemia. Thalassemia is most common in children of Mediterranean origin (McCormack 1979).

Children with Severe Anemias
Nursing Implications. Both sickle cell anemia and thalassemia major are chronic conditions for which there is no cure. The child and the family need a lot of help in coping with

the disease. Families who have one child with the disease may greatly fear another pregnancy.

At the present time, sickle cell anemia or thalassemia cannot be predicted just by an amniocentesis. Even with screening of the fetal blood, definite diagnosing may not be possible due to the high degree of fetal hemoglobin present. Newer methods of electrophoresis are improving the ability to definitely diagnose sickle cell anemia, at birth or before. Couples who have had one child with any genetic disease are usually referred to research centers that can offer the latest techniques for prenatal diagnosis. What wasn't possible during a first pregnancy may have become possible when a second pregnancy is contemplated. (See the listing of clinical genetic service centers in DHSS 1980, 5135.)

Children with hemolytic anemias have lowered hemoglobin and hematocrit counts, elevated reticulocyte counts, and, in some cases, abnormal red blood cells on a periphereal smear. (See Chapter 2 for a discussion on these tests and on the general nursing implications for a patient with anemia.) Children with hemolytic anemias also have elevated *indirect* bilirubin levels. (See Chapter 11 for a discussion on indirect bilirubin as an indicator of hemolytic diseases.)

TAY-SACHS DISEASE

Tay-Sachs, another inherited autosomal recessive condition, is most commonly found in Ashkenazi Jews who are of Eastern European origin (McCormack 1979). As with all other recessive diseases, both parents must have the gene to produce a child with the disease. Tay-Sachs causes mental retardation and eventual death of the child by around age 3 or 4. There is no cure at the present time. It is evidenced by an absence of the enzyme hexoaminidase A.

There is a simple blood test to screen for carriers of Tay-Sachs, and it requires only a venous blood sample. The carriers of the recessive gene have lowered levels of the enzyme hemosaminidase A. The Tay-Sachs test is done on Jewish couples to see whether both are carriers. If needed, the Tay-Sachs test can then be done on amniotic fluid. Unless both parents have the gene, however, there is no need to test the amniotic fluid because the infant will not have the disease. Although the rate of Tay-Sachs is much lower in the non-Jewish population, Tay-Sachs can be done for non-Jewish couples who are concerned about all possible risks. Mass screening programs are planned for Jewish populations who may need to know if the trait is in their family. For example, in San Francisco, various synagogues, in conjunction with the genetic counseling center at the University of California at San Francisco, offer mass screenings for a nominal fee.

PHENYLKETONURIA

Phenylketonuria (PKU), another autosomal recessive disease, may be detected in the carrier state. Suspected carriers are given a test dose of phenylalanine, which is an amino acid. Carriers demonstrate higher levels of phenylalanine in the serum. PKU is discussed in detail at the end of this chapter.

TESTS TO MONITOR FETAL WELL-BEING

ESTRIOL LEVELS IN THE URINE AND PLASMA

During pregnancy, the fetus and the placenta function as a unit to produce estrogens, of which estriol (E_3) is the major estrogenic compound. (See Chapter 15 for a discussion on other tests of estrogen compounds.) Estriol levels begin to increase about the eighth week of pregnancy and continue at high levels to term (Hytten 1975). Consistently high levels of estriol indicate a normally functioning fetal-placental unit. Measurement of estriol may be done on either the plasma or the urine of the pregnant woman.

Toxemia, suspected intrauterine growth retardation (IUGR), chronic hypertension, diabetes, and post maturity are the common reasons for monitoring a pregnancy through estriol levels (Olds 1980). To recognize a trend, however, there must be more than one serum or urine estriol. A decrease over two or three samples, either as a slow downward trend or as an abrupt drop, is evidence of potential fetal distress because the placenta is not functioning normally. Some authors suggest a baseline should be done at 26 weeks for women who are high risk. Diabetic women may have weekly estriol levels after 30 weeks gestation, biweekly after 34 weeks and every other day after 36 weeks (Schuler 1979: 450).

Preparation of Patient
And Collection of Sample
If the urine levels are to be monitored, the patient must collect all urine for 24 hours. (See Chapter 3 for the key points to tell a patient about a 24-hour urine specimen.)

If the estriol level is to be monitored by serum levels, there is no special preparation of the patient. The test requires 2 ml of venous blood. Due to the ease of collecting the blood sample and the lower chance of error than with a 24-hour urine collection, serum levels are a more desirable way to monitor the pregnancy. Due to considerable diurnal variation, the laboratory may do more than one sample a day.

Reference Values

Plasma	Varies with time of gestation. Level continues to rise during pregnancy.
Urine (24-hour specimen)	In the last 6 weeks of pregnancy, the average excretion is between 10 to 24 mg/day, with a mean of 16 mg. Interpretation of the values for an individual patient must be done on a series of tests to see whether there is a downward trend (Diamond, 1979).

NEWBORN SCREENING

For many newborns, the symptoms of serious inborn errors of metabolism are evident at birth. Nurses who work with newborns need to be on the alert for any symptoms or signs that require medical assessment. Some of these characteristics may also be noted by the parents. McCormack has listed nine clinical hints for the diagnosis of inborn errors of metabolism:

1. unexplained metabolic alterations in electrolytes with acidosis or dehydration,
2. progressive downhill course with central nervous system deterioration,
3. unexplained renal or cardiac failure,
4. unexplained large viscera,
5. abnormal urine odor,
6. marked change in features, large tongue, coarse features,
7. thrombocytopenia, neutropenia, and/or anemia,
8. renal colic or calculus, and
9. idiosyncratic or unusual reaction to drugs (McCormack 1979:150).

Different inborn errors of metabolism, of course, cause different symptoms. For example, the only symptom of PKU is a musty odor of the urine, which may not be noticed. Several other inborn defects give urine an odor that has been described as smelling like rotten cabbage, sweaty feet, stale fish, or burned sugar (Thomas 1973).

Although some genetic diseases have symptoms at birth, others do not. Some of these "hidden" defects can cause serious damage if treatment is not begun early. Many tests can be done to detect genetic abnormalities in the newborn, but doing a large number of screening tests on all apparently healthy newborns is simply not feasible. A few genetic diseases are common enough, however, to warrant mass screening for all newborns. For a test to be used as a screening device in healthy newborns, the test must be accurate and highly reliable, it must be easy to do in mass volume, and it must measure a genetic disease that is common enough to warrant the cost of mass screening and for which treatment is available.

For example, at the present time, there is a screening test neither for cystic fibrosis, which is an autosomal recessive genetic disease, nor for the carrier state. But if cystic fibrosis is suspected, the physician will order a sweat test. The sweat test is expensive and technically difficult to interpret, but it is warranted for specific cases. (The sweat test is discussed at the end of this chapter.)

Another newborn test that is not done routinely is a test for a lack of an enzyme to manufacture cortisol, which is called the adrenogenital syndrome. If a physician suspected the disease, she or he would order tests for various enzyme defects. (See Chapter 15 for a detailed description of the tests for adrenogenital syndrome.)

The tests for sickle cell anemia are being perfected so that large-scale screening of newborns is feasible. Refer to the DHSS publications in the references for information from the National Clearinghouse for Genetic Diseases on the latest advances in the testing, diagnosis, counseling, and treatment of all genetic diseases. The Clearinghouse has been in existence since October of 1978.

Newborn Screening Tests Required by Law

Different states may require one or more tests for newborns as a general screening program. Since the sixties, most states have required a test for phenylketonuria (PKU). Any *mandatory* tests for newborn screening must be not only accurate and suitable for mass screening, but they must also detect diseases that can be controlled if early treatment is begun. For example, California requires three screening tests for newborns: galactosemia and hypothyroidism, besides PKU. All three use capillary blood placed on a filter paper. The hospital is also authorized by state law to charge a fee for the tests. An information sheet is given to all new parents that explains in lay terms the reason for the three tests. If the parents do not wish their child to have the tests, they must sign a statement relieving the physician and hospital of any liability for damages that may result from the lack of early detection of the three disorders (Cunningham 1980). Parents are told that if they refuse the tests now, they can request the tests from a physician or a public health nurse later. The nurse can often be useful in further explaining how these tests are very beneficial in helping the newborn get off to the best start possible. The reader is encouraged to discover what screening tests are mandatory in a particular state.

SCREENING TEST FOR PHENYLKETONURIA

Phenylalanine is an amino acid found in all protein foods. The infant with phenylketonuria (PKU) has a build-up of phenylalanine in the serum due to the lack of an enzyme needed for the normal metabolism of this amino acid. Since the phenylalanine spills into the urine, the condition is called phenylketonuria (PKU). PKU is dangerous because the high levels of phenylalanine in the serum can cause brain damage and mental retardation. Originally, screening tests for PKU were done on the urine, but the blood test (Guthrie test) is more valuable. PKU is more common in Caucasians.

Serum PKU Levels
Preparation of Patient and Collection of Sample. The serum level may be abnormally elevated within 24 hours after the infant begins a milk diet. If the infant is not taking milk well, the test should be delayed. (See the discussion on the urine test that can be done later at home.) The laboratory needs to know the date and time of birth, as well as the date and time of the first milk feeding.

    The usual procedure is to do the PKU on the third day. If the baby is breast feeding, a second PKU may be done after the milk supply is abundant. A screening test for PKU can be done on capillary blood drawn from a heel stick. (Chapter 1 describes the procedure for heel sticks for infants.) Serum levels are followed if there is a positive first test. Some babies may have increased phenylalanine levels due to immaturity of the liver.

Reference Values

Serum phenylalanine	1–3 mg/dl

Urine PKU Levels
Although PKU is better detected through the Guthrie blood test, urine can be used when blood testing is not feasible. The child's urine can be tested by a dip and read stick (Phenistix by Ames). Since the recommended times for urine checks for PKU are during the second, fourth, and sixth weeks of life (Ames Product Information 1980), the urine screening may detect cases missed by too early blood screening in the hospital. Any positive discoveries, indicated by a green color, should be followed up with serum testing.

Urine tests may also be used to monitor the effectiveness of dietary management of PKU when it is not feasible to do serum levels.

Since the Phenistix also detect the presence of p-aminosalicylates (PAS), they are used to monitor patients who are taking PAS as treatment for tuberculosis. (A special color chart is used if the Phenistix are used to see if the patient is taking PAS.) Since Phenistix also react with aspirin metabolites and with phenothiazines, they may be of value in revealing or checking for the presence of aspirin or phenothiazines in cases of possible drug overdosage. (See Chapter 17 for more information on toxicology testing.)

Preparation of Patient
And Collection of Sample

Phenistix may be used on any urine specimen either by dipping the stick into the urine or pressing it against a wet diaper. Because salicylates and phenothiazines also cause positive reactions to the test, these drugs invalidate Phenistix as a test for PKU.

Possible Nursing Implications. The treatment for PKU consists of limiting the intake of phenylalanine to a level that is appropriate for each child. Commercial products, such as Lofenalac, contain the essential amino acids with only a small amount of phenylalanine.

A restricted diet, tailored to the serum levels of phenylalanine, makes it possible for the child to develop normally without any mental retardation. The nurse may have a major role in helping the family to adjust their dietary needs for the infant with PKU. Reyzer (1978), a nurse, and a mother of a boy with PKU, has explained in detail how to plan diets that contain a precise amount of phenylalanine. The National Foundation of the March of Dimes gives a free copy of a *Low Protein Cookery for Phenylketonuria* to any family with a child with PKU.

PKU is an autosomal recessive genetic disease. So if a couple have one child with the disease, they have a one-in-four chance of having another child with the disease (refer to Table 18–3). At the present time, PKU cannot be detected by amniocentesis. Parents may opt for a second child, however, even with the known risk, if they see that a first child is progressing well on dietary control. People who have a history of PKU in their families can also be tested for the carrier state since a diet high in phenylalanine causes higher-than-usual serum levels in people who have the one recessive gene (Jensen 1981). The test for PKU carriers, however, is not a common test.

SCREENING TESTS FOR HYPOTHYROIDISM

The pilot program for screening for hypothyroidism in newborns began in North America in 1972. The screening of over 1 million infants resulted in the recommendation to use the T_4 filter paper test for screening and a follow-up of TSH (thyroid-stimulating hormone) for the 3 to 5% of low T_4 results (Fisher 1979). The T_4 filter paper test requires only a drop of capillary blood. (See Chapter 1 for the discussion about heel sticks of infants.)

The tests used for hypothyroidism are discussed in Chapter 15. See the sections on hypothyroidism of the newborn for the symptoms of the disorder, on the medical treatment, and on the nursing implications.

SCREENING TESTS FOR GALACTOSEMIA

The test used to detect this inborn metabolism of galactose is discussed in detail at the end of Chapter 8, where the treatment of the disease and the nursing implications are also covered. Like PKU and hypothyroid tests of the newborn, galactosemia tests can be done via a heel stick to obtain capillary blood for a filter paper. (Chapter 1 discusses heel sticks of infants.)

SWEAT TEST FOR CYSTIC FIBROSIS (CF)

Cystic fibrosis (CF) is a hereditary disease, caused by an autosomal recessive gene. (See Table 18–3), that affects the exocrine glands of the body. Since in this disease the mucous glands produce very thick mucus, its other name is mucoviscidosis. The thick mucus is the most troublesome in the lungs. The other major problem in cystic fibrosis is the partial destruction and malfunction of the exocrine glands in the pancreas. Although CF occurs in one of every 1,500 to 2,000 live births in most Caucasian populations (Kruger 1980:67), there is no genetic screening test for CF at the present time. Because CF also affects exocrine glands, such as the sweat glands, the tests for its detection are based on determining the amount of sodium (Na) and chloride (Cl) in the sweat. The volume of sweat is not increased, even though the Na and Cl content is increased. (Ravel 1978:421)

Preparation of Patient
And Collection of Sample

The screening test may involve placing the patient's hand on a special plate or paper. If the screening test indicates an abnormally high amount of NaCl, more definitive tests are done. The more elaborate tests may include various methods to induce sweat. The exact preparation of the patient is specified by the laboratory.

Reference Values

Children	up to age 15 60 mEq of Na or Cl is the upper limit of normal.
Adults	May have higher levels.

Clinical Significance. The sweat test is used in the diagnosis of cystic fibrosis. Presently, there is no test for the carrier state of the recessive gene for CF.

Possible Nursing Implications. Refer to a pediatric textbook for the very detailed care needed for a child with CF. The malabsorption problems may be partially overcome by the use of oral preparations of pancreatic enzymes. The problem with mucus in the lungs requires diligent and daily respiratory care.

HELPING THE FAMILY WITH A GENETICALLY DEFECTIVE CHILD: GENERAL NURSING IMPLICATIONS

The family who has a child with a genetic defect needs help and encouragement to adjust to the changes that the disease requires. Since hypothyroidism can be controlled by the administration of thyroid, and galactosemia and PKU by diet restrictions, the family can be assured of a normal healthy child. Still, the family needs time to mourn the ''loss'' of the perfect child.

In the case of other defects, such as sickle cell anemia and cystic fibrosis, parents have no assurance that the child will be normal and healthy. When a child is born with any disorder treatable or not so treatable, nurses are in a key position to focus their attention on the total needs of the family unit. They can, for example, be part of a team that does follow-up studies of the family. Johnson (1980) describes how nurses can be involved in self-instruction for the family who has a child with cystic fibrosis. Kruger *et al.* (1980) studied the reaction of families to cystic fibrosis and summarized five methods of assistance used by nurses and other health professionals to help families cope. These five measures are:

1. offering support, including the role of a listener,
2. guiding the parents, which involves use of available resources,
3. teaching so that all family members really understand the disease,
4. the physical care during bouts of illness, and
5. providing an environment that promotes personal development to meet the demands of the situation (Kruger *et al.* 1980:71).

One final important point in helping the family to adjust to the birth of a child with a genetic defect is the availability of genetic counseling to help the couple make a decision about future children. Tishler (1981) has stated that, during the presentation of genetic information, families often first experience denial of the problem, followed by anger and blame. The desirable final phase is integration and insight into the problem. The couple can then make their own decision about future pregnancies.

As nurses take on expanded roles, they may be able to do more and more of this type of care. Surely the development of nursing needs to progress to match the technical advances that make it possible for children with defects to receive sophisticated medical interventions. Medical technology has certainly made it possible to increase the quantity of life. Nurses surely have a role of helping to improve the quality of life.

Questions

18-1. Mrs. Fannin is 6 months pregnant. Which one of these following laboratory reports is *not expected* in a normal pregnancy? (Increases or decreases refer to her prepregnancy values.)

    a. An increase of the neutrophils on a WBC.

    b. A slight increase in both Hgb and Hct levels.

    c. A decrease in pCO_2 levels.

    d. An increase in serum alkaline phosphatase levels.

18-2. The month after Mary had a hystosalpingogram, she missed her period. When menses still had not occurred after two weeks, Mary bought a home pregnancy test kit of the direct agglutination type. If Mary is pregnant, then:

    a. the human chorionic gonadotrophin (HCG) in her urine will react with sensitized cells in the test sample.

    b. the test will be negative because it is only 14 days after an expected period.

    c. the HCG antibodies in her urine will agglutinate the HCG in the test sample.

    d. the gonadotrophins LH and FSH may cause a false *negative* result because the test is the direct agglutination type.

18-3. A quantitative HCG measurement may be used to follow all of the following conditions *except* which?

    a. Hydatidiform moles.   **c.** Choriocarcinoma.

    b. Testicular cancer.   **d.** Normal pregnancy.

18-4. All of the following are tests for carrier states of specific autosomal recessive genetic diseases. Which one is done as a screening test for Jewish people who are of Eastern European origin?

    a. Sickledex for sickle cell anemia.   **c.** Tay-Sachs blood test.

    b. Thalassemia blood test.   **d.** PKU urine test.

18-5. Mr. and Mrs. Green are both carriers of the autosomal recessive genes that cause sickle cell anemia. They have one child who has sickle cell anemia. What is the probability that a second pregnancy will produce a child who does not receive the defective gene from either parents (i.e., no sickle cell anemia or even sickle cell trait)?

    a. one-in-four chance.

    b. one-in-two chance.

    c. All children will have the trait.

    d. Risk cannot be stated because one child has the disease.

18-6. Mrs. Sommers is pregnant and two weeks past her due date. She is having serial determinations of serum estriol levels. A consistently high level on several samples would be evidence of which of the following?

    a. No congenital defects in the fetus.

    b. Possible fetal distress.

    c. An intact and functioning fetal-placental unit.

    d. Maturity of the fetus.

18-7. The rationale for doing PKU, galactesemia, and hypothyroid screening on all newborns is based on all the following principles *except* which?

    a. Mass screening tests for all three disorders are accurate, technically easy to do, and considered cost-effective.

    b. All three genetic defects cause mental retardation if treatment is not begun within weeks or months after birth.

    c. All these diseases may cause symptoms within a day or two after birth.

    d. All three diseases can be effectively controlled by either dietary restrictions or hormone replacement.

18-8. Phenistix (Ames Company), urine dip sticks, are used for all the following purposes *except* which?

    a. Detecting salicylate overdosage.

    b. Detecting phenothiazine overdosage.

    c. Confirmatory diagnosis of PKU.

    d. Assessment of the effectiveness of a low phenylalanine diet.

18-9. Which of the following is not an appropriate role for the community nurse who is following a family that has a child with a genetic defect?

    a. Helping the family find and use available community resources.

    b. Teaching the family about the effects of the disease.

    c. Encouraging the family not to risk having another child.

    d. Assisting with some physical care if the child is ill.

REFERENCES

Ames Product Information. "Phenistix, Semi-Quantitative Dip and Read Test for Phenylketones in Urine," Elkart, Ind.: Ames Laboratories, 1980.

Chedd, Graham. "The New Age of Genetic Screening," *Science* 81 (January–February 1981). 32–40.

Cunningham, George. "Important Information for Parents" (Letter given to all parents of newborns), Maternal and Child Health Branch, Department of Health Services, Sacramento, California, 1980.

"Daisy 2 In-Home Pregnancy Test Kit," Information Booklet. Indianapolis: BioDynamic Home Healthcare, Inc., 1979.

Department of Health and Human Services, *Human Genetics: Informational and Educational Materials* 1:1 1979. DHSS Publication 79-5132. Free.

Department of Health and Human Services. *Clinical Genetic Service Centers. A National Listing* 1980. DHSS Publication 80-5135. Free.

Diamond, Frayda. "High Risk Pregnancy Screening Techniques," *JOGN* 7 (November–December 1979): 15–19.

Fisher, Delbert *et al.* "Screening for Congenital Hypothyroidism: Results of Screening One Million North American Infants," *Journal of Pediatrics* 94 (May 1979): 700–705.

Heagarty, Margaret *et al. Child Health: Basics for Primary Care.* New York: Appleton-Century-Crofts, 1980.

Hytten, Frank and Lind, Tom. *Diagnostic Indices in Pregnancy.* Summitt, N.J.: Ciba-Geigy Corporation, 1975.

Jensen, Margaret *et al. Maternity Care: The Nurse and the Family,* 2nd ed. C. V. Mosby Co., St. Louis, Mo.: 1981.

Johnson, Mary. "Self-Instruction for the Family of a Child with Cystic Fibrosis," *Maternal Child Nursing* 5 (September–October 1980): 345–348.

Kimball, Margaret *et al.* "Prenatal Diagnosis of Neural Tube Defects: A Re-Evaluation of the Alpha Fetoprotein Assay," *Obstetrics and Gynecology* 49 (May 1977): 532–536.

Kruger, Susan *et al.* "Reactions of Families to the Child with Cystic Fibrosis," *Image* 12 (October 1980): 67–72.

McCormack, Michael. "Medical Genetics and Family Practice," *American Family Physician* 20 (September 1979): 143–154.

Olds, Sally *et al. Obstetric Nursing.* Menlo Park, Cal.: Addison-Wesley Publishing Co., 1980.

Ravel, Richard. *Clinical Laboratory Medicine.* Chicago: Year Book Medical Publishers, Inc., 1978.

Reyzer, Nancy. "Diagnosis: PKU," *American Journal of Nursing* 78 (November 1978): 1895–1898.

Schuler, Katherine. "When a Pregnant Woman is Diabetic: Antepartal Care," *American Journal of Nursing* 79 (March 1979): 448–452.

"Testing Fetuses, A Checkup in the Womb," *Time* 115 (March 24, 1980): 48.

Thomas, G. and Scott, G. "Laboratory Diagnosis of Genetic Disorders," *Pediatric Clinics of North America* 20 (February 1973): 105–119.

Tishler, Carl. "The Psychological Aspects of Genetic Counseling," *American Journal of Nursing* 81 (April 1981): 733–734.

Widmann, Frances. "Chapter 16: Pregnancy," in *Clinical Interpretation of Labortory Tests,* 8th ed. Philadelphia: F. A. Davis Co., 1979.

Reference Values
And Other Information

As stressed in Chapter 1, laboratory books such as this one cannot provide a table of *normal* values for laboratory tests because each laboratory must provide its own normal range for the particular technique that it uses and for the unique population it serves. Values that are listed in a book are only *reference* values, and they must be adapted to a particular setting. The primary source for reference values used in this text are those printed periodically in the *New England Journal of Medicine,* with whose permission the tables in Appendix A are reprinted. Reprints and updates of the normal reference values are available (at $2.50 each) by ordering from:

Normal Reference Values
New England Journal of Medicine
1172 Commonwealth Avenue
Boston, Massachusetts, 02134

In addition to the specific reference values listed in Appendix A, Appendix B contains a summary of the changes in newborns and in children. Appendix D presents the changes in pregnancy, and Appendix C, those in the elderly. Documentations for the changes in various populations are included with the tables and throughout the text.

The collection of blood is most often done with the Vacutainer system, which has different-colored tops on the collection tubes to note the additive present. Table A–7 lists the meaning of the color coded tops. The type of additive needed is listed in the fifth column of these tables. The vast majority of serum blood samples require no additives, so blood is collected in a red-top tube.

The tables of reference values also contain the values in SI units, which are explained in Chapter 1. Since reference tables contain many abbreviations and measurement terms, there is a list of common abbreviations included in Appendix E and measurements to help the reader decipher laboratory reports in Appendix F.

APPENDIX A

TABLE A-1. BLOOD, PLASMA, OR SERUM VALUES

Determination	Reference Range		Minimal ML Required	Note	Explanation of Test and Possible Nursing Implications
	Conventional	SI			
Acetoacetate plus actone	0.3–2.0 mg/100 ml	3–20 mg/l	2-S		Chap. 8
Aldolase	1.3–8.2 mU/ml	12–75 nmol·s^{-1}/l	2-S	Use fresh, unhemolyzed serum	Chap. 12
Ammonia	80–110 μg/100 ml	47–65 μmol/l	2-B	Collect in heparinized tube; deliver *immediately* packed in ice	Chap. 10
Amylase	4–25 U/ml	4–25 arb. unit	3-S		Chap. 12
Barbiturate	0 Coma level: phenobarbital, approximately 10 mg/100 ml; most other drugs, 1–3 mg per 100 ml	0 μmol/l	5-S		Chap. 17
Bilirubin (van den Bergh test)	One minute: 0.4 mg/100 ml Direct: 0.4 mg/100 ml. Total: 1.0 mg/100 ml Indirect is total minus direct	up to 7 μmol/l up to 17 μmol/l	3-S		Chap. 11
Bromide	0 Toxic level: 17 mEq/l	0 mmol/l	3-S		Chap. 17

Determination	Normal value	SI value	Specimen	Special instructions	Chapter
Bromsulfalein (BSP)	Less than 5% retention	<0.05 l	3-S	Inject intravenously 5 mg of dye/kg of body weight; draw blood 45 min later	Chap. 11
Calcium	8.5–10.5 mg/100 ml (slightly higher in children)	2.1–2.6 mmol/l	3-S	BSP dye interferes	Chap. 7
Carbon dioxide content	24–30 mEq/l 20–26 mEq/l in infants (as HCO_3^-)	24–30 mmol/l	3-S	Draw without stasis under oil or fill tube to top	Chap. 6
Chloride	100–106 mEq/l	100–106 mmol/l	1-S		Chap. 5
Creatine phosphokinase (CPK)	Female 5–35 mU/ml Male 5–55 mU/ml	0.08–0.58 μmol·s^{-1}/l	3-S	Immediately separate and freeze serum	Chap. 12
Creatinine	0.6–1.5 mg/100 ml	60–130 μmol/l	1-S		Chap. 4
Doriden (Glutethimide)	0 mg/100 ml	0 μmol/l	5-S		Chap. 17
Ethanol	0.3–0.4%, marked intoxication; 0.4–0.5% alcoholic stupor; 0.5% or over, alcoholic coma	65–87 mmol/l 87–109 mmol/l >109 mmol/l	2-B	Collect in oxalate and refrigerate	Chap. 17
Glucose	Fasting: 70–110 mg/100 ml	3.9–5.6 mmol/l	2-P	Collect with EDTA-fluoride mixture	Chap. 8
Iron	50–150 μg/100 ml (higher in males)	9.0–26.9 μmol/l	5-S	Shows diurnal variation higher in a.m.	Chap. 2
Iron-binding capacity	250–410 μg/100 ml	44.8–73.4 μmol/l	5-S		Chap. 2
Lactic dehydrogenase	60–120 U/ml	1.00–2.00 μmol·s^{-1}/l	2-S	Unsuitable if hemolyzed	Chap. 12
Lead	50 μg/100 ml or less	up to 2.4 μmol/l	2-B	Collect with oxalate fluoride mixture	Chap. 17
Lipase	2U/ml or less	up to 2 arb. unit	3-S		Chap. 12

(continued)

TABLE A-1. *Continued*

Determination	Reference Range		Minimal ML Required	Note	Explanation of Test and Possible Nursing Implications
	Conventional	SI			
Lipids Cholesterol	120–220 mg/100 ml	3.10–5.69 mmol/l	2-S	Fasting	Chap. 9
Cholesterol esters	60–75% of cholesterol		2-S	Fasting	Chap. 9
Triglycerides	40–150 mg/100 ml	0.4–1.5 g/l	2-S	Fasting	Chap. 9
Lipoprotein electrophoresis (LEP)			2-S	Fasting; do not freeze serum	Chap. 9
Lithium	Toxic level 2 mEq/l	2 mmol/l	1-S		Chap. 17
Magnesium	1.5–2.0 mEq/l	0.8–1.3 mmol/l	1-S		Chap. 7
Methanol	0		5-B	May be fatal as low as 115 mg per 100 ml; collect in oxalate	Chap. 17
Osmolality	285–295 mOsm/kg water	285–295 mmol/kg	5-S		Chap. 4
Oxygen saturation (arterial)	96–100%	0.96–1.001	3-B	Deliver in sealed heparinized syringe packed in ice	Chap. 6
PCO_2	35–45 mm Hg	4.7–6.0 kPa	2-B	Collect and deliver in sealed heparinized syringe	Chap. 6
pH	7.35–7.45	same	2-B	Collect without stasis in sealed heparinized syringe; deliver packed in ice	Chap. 6

Determination	Conventional	SI	Code	Notes	Reference
PO$_2$	75–100 mm Hg (dependent on age) while breathing room air Above 500 mm Hg while on on 100% O$_2$	10.0–13.3 kPa	2-B		Chap. 6
Phenylalanine	0–2 mg/100 ml	0–120 μmol/l	0.4-S		Chap. 18
Phenytoin (Dilantin)	Therapeutic level, 5–20 μg/ml	19.8–79.5 μmol/l	3-S		Chap. 17
Phosphatase (acid)	Male—Total: 0.13–0.63 Sigma U/ml Female—Total: 0.01–0.56 Sigma U/ml Prostatic: 0–0.7 Fishman-Lerner U/100 ml	36–175 nmol·s^{-1}/l 2.8–156 nmol·s^{-1}/1	1-S	Must always be drawn just before analysis or stored as frozen serum; avoid hemolysis	Chap. 12
Phosphatase (alkaline)	13–39 IU/l; infants and adolescents up to 104 IU/l	0.22–0.65 μmol·s^{-1}/l up to 1.26 μmol·s^{-1}/l	1-S	BSP dye interferes; for Bodansky U multiply IU/l by 0.15 up to 90 U; 0.13 to 256 U	Chap. 12
Phosphorus (inorganic)	3.0–4.5 mg/100 ml (infants in 1st year up to 6.0 mg/100 ml)	1.0–1.5 mmol/l	2-S	Obtain blood in fasting state; serum must be separated promptly from cells.	Chap. 7
Potassium	3.5–5.0 mEq/l	3.5–5.0 mmol/l	2-S	Serum must be separated promptly from cells (within 1 hr)	Chap. 5
Primidone (Mysoline)	Therapeutic level 4–12 μg/ml	18–55 μmol/l	3-S		Chap. 17

(continued)

TABLE A-1. *Continued*

Determination	Reference Range		Minimal ML Required	Note	Explanation of Test and Possible Nursing Implications
	Conventional	SI			
Protein: Total	6.0–8.4 g/100 ml	60–84 g/l	1-S	Patient should be fasting; avoid BSP dye	Chap. 10
Albumin	3.5–5.0 g/100 ml	35–50 g/l	1-S		
Globulin	2.3–3.5 g/100 ml	23–35 g/l		Globulin equals total protein minus albumin	
Electrophoresis Albumin	% of total protein 52–68	0.52–0.68 l	1-S	Quantitation by densitometry	Chap. 10
Globulin: Alpha₁ Alpha₂ Beta Gamma	4.2–7.2 6.8–12 9.3–15 13–23	0.042–0.072 l 0.068–0.12 l 0.093–0.15 l 0.13–0.23 l			Chap. 10
Quinidine	Therapeutic: 1.5–3 µg/ml Toxic: 5–6 µg/ml 0	4.6–9.2 µmol/l 15.4–18.5 µmol/l	1-S		Chap. 17
Salicylate:			5-P	Collect in heparin or EDTA	Chap. 17
Therapeutic	20–25 mg/100 ml; 25–30 mg/100 ml to age 10 yrs. 3 h post dose	1.4–1.8 mmol/l 1.8–2.2 mmol/l			
Toxic	Over 30 mg/100 ml; over 20 mg/100 ml after age 60	over 2.2 mmol/l over 1.4 mmol/l			

Sodium	135–145 mEq/l	135–145 mmol/l	2-S		Chap. 5
Sulfonamide	0 mg/100 ml Therapeutic: 5–15 mg/ 100 ml	0 mmol/l	2-S,B	Value given as unconjugated total is requested	Chap. 16
Transaminase (SGOT) (aspartate aminotransferase)	10–40 U/ml	0.08–0.32 μmol·s^{-1}/1	1-S		Chap. 12
Urea nitrogen (BUN)	8–25 mg/100 ml	2.9–8.9 mmol/l	1-S,B	Urea = BUN $\times$ 2.14. Use oxalate as anticoagulant	Chap. 4
Uric acid	3.0–7.0 mg/100 ml	0.18–0.42 mmol/l	1-S	Serum must be separated from cells at once and refrigerated	Chap. 4

Reprinted from the New England Journal of Medicine, *with permission.*

These values are in common use in the laboratories at the Massachusetts General Hospital and were compiled with the aid of Sidney V. Rieder, Ph.D., the Chemistry Laboratory, Leonard Ellman, M.D., the Clinical Laboratories, Bernard Kliman, M.D., the Endocrine Laboratories and Kurt J. Bloch, M.D., the Clinical Immunology Laboratory.

†*The SI for the Health Professions. World Health Organization: Office of Publications, Geneva, Switzerland, 1977.*

‡*Abbreviations used: SI, Système international d'Unités; d, 24 hours; P, plasma; S, serum; B, blood; U, urine; l, liter; h, hour; and s, second.*

TABLE A-2. URINE VALUES

| Determination | Reference Range | | Minimal Quantity Required | Note | Explanation of Test and Possible Nursing Implications |
	Conventional	SI			
Acetone plus acetoacetate (quantitative)	0	0 mg/l	2 ml	Keep cold	Chap. 3
Amylase	24–76 U/ml	24–76 arb. unit			Chap. 12
Calcium	150 mg/d or less	3.8 or less mmol/d	24-h specimen	Collect in special bottle with 10 ml of concentrated HCl	Chap. 7
Catecholamines	Epinephrine: under 20 μg/d Norepinephrine: under 100 μg/d	<55 nmol/d <590 nmol/d	24-h specimen	Should be collected with 12 ml of concentrated HCl (pH should be between 2.0 and 3.0)	Chap. 15
Chorionic gonadotropin	0	0 arb. unit	1st morning voiding		Chap. 18
Coproporphyrin	50–250 μg/d Children under 80 lb 0–75 μg/d	80–380 nmol/d 0–115 nmol/d	24-h specimen	Specific gravity should be at least 1.015	Chap. 3
Creatinine	15–25 mg/kg of body weight/d	0.13–0.22 mmol·kg⁻¹/d	24-h specimen	Collect with 5 g of sodium carbonate	Chap. 3
Creatinine clearance	150–180 l/d (104–125 ml/min) per 1.73 m² of body surface	1.7–2.1 ml/s	24-h specimen	Order serum creatinine also	Chap. 4

Test			Specimen	Instructions	
Follicle-stimulating-hormone:			24-h specimen		Chap. 15
Follicular phase	5–20 IU/d	same			
Mid-cycle	15–60 IU/d				
Luteal phase	5–15 IU/d				
Menopausal	50–100 IU/d				
Men	5–25 IU/d				
Hemoglobin and myoglobin	0		Freshly voided sample	Chemical examination with benzidine	Chap. 2
5-Hydroxyindole acetic acid	2–9 mg/d (women lower than men)	10–45 μmol/l	24-h specimen	Collect in special bottle with 10 ml of concentrated HCl	Chap. 3
Lead	0.08 μg/ml or 120 μg or less/d	0.39 μmol/l or less	24-h specimen		Chap. 17
Phenosulfonphthalein (PSP)	At least 25% excreted by 15 min; 40% by 30 min; 60% by 120 min	0.25 l	Total output of urine collected 15, 30 and 120 min after injection	Inject 1 ml (6 mg) intravenously, BSP interferes	Chap. 4
Phosphorus (inorganic)	Varies with intake; average 1 g/d	32 mmol/d	24-h specimen	Collect in special bottle with 10 ml of concentrated HCl	Chap. 7
Porphobilinogen	0	0	10 ml	Use freshly voided urine	Chap. 3
Protein:					
Quantitative	<150 mg/24 h	<0.15 g/d	24-h specimen		Chap. 3
Electrophoresis					Chap. 3

(continued)

TABLE A-2. *Continued*

Determination	Reference Range Conventional	Reference Range SI	Minimal Quantity Required	Note	Explanation of Test and Possible Nursing Implications
Steroids:					
17-Ketosteroids (per day)	Age 10: Male 1–4 mg, Female 1–4 mg 20: 6–21, 4–16 30: 8–26, 4–14 50: 5–18, 3–9 70: 2–10, 1–7	Male $\mu mol/d$ 3–14, 21–73, 28–90, 17–62, 7–35 Female $\mu mol/d$ 3–14, 14–56, 14–49, 10–31, 3–24	24-h specimen	Not valid if patient is receiving meprobamate	Chap. 15
17-Hydroxysteroids	3–8 mg/d (women lower than men)	8–22 $\mu mol/d$ as hydrocortisone	24-h specimen	Keep cold; chlorpromazine and related drugs interfere with assay	Chap. 15
Sugar:					
Quantitative glucose	0	0 mmol/l	24-h or other timed specimen	Collect with toluene; refrigerate	Chap. 3, 8
Identification of reducing substances			50 ml	Use freshly voided urine; no preservatives	
Fructose	0	0 mmol/l	50 ml	Use freshly voided urine; also quantitate total reducing substances	
Pentose	0	0 mmol/l	50 ml	Use freshly voided urine	
Urobilinogen	Up to 1.0 Ehrlich U	to 1.0 arb. unit	2-h sample (1–3 p.m.)		Chap. 11
Uroporphyrin	0	0 nmol/d	See Coproporphyrin		Chap. 3
Vanilmandelic acid (VMA)	Up to 9 mg/24 h	up to 45 $\mu mol/d$	24-h specimen	Collect as for catecholamines	Chap. 15

Reprinted from the New England Journal of Medicine, *with permission.*

TABLE A-3. SPECIAL ENDOCRINE TESTS

Determination	Reference Range		Minimal ML Required	Note	Explanation of Test and Possible Nursing Implications
	Conventional	SI			
	a. Steroid Hormones				
Aldosterone	Excretion: 5-19 μg/24 h	14-53 nmol/d	5/d	Keep specimen cold	Chap. 15
	Supine: 48 ± 29 pg/ml	133 ± 80 pmol/l	3-S,P	Fasting, at rest, 210 meq sodium diet	
	Upright: (2 h) 65 ± 23 pg/ml	180 ± 64 pmol/l		Upright, 2 h, 210 meq sodium diet	
	Supine: 107 ± 45 pg/ml	279 ± 125 pmol/l		Fasting, at rest, 110 meq sodium diet	
	Upright: (2 h) 239 ± 123 pg/ml	663 ± 341 pmol/l		Upright, 2 h, 110 meq sodium diet	
	Supine: 175 ± 75 pg/ml	485 ± 208 pmol/l		Fasting, at rest, 10 meq sodium diet	
	Upright: (2 h) 532 ± 228 pg/ml	1476 ± 632 pmol/l		Upright, 2 h, 10 meq sodium diet	
Cortisol	8 a.m.: 5-25 μg/100 ml	0.14-0.69 μmol/l	1-P	Fasting	Chap. 15
	8 p.m.: Below 10 μg/100 ml	0-0.28 μmol/l	1-P	At rest	
	4 h ACTH test: 30-45 μg/100 ml	0.83-1.24 μmol/l	1-P	20 U ACTH, IV per 4 h	
	Overnight suppression test: Below 5 μg/100 ml	<0.14 nmol/l	1-P	8 a.m. sample after dexa-methasone midnight	
	Excretion: 20-70 μg/24 h	55-193 nmol/d	2-d	Keep specimen cold	

(continued)

TABLE A-3. *Continued*

| Determination | Reference Range | | Minimal ML Required | Note | Explanation of Test and Possible Nursing Implications |
	Conventional	SI			
11-Deoxycortisol	Responsive: Over 7.5 μg/100 ml	>0.22 μmol/l	1-P	8 a.m. sample, preceded by 4.5 g of metyrapone PO per 24 h or by single dose of 2.5 g PO at midnight	Chap. 15
Testosterone	Adult male: 300–1100 ng/100 ml Adolescent male: Over 100 ng/100 ml Female: 25–90 ng/100 ml	10.4–38.1 nmol/l >3.5 nmol/l 0.87–3.12 nmol/l	2-P	a.m. sample	Chap. 15
Unbound testosterone	Adult male: 3.06–24.0 ng/100 ml Adult female: 0.09–1.28 ng/100 ml	106–832 pmol/l 3.1–44.4 pmol/l	2-P	a.m. sample	Chap. 15
b. Polypeptide Hormones					
Adrenocorticotropin (ACTH)	15–70 pg/ml	3.3–15.4 pmol/l	5-P	Place specimen on ice and send promptly to laboratory	Chap. 15
Calcitonin	Undetectable in normals. >100 pg/ml in medullary carcinoma	0 >29.3 pmol/l	5-P	Test done only on known or suspected cases of medullary carcinoma of the thyroid	Chap. 7, 15

Test	Conventional values	SI values	Sample	Conditions	Reference
Growth hormone	Below 5 ng/ml	<233 pmol/l	1-S	Fasting, at rest	Chap. 15
	Over 10 ng/ml	>465 pmol/l		After exercise	
	Children:				
	Male: Below 5 ng/ml	<233 pmol/l			
	Female: Up to 30 ng/ml	0–1395 pmol/l		After glucose load	
	Male: Below 5 ng/ml	<233 pmol/l			
	Female: Below 10 ng/ml	0–465 pmol/l			
Insulin	6–26 μU/ml	43–187 pmol/l	1-S	Fasting	Chap. 8
	Below 20 μU/ml	<144 pmol/l		During hypoglycemia	
	Up to 150 μU/ml	0–1078 pmol/l		After glucose load	
Luteinizing hormone	Male: 6–18 mU/ml	6–18 u/l	2-S,P	Pre- or post-ovulatory	Chap. 15
	Female: 5–22 mU/ml	5–22 u/l		Mid-cycle peak	
	30–250 mU/ml	30–250 u/l			
Parathyroid hormone	<10 μl equiv/ml	<10 ml equiv/l	5-P	Keep blood on ice, or plasma must be frozen if it is to be sent any distance; a.m. sample	Chap. 7
Prolactin	2–15 ng/ml	0.08–6.0 nmol/l	2-S		Chap. 15
Renin activity	Supine: 1.1 ± 0.8 ng/ml/h	0.9 ± 0.6 (nmol/l)h	4-P	EDTA tubes, on ice; normal diet	Chap. 15
	Upright: 1.9 ± 1.7 ng/ml/h	1.5 ± 1.3 (nmol/l)h			
	Supine: 2.7 ± 1.8 ng/ml/h	2.1 ± 1.4 (nmol/l)h		Low sodium diet	
	Upright: 6.6 ± 2.5 ng/ml/h	5.1 ± 1.9 (nmol/l)h			
	Diuretics: 10.0 ± 3.7 ng/ml/h	7.7 ± 2.9 (nmol/l)h		Low sodium diet	

(continued)

TABLE A-3. *Continued*

Determination	Reference Range		Note	Minimal ML Required	Explanation of Test and Possible Nursing Implications
	Conventional	SI			
	c. Thyroid Hormones				
Thyroid-stimulating-hormone (TSH)	0.5–3.5 μU/ml	0.5–3.5 mU/l		2-S	Chap. 15
Thyroxine-binding globulin capacity	15–25 μg T_4/100 ml	193–322 nmol/l		2-S	Chap. 15
Total tri-iodothyronine by radioimmunoassay (T_3)	70–190 ng/100 ml	1.08–2.92 nmol/l		2-S	Chap. 15
Total thyroxine by RIA (T_4)	4–12 μg/100 ml	52–154 nmol/l		1-S	Chap. 15
T_3 resin uptake	25–35%	0.25–0.35		2-S	Chap. 15
Free thyroxine index (FT_4 I)	1–4 ng/100 ml	12.8–51.2 pmol/l		2-S	Chap. 15

Reprinted from the New England Journal of Medicine, *with permission.*

TABLE A-4. HEMATOLOGIC VALUES

| Determination | Reference Range | | Minimal ML Required | Note | Explanation of Test and Possible Nursing Implications |
	Conventional	SI			
Coagulation factors:					
Factor I (fibrinogen)	0.15–0.35g/ 100 ml	4.0–10.0 μmol/1	4.5-P	Collect in Vacutainer containing sodium citrate	Chap. 13
Factor II (prothrombin)	60–140%	0.60–1.40	4.5-P	Collect in plastic tubes with 3.8% sodium citrate	Chap. 13
Factor V (accelerator globulin)	60–140%	0.60–1.40	4.5-P	Collect as in factor II determination	Chap. 13
Factor VII-X (proconvertin-Stuart)	70–130%	0.70–1.30	4.5-P	Collect as in factor II determination	Chap. 13
Factor X (Stuart factor)	70–130%	0.70–1.30	4.5-P	Collect as in factor II determination	Chap. 13
Factor VIII (antihemophilic globulin)	50–200%	0.50–2.0	4.5-P	Collect as in factor II determination	Chap. 13
Factor IX (plasma thromboplastic cofactor)	60–140%	0.60–1.40	4.5-P	Collect as in factor II determination	Chap. 13
Factor XI (plasma thromboplastic antecedent)	60–140%	0.60–1.40	4.5-P	Collect as in factor II determination	Chap. 13
Factor XII (Hageman factor)	60–140%	0.60–1.40	4.5-P	Collect as in factor II determination	Chap. 13

(continued)

465

TABLE A-4. *Continued*

Determination	Reference Range		Minimal ML Required	Note	Explanation of Test and Possible Nursing Implications
	Conventional	SI			
Coagulation screening tests:					
Bleeding time (Simplate)	3–9 min	180–540 s			Chap. 13
Prothrombin time	Less than 2-s deviation from control	Less than 2-s deviation from control	4.5-P	Collect in Vacutainer containing 3.8% sodium citrate	Chap. 13
Partial thromboplastin time (activated)	25–37 s	25–37 s	4.5-P	Collect in Vacutainer containing 3.8% sodium citrate	Chap. 13
Fibrinolytic studies:					
Euglobin lysis	No lysis in 2 h	0 (in 2 h)	4.5-P	Collect as in factor II determination	Chap. 13
Fibrinogen split products:	Negative reaction at greater than 1:4 dilution	0 (at >1:4 dilution)	4.5-S	Collect in special tube containing thrombin and epsilon amino caproic acid	Chap. 13
"Complete" blood count:					
Hematocrit	Male:45–52% Female:37–48%	Male:0.42–0.52 Female:0.37–0.48	1-B	Use EDTA as anticoagulant; the seven listed tests are performed automatically on the Coulter counter Model S, which directly determines cell counts, hemoglobin (as the cyanmethemoglobin	Chap. 2
Hemoglobin	Male:13–18 g/100 ml Female:12–16 g/100 ml	Male:8.1–11.2 mmol/l Female:7.4–9.9 mmol/l			
Leukocyte count	4300–10,800/mm^3	4.3–$10.8 \times 10^9/1$			
Erythrocyte count	4.2–5.9 million/mm^3	4.2–$5.9 \times 10^{12}/1$			
Mean corpuscular volume (MCV)	80–94 μm^3	80–94 fl			

Test	Conventional	SI units	Specimen	Remarks	Reference
Mean corpuscular hemoglobin (MCH)	27–32 pg	1.7–2.0 fmol		derivative) and hematocrit and computes MCV, MCH and MCHC	
Mean corpuscular hemoglobin concentration (MCHC)	32–36%	19–22.8 mmol/1			
Erythrocyte sedimentation rate	Male:1–13 mm/h Female:1–20 mm/h	Male:1–13 mm/h Female:1–20 mm/h	5-B	Use EDTA as anti-coagulant	Chap. 2
Erythrocyte enzymes: Glucose-6-phosphate dehydrogenase	5–15 U/g Hb	5–15 U/g	9-B	Use special anticoagulant (ACD solution)	Chap. 2
Ferritin (serum) Iron deficiency	0–20 ng/ml	0–20 µg/1			Chap. 2
Iron excess	Greater than 400 ng/1	>400 µg/1			
Folic acid Normal	Greater than 1.9 ng/ml	>4.3 mmol/1	1-S		Chap. 2
Borderline	1.0–1.9 ng/ml	2.3–4.3 mmol/1	1-S		
Haptoglobin	100–300 mg/100 ml	1.0–3.0 g/1	1-S		Chap. 14
Hemoglobin studies: Electrophoresis for abnormal hemoglobin			5-B	Collect with anticoagulant	Chap. 2
Electrophoresis for A₂ hemoglobin	1.5–3.5%	0.015–0.035	5-B	Use oxalate as anti-coagulant	Chap. 2
Hemoglobin F (fetal hemoglobin)	Less than 2%	<0.02	5-B	Collect with anticoagulant	Chap. 18
L.E. (lupus erythematosus) preparation: Method I	0	0	5-B	Use heparin as anti-coagulant	Chap. 14
Method II	0	0	5-B	Use defibrinated blood	

(continued)

TABLE A-4. *Continued*

| Determination | Reference Range | | Minimal ML Required | Note | Explanation of Test and Possible Nursing Implications |
	Conventional	SI			
Platelet count	150,000–350,000/ mm³	150–350×10⁹/1	0.5-B	Use EDTA as anti-coagulant; counts are performed on Clay Adams Ultraflow; when counts are low, results are confirmed by hand counting	Chap. 13
Platelet function tests:					
Clot retraction	50–100%/2 h	0.50–1.00/2 h	4.5-P	Collect as in factor II determination	Chap. 13
Platelet aggregation	Full response to ADP, epinephrine and collagen	1.0	18-P	Collect as in factor II determination	Chap. 13
Reticulocyte count	0.5–1.5% red cells	0.005–.015	0.1-B		Chap. 2
Vitamin B₁₂	90–280 pg/ml (borderline:70–90)	66–207 pmol/1 (borderline:52–66)	12-S		Chap. 2

Reprinted from the New England Journal of Medicine, with permission.

TABLE A-5. MISCELLANEOUS VALUES

| Determination | Reference Range | | Minimal ML Required | Note | Explanation of Test and Possible Nursing Implications |
	Conventional	SI			
Autoantibodies Thyroid colloid and microsomal antgens	Absent		2-S	Low titers in some elderly normal women	Chap. 14
Carcinoembryonic antigen (CEA)	0–2.5 ng/ml, 97% healthy non-smokers	0–2.5 µg/l 97% healthy non-smokers	20-P	Must be sent on ice	Chap. 10
Digitoxin	17±6 ng/ml	22±7.8 nmol/l	1-S	Medication with digitoxin or digitalis	Chap. 17
Digoxin	1.2±0.4 ng/ml	1.54±0.5 nmol/l	1-S	Medication with digoxin 0.25 mg per day	Chap. 17
	1.5±0.4 ng/ml	1.92±0.5 nmol/l	1-S	Medication with digoxin 0.5 mg per day	
Immunologic tests: Alpha-feto-globulin	Abnormal if present		5-clotted blood		Chap. 14
Alpha 1-Antitrypsin	200–400 mg/100 ml	2.0–4.0 g/1	10-B		Chap. 10
Antinuclear antibodies	Positive if detected with serum diluted 1:10		10-clotted blood	Send to laboratory promptly	Chap. 14
Anti-DNA antibodies	Less than 15 units/ml		10-B		Chap. 14
Bence-Jones protein	Abnormal if present		100-U		Chap. 10
Complement, total hemolytic	150–250 U/ml		10-B	Must be sent on ice	Chap. 14

(continued)

TABLE A-5. *Continued*

Determination	Reference Range		Minimal ML Required	Note	Explanation of Test and Possible Nursing Implications
	Conventional	SI			
C3	Range 55–120 mg/100 ml	0.55–1.2 g/1	10-B		Chap. 14
C4	Range 20–50 mg/100 ml	0.2–0.5 g/1	10-B		Chap. 14
Immunoglobulins:					
IgG	1140 mg/100 ml Range 540–1663	11.4 g/1 5.5–16.6 g/1			Chap. 10
IgA	214 mg/100 ml Range 66–344	2.14 g/1 0.66–3.44 g/1			
IgM	168 mg/100 ml Range 39–290	1.68 g/1 0.39–2.9 g/1			
Viscosity	1.4–1.8		10-B	Expressed as the relative viscosity of serum compared to water	Chap. 10
Propranolol (includes bio-active 4-OH metabolite)	100–300 ng/ml	386–1158 nmol/1	1-S	Obtain blood sample 4 h after last dose of beta blocking agent	Chap. 17
Stool fat	Less than 5 g in 24 h or less than 4% of measured fat intake in 3-d period	<5 g/d	24-h or 3-day speci-men, prefer-ably with markers		Chap. 16

Reprinted from the New England Journal of Medicine, with permission.

TABLE A-6. VACUTAINER COLLECTION SYSTEM*

Color of Tube	Meaning
Red	No additives
Green	Contains heparin
Lavender	Contains EDTA
Blue	Contains sodium citrate
Black	Contains sodium oxalate
Gray	Contains glycolytic inhibitor
Yellow	Sterile interior
Brown	Minimal lead content

*See Chapter 1 for tips on drawing venous blood.

APPENDIX B:
REFERENCE VALUES FOR NEWBORNS AND CHILDREN COMPARED TO ADULT VALUES

Name of Test	Change in Value	Explanation for Change Found in
Acid phosphatase	Higher in newborn	Chap. 12
Aldorase	Higher in newborns and children	Chap. 12
Alkaline phosphatase	Higher until puberty	Chap. 12
ALT (SGOT)	Higher in newborns	Chap. 12
Ammonia	Higher in newborns, particularly prematures. Also higher in children	Chap. 10
Amylase	Low or absent in newborns	Chap. 12
Bicarbonate	Lower in newborns and slightly lower in children	Chaps. 5-6
Bilirubin	Higher until 1 month old	Chap. 11
BUN	Slightly lower in newborns	Chap. 4
Calcium	Lower in newborns first few days. Slightly higher in children	Chap. 7
Carbon dioxide content	Lower in infants and children	Chap. 6
Cholesterol	Lower in children	Chap. 9
Creatinine	Lower in children. Increases with age. Higher in males after puberty	Chap. 4
Fibrinogen	Lower in newborns	Chap. 13
Gonadotropins (FSH and LH)	Lower in children	Chap. 15
Glucose	Lower in newborns	Chap. 8

(continued)

Name of Test	Change in Value	Explanation for Change Found in
Growth hormone (GH)	Higher in newborns and children	Chap. 15
Hemoglobin, hematocrit, and RBC	High in newborn, lower by age 1 and adult levels by 8–13 years	Chap. 2
Immunoglobulins— IgG, IgA, etc.	Newborn contains some from mother, varies with age	Chap. 10
17-ketogenic steroids	Low in newborns and increases with age	Chap. 15
LDH	Very high in newborn, adult level by age 14	Chap. 12
Magnesium	Slightly lower?	Chap. 7
Metanephrines (urine)	Higher in infants	Chap. 15
pH	Lower in newborns	Chap. 6
pO₂	Lower in newborns	Chap. 6
Phosphorus	Highest in newborns, levels decline by puberty	Chap. 7
Potassium	Slightly higher in newborn?	Chap. 5
Pregnanediol	Lower in children	Chap. 15
Pregnantriol	Lower in children	Chap. 15
PT (prothrombin time)	Higher in newborns	Chap. 13
PTT (partial thromboplastin time)	Higher in newborns	Chap. 13
Reticulocytes	Higher in newborn	Chap. 2
SGOT (see ALT)	Higher in infants	Chap. 12
Specific gravity	Lower until age 2	Chap. 3
Testosterone	Much lower in children	Chap. 15
Total protein	Slightly lower in children	Chap. 10
Triglycerides	Lower in children	Chap. 9
Uric acid	Lower values until puberty	Chap. 4
WBC	Extremely high in newborns, differential also different in children	Chap. 2

References for Appendix B

Cherian, George and Hill, Gilbert. "Percentile Estimates of 14 Chemical Constituents in Sera of Children and Adolescents," *American Journal of Clinical Pathology* 69 (January 1978): 24–31.

Jensen, Margaret *et al. Maternity Care, the Nurse and the Family.* 2nd ed., p. 908. St. Louis, Mo.: C. V. Mosby, Co., 1981

Meites, Samuel, ed. *Pediatric Clinical Chemistry. A Survey of Normals, Methods and Instrumentation with Commentary.* Washington, D.C.: American Association for Clinical Chemistry, Inc., 1977.

"Pediatric Values," Children's Hospital, San Francisco, California, 1981.

"Pediatric Values," Kaiser Hospital, San Francisco, California, 1981.

* Also see other references for specific tests in each chapter. Note that the values for premature infants are not the same as for newborns at term. Consult a speciality text for high risk neonate care.

APPENDIX C:
POSSIBLE ALTERATIONS IN REFERENCE VALUES
FOR THE AGED

	Possible Change in Value	Explanation for Change Found in
Alkaline phosphatase	Decrease?	Chap. 12
Antinuclear antibodies (ANA)	May be present	Chap. 14
Blood sugar, fasting and 2 hr pc	Increase	Chap. 8
BUN	Increase	Chap. 4
Calcium	May lower but this not well documented?	Chap. 7
Cholesterol	Increase	Chap. 9
Creatinine clearance	Decrease	Chap. 4
Glucose tolerance test (GTT)	Change in curve	Chap. 8
Gonadotropins (LH, FSH)	Eventually decrease but increase postmenopausal	Chap. 15
Immunoglobulins	Decreases and alterations	Chap. 10
17-ketosteroids	Decrease	Chap. 15
pO_2	Decrease	Chap. 6
Phosphorus	May lower with age?	Chap. 7
Pregnanediol	Decrease in woman	Chap. 15
Rheumatic factor (RF)	May be present	Chap. 14
Sedimentation rate (ESR)	Increases	Chap. 2
T_3 RIA	Decrease?	Chap. 15
Triglycerides	Increase	Chap. 9
Uric acid	Slightly higher values	Chap. 4
VDRL	May become reactive?	Chap. 14

References for Appendix C*

Gerboes, K. *et al.* "Is the Elderly Patient Accurately Diagnosed?" *Geriatrics* 34 (May 1979): 91–96

Harnes, Jack. "Normal Values with Increasing Age," *Journal of Chronic Diseases* 33 (September 1980): 593–594

Ravel, Richard. "Effects of Age on Laboratory Tests," in *Clinical Laboratory Medicine,* 3rd ed., Chicago, Ill.: Year Book Medical Publishers Inc., 1978

* Also see the reference values for specific tests in each chapter. Note that the effect of age on many tests is not known. The figures used for normals may sometimes be more reflective of the common underlying chronic diseases of the elderly rather than of a normal healthy stage. For example, hypertension affects many elderly patients, and it can cause some renal changes that in turn can change the values of various laboratory tests. Ravel (1978) has a concise review of the literature that best supports changes in laboratory values for persons over fifty.

APPENDIX D:
ALTERED REFERENCE VALUES FOR
COMMON LABORATORY TESTS IN NORMAL PREGNANCIES*
AND WITH ORAL CONTRACEPTIVES**

Name of Test	Change in Value	Explanation for Change Found in
(Increases or decreases are in relation to the woman's prepregnancy values.)		
Aldosterone**	Increase	Chap. 15
Alkaline phosphatase	Marked increase	Chap. 12
Albumin**	Decrease	Chap. 10
B_{12}	Decrease	Chap. 2
Bilirubin**	Occasional increase	Chap. 11
Bicarbonate	Decrease	Chap. 6
Blood glucose**	Variations in trimesters	Chap. 8
BSP retention	Increase	Chap. 11
BUN	Slight decrease	Chap. 4
C-reactive protein	Increase	Chap. 14
Calcium	Decreases with albumin levels	Chap. 7
pCO_2	Decrease	Chap. 6
Cholesterol	Increase	Chap. 9
Cortisol	Increase	Chap. 15
Creatinine clearance	Increase	Chap. 4
Creatinine (serum)	Decrease	Chap. 4
Fibrinogen levels**	Increase	Chap. 13
Folic acid levels**	Decrease	Chap. 2
Hemoglobin, hematocrit	Decrease	Chap. 2
Iron	Decrease	Chap. 2
Lipase	Increase	Chap. 12
Magnesium**	May decrease	Chap. 7
Phosphorus	May decrease	Chap. 7
Protein electrophoresis	Change in pattern	Chap. 10
PT	May decrease	Chap. 13
PTT	May decrease	Chap. 13
Platelets	Increase after delivery	Chap. 13
Sed rate	Increase	Chap. 2

APPENDIX D   (*Continued*)

Name of Test	Change in Value	Explanation for Change Found in
T_3-T_4 and thyroid-binding** globulin	Altered values	Chap. 15
Triglycerides**	Increase	Chap. 9
Uric acid	Decrease in early pregnancy	Chap. 4
WBC	Increase in total and in neutrophils	Chap. 2

References for Appendix D*

Jensen, Margaret *et al. Maternity Care, the Nurse and the Family.* 2nd ed., p. 888. St. Louis, Mo.: C. V. Mosby, Co., 1981

Hytten, Frank and Lind, Tom. *Diagnostic Indices in Pregnancy.* Summitt, N.J.: Ciba-Geigy Corp. 1975

Milne, J. A., ed. ''Physiological Response to Pregnancy in Health and Disease,'' *Post Graduate Medical Journal* 55 (May 1979): 293–367

* Also see references for specific tests discussed in each chapter.
** Note that many of the effects of oral contraceptives on laboratory tests are similar to those found in pregnancy. See the Medical Letter on Drugs and Therapeutics 21: 55–56 June 29, 1979 for 32 references about the effects of oral contraceptives.

APPENDIX E: ABBREVIATIONS*

ABG	Arterial blood gases
ABO	Blood types
ACD	Acid citrate dextrose (anticoagulant)
ACTH	Adrenocorticotrophic hormone
ADH	Antidiuretic hormone
AFB	Acid-fast bacillus
AHG	Antihemophilia globulin
AFP	Alpha-fetoprotein
A/G ratio	Albumin/globulin ration (outdated)
ALA	(delta) aminolevulinic acid
ALT	Alanine amino transferase (new term for SGPT)
APPT	Activated partial thromboplastin time (also PTT)
ANA	Antinuclear antibodies
ASO	Antistreptolysin O titer
AST	Asparate amino transferase (new name for SGOT)
BC	Blood culture
BCP	Biochemical profile; also, birth control pills
BMR	Basal metabolic rate
Br	Bromide
BS	Blood sugar
BSP	Bromsulphalein (dye for liver function test)
BUN	Blood urea nitrogen

(continued)

APPENDIX E   (*Continued*)

C_3, C_4	Complement factors
C&S	Culture and sensitivity
Ca++	Calcium
CBC	Complete blood count
CEA	Carcinoembryonic antigen
CF	Complement fixation
Cl^-	Chloride
CO_2	Carbon dioxide (pCO_2 = partial pressure)
CPK	Creatine phosphokinase
Cr	Chromium
CRP	C-reactive protein
Crit	Hematocrit
CSF	Cerebrospinal fluid
Cu	Copper
CUA	Clean urinalysis
Diff	Differential (white blood cell count)
EDTA	Ethylenediaminotetracetate (anticoagulant for blood samples)
ESR	Erythrocyte sedimentation rate
Fe	Iron
FBS	Fasting blood sugar
FEP	Free erythrocyte porphyrins
FSH	Follicle-stimulating hormone
FTA	Fluorescent treponemal antibodies
GC	Gonococcus
GFR	Glomerular filtration rate
GH	Growth hormone
G-6-PD	Glucose-6-phosphatase dehydrogenase
GTT	Glucose tolerance test
HAA	Hepatitis-associated antigen
HAT	Heterophile antibody titer
Hb (Hgb)	Hemoglobin
HBD	Hydroxybutyric dehydrogenase
$HB_S Ag$	Hepatitis B surface antigen
HCG	Human chorionic gonadotropin
Hct	Hematocrit
Hg	Mercury
5HIAA	5-hydroxyindoleacetic acid
ICSH	Interstitial cell-stimulating hormone (LH in female)
IFA	Immunofluorescence antibody test (may be direct or indirect)
Ig	Immunoglobulin (such as IgA, IgM, etc.)
K++	Potassium
17-KGS	17-ketogenic steroids
17-KS	17-ketosteroids
LDH	Lactic dehydrogenase
LDL	Low-density lipoprotein
LE Prep	Lupus erythematous test
LFT	Liver function tests
LH	Luteinizing hormone (ICSH in male)
Li	Lithium
lytes	Electrolytes (Na, K, Cl, bicarbonate)
MCH	Mean corpuscular hemoglobin (erythrocyte indices)
MCHC	Mean corpuscular hemoglobin concentration (erythrocyte indices)
MCV	Mean corpuscular volume (erythrocyte indices)

APPENDIX E (*Continued*)

MHA	Microhemagglutination test
Mg	Magnesium
MIC	Minimal inhibitory concentration
N	Nitrogen
Na++	Sodium
NC	Normal color
NL	Normal
NPN	Nonprotein nitrogen
O_2	Oxygen (pO_2 = partial pressure)
O&P	Ova and parasites
17-OH	17-hydroxysteroids
OTC	Over-the-counter (drugs)
P	Phosphorus
Pb	Lead
PBI	Protein-bound iodine (outdated)
PCV	Packed cell volume (hematocrit)
pH	Hydrogen-ion concentration
PKU	Phenylketonuria
Pl.ct.	Platelet count
PMNs	Polymorphonuclear (type of WBC)
PSP	Phenolsulfonphthalein (dye for renal excretion test)
PPLO	Pleuropneumonia-like organism (has characteristics between virus and bacteria)
PT	Prothrombin time
PTH	Parathyroid hormone or parathormone
PTT	Partial thromboplastin time (*see also* APTT)
PP or PC	Postprandial (or after meals)
QNS	Quantity not sufficient
RAST	Radioallergosorbent test
RAI	Radioactive iodine
RBC	Red blood cell
Retic	Reticulocyte count
RF	Rheumatoid factor (also called RA factor)
Rh	Rhesus; Rh factor in blood
RIA	Radioimmunoassay
R/O	Rule out
RPR	Rapid plasma reagin
segs	Segmented neutrophils of WBC
S&A	Sugar and acetone
SG	Specific gravity
SGOT	Serum glutamic-oxaloacetic transaminase (newer name is AST)
SGPT	Serum glutamic-pyruvic transaminase (newer name is ALT)
SMA	Sequential multiple analyzer (SMA-6 does 6 tests, SMA-12,12 tests)
Stat	Immediately
STS	Serologic test for syphilis
T-C	Type and cross match
T&S	Type and screen
T_3	Triiodothyronine
T_4	Thyroxine
TPI	Treponema pallidum immobilization
TBG	Thyroid-binding globulin
TIBC	Total iron-binding capacity
TP	Total protein

(*continued*)

APPENDIX E   *(Continued)*

TRH	Thyroid-releasing hormone
TSH	Thyroid-stimulating hormone (thyrotropin)
TSP	Total serum proteins
UA	Urinalysis
UC	Urine culture
UrAc	Uric acid
VDRL	Venereal Disease Research Laboratory (test for syphilis)
VLDL	Very low-density lipoprotein
VMA	Vanillylmandelic acid
WBC	White blood cell; white blood count
WNL	Within normal limits
WNR	Within normal range
X match	Cross match (of blood)
X	Female chromosome
Y	Male chromosome

*Compiled from various sources. Same abbreviations are common in Canada. See Watson, E. M. "Clinical Laboratory Procedures," Canadian Nurse 70 (February 1974): 25-44

APPENDIX F:
UNITS OF MEASUREMENT

cc	cubic centimeter (same as ml, 1/1,000 liter, which is the preferred term).
cm	centimeter
cu mm or mm³	cubic millimeter
d or dl	deciliter (1/10 of a liter)
g or gm	gram (1/1,000 of a kilogram, 15 grains)
hpf	high power field microscope
G%	grams in 100 ml
IU	international unit
kg, K, or k	kilogram (1,000 grams, or 2.2 pounds)
l	liter (1,000 ml or 1,000 cc)
lpf	low power field microscope
mcg or μg	micrograms (1/1,000 milligram)
mc	millicurie
mEq or meq	milliequivalent (see Chapter 5 for formula)
mg or mgm	milligram (1/1,000 gram)
mg%	milligrams in 100 milliliters (same as dl)
mIU	milliinternational unit (1/1,000 IU)
ml	milliliter (1/1,000 liter, same as cc)
mm	millimeter (1/10 centimeter)
mm³ or cu mm	cubic millimeter (see RBC count, Chapter 2)
mmHg	millimeters of mercury (see blood gases, Chapter 6)
mmol	millimoles (see Chapter 1 on SI units)
mOsm	milliosmoles (see Chapter 3)
ng	nanogram (1/1,000 microgram, see Chapter 15)
pg	picogram (1/1,000 nanogram, see Chapter 15)
QNS	quantity not sufficient
SI	international system, see Chapter 1
u	international enzyme unit
μ	micro
μg (mcg)	microgram (1/1,000 milligram)
w/v	weight/volume
μc	microcurie (1/1,000 of a millicurie)
WNL	within normal limits
WNR	within normal range
<	less than
>	greater than

APPENDIX G:
ANSWERS TO QUESTIONS

Chapter 1
1-1. c
1-2. d
1-3. b
1-4. c
1-5. d
1-6. a
1-7. c
1-8. a
1-9. d

Chapter 2
2-1. a
2-2. d
2-3. c
2-4. b
2-5. d
2-6. a
2-7. c
2-8. c
2-9. d
2-10. c
2-11. c
2-12. a
2-13. d
2-14. b
2-15. b
2-16. a
2-17. d
2-18. a
2-19. c
2-20. d
2-21. d
2-22. b
2-23. b
2-24. d

Chapter 3
3-1. c
3-2. d
3-3. a
3-4. a
3-5. d
3-6. c
3-7. b
3-8. d
3-9. c
3-10. d
3-11. d
3-12. a
3-13. c
3-14. b

Chapter 4
4-1. c
4-2. c
4-3. a
4-4. b
4-5. d
4-6. d
4-7. c
4-8. b
4-9. b
4-10. c
4-11. b
4-12. b
4-13. a
4-14. d
4-15. d

Chapter 5
5-1. d
5-2. a
5-3. d
5-4. a
5-5. b
5-6. b
5-7. b
5-8. b
5-9. d
5-10. c
5-11. a
5-12. a
5-13. c
5-14. a
5-15. c
5-16. c
5-17. d
5-18. c
5-19. d
5-20. d
5-21. b
5-22. c
5-23. c
5-24. b
5-25. d
5-26. c
5-27. a

Chapter 6
6-1. b
6-2. b
6-3. d
6-4. a
6-5. c
6-6. d
6-7. d
6-8. d
6-9. d
6-10. b
6-11. b
6-12. d
6-13. b
6-14. a
6-15. b
6-16. d
6-17. c
6-18. a
6-19. a
6-20. b
6-21. d
6-22. c
6-23. c
6-24. b
6-25. d
6-26. b
6-27. c

Chapter 7
7-1. a
7-2. c
7-3. a
7-4. a
7-5. a
7-6. c
7-7. d
7-8. b
7-9. c
7-10. c
7-11. d
7-12. b
7-13. d
7-14. a
7-15. a
7-16. a
7-17. d
7-18. c
7-19. b

Chapter 8
8-1. c
8-2. d
8-3. d
8-4. c
8-5. d
8-6. a
8-7. b
8-8. c
8-9. b
8-10. c
8-11. c
8-12. a
8-13. a
8-14. b
8-15. d
8-16. d

Chapter 9
9-1. d
9-2. b
9-3. d
9-4. b
9-5. c
9-6. a
9-7. d
9-8. c
9-9. b
9-10. a
9-11. d
9-12. a

Chapter 10

10-1. a
10-2. c
10-3. b
10-4. c
10-5. d
10-6. b
10-7. d
10-8. b
10-9. b
10-10. a
10-11. a
10-12. b
10-13. b
10-14. a
10-15. c
10-16. c
10-17. d
10-18. c
10-19. d

Chapter 11

11-1. d
11-2. d
11-3. c
11-4. b
11-5. c
11-6. b
11-7. a
11-8. a
11-9. d
11-10. c
11-11. d
11-12. d
11-13. a
11-14. d
11-15. c
11-16. c

Chapter 12

12-1. c
12-2. a
12-3. d
12-4. a
12-5. a
12-6. c
12-7. a
12-8. a
12-9. b
12-10. a
12-11. a
12-12. c
12-13. d
12-14. b
12-15. a
12-16. b

Chapter 13

13-1. b
13-2. d
13-3. a
13-4. a
13-5. b
13-6. d
13-7. d
13-8. a
13-9. d
13-10. b
13-11. c
13-12. b
13-13. c
13-14. b
13-15. a
13-16. d
13-17. c

Chapter 14

14-1. d
14-2. b
14-3. c
14-4. b
14-5. a
14-6. b
14-7. d
14-8. c
14-9. d
14-10. d
14-11. b
14-12. a
14-13. d
14-14. a
14-15. d
14-16. c
14-17. d
14-18. b
14-19. a
14-20. b
14-21. d
14-22. c

Chapter 15

15-1. c
15-2. a
15-3. a
15-4. d
15-5. a
15-6. b
15-7. b
15-8. d
15-9. d
15-10. b
15-11. d
15-12. b
15-13. b
15-14. d
15-15. a
15-16. c
15-17. b

Chapter 16

16-1. c
16-2. c
16-3. d
16-4. a
16-5. b
16-6. d
16-7. c
16-8. c
16-9. a
16-10. b
16-11. d
16-12. a
16-13. b
16-14. d
16-15. d
16-16. b
16-17. b
16-18. a

Chapter 17

17-1. a
17-2. d
17-3. d
17-4. b
17-5. c
17-6. b
17-7. c
17-8. d
17-9. b
17-10. a
17-11. b
17-12. c
17-13. a
17-14. b
17-15. a
17-16. c
17-17. b
17-18. c
17-19. d
17-20. b

Chapter 18

18-1. b
18-2. a
18-3. d
18-4. c
18-5. a
18-6. c
18-7. c
18-8. c
18-9. c

Author Index

Italic entries indicate reference or bibliographic material.

Subject Index

Italic entries indicate reference or bibliographic material.